Y0-AQS-242

SOFT AND HARD TISSUE REPAIR

Surgical Science Series, Volume 2

OTHER VOLUMES IN THE SERIES

Karran: Controversies in Surgical Sepsis

SOFT AND HARD TISSUE REPAIR

Biological and Clinical Aspects

Edited by
Thomas K. Hunt, M.D.
R. Bruce Heppenstall, M.D.
Eli Pines, Ph.D.
David Rovee, Ph.D.

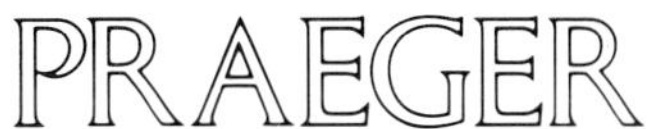

PRAEGER SPECIAL STUDIES • PRAEGER SCIENTIFIC

New York • Philadelphia • Eastbourne, UK
Toronto • Hong Kong • Tokyo • Sydney

Library of Congress Cataloging in Publication Data
Main entry under title:

Soft and hard tissue repair.

(Surgical science series ; v. 2)
Includes bibliographies and index.
1. Wounds and injuries--Congresses. 2. Wound healing--Congresses. I. Hunt, Thomas K. II. Series. [DNLM: 1. Wound healing--Congresses. 2. Regeneration--Congresses. 3. Implants, Artificial--Congresses. 4. Skin--Transplantation--Congresses. W1 SU767LM v.2 / WO 185 S681 1983]
RD94.S64 1984 617'.1 83-24595
ISBN 0-03-063666-3 (alk. paper)

Magnifications used for figures in this book are original, prepress magnifications. Photographs have been reduced to fit house specifications.

Published in 1984 by Praeger Publishers
CBS Educational and Professional Publishing
a Division of CBS Inc.
521 Fifth Avenue, New York, NY 10175 USA

456789 052 987654321

Printed in the United States of America
on acid-free paper

Preface

Wound healing is a unique summation of natural processes—a fascinating, though frustrating, pursuit for those who try to understand it. Unfortunately, in those first few hours after injury a bewildering array of responses occurs, and it is difficult to understand them all. Detailed knowledge of the complement cascade, coagulation, inflammation, intracellular messengers, cell receptors, circulatory dynamics, cell cycles, collagen and proteoglycans synthesis and lysis, cell-mediated immunity, natural immunity, regeneration, among others, is needed even to describe these processes, much less understand them.

In May 1983, a group of international investigators gathered, with the support of Johnson & Johnson Products, Inc., to share expertise in various areas of biology and to consider their accumulated knowledge of technical achievements, medical and veterinary skills (and needs) on the subject of wound repair.

Similar conferences have been held every three or four years. For decades, they have centered about fibroblasts and collagen, and were dominated by collagen biochemists and surgeons. At this conference, the organizers, aware of the importance of the explosion of data in cell biology to wound-healing science, placed the emphasis on cells and cell-to-cell messengers.

This book is unique, with its emphasis on bone as well as soft tissue repair, its discussions of macrophages, cell growth factors and chemoattractants, and its discussion of the practical and theoretical. Perhaps for the first time, serious and successful attempts to encourage one aspect of repair over another were discussed. In particular, the participants seem to have forgotten the traditional "<u>ne plus ultra</u>" of wound healing. Almost everyone discussed some way of modifying repair—even accelerating it. The old, "I dressed the wound, God healed it," philosophy was not heard. We postulated that healing can be made faster or slower. We resolved that hypertrophic scar, for instance, can be controlled and perhaps eliminated. Everyone agreed that ways will be found.

Cells were the focus. We considered the conditions that make them adopt reparative behavior, that make them stop repairing, the signals that lead them to move, make collagen, form new blood vessels, calcify bone, and reepithelize. We exchanged practical information, theories, and techniques; we achieved a great amount of consensus.

This book is the formal report; it is the distillate of the facts. The smell of the pines and the greens at Tarpon Springs is gone. But the gleam in the eye from new insight, scientific fellowship, and broadened understanding remains.

R. Bruce Heppenstall
Thomas K. Hunt
E. Pines
David T. Rovee

Contents

Chapter Page

PART III
INDUCTION OF REPAIR

PART IV
SKIN REPLACEMENT

Chapter		Page

Chapter		Page

Chapter		Page

SOFT AND HARD TISSUE REPAIR

PART I
Internal/External Environment in Wounded Tissue

1
Cellular Control of Repair

Thomas K. Hunt, David R. Knighton,
K. K. Thakral, Walter Andrews
and Dov Michaeli

INTRODUCTION

This book was conceived several years ago when we began to realize that the cells involved in wound healing send and receive important, controlling, chemical messages, and when we recognized that our concepts of soft tissue and bone repair were becoming more and more one body of knowledge. We tried to design it in such a way that it would at once encompass soft tissue and bone repair. We wanted to share new information on how repair is modulated by controlling cells, and how those cells are themselves stimulated to exert their control. We tried to assemble investigators who are working on controlling mechanisms of soft and hard tissue healing, and to team them with the clinically-oriented in order to develop insights into how this new information can be translated into clinically useful knowledge.

The contributors to the section on cellular control have their own reasons for arriving at their present perspectives. My colleagues and I arrived at ours more or less as follows: we observed that healing wounds are "intelligent" tissues. Healing starts only after tissue is injured, with rare exceptions. Healing normally stops when its task is done. It respects boundaries of epithelia, implanted prostheses, etc. Its dimensions are appropriate, in general, to the scope of the injury. Simple injuries, by and large, are repaired simply. Complex inuuries incite a much more complex repair. However, wounds clearly respond to many stimuli. About twelve years ago, we concluded that the control of repair must, therefore, rest in "intelligent" responders; that is, cells. From that time to now, our work has rested on the framework of cell biology. We have searched for connections between injury and reparative cell behavior, on the one hand, and between the various reparative cells, on the other hand.

This seems only common sense now, but it took some courage to draw away from the prior emphasis on fibroplasia and collagen synthesis, deposition, polymerization, calcification, and lysis, which comprised almost the entirety of wound healing research just a decade ago. Though these processes are important, we must now acknowledge that even the fibroblast takes its marching orders from a higher authority.

In a grant application written soon after we resolved to "follow the cells," we wrote:

> It seems time to pursue once again the Holy Grail of wound healers, what starts and what stops wound healing. We are aware, of course, that many distinguished careers in wound healing research ended in frustrating and fruitless assaults on these two simple questions. Now, however, new knowledge in cell biology seems already to have laid out the beginning of repair for us, in the complement system, and somewhere in the inflammatory cells we can see emerging the major director of the extent and duration of repair. Furthermore, when wound healing ignores its usual mandate, when repair becomes excessive or fails entirely, the concept that overactivity or failure of cells to perform their usual functions provides us with far more appealing targets for trouble shooting than looking for defects in collagen synthesis, structure or polymerization. Failed repair most often occurs in the milieu of disordered inflammation. Excessive repair often relates to further injury and apparently to immune disorders. Disorders of collagen structure seem now to apply mainly to genetic disorders of connective tissue.

We will be discussing environmental messengers to cells which cause them to move, divide, secrete "growth factors," synthesize collagen, and attract new blood vessels. As a stimulus for discussion I have set up a schema of wound healing. (See Figure 1.1.)

MECHANISMS OF TISSUE REPAIR

Injury, whether mechanical, thermal, chemical, immunologic or ischemic, activates tissue complement which in turn attracts

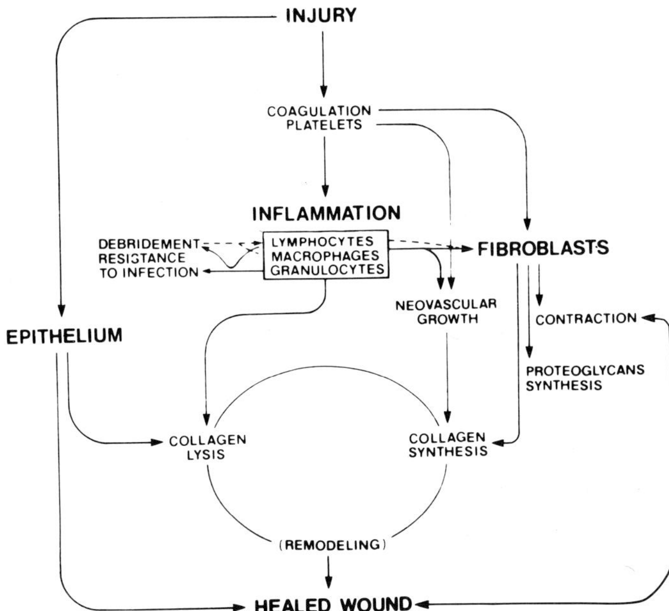

FIGURE 1.1 Schematic concept of wound healing.

inflammatory cells. When the injury involves blood vessels (repair is much simpler if it does not), the coagulation cascade is also activated. Though tests have not been comprehensively exhaustive, fibrin polymerization and lysis, and platelet activation stand out as relevant to repair. Fibronectin will be discussed in Chapter 2.

Fibrin polymerization and lysis produce chemoattractant peptides which in turn attract mononuclear cells. Fibrin may stimulate macrophages, as noted below. Therefore, these steps act as a reinforcing "loop" to tissue complement.

Platelet activation releases substances which stimulate cell replication and angiogenesis, as will be discussed by Dr. Samuel Joseph Leibovich in Chapter 18 and by Dr. Dov Michaeli et al., in Chapter 21. By twelve hours or so after injury, an inflammatory response is established; local pH and pO_2 falls, pCO_2 rises, glucose is utilized rapidly, and lactate accumulates. (See Chapter 4.)

We know from the works of Stein and Levenson,[1] as well as Leibovich and Ross and their colleagues,[2] that granulocytes and lymphocytes seem to play mostly a defensive role against infection. Later, Dr. Thomas K. Hunt will discuss the interaction of the wound environment and the efficiency of the granulocyte defense. (See Chapter 24.)

Macrophages seem to take over the direction of repair at this time, secreting substances which cause: 1) fibroblasts to replicate (so-called "MDGF"—macrophage-derived growth factor); and 2) blood vessels to approach the wound ("WAF"—wound angiogenesis factor). Somehow, these same cells stimulate fibroblasts to secrete collagen as well, although the mechanism is not known. Lymphocytes may have a similar but lesser role.[18]

A few days after the injury, wound cells begin to be arranged in a characteristic pattern, which will be described by Dr. Ian Silver in Chapter 4. Granulation tissue, or rather tissue progressively filling a dead space, is arranged with macrophages lining the dead space and covering a layer of immature fibroblasts (with the replicating cells nearest the new capillary), which in turn cover a layer of budding capillaries, which make a band of intense angiogenesis. Behind this is an area of collagen synthesis, and behind this, an area of resolution in which excess vessels and collagen are removed. This unit, the "_healing module_," as I call it (Figure 1.2), moves toward the dead space by means which we hope will become clearer later in this book. Fibroblasts within the module are stimulated to make collagen in support of blood vessel growth. By means that I suspect will remain unclear for some time, a few—but only a few—of the myriad new capillaries remain and enlarge, and the vessels which bring blood to the wound module soon condense into a few major feeding vessels. Dr. Silver, more than anyone, has characterized the module; and as this book proceeds, it should become apparent that when healing is regarded in this manner, strong similarities appear between the "module" of soft tissue healing and the "cutting cone" of fracture repair. Our own conviction is that the energy-deficient space just beyond the reach of the growing circulation is probably the ultimate source of the major stimuli to angiogenesis and collagen synthesis. This will become apparent in contributions to be made by Drs. Silver and David Knighton. The primarily repairing wound is simpler than the "granulating" one, but the general architecture of the wound module can be found there as well.

These remarks crystallize the work of many investigators using many model systems. Numerous _in vivo_ and _in vitro_ models of reparative phenomena have appeared in the last decade. One of the most useful to us is the rabbit cornea, and I will use it to illustrate one experimental base on which these concepts rest.

Cornea is a highly defined tissue, with anatomically defined borders, in which angiogenesis and fibroplasia can be initiated

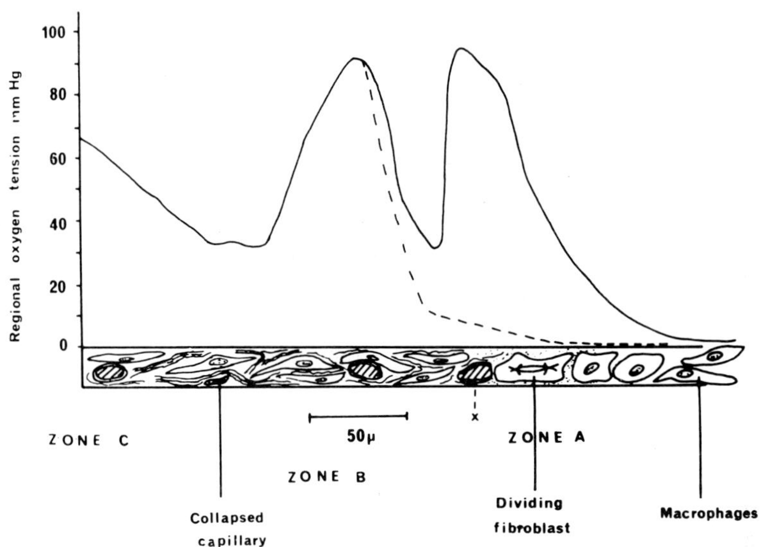

FIGURE 1.2 Cross-section of rabbit ear chamber showing the typical architecture of the healing wound. The "space" is on the right and the normal tissue out of sight to the left. The lactate concentration in the space is = 10 mM, a ten-to-one gradient to the vessels. The fibroblasts and new capillaries ("x") divide in a zone of pO_2, from about 80 to 40 mm Hg. The new fibroblasts are "born" on the right, in high lactate and low pO_2. Later, when a new capillary loop grows out to the right toward the space, the fibroblasts will be in higher pO_2 and lower lactate, characteristic of zones B and C. There, unneeded capillaries are regressing and fibroblasts have the requisite oxygen to synthesize collagen—if perfusion is adequate. The dotted line shows the pO_2 pattern measured in hypovolemia.

and observed easily (Figure 1.3). The cornea can heal small incised wounds without producing visible angiogenesis or scar. One can just as easily burn it with silver nitrate and produce overt angiogenesis and scar. One can inject cells into its substance. Some cells will initiate the complex pattern of healing in it, while others will not. One can insert slips of Hydron™ plastic without inducing angiogenesis or scar unless certain chemicals are incorporated into the Hydron™ in advance. With this model we can separate the fact of injury from the conditions and cells which cause angiogenesis and scar. The following

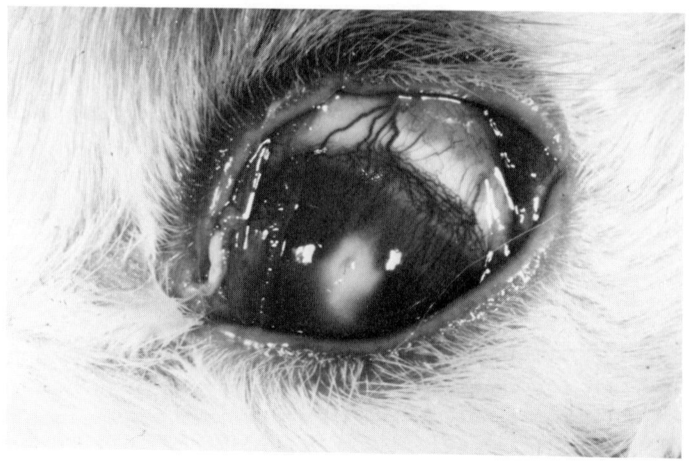

FIGURE 1.3 An example of corneal scar and angiogenesis. This is 3+ angiogenesis and 3+ scar. It is the result, after ten days, of injection of more than 10^6 autologous 21-day old wound cells.

experiments were meant to explore the connection between inflammatory cells and collagen synthesis.

METHODS

Studies in the Rabbit Model

Wounds were made under the dorsal skin of rabbits by inserting wire-mesh cylinders.[3] Fluid aspirated from these cylinders seven days later, contains a mixture of granulocytes (approximately 85%), lymphocytes and macrophages. Twenty-one days after implantation the fluid contains 95% macrophages, as demonstrated by alpha-naphthylbutyl esterase staining. This fluid and its cells were aspirated by a hypodermic syringe. The cells were concentrated by centrifugation, washed with Earl's balanced salt solution (EBSS), and transplanted by injection into the substance of the cornea of the same animal.

In our early experiments, we injected approximately 5×10^6 of these cells, in 0.2 ml of fluid, into the central cornea and

TABLE 1.1

Reparative Effects of Cell Components and Suitable Controls on Angiogenesis and Scar

Number of Animals	Injections	Neovascularization Day 4	Day 8	Day 20	Scar
20	EBSS, wound fluid, endotoxin, or resting peritoneal macrophages	0	0	0	0
9	Wound granulocytes and lymphocytes	0	0	0	0
6	Stimulated peritoneal macrophages	1	2	0	1+
10	Wound macrophages from 4- or 10-day old wounds	1	1	0	1+
4	Endotoxin-stimulated macrophages from 4-day old wounds	1	2	2.5	2+
20	Endotoxin-stimulated macrophages from 21-day old wounds, or sonicated, stimulated cells	1	2.5	4.0	2+

produced angiogenesis and scar[5] (Table 1.1). From this data, we concluded that macrophages are conditioned to behave in a reparative role by residence in a wound. The fact that these cells initiated several times more angiogenesis and scar when exposed to small amounts of E. coli endotoxin led us to conclude that wounding is not a maximum stimulus to macrophages. Since 5×10^6 macrophages almost always induced healing, while granulocytes in even hundredfold greater numbers rarely did, we concluded that macrophages are far more powerful directors of repair than granulocytes and lymphocytes.

Studies of the Coagulation System

In a brief survey of the coagulation system (once again using autologous materials, except where otherwise specified),

0.2 ml-volumes were again injected into the central cornea. Injection of 10^8 platelets into the substance of the central cornea in 15 eyes produced no angiogenesis or scar, nor did control injections of thrombin (three positives in 11 injected corneas). However, combination of these two elements excited both angiogenesis and scar in all 17 corneas tested. Histologic examination of the corneas showed a mononuclear infiltrate, fibroplasia, collagen deposition and hypertrophic corneal epithelium. These observations have been refined by Dr. Knighton et al.[5] and will be reported among other studies by Dr. Michaeli in Chapter 21. Injection of whole autologous blood clot produced angiogenesis in only one of ten corneas, whereas injection or implantation of autologous fibrin clot produced angiogenesis and scar in three of four corneas.

Control implants and injections for these experiments were 5μ latex beads and washed Hydron polymer. All gave suitably negative results (0+/4 for latex, and 1+/10 for Hydron).

More recently, using more refined techniques, components of the coagulation system, wound inflammatory cells, cultured cells and their conditioned medium, and derivatives of all these have been assayed for their ability to produce angiogenesis, fibroplasia and, in some cases, collagen synthesis using the rabbit cornea assay.

In this assay, various concentrations of the above materials were injected in 0.05-ml volumes (sometimes suspended in EBSS) into the peripheral substance of the cornea.

Rabbits were anesthetized with intravenous pentobarbital and their corneas further anesthetized with topical xylocaine. Test solutions were injected with a 30g needle in the junction between the superficial and deep thirds of the cornea, so that the center of the injection was 3 mm and the peripheral border of the injection approximately 2 mm from the limbal margin.

The corneas were inspected every other day, using 2.5 x optical magnification. Photographs were taken by hand-held cameras, using a macro-lens and standard photographic techniques. Corneal neovascularization was graded from 0 to 4+. Zero denoted no ingrowth of limbal capillaries into the corneal stroma; 1+ denoted 0-1 mm capillary ingrowth in a localized arc adjacent to the injection site; 2+ denoted 1-2 mm ingrowth in a localized arc adjacent to the injection site; 3+ denoted 2-3 mm ingrowth of vessels adjacent to the injection site; and 4+ denoted 4 mm or greater vessel ingrowth in a wide arc along the limbal edge. The degree of corneal opacification, a measure of collagen deposition in the cornea, was measured and expressed by its greatest diameter in millimeters.

Coagulation

Whole blood was injected, both clotted and heparinized. Serum and red cells were separated and injected. Autologous fibrin clot was implanted after exhaustive washing in EBSS. Purified bovine thrombin was injected in EBSS. Suspensions of autologous platelets alone, platelets activated with 0.1 U thrombin, and activated and washed platelets were all injected in EBSS.

Leukocytes

Peritoneal macrophages were injected into the cornea in various numbers and were compared with macrophages derived by aspiration of the dead-space fluid of 20-day old, wire mesh cylinder wounds. In this case, the cell count was approximately 95% macrophages and 5% other cells, as determined by nonspecific esterase staining. Wound-derived granulocytes were similarly injected by aspirating seven-day old wounds in which granulocytes predominated. Wound inflammatory cells were obtained by implanting four stainless steel wire mesh cylinders, each 2 cm in diameter and 5 cm long, under the panniculus carnosus on the dorsal surface of New Zealand white rabbits.[6] Wound fluid, with its inflammatory cells was harvested at seven and 21 days by aspirating fluid from one end of the cylinder with an 18g hypodermic needle. Aspirated fluid was centrifuged at 2000 rpm for 15 minutes. The supernatant was discarded and the cell pellet resuspended in 5 ml EBSS. Fifteen milliliters of sterile distilled water was added for 45 seconds, and isotonicity was restored by adding 5 ml of 3.5% sterile NaCl. The cells were centrifuged at 800 rpm for 12 min, and the supernatant discarded. The cell pellet was resuspended in 5 ml EBSS and the total cell count determined. The differential count was obtained on a small sample by staining a thin smear with Wright's stain. The cell suspension was then centrifuged again at 800 rpm for 20 min, the supernatant discarded and the desired concentration of cells obtained by dilution with EBSS, so that 0.05 ml contained the appropriate number of cells.

In some cases, macrophages obtained from 21-day old wounds were incubated in 1 μg/ml *E. coli* endotoxin (055:B5). The cells were then washed with EBSS, resuspended and injected.

In all, five groups of wound cells were tested. Group I was largely granulocytes from seven-day-old cylinders; groups II-IV were varying numbers of macrophages from 21-day old wounds; and group V was cells from 21-day-old wounds stimulated by endotoxin. Controls consisted of 0.05-ml injections of endotoxin (1 μg/ml in EBSS) and 0.05 ml EBSS alone.

Wound Fluid

As controls to these experiments, whole rabbit wound fluid was centrifuged free of cells. Ten μl was mixed with an equal volume of Hydron™[7] on a polyethylene sheet, then dried under reduced pressure. The resulting pellets were implanted into rabbit corneas, to lie with the nearest edge 3 mm from the corneal limbus, analogous to the injection of cells as described earlier. Corneas were observed as described above.

Studies of Collagen Synthesis

In some experiments, collagen synthetic capacity was measured by the method of Uitto, Prockop and Udenfriend.[8,9] At eight days after injection of wound fluid, a 6-mm diameter corneal button centered on the injection site was excised with a corneatome. The buttons were incubated in 1 mC of ^{14}C-proline in phosphate-free, Kreb's-Ringer's solution with 20 mM HEPES buffer, 20 mM glucose, and 0.5 mg/ml Ampicillin. After incubation was stopped, the corneal tissue was homogenized in cold tap water and hydrolyzed in 6N HCl. Hydrolyzed samples were dried over a vacuum and reconstituted in distilled water and the total radioactive proline measured by the methods of Prockop and Udenfriend.[10] Hydroxyproline values are expressed as counts/min/sample, plus or minus one standard deviation of the mean.

RESULTS

Whole heparinized blood produced no significant angiogenesis or scar in four corneas, where clotted blood produced 3-4+ angiogenesis and 2-3 mm scar in all four corneas tested. When whole blood was quickly centrifuged before coagulation occurred and the red cells placed into the cornea, three out of five corneas demonstrated 1-3+ angiogenesis and small scars, a finding we have recently traced to derivatives of heme. Fibrin clot was positive in nine out of ten corneas with 4+ angiogenesis and 3-4 mm scars.

Results with platelets will be discussed more fully by Dr. Michaeli in Chapter 21. In general, however, whole anticoagulated platelets produced neither angiogenesis nor scar. Platelets activated with a small amount of thrombin produced both angiogenesis and mild scar. Washed platelet skeletons produced neither angiogenesis nor scar, and corneal explants incubated with ^{14}C-proline demonstrated a significant elevation of collagen production after injection of thrombin-activated platelets.[5]

Control injection of EBSS produced no corneal opacification nor capillary proliferation in any of six corneas. In various series of experiments, resident peritoneal macrophages produced neither angiogenesis nor scar. Of 18 corneas injected with seven-day-old wound cells (mostly granulocytes), only six gave a positive angiogenic response and 2-3 mm opacification. All six of these responding corneas in the series received more than 10^6 macrophages in the cell preparations, along with the granulocytes. Corneas which showed no response contained from three to 17 × 10^6 granulocytes and 1 × 10^5 to 3 × 10^6 macrophages (Table 1.2).

Corneas injected with cells obtained from 21-day old wounds were positive 19 times out of 23 for angiogenesis and significant corneal opacification. In general, corneas in which angiogenesis developed had been injected with more than 2 × 10^6 macrophages. Eleven corneas injected with 2 × 10^6 cells produced 1-2+ neovascularization and 1-2 mm opacification. Corneas injected with 5 × 10^6 cells had a 2-3+ neovascular response and 2-3 mm opaci-

TABLE 1.2

Response of Angiogenesis and Scar to Varying Numbers of Wound Cells

Number of Corneas	Number 21-day old Cells (75-90% macrophages) Injected	Opacification (scar)	Angiogenesis
11	2 × 10^6	1-2 mm	1-2+
5	5 × 10^6	2-3 mm	2-3+
6	6-7 × 10^6	4-5 mm	3+
5	2 × 10^6 (endotoxin-activated)	4-5 mm	4+
6	1 μg (endotoxin alone)	(2/6) 1-2 mm (4/6) 0	(2/6) 1+ (4/6) 0

fication. Corneas injected with 6-7 × 10^6 cells produced 3+ neovascularization and 4-5 mm opacification.

Endotoxin-activated 21-day old wound cells (2 × 10^6) produced 4+ angiogenesis and 4-5 mm opacification in all five corneas injected. Controls in which the same amount of endotoxin alone had been injected, produced 1+ angiogenesis in two corneas and none in four. A one- to two-mm area of opacification resulted in the two positive corneas. These corneas contained many inflammatory cells on histologic analysis.

In general, histologic examination showed the injected macrophages, new collagen deposition, and fibroblast proliferation throughout the surrounding stroma. There was no epithelial proliferation over the injection sites. Capillaries extended from the limbus to the injection sites.

Control corneas injected with EBSS alone produced labeled collagen to the extent of 431 ± 29 cpm (one SDM). This is a degree of synthesis similar to that previously found in uninjected control corneas. Eleven corneas injected with 21-day old wound cells (2 × 10^6 cells, 75-90% macrophages) produced labeled collagen of 457 ± 29 cpm. This group is not statistically distinct from the control group.

On the other hand, five corneas injected with 5 × 10^6 21-day old wound cells produced 596 ± 73 cpm labeled collagen, and six corneas injected with 6-7 × 10^6 such cells produced 686 ± 97 cpm. Both of these groups are significantly distinct from the control corneas and those injected with 2 × 10^6 cells at a confidence level of $p < 0.005$. Corneas injected with endotoxin alone produced an average of 723 ± 30 cpm, while 2 × 10^6 21-day-old wound cells activated with endotoxin produced 1260 ± 199 cpm. Endotoxin-stimulated wound cells are statistically distinct from control endotoxin injections and from all the nonendotoxin-activated wound cell injections, at a confidence level of $p < 0.001$.

Corneas into which wound fluid was implanted in Hydron™ pellets demonstrated only 3 and 4+ angiogenesis. No scar ever became visible. The same was true of other experiments in which we implanted fibroblast growth factor, epidermal growth factor, and urogastrone. Some fibroplasia was noted, but visible collagen deposition was notably absent in these cell-free preparations.[11]

DISCUSSION

Clearly, a number of signals arise from the injured areas and influence cells which ordinarily perform other functions, to behave in a reparative mode when they enter damaged tissue. The first signals undoubtedly come from tissue complement and are soon joined by signals originating from the coagulation system (fibrin polymers and platelet factors). The end result is an inflammatory exudate rich in mononuclear cells, from which further messengers arise.

Almost immediately after injury, thrombin-activated platelets release one or more substances which have the potential to be reparative, in that they cause fibroblasts to replicate and may well be able to cause endothelial cells to move and replicate. This is a new development in wound-healing theory. Its biologic role is difficult to assess as yet, but we are inclined to believe that it is important, though not absolutely critical, because inflammatory cell functions duplicate platelet functions. We suspect that platelets give repair a quicker start than would occur if macrophages were forced to act alone. We have seen patients with thrombocytopenia, leukopenia and stalled repair who healed after systemic or local platelet therapy. Almost simultaneously, fibrin-derived peptides attract mononuclear cells, and fibrin itself may stimulate macrophages, a double amplification mechanism. Fibrin-treated corneas soon exhibit a rich mononuclear infiltrate and develop angiogenesis and scar.[4]

Presumably, the macrophage and platelet signals act together. Data presented above suggest that the macrophage may be activated by fibrin and perhaps foreign substances in the wound. Data to be presented later by Dr. Knighton in Chapter 3 suggest that the characteristic wound hypoxia activates macrophages to produce angiogenesis factor and possibly macrophage-derived growth factor (which stimulates the replication rate of fibroblasts). Though the oxygen tension in the injected macrophages has not yet been measured, transcorneal oxygen tension has been mapped. In our techniques, the cells are injected in a layer of cornea in which oxygen tension is normally about 40 mm Hg. Since the injected cells increase cell population and consume oxygen, pO_2 in the area of these cells will fall, certainly to the range of oxygen availability which stimulates secretion of angiogenesis factor (10-35 mm Hg).

The angiogenic substance we have isolated from wound fluid (presumably, but not necessarily, produced by macrophages) is a chemoattractant and not a mitogen.[16] Thus, there are a combination of growth-directors and growth-stimulators being produced at the same time, whose targets are both fibroblasts and endothelial cells.

Almost lost in this data are interesting observations on initiation of collagen synthesis. In countless experiments we have seen collagen deposition after injection of cells, but not after injection of cell products, wound fluid, fibroblast growth factor or epidermal growth factor. We have seen angiogenesis in both cases, but pronounced collagen synthesis seems to occur only when living cells or platelet factors are present. This could be interpreted in many ways, but we favor the explanation that cells consume oxygen, leaving a local hypoxia and high local lactate concentration. Both of these conditions have been shown to stimulate prolyl hydroxylase activity and collagen synthesis.[12,13,14] We postulate, therefore, that three types of signal are needed to bring fibroblasts and endothelial cells into action: 1) a mitogen, 2) a chemoattractant, and 3) a deficiency of energy to induce the collagen synthetic mechanism to action.

According to Silver's highly detailed observations of wound healing in the rabbit ear chamber,[16] the characteristic position of the macrophage in the wound module is at the head of the advancing module, next to the dead space. Why or how the macrophage selects this position is not known; perhaps it is simply because only the macrophage can live in these marginal conditions. Nevertheless, it is a fortuitous position because these hostile conditions obviously can program it to lead fibroblasts and endothelial cells on into the wound void.

With all these growth and growth-directing factors, it would seem reasonable that some should act upon the epithelial cell. However, to the best of our knowledge, this connection has not yet been made, though epidermal growth factor (EGF) or urogastrone is known to exist in wounds. Much attention has been given, however, to the increased growth rates of squamous epithelium under increasing oxygen concentrations (see Chapter 17).

With this detailed concept of how wounds begin to heal, the solution to the problem of how they stop healing would seem to be almost immediately at hand. When Drs. Silver, Knighton and I exposed healing wounds in ear chambers of rabbits to room-air oxygen tensions, perfused through a thin Teflon membrane covering the wounds, healing dramatically stopped.[17] Within the next 48 hours, angiogenesis ceased to move forward into the dead space and new vessels disappeared. At this time, of course, there remained very little of the initial stimulators, that is, dead and dying cells, denatured collagen, foreign body, bacteria, etc. It seems, therefore, that in uncomplicated healing, when the initial damage is cleared and the contribution from the coagulation system diminishes, the major contributor to the continuation of macrophage signals may be the energy deficit present at the center of the wound. In Chapter 24, Dr. Knighton will suggest that healing will continue until that energy deficit is overcome by assembly of a new vascular supply.

Growth directors and growth regulators are very close to being manufacturable in sizeable quantities. An era of practical application of this kind of information is extremely close. We now find ourselves with many, often redundant "growth producers," a common situation in nature, and it remains to find those which are most efficacious, safest, and most inexpensive to produce in order to apply these findings to practical applications such as failures and excesses of healing, artificial skin for burn patients, small artificial arteries for neuro- and neonatal surgery, means of controlling the tendency of the common bile duct to stricture after injury and repair, and so forth. It seems inevitable to conclude that we are at the very beginning of an explosion of practical understanding of healing and scarring phenomena. This information should have wide practical application in medicine.

NOTES

1. Stein J, Levenson SM. Effect of the inflammatory reaction in subsequent wound healing. Surg Forum 17:484-485, 1966.

2. Leibovich SJ, Ross R. A macrophage-dependent factor that stimulates the proliferation of fibroblasts in vitro. Am J Pathol 84:501-513, 1976.

3. Greenburg GB, Hunt TK. The proliferative response in vitro of vascular endothelial and smooth muscle cells exposed to wound fluids and macrophages. J Cell Physiol 97:353-360, 1978.

4. Hunt TK, Andrews WS, Halliday B, Greenburg GB, Knighton DR, Clark RA, Thakral KK. Coagulation and macrophage stimulation of angiogenesis and wound healing. In The Surgical Wound, Dineen P, Hildick-Smith G (eds), pp. 1-18. Philadelphia: Lea & Febiger, 1981.

5. Knighton DR, Thakral KK, Hunt TK. Platelet-derived angiogenesis: Initiator of the healing sequence. Surg Forum 31: 226-227, 1980.

6. Hunt TK, in preparation, 1983.

7. Polverini PJ, Cotran RS, Gimbrone MA Jr, Unanue ER. Activated macrophages induce vascular proliferation. Nature 269:804-806, 1977.

8. Uitto J. A method for studying collagen biosynthesis in human skin biopsies in vitro. Biochem Biophys Acta 201: 438-445, 1970.

9. Prockop DJ, Udenfriend S. A specific method for the analysis of hydroxyproline in tissues and urine. Anal Biochem 1:228-239, 1960.

10. Ibid.

11. Gospodarowicz D, Bialecki H, Thakral KK. Exp Eye Res 28:501, 1979.

12. Langness U, Udenfriend S. Collagen proline hydroxylase activity and anaerobic metabolism. In Biology of Fibroblast, Kulonen E, Pikkarainen J (eds), pp 373-378. London and New York: Academic Press, 1973.

13. Green H, Goldberg B. Collagen and cell protein synthesis by an established mammalian fibroblast line. Nature 204:347, 1964.

14. Levene CK, Bates CJ. The effect of hypoxia on collagen synthesis in cultured 3T6 fibroblasts and its relationship to the mode of action of ascorbate. Biochem Biophys Acta 444:446-452, 1976.

15. Banda MJ, Knighton DR, Hunt TK, Werb Z. Isolation of a nonmitogenic angiogenesis factor from wound fluid. Proc Natl Acad Sci USA (Cell Biol) 79:7773-7777, 1982.

16. Silver IA. The measurement of oxygen tension in healing tissue. Progr Resp Res 3:124-135, 1969.

17. Knighton DR, Silver IA, Hunt TK. Regulation of wound healing angiogenesis—effect of oxygen gradients and inspired oxygen concentration. Surgery 90:262-270, 1981.

18. Wahl SM. Role of mononuclear cells in the wound repair process. In The Surgical Wound, Dineen P, Hildick-Smith G (eds), pp. 63-74. Philadelphia: Lea & Febiger, 1981.

2
Molecular Mediators of Tissue Repair

Gary R. Grotendorst, Dobromir Pencev,
George R. Martin and Jaro Sodek

ABSTRACT

Our studies show that trauma activates a cascade of chemoattractants and mitogens that recruit phagocytes, fibroblasts and endothelial cells into the wound and cause the proliferation of fibroblasts and endothelial cells. The chemoattractants are produced during the clotting of blood by degradation of the surrounding tissue and by the cells entering the wound. Such factors regulate the numbers and types of cells in the wound and in this way control the rate of wound healing. One such factor, the platelet-derived growth factor (PDGF), is released only at sites of injury and has both chemotactic and mitogenic activity toward fibroblasts and smooth muscle cells. PDGF appears to be a wound hormone. Addition of PDGF to an experimental wound model in rats increased the entry and proliferation of cells and the rate at which collagen was deposited. These studies suggest that the levels of chemoattractants and mitogens in the wound are limiting and that wound healing may be improved by the administration of such factors.

This work was supported in part by a grant from the Collagen Corporation, Palo Alto, California.

INTRODUCTION

The repair of damaged tissue requires the concerted action of many specialized cell types to rebuild the tissue (for review see Ross, 1969, Howes & Hoopes, 1977; Gabbiani, 1981; Shoshan, 1981). In part, the process resembles the morphogenetic development of the original tissue or regeneration. The cells involved include blood cells such as leucocytes, monocytes and platelets as well as fibroblastic cells, smooth muscle cells, endothelial cells and parenchymal cells in the case of internal organs. The cells invade the wound in a precise sequence and each has specific functions. For example, some resorb damaged tissue whereas others deposit new extracellular matrix which helps to repair the tissue. It is likely that the migration of the cells is the limiting event in tissue repair and that the migration and proliferation of the cells in the wounds are controlled by chemical factors present at the wound site. These factors include factors produced during the coagulation of the blood, others formed during tissue breakdown and some which are secreted by the cells which enter the wound.

This chapter will deal with the molecular factors which are involved in wound repair including chemoattractants, growth factors and extracellular matrix components. In addition, we will discuss how these factors may arise and function during repair reactions. Some of these factors may function as wound hormones. The levels of these factors may be limiting in wound healing and occur in excessive amounts in conditions where chronic injury leads to fibrosis.

FACTORS CONTROLLING CELLULAR MIGRATIONS: "CHEMOATTRACTANTS"

Most cells respond to chemical signals in their environment either by alterations in their metabolism, movement, growth or differentiation. When a cell responds by directed migration along a gradient toward the source of a chemical, the process is referred to as chemotaxis. Chemotaxis has been described in microorganisms (Adler, 1975) as well as in various cells from higher vertebrates (Schiffmann and Gallin, 1979). For microorganisms, the attractant molecules are typically nutrients, such as glucose or amino acids, and the chemotactic process serves to lead the microorganism to sites of food. For cells of higher organisms, chemotaxis has developed for host defense from infection, morphogenesis and wound repair.

After trauma, the damaged tissue is sequentially invaded by specialized cell types which repair the tissue. It is likely that the migrations of these cells into the wound tissue are controlled by chemotactic factors present in the wound. A number of chemotactic factors have been identified by in vitro studies with animal cells. Many of these factors are the products of the blood clotting reactions (Snyderman et al, 1970), complement activation (Postlethwaite et al, 1979), and inflammation (Postlethwaite et al, 1976), indicating that they have the potential to act in vivo during wound repair. Chemotactic factors are probably specific for a particular cell type and regulate the sequence and the magnitude of the cellular response (Table 2.1).

Leucoattractants

Phagocytic cells (leucocytes and macrophages) are the first cells to accumulate in the wound. The response of these cells to various chemoattractants which are present in wounds was studied in vitro. Leucocytes arrive first at the wound site probably due to their high motility and to the fact that these chemoattractants are produced immediately after injury. Although leucocytes arrive at least 24 hours before the slower migrating macrophages, these cells are attracted to the same factors, including C5a (Snyderman et al, 1970) bacterial products (Ward et al, 1968; Schiffmann et al, 1975), and platelet-factor 4 (Deuel et al, 1981). Studies with synthetic N-formylmethionyl peptides, which are to be related to the bacterial chemoattractants, and C5a indicate that the responding cells have specific surface receptors which bind the chemoattractants. Nonresponding cells (fibroblasts, endothelial cells, etc) lack these receptors.

Connective Tissue Cell Attractants

Fibroblasts and smooth muscle-like cells begin to appear on the third or fourth day after injury. In vitro tests show that fibroblasts are attracted to collagen, collagen α-chains, and collagenous peptides (Postlethwaite et al, 1978) as well as fibronectin (Gauss-Müller et al, 1980) and fibronectin-fragments (Postlethwaite et al, 1981; Seppä et al, 1981). In addition, a factor secreted by platelets, the platelet-derived growth factor (PDGF), is highly active in attracting fibroblasts and smooth muscle cells (Grotendorst et al, 1981; 1982A, Seppä et al, 1982). The potency of the various factors varies markedly. Whereas collagen fragments show activity at 10^{-3}M, PDGF is active at 10^{-10}M. Although chemoattractant activity can be demonstrated in vitro for collagen and fibronectin, in situ such molecules would

TABLE 2.1

Chemoattractants Present during Wound Repair

Chemoattractants	Target Cells	Functions of Target Cells
C5A, Platelet Factor 4, Elastin Peptides, F-Met Peptides	Neutrophils, Monocytes	Phagocytes
Fibronectin, PDGF	Fibroblasts, Smooth Muscle Cells	Matrix Producing Cells
Lymphokines, Monokines Complement Peptides		
Fibronectin, Laminin Monokines	Endothelial Cells	Vascular System

TABLE 2.2

Target Cell Specificity of PDGF Chemotactic Activity

Cell Type	Migratory Response Stimulation Above Control[a]
Fibroblast	590
Smooth Muscle Cell	400
Endothelial Cell	25
Monocyte	30
Neutrophil	30

[a]The migratory response of the various cells was determined using modified Boyden chambers. The data are presented as the percent increase in migration above the control where no attractant is present. Both monocytes and neutrophils as well as endothelial cells which do not respond to PDGF exhibit a 4-7 fold increase in migration to their respective chemotactic factors.

have to diffuse into the surrounding tissue to reach the cells. It is unlikely that these molecules would penetrate far into tissues due to low solubility in the case of collagen, or due to fibronectin's large size and affinity for other matrix components. Fragments produced by the degradation of collagen or fibronectin could attract fibroblasts although rather high levels of these peptides are required (Postlethwaite et al, 1978, 1981; Seppä et al, 1981).

Detailed studies showed that the mitogenic activity of serum was due to a factor released by platelets in the clotting process (Ross et al, 1974; Kohler and Lipton, 1974; Westermark and Wasteson, 1976). This factor, PDGF (M_r = 31,000), is present in platelets and is released following their adherence or aggregation. It is not present in plasma but is released only in damaged areas. PDGF causes connective tissue cells to undergo DNA synthesis and cell division in the presence of other factors contained in plasma (Pledger et al, 1977; Vogel et al, 1978) such as somatomedin and insulin (Stiles et al, 1980). Fibroblasts and smooth muscle cells respond to PDGF and possess specific PDGF cell receptors whereas cells lacking these receptor (endothelial and epithelial cells) are not responsive to PDGF as either a mitogen or a chemoattractant (Table 2.2). These observations suggest that PDGF is a wound hormone for fibroblastic cells and is active in recruiting fibroblasts to the trauma site.

Although PDGF is a potent chemoattractant, other growth factors (i.e. insulin, the somatomedins, epidermal growth factor, and fibroblast growth factor) are not chemotactic (Grotendorst et al, 1982A; Seppä et al, 1982). In fact, the chemotactic activity of PDGF is not dependent on DNA synthesis or mitosis and is unaffected by hydroxyurea or cytosine arabinoside. Further, chemotaxis occurs within four hours which is before any change in DNA synthesis is detected and probably requires fewer PDGF molecules to be bound to cell surface receptors. The dual activity of PDGF could serve to attract cells from the surrounding tissue into the wound and then stimulate their proliferation.

Endothelial Cell Chemoattractants

Soon after the arrival of fibroblastic cells, new capillaries and other blood vessels begin to develop and invade the wound. Vascularization has been investigated in a number of conditions and particularly in tumors. It has been shown that capillaries and endothelial cells show orientation toward tumor tissues. "Angiogenic factors" have been extracted from normal tissue

(Glaser et al, 1980), the media of 3T3 L1 adipocytes (Cästellot et al, 1982), and from tumor cell-conditioned media (Zetter, 1980) and have been shown to induce vascularization in vivo. Recent studies have shown a good correlation between chemotactic activity in such extracts and their angiogenic activity (Glaser et al, 1980; Seppä et al, 1983, in press). Wound exudates also contain a factor which elicits the directed migration of endothelial cells but does not cause their proliferation (Banda et al, 1982). Other cells in the wound may also produce endothelial cell attractants but this has not yet been established.

Studies in model systems suggest that the type of matrix in contact with the endothelial cells determines their phenotype (Maciag et al, 1982; Madri and Stenn, 1982). For example, when capillary endothelial cells are plated in culture on type I collagen, they proliferate and form a continuous sheet. When plated on type IV collagen, the cells stop proliferating and form tube-like structures. The ability to alter the cell phenotype as it passes through different matrices may ensure the recruitment of the capillary cells. Such phenomena may also be important in initiating the spread of capillaries through the wound and integrating capillaries into other tissue elements.

A CASCADE OF CHEMOATTRACTANTS REGULATING THE ENTRY OF CELLS INTO WOUNDS

Clearly the critical factor in restoration of the wound is attracting the cells that debride the wound, produce the extracellular matrix and restore tissue structure. It is likely that specific chemoattractants regulate the various cell types entering the wound. Thus, the phagocytic cells, neutrophils, and macrophages show similar responsiveness. Fibroblasts and smooth muscle cells also respond to common factors different from the phagocyte factors whereas endothelial cells answer to only their own signals. Presumably, key factors in this process are the time of appearance, level of chemoattractant, and the length of time that the attractant is produced. Clearly, the level of chemoattractant is carefully regulated and the production of chemoattractants is probably under some type of negative feedback control.

The fact that the cells appear in an ordered sequence suggests that the chemoattractants are also produced in series. One possibility is that each cell type entering the wound produces an attractant that induces the migration of a subsequent population of cells. The extreme range of potency of chemoattractants suggests that they may serve different functions in the wound. Further, because there are many attractants for each cell type, all of the chemoattractants may not be present in every wound, and some may predominate in certain situations but not in others.

GROWTH FACTORS INVOLVED IN WOUND REPAIR

After connective tissue cells migrate into the wound, they rapidly proliferate. Although the growth of connective tissue cells is influenced by many factors, polypeptide growth factors are probably the most important promoters of fibroblast and smooth muscle cell proliferation (Table 2.3). The polypeptides can be separated into two distinct groups which act synergistically (Pledger et al, 1977; Vogel et al, 1978; Stiles et al, 1980). The first group, called competence factors, activates quiescent cells in the G_0 phase of the cell cycle enabling them to respond to the

TABLE 2.3

Growth Factors Present during Wound Repair

Factor	Source	Time of Appearance	Responsive Cells
PDGF[1]	Platelets	Within Minutes in Smooth Muscle	Fibroblasts
MDGF[2]	Monocytes	24-48 hours	Fibroblasts
AMDGF[3]	Alveolar Macrophages		
MDECGF[4]	Macrophages	24-48 hours	Endothelial Cells
ECDGF[5]	Endothelial Cells	5-7 days	Fibroblasts

[1] Platelet-derived growth factor.
[2] Monocyte-derived growth factor.
[3] Alveolar macrophage-derived growth factor.
[4] Macrophage-derived endothelial cell growth factor.
[5] Endothelial cell-derived growth factor.

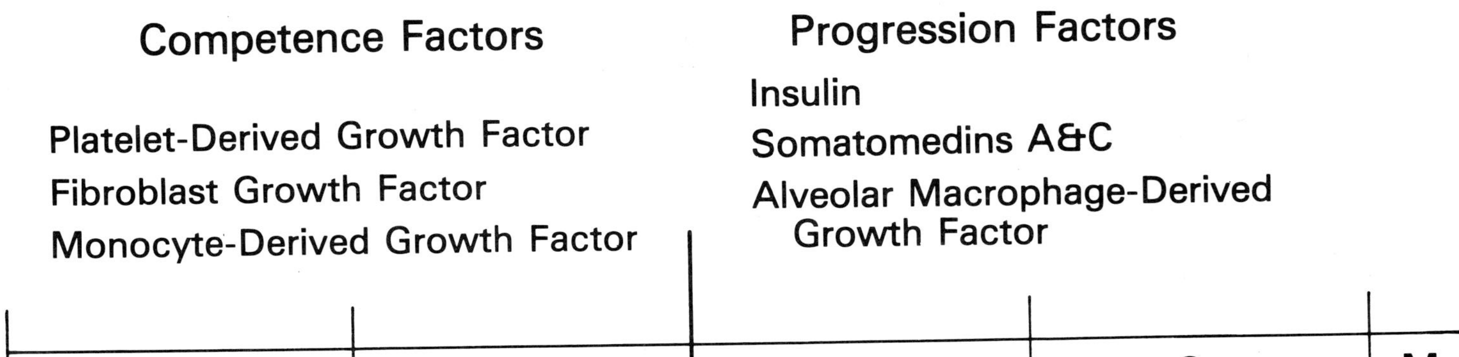

FIGURE 2.1 The growth of connective tissue cells is regulated by polypeptide growth factors which act through specific cell surface receptors. Two classes of these factors have been described; "Competence" and "Progression" factors. Competence factors act during the G_0-G_1 phase of the cell cycle preparing the cell to enter S-phase. However, the cells cannot enter S-phase unless progression factors are present. Factors from both classes must be present in order for cell replication to occur.

second group of growth factors, called progression factors (Figure 2.1).

The primary competence factor present during the initial phases of wound healing is the platelet-derived growth factor (PDGF). It is released from the α-granules of platelets when platelets aggregate. Thus, PDGF is not present normally in body fluids but is found only at sites of tissue injury. PDGF acts to stimulate cell growth by binding to specific cell surface receptors (Heldin et al, 1981; Bowen-Pope et al, 1982; Huang et al, 1982) which are present on connective tissue cells such as fibroblast, smooth muscle cells and glial cells. These receptors are absent from endothelial and epithelial cells (Heldin et al, 1981).

Recently, macrophages have been shown to produce both competence and progression factors. A macrophage-derived competence factor was described by Glenn and Ross (1981). This factor is not produced by peripheral blood monocytes unless they have been activated by substances such as lipopolysaccharide. This factor would thus be secreted by macrophages at sites of inflammation. Alveolar macrophages also produce growth factors which act as progression factors (Bitterman et al, 1982). These results indicate that activated macrophages may produce both competence and progression factors. Thus, connective tissue cell proliferation can be stimulated by macrophages in the absence of any other blood-derived growth factors.

The factors which regulate the growth of endothelial cells are less understood then those for connective tissue cells. These cells do not show any response to PDGF, but are stimulated to grow by factors present in extracts of brain (Gospodarawicz et al, 1975), retina (Glaser et al, 1980), tumors (Zetter, 1980; Seppä et al, 1983 in press), and serum (Clemons et al, 1983). The angiogenic response requires both migration and proliferation by endothelial cells. Whether the growth of these cells is controlled by a similar system as the competence and progression factors which regulate connective tissue cell growth is not presently known. One might predict that there might be factors possessing both chemotactic and mitogenic activities that act on endothelial cells. Several of the endothelial cell chemoattractants produced by tumor cells (Zetter, 1980), and found in normal tissue extracts (Glaser et al, 1980), appear to act as both chemoattractants and mitogens, although these factors have yet to be purified to homogeneity and characterized.

EXTRACELLULAR MATRIX COMPONENTS IN WOUND REPAIR

The extracellular matrix is composed of collagens, glycoproteins, and proteoglycans molecules which interact in a specific manner with each other, and with the cells of that particular tissue (Kleinman et al, 1980) (Table 2.4). Each of these components has a specific function in their respective tissues. Thus, collagens are the structural components, whereas the major glycoproteins present function as cell attachment factors and link the cells to their collagenous matrix. Proteoglycans appear to play diverse roles in tissue functions ranging from hydration for cushioning in cartilage to filtration barriers in basement membranes. During wound repair, the type and amount of matrix produced determines the integrity of the restructured tissue.

At present there are at least five, well-described collagens which occur in different tissues. With the exception of basement membrane collagen, these collagens occur in fibers in the tissue (Bornstein and Sage, 1980). Basement membrane collagen forms a loose meshwork where the molecules are joined end to end (Timpl et al, 1981). Collagens act to give added strength and

TABLE 2.4

Matrix Sets

Cell Type	Collagen	Glycoprotein	Proteoglycan
Fibroblast	Type I, III	Fibronectin (small)	Chondroitin SO_4
Smooth Muscle	Types I, III, V[a] Laminin	Fibronectin (large and small)	Chondroitin SO_4
Chondrocyte	Type II Link Protein	Chondronectin (large)	Chondroitin SO_4
Epithelial	Type IV Fibronectin	Laminin (large)	Heparan SO_4

[a] The attachment protein which functions with type V collagen is not known but is distinct from fibronectin, laminin and other known proteins.

support to tissues and also function as specific substrates for cell adhesion and migration.

Cells do not bind directly to collagen but interact via glycoproteins called attachment factors (Kleinman et al, 1981). These factors are large glycoproteins which contain specific binding sites for collagens, proteoglycans and cell surface receptors. Three different attachment factors have been described to date. The best characterized of these factors is fibronectin. Fibronectin is a large glycoprotein (M_r = 450,000) composed of two similar if not identical peptide chains. Fibronectin is found in many tissues and in plasma (Mosher, 1980). It functions as an attachment protein for fibroblasts and smooth muscle cells to collagen types I and III. It also may function in the attachment of macrophages to collagen and to debris during phagocytosis (Hopper et al, 1976; Saba et al, 1978).

Fibronectin may participate in a variety of steps in wound healing. During the blood clotting reaction, fibronectin is enzymatically crosslinked to fibrin by transglutaminase (Mosher, 1980). This complex may help maintain the clot bound to the margins of the wound. In addition, fibronectin as well as proteolytic fragments of fibronectin have been found to act as chemoattractants for fibroblasts (Gauss-Müller et al, 1980; Postlethwaite et al, 1981; Seppä et al, 1981). Thus, fibronectin serves not only as an attachment factor in connective tissue, but attracts cells (macrophages and fibroblasts) to the wound site. It also aids macrophages in cleaning the wound site by its opsonic activity.

The attachment of epithelial or endothelial cells to basement membrane collagen is mediated by laminin. Laminin is a large molecule (M_r = 1,000,000) containing four chains, an A-chain (M_r = 400,000) and three B-chains (M_r = 200,000) (Timpl et al, 1979). These are organized in the form of a cross. Laminin is produced by epithelial cells (Foidart et al, 1980A) and by both striated and smooth muscle cells. It is found only in basement membranes (Foidart et al, 1980B). During wound repair, laminin is probably first produced in the wound site by myofibroblasts which are the first connective tissue cells to arrive. The deposition of laminin by these cells could aid the ingrowth of new blood vessels by supporting the attachment of endothelial cells.

Chondrocytes utilize a different attachment factor, chondronectin (Hewitt et al, 1980). This glycoprotein is smaller than both fibronectin and laminin (176,000 MW) and is composed of three apparently identical subunits (M_r = 55,000) (Varner et al, in press). Chondronectin is found in cartilage, in the vitreous of the eye and in serum. It does not appear to have any chemotactic activity but it does promote the growth and production of matrix by chondrocytes (Grotendorst et al, 1982B).

The attachment factors appear to affect the phenotypic expression of the cells with which they contact. For example, epithelial cells are stimulated to synthesize new basement membrane components in the presence of fibronectin (Foidart et al, 1980A; Brownell et al, 1981). Fibronectin has also been shown to alter the phenotype of chondrocytes causing them to assume a more fibroblastic morphology and to switch from the production of cartilage-specific proteins to fibroblast proteins (Pennypacker et al, 1979). In this manner, the distribution of specific attachment factors in a wound site could alter the types of cells which invade the area as well as the functional activities of those cells.

Excessive Matrix Production: Fibrotic Lesions

Excessive matrix production in response to trauma is thought to underly certain fibrotic disorders. In this case, recruitment of fibroblasts or smooth muscle cells and matrix deposition may not always be of benefit to the host. Clearly, fibroblasts are present and active in healing skin wounds. The types of collagen produced under these conditions are those associated with fibroblasts (Types I, III). However, in sites where fibrotic reactions occur due to trauma, toxins or disease, such as the liver (Rauterberg et al, 1981), blood bessels (Ooshima, A. 1981), skin (Gay et al, 1980), or tumor capsules (Barsky et al, 1982), type V collagen, a product of smooth muscle cells, is deposited. Possibly the collagen deposited in these sites is produced by smooth muscle cells recruited by chemoattractants from blood vessels. The nature of this matrix may differ significantly from that produced by fibroblasts and could be responsible for adhesions and contractions. In burns, smooth muscle cells could be present as a major portion of the reparative cells in the skin due to damage to fibroblasts and account for the unusual properties of the scarring encountered under these conditions.

RATE-LIMITING STEPS IN WOUND HEALING

The assessment of wound healing is often based on measurements of collagen content of the tissue or on tensile strength. Studies show that the deposition of crosslinked collagen fibers parallels the regaining of tissue tensile strength (Peacock and Madden, 1966). Even under optimal conditions, however, this

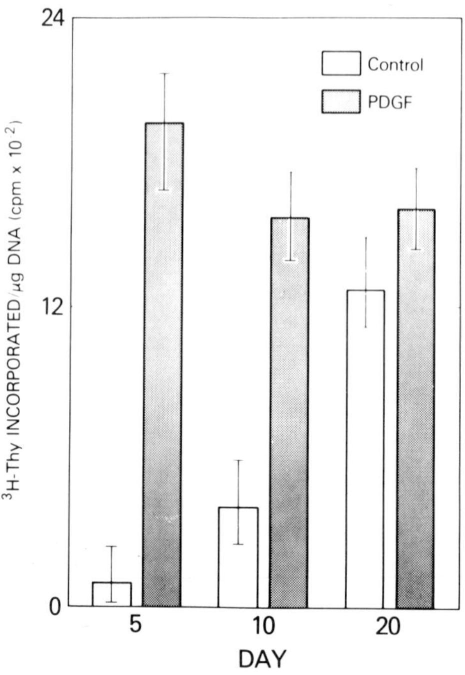

FIGURE 2.2 Stimulation of DNA synthesis in PDGF treated wounds. Stain-steel mesh chambers (1 cm dia) were filled with a collagen gel with or without PDGF (50 ng/ml). The chambers were surgically implanted subcutaneously in rats. After 5, 10 and 20 days, the chambers were removed and the level of DNA synthesis was determined by incubating the chambers in serum free DMEM containing 2 μCi/ml of ^{3}H-Thymidine. After 2 hours, the reaction was stopped by extracting the total DNA with 0.1N NaOH in 0.1% Triton X-100. The DNA content of the chamber and the amount of ^{3}H-Thymidine incooperated into TCA precipitable material was determined. The data are expressed as cpm/μg of DNA and are the mean values of six individual experiments.

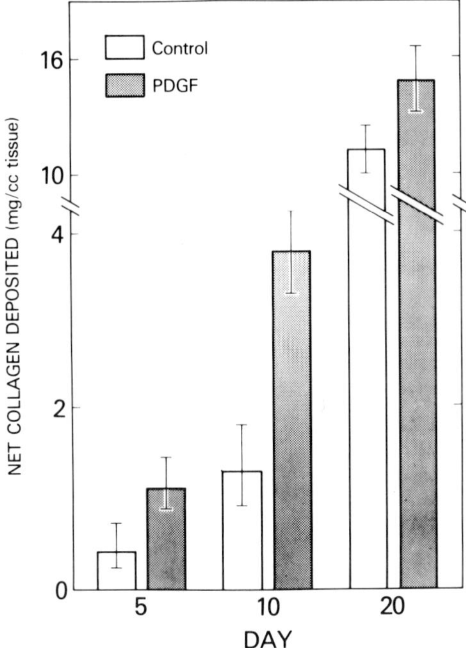

FIGURE 2.3 Stimulation of collagen deposition by PDGF. The collagen content of chambers similar to those described under Figure 2.2 was determined by amino acid analysis using hydroxyproline content as a measure for collagen. The data are the mean values of six individual experiments.

is a relatively slow process. The migration of cells into the wound site regulates the rate of repair since the numbers of cells in the wound, including fibroblasts and endothelial cells, govern the rate of healing. It is possible that several of the factors present during normal wound repair might be present at suboptimal levels.

We measured the rate of wound repair in stainless steel mesh chambers (Schilling-Hunt) (Hunt et al, 1967) which were implanted subcutaneously in rats. The implantation of these chambers induces a wound repair response (Hunt et al, 1967). Sporn et al (1983) have shown that injection of transforming growth factors into the wound chamber stimulates the growth of connective tissue cells in and around the chamber. We used chambers which were filled with a collagen gel (3 mg/ml), either alone or containing the platelet-derived growth factor (50 ηg/ml). The collagen gel alone did not change the amount of DNA synthesis or collagen deposition when compared to empty chambers. However, addition of PDGF to the chamber caused a marked increase in DNA synthesis during the first days after implantation (Figure 2.2). In addition, there was a parallel increase in collagen deposition in the wound chambers containing PDGF (Figure 2.3). It appears that both the cell division and collagen deposition in the chambers containing PDGF and collagen eventually reach the same level as the control chambers indicating that the termination of the healing response appears to be normal.

These data suggest that the rate of wound repair in normal animals can be increased by supplementation of the wound area with chemotactic and mitogenic factors. Many conditions are known where wound healing is impaired. It may be possible to improve wound healing in these situations by utilizing factors which stimulate the migration and proliferation of connective tissue cells. Potent natural products are available for such tests.

REFERENCES

Adler, J (1975) Chemotaxis in bacteria. Ann. Rev. Biochem. 44:341-356.

Banda, MJ, Knighton, DR, Hunt, TK and Werb, Z (1982) Isolation of a nonmitogenic angiogenesis factor from wound fluid. Proc. Natl. Acad. Sci., USA 79:7775-7777.

Barsky, SH, Rao, CN, Grotendorst, GR and Liotta, LA (1982) Increased content of type V collagen in desmoplasia of human breast carcinoma. Am. J. Pathol. 108:276-283.

Bitterman, PB, Rennard, SI, Hunninghake, GW and Crystal, RG (1982) Human alveolar macrophage growth factor for fibroblasts: Regulation and partial characterization. J. Clin. Invest. 70:806-822.

Bornstein, P and Sage, H (1980) Structurally distinct collagen types. Ann. Rev. Biochem. 49:957-1003.

Bowen-Pope, DF and Ross, R (1982) Platelet-derived growth factor II. Specific binding to cultured cells. J. Biol. Chem. 257:5161-5171.

Brownell, AG, Bessen, CC and Slavkin, HC (1981) Possible functions of mesenchyme cell-derived fibronectin during formation of basal lamina. Proc. Natl. Acad. Sci. USA 78: 3711-3715.

Cästellot, JJ, Karnovsky, MJ and Speigelman, BM (1982) Differentiation-dependent stimulation of neovascularization and endothelial cell chemotaxis by 3T3 adipocytes. Proc. Natl. Acad. Sci. USA 79:5597-5601.

Clemons, DR, Isley, WL and Brown, MT (1983) Dialyzable factor in human serum of platelet origin stimulates endothelial cell replication and growth. Proc. Natl. Acad. Sci. USA 80: 1641-1645.

Deuel, TF, Senior, RM, Chang, D, Griffin, G, Hemilsson, RL, and Kaiser, ET (1981) Platelet factor 4 is chemotactic for neutrophils and monocytes. Proc. Natl. Acad. Sci. USA 78: 4584-4587.

Foidart, JM, Berman, JJ, Paglia, L, Rennard, S, Abe, S, Perantoni, A, and Martin, GR (1980A) Synthesis of fibronectin, Laminin, and several collagens by a liver-derived epithelial line. Lab. Invest. 42:525-532.

Foidart, JM, Bere, EW, Yaar, M, Rennard, SI, Gullino, M, Martin, GR, and Katz, SI (1980B) Distribution and immunoelectron microscopic localization of laminin, a noncollagenous basement membrane glycoprotein. Lab. Invest. 42:336-342.

Gabbiani, G (1981) The myofibroblast: A key cell for wound healing and fibrocontractive diseases. Prog. Clin. Biol. Res. 54:183-194.

Gauss-Müller, V, Kleinman, HK, Martin, GR, and Schiffmann, E (1980) Role of attachment factors and attractants in fibroblast chemotaxis. J. Lab. Clin. Med. 96:1071-1080.

Gay, RE, Buckingham, RB, Prince, RK, Gay, S, Rodan, GR and Miller, EJ (1980) Collagen types synthesized in dermal fibroblast cultures from patients with early progressive systemic sclerosis. Arthritis and Rheumatism 23:190-196.

Glaser, BM, D'Amore, PA, Seppä, HEJ, Seppä, SI, and Schiffmann, E (1980) Adult tissues contain chemoattractants for vascular endothelial cells. Nature 288:483-484.

Glenn, KC and Ross, R (1981) Human monocyte-derived growth factor(s) for mesenchymal cells: Activation of secretion by endotoxin and concanavalin A. Cell 25:603-615.

Gospodarowicz, D, Moran, JS and Braum, DL (1975) Control of proliferation of bovine vascular endothelial cells. J. Cell Physiol. 91:377-386.

Grotendorst, GR, Seppä, HEJ, Kleinman, HK, and Martin, GR (1981) Attachment of smooth muscle cells to collagens and their migration toward platelet-derived growth factor. Proc. Natl. Acad. Sci. USA 78:3669-3672.

Grotendorst, GR, Chang, T, Seppä, HEJ, Kleinman, HK and Martin, GR (1982A) Platelet-derived growth factor is a chemoattractant for vascular smooth Muscle cells. J. Cell. Physiol. 113:261-266.

Grotendorst, GR, Kleinman, HK, Rohrbach, DH, Hewitt, AT, Varner, HH, Horigan, EA, Hassell, JR, Terranova, VP, and Martin, GR (1982B) Role of attachment factors in mediating the attachment, distribution and differentiation of cells. In Growth of Cells in Hormonally Defined Media, Subasku, Sato, and Pardee (eds), pp. 403-414. New York: Cold Spring Harbor Press.

Heldin, CA, Westermark, B, and Wasteson, A (1981) Specific receptors for platelet-derived growth factor on cells derived from connective tissue and glia. Proc. Natl. Acad. Sci. USA 78:3364-3368.

Hewitt, AT, Kleinman, HK, Pennypacker, JP, and Martin, GR (1980) Identification of an adhesion factor for chondrocytes. Proc. Natl. Acad. Sci. USA 77:385-388.

Hopper, KE, Adelmann, BC, Gentner, G, and Gay, S (1976) Recognition by guinea pig peritoneal exudate cells of conformationally-different states of the collagen molecule. Immunology 30:249-259.

Howes, RM and Hoopes, JE (1977) Current concepts of wound healing. Clin. Plastic Surg. 4:173-179.

Huang, JS, Huang, SS, Kennedy, B, and Deuel, TF (1982) Platelet-derived growth factor: Specific binding to target cells. J. Biol. Chem. 257:8130-8136.

Hunt, TK, Twomey, P, Zederfeldt, B, and Dunphy, JE (1967) Respiratory gas tensions and pH in healing wounds. Am. J. Surg. 114:302-307.

Kleinman, HK, Hewitt, AT, Grotendorst, GR, Martin, GR, Murry, JC, Rohrbach, DH, Terranova, VP, Rennard, SI, Varner, HH, and Wilkes, CM (1980) Role of matrix proteins in the adhesion and growth of cells. In Current Trends in Prenatal Craniofacial Development, Pratt, RM and Christiansen, RL (eds) p. 277-295. Holland, NY: Elsevier-Norok.

Kohler, N and Lipton, A (1974) Platelets as a source of fibroblast growth-promoting activity. Exp. Cell Res. 87:297-301.

Madri, JA and Stenn, KS (1982) Aortic endothelial cell migration I. matrix requirements and composition. Am. J. Pathol. 106: 180-186.

Maciag, T, Kadish, J, Wilkins, L, Sternerman, MB, and Weinstein, R (1982) Organizational behavior of human umbilical vein endothelial cells. J. Cell Biol. 94:511-520.

Mosher, DR (1980) Fibronectin. Prog. Hemostasis Thromb. 5: 111-151.

Ooshima, A (1981) Collagen α, β chain: Increased production in human atherosclerosis. Science 213:666-668.

Peacock, EE and Madden, JW (1966) Some studies on the effect of β-Aminopropionitrite on collagen in healing wounds. Surgery 60:7-12.

Pennypacker, JP, Hassell, JR, Yamada, KM, and Pratt, RM (1979) The influence of an adhesion cell surface protein on chondrogenic expression in vitro. Exp. Cell. Res. 121:411-415.

Pledger, WJ, Stiles, CD, Antoniades, HN, and Scher, CD (1977) Induction of DNA synthesis in Balb/c 3T3 cells by serum components: Reevaluation of the commitment process. Proc. Natl. Acad. Sci. USA 74:4481-4485.

Postlethwaite, AE, Snyderman, R, and Kang, AH (1976) Chemotactic attraction of human fibroblasts to a lymphocyte-derived factor. J. Exp. Med. 144:1188-1303.

Postlethwaite, AE, Seyer, JM, and Kang, AH (1978) Chemotactic attraction of human fibroblasts to type I, II and III collagens and collagen-derived peptides. Proc. Natl. Acad. Sci. USA 75:871-875.

Postlethwaite, AE, Snyderman, R, and Kang, AH (1979) Generation of a fibroblast chemotactic factor in serum by activation of complement. J. Clin. Invest. 64:1379-1385.

Postlethwaite, AE, Keski-Ojá, J, Balian, G, and Kang, A (1981) Induction of fibroblast chemotaxis by fibronectin. Localization of the chemotactic region to a 140,000 molecular weight non-gelatin binding fragment. J. Exp. Med. 153:494-499.

Rauterberg, J, Voss, B, Pott, G, and Gerlach, U (1981) Connective tissue components of normal and fibrotic liver. Klin Wochenschr 59:767-779.

Ross, R (1969) Wound healing. Sci. Am. 220:40-50.

Ross, R, Glomset, J, Kariya, B, and Harlser, L (1974) A platelet-dependent serum factor that stimulates the proliferation of arterial smooth muscle cells in vitro. Proc. Natl. Acad. Sci. 71:1207-1210.

Saba, TM, Blumenstock, FA, Weber, P, and Kaplan, JE (1978) Physiologic role of Cold-Insoluble globulin in systemic host defense: Implications of its characterization as the opsonic α_2-surface-binding glycoprotein. N.Y. Acad. Sci. 312:43-55.

Schiffman, E, Showell, HV, Corcoran, BA, Ward, PA, Smith, E, and Becker, EL (1975) The isolation and partial characterization of neutrophil chemotactic factors from Escherichia coli. J. Immunol. 114:1831-1837.

Schiffmann, E and Gallin, JI (1979) Biochemistry of phagocyte chemotaxis. In Current Topics in Cellular Regulation. Vol 15: p. 203-261. New York: Academic Press.

Seppä, HEJ, Yamada, KM, Seppä, SI, Silver, MH, Kleinman, HK, and Schiffmann, E (1981) The cell-binding fragment of fibronectin is chemotactic for fibroblasts. Cell Biol. Int. Rep. 5:813.

Seppä, HEJ, Grotendorst, GR, Seppä, SI, Schiffmann, E, and Martin, GR (1982) The platelet-derived growth factor is a chemoattractant for fibroblasts. J. Cell Biol. 92:584-588.

Seppä, SI, Seppä, H, Liotta, LA, Glaser, B, Martin, GR, and Schiffmann, E (1983). Cultured tumor cells produce chemotactic factors specific for endothelial cells: A possible mechanism for tumor-induced angiogenesis. Metastases and Invasion. In Press.

Shoshan, S (1981) Wound healing. Int. Rev. of Connect. Tissue Res. Vol 9:1-26.

Snyderman, R, Phillips, J, and Mergenhagen, SE (1970) Polymorphonuclear leukocyte chemotactic activity in rabbit serum and guinea pig serum treated with immune complexes: Evidence for C5a as the major chemotactic factor. Infect. and Immun. 1:521-525.

Sporn, MB, Roberts, AB, Shull, JH, Smith, JM, Ward, JM, and Sodek, J (1983) Polypeptide transforming growth factors isolated from bovine sources and used for wound healing in vivo. Science 219:1329-1331.

Stiles, CD, Pledger, WJ, Tuclah, RW, Martin, RG, and Scher, CD (1980) Regulation of the Balb/c 3T3 cell cycle-effects of growth factors. J. Supramolec. Structure 13:489-499.

Timpl, R, Wiedmann, H, van Delden V, Furthmayr, H, and Kuhn, K (1981) A networks model for the organization of type IV collagen molecules in basement membranes. Eur. J. Biochem. 120:203-211.

Timpl, R, Rohde, H, Gehron-Robey, P, Rennard, SI, Foidart, JM, and Martin, GR (1979) Laminin—a glycoprotein from basement membrane. J. Biol. Chem. 254:9933-9937.

Varner, HH, Furthmayr, H, Nilsson, B, Fietzek, PP, Osborne, JC, DeLuca, S, Martin, GR, and Hewitt, AT (1983) Further characterization of chondronectin, the chondrocyte attachment factor. Arch. Biochem. Biophys. In Press.

Vogel, A, Raines, E, Kariya, B, Rivest, MJ, and Ross, R (1978) Coordinate control of 3T3 cell proliferation by platelet-derived growth factor and plasma components. Proc. Natl. Acad. Sci. USA 75:2810-2814.

Ward, PA, Lepow, IH, and Newman, LJ (1968) Bacterial factors chemotactic for polymorphonuclear leukocytes. Am. J. Pathol. 52:725-736.

Westermark, B and Wasterson, A (1976) A platelet factor stimulating human normal glial cells. Exp. Cell Res. 98:170-174.

Zetter, BR (1980) Migration of capillary endothelial cells is stimulated by tumor-derived factors. Nature 285:41-43.

3
Regulation of Repair: Hypoxic Control of Macrophage Mediated Angiogenesis

David R. Knighton, Sven Oredsson, Michael Banda and Thomas K. Hunt

Wound healing represents an orderly, controlled cellular response to injury. The sequential morphologic and structural changes which occur during repair have been characterized in great detail and in some instances quantified. The mechanisms which regulate the cellular and biochemical responses to injury, on the other hand, are presently under active investigation.

The regulation of repair begins with signals which translate a mechanical injury into biochemical messages which can be recognized by circulating monocytes and neutrophils, and local connective tissue cells. These signals are generated by activation of Hagemann factor, the clotting cascade, the complement cascade, the kinin system, and by-products from platelet release. In response to these signals, circulating neutrophils and monocytes are attracted to the site of injury, fibroblasts are stimulated to move, divide, and produce large amounts of new collagen, and new capillary growth (angiogenesis) is stimulated. The extent of the injury and method of mechanical closure help determine the magnitude of the repair response and the length of time needed to complete repair.

All soft tissue wounds, regardless of size, heal in a similar manner. Injury results in tissue disruption and coagulation of the microvasculature at the edge of the wound. Whether the wound is closed primarily or left open, the cellular response is similar, only the volume of the central wound space varies.

The cellular morphology consists of three distinct zones (see Figure 3.1). The central avascular wound space is hypoxic, acidotic, hypercarbic, and has high lactate levels.[1] Adjacent to the wound space is a gradient zone of ischemia which is populated by dividing fibroblasts. The oxygen gradient depends on the inspired oxygen concentration. For animals breathing room air (21% oxygen) the pO_2 over the capillary is 80 mm Hg and 100-150μ

away, in the dead space, the pO_2 approaches zero. Behind the leading zone is an area of active collagen synthesis characterized by mature fibroblasts and numerous newly formed capillaries. As the wound heals, this "wound module" as described by Dr. Hunt (Chapter 1), advances as a unit until the two edges meet and healing stops.

Repair is one of many biologic or pathologic systems where cellular proliferation and angiogenesis occur in the presence of an oxygen gradient. Most systems are associated with high tissue metabolic demands which create local oxygen and metabolite gradients. There are many examples: malignant neoplasms create an oxygen gradient because of their increased metabolic rates;[2,3] the corpus luteum stimulates a neovascular response when increased steroid synthesis occurs during pregnancy;[4,5] increased capillary density and diameter have been demonstrated in chronically ischemic tissue resulting from atherosclerosis, chronic electrical stimulation of muscle, or hypoxia associated with living at high altitude.[6,7,8,9]

The healing wound offers a unique experimental situation to study this relationship because the oxygen gradient is mechanically formed and the response to experimental manipulation can be easily quantified using a modification of Clark's rabbit ear chamber.[10] The chamber consists of an acrylic disc which is implanted into the rabbit's ear so that the underside of the disc is in contact with the perichondrium of the ear. A wound space is defined in the center of the chamber and holes in the bottom of the disc allow tissue to grow into the wound space.

We utilized three modifications of this chamber to test the effect of raising or lowering the pO_2 in the central wound healing space on the progression of healing and angiogenesis. The first chamber was designed to completely seal the wound space from atmospheric oxygen to maintain physiologic oxygen tension in the chamber. The second chamber was fitted with a cover fashioned from Permanox plastic which has a high permeability to oxygen and is made for tissue culture. The third chamber was fitted with two covers. The inner cover was Permanox plastic and a second outer cover was fashioned from an oxygen-impermeable plastic.

After implantation into New Zealand rabbits, the progression of healing and angiogenesis was quantified by photographing the chambers with a standard dissecting microscope. The total chamber area and the area covered by new vessels was then measured with a planimeter and results were expressed as percent of the total chamber covered with new vessels.

Two experiments were performed to test the effect of manipulating the oxygen gradient from the perfused edge of connective tissue to the wound space. First, rabbits were implanted with ear chambers equipped with oxygen-permeable or impermeable covers. The impermeable cover kept the wound space oxygen near zero, and the permeable cover allowed the wound space to equilibrate with atmospheric oxygen. Photographs were taken every other day. When oxygen impermeable covers were used, connective tissue entered the chamber and proceeded to grow at a uniform rate until the chamber was filled with new vessels.

The advancing capillaries have three distinctive zones. At the leading edge, they had a "brush border" appearance with areas of hemorrhage. Behind this border of actively growing capillaries, the vessels form into a dense network of individual nonhemorrhagic channels. Behind this, the vessels mature into afferent and efferent vessels. The zone of growing capillaries advances until the chamber is completely filled with a mature vascular network.

In chambers fitted with oxygen-permeable covers from implantation, newly-formed capillaries entered the chamber as usual, but as the advancing tissue was exposed to atmospheric oxygen, the brush border disappeared and a mature vessel pattern developed. This mature pattern persisted as long as the chambers were left in place (see Figure 3.2).

The second set of experiments was designed to test whether the effect found in the first experiments was reversible. Chambers equipped with two covers were implanted with the outer oxygen-impermeable cover in place from the outset. The outer, oxygen-impermeable cover was removed at different stages in the healing sequence and the effect on further progression was recorded. In another group of animals, the oxygen-impermeable cover was removed and then replaced immediately to control for the manipulation needed to remove the impermeable cover.

Removing the oxygen impermeable cover arrested vessel growth and caused maturation of the new capillary network. This occurred whether 15%, 30%, 60%, or 70% of the chamber was filled with new vessels. When 80% of the chamber was filled with new vessels, the small remaining wound space was filled in spite of the change in oxygen concentration. Control chambers from which the oxygen-impermeable covers were removed and replaced immediately, continued to grow but at a slower rate than was recorded in chambers where the wound space remained hypoxic throughout the experiment.

These experiments clearly demonstrate that a hypoxic central wound space is required for normal angiogenesis and healing to proceed. The mechanism by which changes in the oxygen tension affected capillary growth and healing was still in question. Previous observations and experiments from various laboratories have shown that the macrophage is the primary cell populating the wound space. Activated wound and peritoneal macrophages also stimulate angiogenesis in various experimental systems. The question was then asked, whether macrophages were sensitive to their oxygen environment, and whether angiogenesis stimulated by macrophages could be stimulated or suppressed by changes in local oxygen tension.

To answer these questions, bone marrow macrophages were cultured from rabbit tibias on oxygen-permeable Permanox tissue culture plates. The macrophages were initially plated and cultured in room air for nine days in standard medium and a combination of rabbit and newborn calf serum. Cultures were then divided into test and control groups. All cultures were washed and serum containing medium was replaced with medium containing 0.2% lactalbumin. Test cultures were made hypoxic by culture in a controlled gas chamber which was continually flushed with a 2% oxygen-5% carbon dioxide-73% nitrogen mixture. Control cultures remained in a room air-carbon dioxide chamber. The cells were exposed to these two oxygen concentrations for 48 hours and then the conditioned supernatant was removed, filtered, and tested for plasminogen activator and rabbit fibroblast mitogenic activity. Conditioned media were also dialysed against acetic acid, lyophilized, concentrated to 10x, and resuspended in media. Twenty microliters was suspended in Hydron™ polymer pellets and implanted into the rabbit cornea to determine the amount of angiogenesis factor contained in the supernatant.

Angiogenesis was graded as a 0 to 4+ response depending on the degree of corneal neovascularization stimulated by the implanted supernatant. Hypoxic macrophages uniformly produced a 4+ response (see Figure 3.3), while supernatants from macrophages cultured in 20% oxygen were uniformly negative (see Figure 3.4). Hypoxic macrophage supernatants also contained 25 U/ml of plasminogen activator activity and a four-fold increase in fibroblast mitogenic activity over controls. Normoxic macrophage supernatants produced 1 U/ml plasminogen activator activity and a three-fold increase in fibroblast mitogenic activity (see Figure 3.5).

Since exposing the cells to hypoxia stimulated angiogenesis and plasminogen activator activity, we then asked whether returning the hypoxic cultures to room air would reverse the responses.

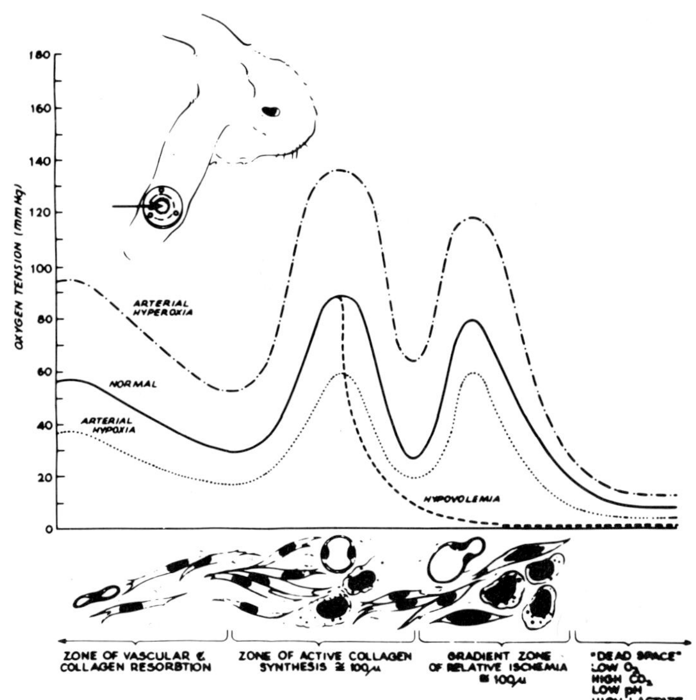

FIGURE 3.1

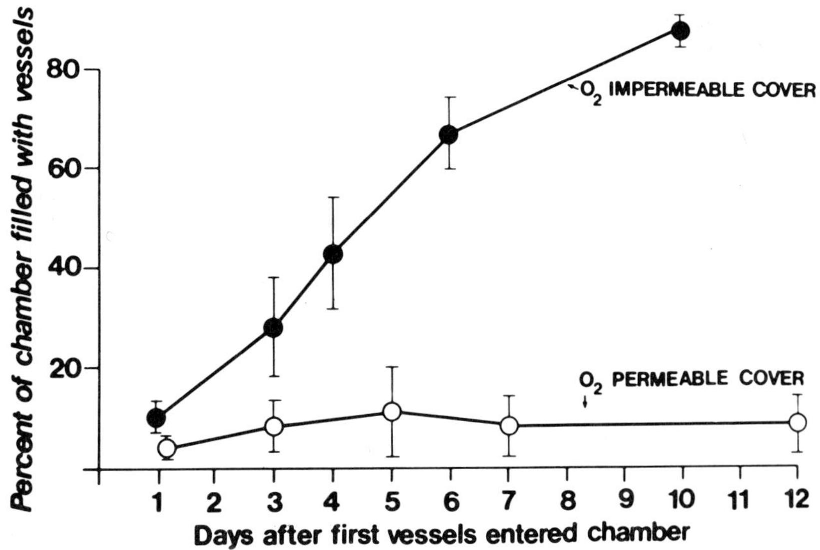

FIGURE 3.2

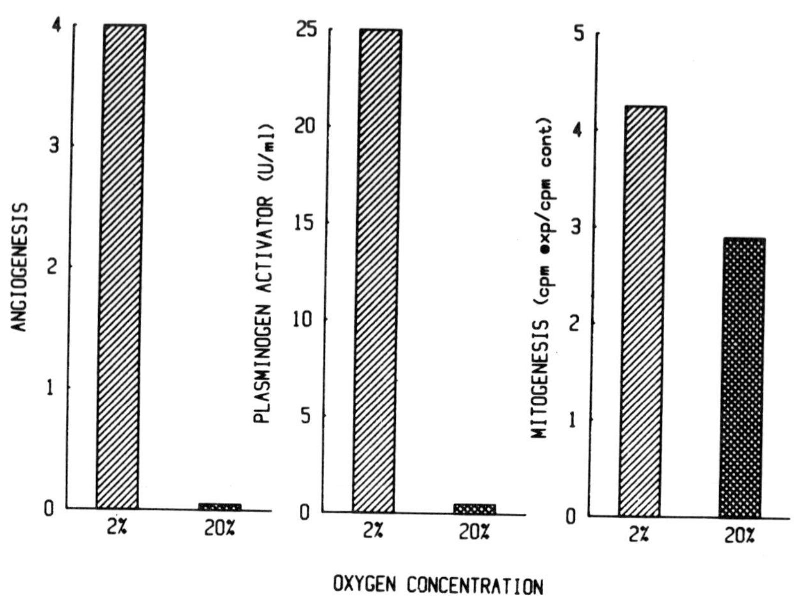

Supernatants from cells cultured in 2% oxygen for 48 hours were removed for testing. The cells were washed with fresh media with lactalbumin, and they were then returned to the room air incubator for a second 48-hour period. This conditioned media was removed and tested. Supernatants from the hypoxic macrophages stimulated angiogenesis, while supernatants from the same macrophages exposed to 20% oxygen produced no angiogenesis.

These experiments demonstrate that macrophage-derived angiogenesis is stimulated by hypoxia and suppressed by increased oxygen tension. The production of plasminogen activator follows a similar pattern while mitogenic activity is affected to a lesser extent.

Putting these results together with the ear chamber experiments we have formulated a possible mechanism which may explain how hypoxic wound gradients stimulate angiogenesis and how the duration of repair is regulated. As described earlier, the mechanical disruption which initiates repair forms a hypoxic wound space which is populated exclusively by macrophages. This hypoxic environment stimulates the macrophages to produce angiogenesis factor(s), plasminogen activator, and to a lesser extent, mitogenesis factor(s). These factors in turn stimulate the surrounding connective tissue to proliferate. When the wound edges become close enough (approximately 200-300μ), the oxygen tension in the wound space will increase, suppressing the secretion of angiogenesis factor(s) by macrophages which in turn stops the connective tissue proliferation.

Any physiologic or pathologic situation where local oxygen tensions are decreased could also stimulate tissue macrophages to secrete angiogenesis factor(s). This may be the mechanism which stimulates capillary proliferation in hypoxic tissue resulting from electrode implantation, arterial insufficiency, exercise or existence at high altitude.

Finally, the high level of angiogenesis activity found in hypoxic macrophage cultures along with previous data that wound macrophages stimulate angiogenesis in the corneal assay system, prompted us to attempt isolation of the angiogenesis factor from wound fluid. Briefly, we collected cell-free 21-day-old wound fluid from wire mesh cylinders implanted in rabbits. The wound fluid was clarified by centrifugation, dialysed in an Mr 2,000-limit dialysis bag for 72 hours, and the retentate was dialysed in a Mr 14,000-limit dialysis bag for 24 hours. The dialysate was then lyophilized, and reconstituted. Chromatography was carried out on a high pressure liquid chromatograph and fractions were suspended in Hydron™ for testing in the rabbit cornea angiogenesis assay. The isolated angiogenesis factor was purified 9,600-fold with a yield of 81%. The purified wound fluid angiogenesis factor contained no mitogenic activity for cultured rabbit brain capillary endothelium, but did stimulate capillary endothelial cell migration.[11]

Supported by NIH Grant GM-27345, AM-32746, and U.S. Department of Energy.

NOTES

1. Silver IA. The measurement of oxygen tension in healing tissue. Progr Resp Res 3:124-135, 1969.

2. Brem S, Cotran R, Folkman J. Tumor angiogenesis: A quantitative method for histologic grading. J Natl Cancer Inst 48:347-356, 1972.

3. Folkman J. Tumor angiogenesis. Adv Cancer Res 10: 331-358, 1974.

4. Gospodarowicz D, Thakral KK. Production of a corpus luteum angiogenic factor responsible for proliferation of capillaries and neovascularization of the corpus luteum. Proc Natl Acad Sci 75:847-851, 1977.

5. Jakob W, Jentzsh KD, Mauersberger D, Oehme P. Demonstration of angiogenesis activity in the corpus luteum of cattle. Exp Pathol 13:231-236, 1977.

6. Hammarsten J, Bylund-Fellenius AC, Holm J, Schersten T, Krotkiewski M. Capillary supply and Muscle fiber types in patients with intermittent claudication: Relationships between morphology and metabolism. Eur J Clin Invest 10: 301-305, 1980.

7. Hudlicka D, Myrhage R, Cooper J. Growth of capillaries in adult skeletal muscle after chronic stimulation. Bibl Anat 15: 508-509, 1977.

8. Makitie J. Ultrastructure and density of skeletal muscle capillaries in atherosclerosis obliterans. Bibl Anat 16: 380-383, 1977

9. Valdivia E. Total capillary bed in striated muscle of guinea pigs native to the Peruvian mountains. Am J Physiol 194:585-589, 1958.

10. Knighton D, Silver I, Hunt T. Regulation of wound-healing angiogenesis - effect of oxygen gradients and inspired oxygen concentration. Surgery 90:262-270, 1981.

11. Hunt T, Andrews W, Halliday B, Greenburg G, Knighton D, Clark R, Thakral K. Coagulation and macrophage stimulation of angiogenesis and wound healing. In The Surgical Wound, Dineen P, Hildick-Smith, G (eds), Philadelphia: Lea and Febiger, 1981.

4
Cellular Microenvironment in Healing and Non-Healing Wounds

Ian A. Silver

INTRODUCTION

Cell behavior may be markedly affected by conditions in the local environment and the cells themselves may alter that environment by changes in their own metabolic activity. While clinical judgments of supposed conditions in wounds have long been commonplace, actual measurement of the wound environment is a relatively recent development pioneered by Hunt and his coworkers (Hunt 1964; Hunt et al. 1967).

Their findings and those of Remensnyder and Majno (1968) and Silver (1965) showed that in many wounds, the cells at the growing edge of the healing tissue exist under conditions of considerable deprivation in relation to oxygen supply (and presumably other nutrients). The environment tends to be acidic, containing high concentrations of lactate, and hypercarbic. Measurements with microprobes (Silver 1965) also showed that there were steep gradients of oxygen tension within the tissue and that these gradients were characteristic of the various zones in which cellular proliferation and maturation were taking place.

The cell population in a wound consists of a structured series extending from the wound cavity to the fully mature tissue, which may be described as a "wound module." At the edge of a wound is an "advance guard" of scavenging cells, the majority of which are macrophages in the noninfected wound. If the wound is infected, these macrophages are accompanied by large numbers of polymorphonuclear neutrophilic leukocytes. Macrophages carry out debridement of any remaining injured tissue or effete cells. They also appear to produce a number of growth-stimulating factors and may be responsible for providing a chemotaxic gradient which encourages growth and migration of other cells in particular directions. The environment of the wound cavity is generated to large extent by this cell population, since phagocytes tend to derive their energy production by glycolysis, in addition to oxygen consumption, especially in hypoxic conditions.

Beneath the phagocytes is a layer of cells of mesenchymal origin, around which collagen Type III can be demonstrated by immunofluorescent techniques. These cells appear to be inactive and may be unable to divide because of the hypoxic local environment. Deep to these again is a group of dividing fibroblasts which are associated with the most distal, perfused capillary arcades. Among these cells are new endothelial sprouts, which are forming but have not yet joined, and are either blind-ending buds or solid cores of cells. It is not clear how these endothelial buds find each other to form loops, but we have shown, using anti-factor VIII immunofluorescence techniques (Strangeways and Silver, unpublished data), that endothelial cells send out long processes randomly, both in culture and in tissue in rabbit ear chambers, and it would appear that when two such processes meet from different arcades the cells subsequently grow down the line of their first contact and thus form a complete loop. This formation of loops occurs at right angles to the environmental gradient down which the endothelial cells grow, and therefore the signal that induces it must be very compelling.

Behind the first perfused capillary loops are usually more dividing fibroblasts which provide cells to form the new tissue. Proximal to these are maturing fibroblasts which have been left behind as the granulation tissue extends into the wound cavity. The characteristic microenvironment of this maturing zone is very different from that at the wound edge. Around these fibroblasts, new collagen stands can be seen, and this collagen becomes progressively more crosslinked with age (Bailey and Etherington 1980). Among these fibroblasts are groups of persistent macrophages and very frequently some lymphocytes and plasma cells, especially when there has been an antigenic component to the injury, such as infection. As the granulation tissue matures, scar collagen becomes predominant and the cell population is reduced. At the same time there is an apparent reduction in vascularization of the tissue; while many blood vessels are present, only a few of them are perfused. In older scar tissue even the paths of the blood vessels are obliterated and a relatively sparse network of patent vessels remains. In maturer scars, the environment is relatively homogeneous, with shallow pO_2 gradients, but in the actively synthetic stage, when the structure is well vascularized, relatively steep oxygen gradients are found, and these persist in hypertrophic scars.

In the successfully healing wound, the process outlined above continues until the cavity is completely filled and the surface covered by epithelium. When this situation is reached, further proliferation ceases and maturation takes place, with the end result that the wound cavity is infiltrated with new collagen, mainly Type III. A scar is formed where the Type III collagen is gradually replaced by Type I, often with concomitant secondary wound contraction.

In the nonhealing wound, which may arise from the persistence of foreign bodies; infiltration by tumor cells; the presence of irritants, parasites or infection; or, more importantly, because of the failure to develop an adequate blood supply due to a variety of hemodynamic factors such as varicose veins or atherosclerosis, the repair process is arrested, either initially or at some stage during its development. This usually results in a persistent open ulcer with little or no active repair tissue, the surface of which is eroded at the same or greater rate than that at which it advances. The base of such ulcers is often highly fibrosed, so that the scarring process extends very close to the healing surface and further reduces blood supply. The epidermal cells in these lesions are apparently unable to move across the open surface. In the early stages, epidermal proliferation may occur, but the migrating cells fail to adhere and detach, or they may die as a result of exposure to an excessively hostile environment which lacks the necessary nutrients or contains toxins. The understanding of why a wound may fail to heal depends on an adequate appreciation of the way in which cells behave and the range of environments which may develop within different types of wounds.

METHODS OF MEASURING CELLULAR MICROENVIRONMENT

Microenvironment is generally taken to indicate the very local conditions which occur at the surface of a cell and to which the cell itself reacts directly. However, this very local environment is often affected by the more general environment of a wound, and for this reason the latter cannot be ignored.

The original methods for measuring wound environment were devised by Hunt et al. (1967), who created artificial wound cavities by the subcutaneous implantation of wire mesh cylinders. Niinikoski and Hunt (1972) later implanted gas-permeable tubing in normal tissue and in wounds. The tubing was perfused slowly with saline, and gas exchange through its walls allowed assessment of the conditions in the wound by analysis of the emerging fluid, while the wire mesh cylinders filled naturally with wound fluid, which could be aspirated and analyzed.

General wound environment may also be examined by the use of mass spectrometer probes or by the insertion of relatively large electrodes. Remensnyder and Majno (1968) made use of polarographic techniques which had been described earlier, for the measurement of tissue environment in wounds (Davis and Brink 1942; Cater, Silver and Wilson 1959). Most investigators have concentrated on the measurement of oxygen tension in wounds or wound fluid, although Hunt et al. (1967), also measured CO_2 and pH.

With the advent of microprobes small enough to be inserted into intact tissue without causing gross damage, it became possible to measure local tissue conditions with respect to oxygen (Cater and Silver 1961; Silver 1965; Whalen, Riley and Nair 1967), ions (Walker 1971), and pH (Khuri 1967; Thomas 1974), and combinations of these. The advent of enzyme-linked substrate electrodes (Clark 1973) and their miniaturization for use in tissues (Silver 1975) allowed much more precise analysis of environment in and around experimental wounds. However, most microprobes are too fragile for use in patients, and new sensors are required which combine robust construction with small size, to achieve clinical acceptability. Some of these have been produced for experimental use, in the form of fiberoptic probes (Peterson, Goldstein and Fitzgerald 1980) to which are bonded microspheres or microcapsules containing dyes which respond to different modalities such as oxygen, pH and ions. There is also a rapid development of chemosensitive photodiodes and other microchips which are small enough to be incorporated either into wound dressings or laid on the surface of wounds and may prove useful in monitoring wound environment and thus give early warning of clinical problems.

An older method of investigating cellular microenvironment is the use of vital dyes and histochemistry which demonstrate localities of differing pH or enzyme activities (Pugh and Walker 1961). While these techniques may be of value in particular experimental or clinical circumstances, and may be useful in the analysis of biopsies, they are not generally applicable, in that they provide evidence about the microenvironment only at a given site at one particular time, and measurements at that site cannot be continued.

In addition to chemical environment, account also has to be taken of the physical environment in which cells find themselves. Electrical gradients of some hundreds of millivolts can be measured with simple, nonpolarizable electrodes between the outer layer of the epidermis and freshly injured connective tissue. These gradients may be important in the exact replacement of whole limbs which is common in some of the lower animals, such as urodele amphibia, and in the regeneration of whole fingertips in young children. Electrical gradients, as well as oxygen and mechanical factors (Bassett and Herrmann 1961), are important in the healing of hard tissue injuries, and it has been demonstrated by Brighton, Black and Pollack (1979), that not only do electrical gradients exist at the site of bone damage, but imposed gradients may accelerate or slow the repair process at these sites. Furthermore, work distortion of bone produces piezoelectric high frequency discharges, and it is reasonable to suppose that the healing of bone fractures is to some extent dependent on the characteristics of such piezoelectric discharges, although as yet there is no evidence for this. Another factor which may be important in wound healing and is almost certainly of importance in the healing of hard tissues, is the degree and direction of stress to which the wounded tissue is subjected. Stretching of a tissue may cause unidirectional migration of cells, and it also appears to affect the way in which these lay down the fibrous proteins.

In relation to epithelial migration the environmental water content is clearly of great importance in determining at what level epithelium will migrate over or through wounded tissue. Thus, measurements of tissue hydration may be of considerable value.

All the factors mentioned above may be measured by physical devices, but there are biological substances affecting the tissue environment which are much more difficult to quantitate. Various growth-promoting or -inhibiting substances have been described in tissue such as "chalones" (Bullough and Laurence 1960). A multiplicity of factors which arise from the activities of macrophages, platelets and lymphocytes stimulate other cells either to divide or to undertake synthesis. So far it has not proved possible to identify these within a wound in vivo, although they can be recognized *in vitro*.

EPIDERMAL HEALING

Epidermis is a "labile" tissue which constantly undergoes replacement and is capable of exact "regeneration" without scar formation. Under normal circumstances, it replaces surface wear and tear to maintain a thickness which is characteristic for each area of the body. It has been suggested that this replacement is controlled by a negative feedback system based on aging products called "chalones" (mitotic inhibitors) (Bullough and Laurence 1960) which leak into the environment of the active basal cells from dying cells at the skin surface. A complex interplay between chalones and other factors has been suggested as maintaining epidermal thickness at the normal level. Decrease in epidermal thickness might be attributable to excessive chalone in the environment, or excessive sensitivity of the cells of the stratum germinativum to chalone. Increase in epidermal thickness might be attributable to a decrease in chalone production or sensitivity to its effects.

If epidermis is damaged, there is normally a lag period of approximately 12 hours before new mitoses appear in the stratum germinativum. Following this, epidermal cells migrate into and across the injured site, but the route which they take depends on a number of environmental conditions. The most important factors appear to be (a) the degree of tissue hydration and (b) oxygen availability. Epidermal cells will only migrate across or through well-hydrated environments. In an open wound, this means that these cells will move across the surface of the lesion only if an occlusive dressing or some other kind of protection prevented evaporation and kept the surface moist. Where a wound surface has dried, epidermis migrates into the dermis and cuts a path through live tissue at a level apparently determined by its degree of hydration. This results in further destruction of tissue in the base of the wound.

The rate of migration may be affected by both hydration and by oxygen supply. Winter (1972) has demonstrated clearly that although the mitotic rate and the speed of migration of epidermis are independent of each other, both respond to similar environmental factors. Unlike connective tissue growth, epidermal proliferation is not inhibited by levels of oxygen up to 100 kPa (760 mm Hg) (Bullough and Johnson 1951), but neither does it appear to grow up or down oxygen gradients. However, the more oxygen that is present in the cellular environment, the greater are the possibilities for oxidative energy production and consequently the greater the potential for increased rates of migration. Environmental factors also are important in ensuring that epidermal cells migrating from multiple sites, such as the edges of wounds, the ends of sweat glands, and hair follicles, meet at the same level and thus form a single continuous layer, rather than a series of overlapping individual layers.

In nonhealing ulcers, there may be a number of environmental factors which cause inhibition of epidermal cell mitosis and/or failure to migrate across, or to adhere to the wound surface. Inadequate energy supply may inhibit either mitosis or migration, and the presence in the wound of toxins from either bacteria or degraded tissue may also be involved. Epithelial adherence to tissue surfaces depends in some unrecognized way on certain adhesive factors such as fibronectin and also possibly on the type of collagen across which the epithelium is migrating. In moist, open wounds epithelium migrates across the surface of granulation tissue, in which the collagen is largely Type III. However, when epithelium migrates through tissue underneath a desiccated scab, it cuts through existing collagen Type I in the dermis, but is later raised from this position by granulation tissue forming under it. On the other hand, epithelium will not cut through granulation tissue, and if the surface of new granulation tissue is allowed to dry, the epithelium is inhibited from either migrating across the surface or cutting through under the scab. The environmental factors which direct epithelial cells to adhere to, or cut through, existing tissue are obscure. Epithelium is resistant to low pH, and it is possible that the lactate which is produced at a wound surface by phagocytic activity may be an important part of the stimulus to epithelial growth. Eisinger et al. (1979), have shown that epidermal keratinocytes can be purified in culture by exposing them to pH as low as 5, which kills Langerhans cells and melanocytes, as well as fibroblasts. This is not surprising in view of the extremely acid pHs which may exist on some keratinized surfaces such as skin and vagina.

CONNECTIVE TISSUE HEALING

Unlike epidermis, connective tissue normally heals by repair and scarring, and this involves the formation of granulation tissue within whatever tissue has been damaged.

In the wound cavity, the oxygen tension is low (0-10 mm Hg) (Hunt et al. 1967; Remensnyder and Majno 1968; Silver 1969), it is at an acid pH (Hunt et al. 1967), and CO_2 is usually slightly above that of normal tissue. Lactate levels are high and extracellular potassium concentration is slightly increased. The population of cells in this region consists almost entirely of macrophages in a clean wound, at a pH of 6.5-6.9, but in an infected wound, where there is a large population of polymorphs, the pO_2 is zero, the pH may drop as low as 3, and potassium concentrations rise to 5.5-7.5 mM, due to release from dying neutrophils.

In addition to physical factors that can be measured, the cell population in the wound produces a number of growth-promoters such as platelet and macrophage fibroblast-stimulating factor and angiogenic factor(s). Also present are inflammatory mediators such as complement fragments, leukotrienes and prostaglandins. In addition to these, there are both neutral and acid proteases which have been released by activated macrophages or disintegrating neutrophils. This general environment, although radically different from that of normal tissue, may be different again from the extremely local conditions which occur at the surfaces of cells attached to tissue debris, invading organisms or foreign bodies. Macrophages which are in the process of degrading fibrous collagen may, even in a neutral or alkaline surrounding, produce an ultramicroenvironment at their attachment sites into which hydrogen ions appear to be secreted selectively, thus providing conditions which permit the extracellular local activity of acid hydrolases (Etherington, Pugh and Silver 1981).

In addition to producing a very local microenvironment, some cells are able to concentrate certain lysosomal enzymes at the attachment site, rather than leave them distributed randomly throughout the cytoplasm. Thus, successful degradation of debris may take place locally in a general environment which is not conducive to the action of the particular group of enzymes that are employed. This strategy may also be used by cells in the presence of certain enzyme-inhibitors or anti-enzyme antibodies and thus frustrate their action.

A particular behavior of macrophages which increases the efficiency of production of very local environments is the phenomenon of "clumping," where a single macrophage starts a phagocytic process, sends out chemotaxic signals, and attracts to itself other macrophages which subsequently form an attached colony and thereby are able to produce a considerable region of specialized environment into which their enzymes can be secreted and from which interfering substances can be excluded.

The wound cavity is essentially an area for "infilling" by normal granulation tissue, and it is at the edge of this tissue that the most profound differences from normal tissue occur in relation to local cellular environment. The cells at the edge of the granulation tissue exist in a relatively hypoxic, acidic and slightly hypercarbic area, with slightly raised potassium concentration. The glucose levels are low (2-4 mM) and lactate levels high (50-90 mM). Under these conditions, the newly formed mesenchymal cells secrete a minimal amount of soluble collagen, which is difficult to demonstrate except by immunohistochemistry with anti-Type III collagen fluorescein-labeled antibody. Deeper within the tissue, toward the first capillary arcades, the oxygen tension rises sharply to high levels (Remensnyder and Majno 1968; Silver 1965), since these new vessels frequently contain arterialized blood. In this zone of high oxygen tension with steep oxygen gradients, there is a population of rapidly dividing fibroblasts. This region is also somewhat acidic in nature, with pHs of the order of 6.9, as opposed to the much lower levels around 6.5 in the wound cavity.

Deeper into the granulation tissue, where maturation is taking place, the oxygen gradients become flatter, with an average reading of approximately 30-40 mm Hg, and although lactate may be detected in this zone there is much less than in the wound cavity. In this area, the glucose levels in the tissue are normal (approximately 7 mM).

As the defect heals, the wound space becomes infilled with new granulation tissue, and existing granulation tissue matures to form collagen fibers and, subsequently, scar. Migration of fibroblasts appears to be dependent to some extent on adhesion tracks, which involve the deposition of fibronectin and possibly other mediators of cellular adhesion. There must also be some feedback influence of the fibrous proteins in the environment onto the fibroblasts which determines how much of any particular type of protein is deposited. This is particularly the case in relation to elastin secretion, although the mechanism of feedback from the protein composition of the environment to the synthetic cell is not understood. However, if it fails, excessive fibrous or elastotic reactions occur. Hypertrophic scars and keloids may be formed, where, despite the presence of an overlying epithelium, fibroblasts continue to divide and synthesize new collagen in excess of what is required for "in-filling" the wound cavity.

If environmental conditions are changed artificially in a wound, healing can be inhibited. The simplest demonstration of this is the inhibition of angiogenesis by increasing the oxygen tension within the wound cavity. This results in the formation of a venous ring at the edge of a growing tissue and no further advance of the tissue into the wound cavity. It is not clear whether this is due to the direct effect of oxygen or whether the presence of excess oxygen inhibits the secretion of an angiogenic factor normally produced by hypoxic macrophages (Knighton Silver and Hunt 1981).

NONHEALING WOUNDS

Indolent wounds, in which healing either fails to take place completely, or starts and subsequently fails to progress, are a major problem in burns, atherosclerotic and varicose ulcers, pressure sores, and injuries in elderly patients (Goodson and Hunt 1979), especially over superficial bony prominences (Crawford and Gipson 1977). However, the commonest cause of nonhealing is probably infection, and the environment in infected wounds can be radically different from that in clean normal wounds.

The environment may be changed in a number of different ways in nonhealing wounds, but it is important to remember that the cell population in a wound is determined partly by the inflammatory response and the aggregation of new cells coming in from the blood and partly by local tissue proliferation. The inflammatory reaction not only brings in large numbers of phagocytes and growth factors, but the new cells increase the metabolic requirements of the tissue and therefore tend to produce hypoxia due to increases in oxygen uptake, especially during the "respiratory burst" of activation, together with possible substrate deprivations because of increased demands.

Since much of their energy production is glycolytic, phagocytes tend to reduce the local pH, especially through the production of lactic acid. This in itself may be beneficial, in that lactate is bacteriostatic (Hunt et al. 1967) and also stimulates the formation of collagen. However, it may be excessive, and purulent wounds are characterized by very low pHs, which may be directly damaging to the surrounding cells. This damage is augmented by the release of cathepsins and other proteolytic enzymes from dead and dying polymorphs. The center of purulent wounds is almost always anoxic, with a pH of approximately 3 and very high levels of lactate. This is an example of excessive inflammatory cellular response producing conditions which are inimical to healing.

At the other end of the scale, burn wounds frequently elicit an inflammatory response which is primarily vascular in nature and has a very small cellular component. Very few macrophages appear in the area and those that do, have difficulty in removing the heat-coagulated tissue. In addition, there is a lack of angiogenesis, which may arise from scarcity of appropriately activated macrophages. The probability that there is a deficiency of angiogenic factors rather than a lack of responsiveness in the local blood vessels can be demonstrated by seeding the burn area with activated macrophages from another source (Silver, unpublished data), since this promotes rapid angiogenesis and ingrowth of new blood vessels.

A second feature of burns is that the environment is not sharply changed at the edge of the damaged tissue. In a traumatic wound there is usually a very rapid gradation from normal tissue through the wound edge into the wound cavity. In a burn, the central part is dead and the tissue coagulated. This abuts an area in which the tissue is dying or severely affected by degradation products from the burnt tissue, in which cells are nonviable but not yet dead. Abutting this is an area of viable but damaged tissue in which there is an inflammatory response, usually mainly of a vascular nature. Beyond this again there is an area of normal tissue. If measurements of microenvironment are made through these zones it is found that there is a gradual change from well-oxygenated, normal tissue through a hyperoxygenated, inflamed zone into a region in which oxygen concentration gradually falls the further the electrode is moved from the last functional blood vessel. This gradation is much shallower than that seen in a traumatic wound, presumably because the oxygen uptake of the burnt tissue is relatively low, the number of surviving cells is small, and there are few inflammatory cells.

A third feature of a burn is that fluid is rapidly lost through it, and the water-impermeable characteristic of the epidermis is lost, resulting in rapid evaporation of fluid from the surface and a constant seeping of serum from the damaged blood vessels out onto the surface of the tissue. The tissue fluid becomes relatively protein-rich, and the ionic concentration approximates that of blood. Nevertheless, if a burn is removed surgically, leaving a bed which is, to all intents and purposes, the same as that formed by any excised surgical or traumatic wound, healing starts immediately and without the complications mentioned above.

NONHEALING ULCERS

In the typical ulcer there is a rim of inflamed tissue which is closely adjacent to fibrosed scar and covered only by an exudate of inflammatory cells or at best a thin layer of inactive granulation tissue. The blood supply is poor, and the oxygen tension at the growing surface is usually low, under the exudate. In addition, this exudate is frequently rich in proteolytic enzymes and harbors low-grade infection. As a result there is slow epidermal migration and what few cells are produced are cast adrift after they have moved out onto the surface of any granulation tissue that may be present.

Conversely, in some ulcers the oxygen tension is extremely high throughout and there is a great scarcity of macrophages. Under these circumstances, it appears that there may be no stimulus to angiogenesis, since Knighton et al. (1981), have shown that it is probably hypoxic macrophages which produce angiogenic factors. There is, however, a curious anomaly. Bacterial endotoxins which are usually present in ulcers cause priming and activation of macrophages, which would be expected to increase their ability to release angiogenic and other growth factors. It appears that there is something in the environment of ulcers which prevents either this priming being successful or the results of activation acting on other cells.

A feature of nonhealing ulcers is the frequent presence of necrotic tissue. Where this has not been invaded by active macrophages, the pH eventually becomes alkaline. During early necrosis in tissues that contain a large amount of glycogen, there is first a rapid fall in the pH at the time of cell death, but conditions then slowly change as the $-NH_2$ endings of the proteins become exposed during denaturation. It is this change which causes necrotic tissue to be eosinophilic in standard hematoxylin and eosin preparations.

FOREIGN BODIES

Foreign bodies in wounds create different environments, according to whether they are irritant or biocompatible. All foreign bodies are rapidly clothed by macrophages and become almost completely anoxic, but some inert substances such as carbon may remain in a wound without causing problems. However, those that are mildly soluble and of an irritant nature, such as silica, cause the local macrophage population to secrete cell-stimulating factors or to die. The presence of silica in wounds often leads to nonhealing or excessive fibrosis. Infected foreign bodies form a focus for bacterial activity which is difficult for phagocytes to control. Recurrent abscesses tend to form around these, but the most striking feature of the environment of irritant foreign bodies is the persistence of extreme hypoxia which is induced within them. Non-irritant substances such as titanium attract a fleeting coat of macrophages for a few days only, after which the phagocytes move away, and this is one of the features which makes for biocompatibility.

CELLULAR SUCCESSION

The successful healing of a wound depends on the right sequence of cells invading the tissue. It is possible that under some circumstances, environmental factors may provide an inappropriate stimulus and encourage the development of a cell population in an inappropriate sequence. This could occur because of suppression of one series of cells or because of a lack of stimulus, but our understanding of these factors is still very obscure.

Aging is another general feature which is involved in the nonhealing of wounds. In young patients and young animals, healing is usually uneventful and rapid, but as the individual gets older the healing process slows (Leaming 1963) and finally may cease altogether. This appears to be associated with the number of divisions cells have undergone in the body during the life of the organism, but it may also be due to development of suboptimal environmental conditions in the older animal. However, it seems likely that at least part of slow healing in old age is due to the cells themselves, since those from older individuals transplanted into tissue culture divide more slowly even in an "ideal" environment.

HYPOVOLEMIA AND SHOCK

Wounds in patients who have been subjected to hypovolemia or true shock may heal slowly. This is particularly the case when healing has started before hypovolemia develops. If hypovolemia occurs, as it commonly does, in the early stages of injury, before fibroblast proliferation has started, there is little inhibition of healing, provided that normovolemia is restored immediately. However, if a patient is allowed to suffer insidious loss of blood volume after 24 to 36 hours, when healing will have started, there is withdrawal of blood from the granulation tissue and the wound area becomes severely hypoxic and acidic (Silver 1973). These conditions are damaging to young fibroblasts, so the new cells may die or become severely injured and the healing process is delayed. Even mild hypovolemia will cause such problems to occur. Conversely, excessive rehydration of a patient, particularly with low osmotic pressure solutions, may cause edema, and this again particularly affects healing tissue. Very slight increases in intercapillary distances due to increases in the extracellular fluid volume may cause changes in diffusion distances which lead to hypoxia and cell damage (Heughan, Niinikoski and Hunt 1972).

CONCLUSION

Cellular microenvironment in wounds is normally kept within very narrow limits, and within these limits cells proliferate and fill in the defect. If there are changes in the microenvironment produced either by the cells themselves or by external factors, they may inhibit normal wound healing and result in incomplete closure or excessive cellular proliferation.

REFERENCES

Bailey AJ, Etherington DJ. 1980. Metabolism of collagen and elastin. In Comprehensive Biochemistry, 19B, Protein Metabolism, edited by M. Florkin and E. M. Stotz, pp 299-460. The Netherlands: Elsevier-North Holland-Excerpta Medica.

Bassett CAL, Herrmann I. 1961. Influence of oxygen concentration and mechanical factors on differentiation of connective tissue in vitro. Nature (London) 190:460.

Brighton CT, Friedenberg ZB, Black J. 1979. Evaluation of the use of constant current DC in treatment of non-unions. In Electrical Properties of Bone and Cartilage, pp 519-545, edited by Brighton CT, Black J, and Pollack SR. New York: Grune and Stratton.

Bullough WS, Johnson M. 1951. Epidermal mitotic activity and oxygen tension. Nature (London) 167:488.

Bullough, WS, Laurence EB. 1960. The control of epidermal mitotic activity in the mouse. Proc Roy Soc Lond B 151: 517-536.

Cater DB, Silver IA, Wilson GM. 1959. Apparatus and technique for the quantitative measurement of oxygen tension in living tissues. Proc Roy Soc Lond B 151:256-276.

Cater DB, Silver IA. 1961. Microelectrodes and electrodes used in biology. In Reference Electrodes, edited by JG Janz and DJG Ives, pp 464-523. New York: Academic Press.

Clark LC. 1973. A polarographic enzyme electrode for the measurement of oxidase substrates. In Oxygen Supply, edited by M. Kessler et al, pp 120-132. Munich: Urban and Schwarzenberg.

Crawford BS, Gipson M. 1977. The conservative management of pretibial lacerations in elderly patients. Br J Plasts Surg 30:174-176.

Davis PW, Brink F. 1942. Microelectrodes for measuring local oxygen tension in animal tissues. Rev Sci Instrum 13:524-533.

Eisinger M, Lee JS, Hefton JM, Darzynkiewicz Z, Chiao JW, DeHarven E. 1979. Human epidermal cell cultures: Growth and differentiation in the absence of dermal components or medium supplements. Proc Natl Acad Sci USA 76:5340-5344.

Etherington DJ, Pugh D, Silver IA. 1981. Collagen degradation in an experimental inflammatory lesion. Studies on the role of the macrophage. Acta Med Biol Germ 40:1625-1636.

Goodson WH III, Hunt TK. 1979. Wound healing and aging. J Invest Dermatol 73:88-91.

Heughan C, Niinikoski J, Hunt TK. 1972. Effect of excessive infusion of saline solution on tissue oxygen transport. Surg Gynec Obst 135:257-260.

Hunt TK. 1964. A new method of determining tissue oxygen tension. In Hyperbaric Oxygenation, Proceedings of the Second International Congress, Glasgow, p 432. Edinburgh: Livingstone.

Hunt TK, Twomey P, Zederfeldt B, Dunphy JE. 1967. Respiratory gas tension and pH in healing wounds. Am J Surg 114: 302-308.

Khurie RN. 1967. pH glass microelectrode for in vivo applications. Rev Sci Instrum 39:730-732.

Knighton DR, Silver IA, Hunt TK. 1981. Regulation of wound healing angiogenesis--Effect of oxygen gradient and inspired oxygen concentration. Surgery 90:262-270.

Leaming DB. 1963. The influence of age on wound healing. J Surg Res 3:43-47.

Niinikoski J, Hunt TK. 1972. Measurement of wound healing with implanted Silastic[R] tube. Surgery 71:22-26.

Peterson JI, Goldstein SR, Fitzgerald RV. 1980. Fiberoptic probe for physiological use. Anal Chem 52:864-869.

Pugh D, Walker PG. 1961. Histochemical localization of beta-glucosuronidase and N-acetyl-D-glucosaminadase. J Histochem Cytochem 9:105-116.

Remensnyder JP, Majno G. 1968. Oxygen gradients in healing wounds. Am J Pathol 52:301-308.

Silver IA. 1965. Some observations on the cerebral cortex with an ultramicro, membrane covered, oxygen electrode. Med Electron Biol Eng 3:377-387.

Silver IA. 1975. Ionic composition of pericellular sites. Phil Trans Roy Soc Lond B 271:261-272.

Silver IA. 1973. Local and systemic factors which affect the proliferation of fibroblasts. In The Biology of Fibroblast, edited by E. Kulonen and J. Pikkarainen, pp 507-520. New York: Academic Press.

Thomas RC. 1974. Intracellular pH of snail neurones measured with a new pH sensitive glass microelectrode. J Physiol (Lond) 210:82-83P.

Walker JL. 1971. Ion-specific ion exchanger, microelectrodes. Anal Chem 43:89-91.

Whalen W, Riley J, Nair PL. 1967. A microelectrode for measuring intracellular pO_2. J Appl Physiol 23:798-801.

Winter GD. 1972. Oxygen and wound healing. In Epidermal Wound Healing, edited by H. I. Maibach and D. T. Rovee, pp 163-170. Chicago: Yearbook Medical Publishers.

5
Glycosaminoglycan Interactions in Early Wound Repair

Charles N. Bertolami

INTRODUCTION

The presence of extracellular, high molecular weight, anionic polysaccharides in open wound granulation tissues has been acknowledged since the work of Balazs and Holmgren (1949; 1950), but the exact function of such substances has remained a subject of speculation. These wound carbohydrates are now known to be glycosaminoglycans (Dunphy and Udupa 1955; Jackson, Flickinger and Dunphy 1960; Bentley 1967; Bertolami and Donoff 1982; 1978) and their behavior in solution appears to explain many of the physical properties of various connective tissues (Toole 1976; Jeanloz 1970); however, current interest relates less to their purely structural contributions to tissue integrity than to their hypothetical capacity for actively directing tissue development (Toole 1976; 1972; Toole and Gross 1971; Toole and Trelstad 1971; Toole, Jackson and Gross 1972; Orkin and Toole 1978; 1980a; 1980b; Polansky, Toole and Gross 1974). This expanded perception of glycosaminoglycan function has evolved from the observation that distinct parallels exist between wound healing and embryogenesis (Bertolami and Donoff 1978; 1982). Tissue formation in both systems requires cellular proliferation, migration, differentiation, matrix synthesis/resorption, and programmed cellular death; however, only recently have repair processes been systematically examined from a developmental perspective (Bertolami and Donoff 1978; 1979a,b; 1982). It is within this developmental context that glycosaminoglycans have assumed importance during early wound repair. This chapter will review evidence for a potentially direct role for glycosaminoglycans in modulating cellular behavior during healing.

MUCOPOLYSACCHARIDES, GLYCOSAMINOGLYCANS, AND PROTEOGLYCANS

The term "acid mucopolysaccharide" has never been rigorously defined (Silbert 1982) but was originally applied by Meyer (1938) to a category of connective tissue carbohydrates possessing similar physical and chemical properties. As understanding of the chemistry of such substances increased, the name "glycosaminoglycan" was considered more descriptive and has now supplanted the older term (Jeanloz 1970; Silbert 1982).

Glycosaminoglycan solutions are characteristically viscous, readily form gels, and appear to be important in maintaining animal tissue rigidity (Jeanloz 1970; Sharon 1975). Chemically, these polysaccharides are usually composed of an amino sugar, 2-amino-2-deoxy-D-glucose (D-glucosamine) or 2-amino-2-deoxy-D-galactose (D-galactosamine) and a uronic acid (either D-glucuronic acid or L-iduronic acid). N-acetyl, O-, or N-sulfate groups may be present (Jeanloz 1970). Exceptions to this general description are notable and explain the characteristic heterogeneity of glycosaminoglycans at all levels of their organization.

Glycosaminoglycans that have been studied in detail include: hyaluronic acid, chondroitin, chondroitin-4-sulfate, chondroitin-6-sulfate, dermatan sulfate, keratan sulfate, heparan sulfate, and heparin (Figure 5.1).

Most of these large, polyanionic molecules are composed of a repeating uronic acid-hexosamine disaccharide possessing β-(1→4) and β-(1→3) linkages (Toole 1976; Jeanloz 1970; Sharon 1975). Intact molecules usually range from 1-2 × 10^4 daltons for sulfated forms to 1-2 × 10^7 daltons for hyaluronate; the frequent presence of carboxyl and sulfate groups accounts for their highly anionic character (Table 5.1).

Except for hyaluronic acid, glycosaminoglycans are not naturally found as isolated polysaccharide chains (Toole 1976); instead, they are covalently linked to a protein core by a characteristic linkage region consisting of: serine-xylose-galactose-galactose-uronic acid-hexosamine. The term "proteoglycan" is reserved for the resulting protein-glycosaminoglycan complex (Silbert 1982; Sharon 1975) (Figure 5.2).

Hyaluronic Acid

The disaccharide Δ4, 5-glucuronyl-β-(1→3)-N-acetylgludosamine is the repeating unit of which polymeric hyaluronic acid is composed (Sharon 1975) (Figure 5.1). While often portrayed as the archetypic glycosaminoglycan, hyaluronic acid differs from

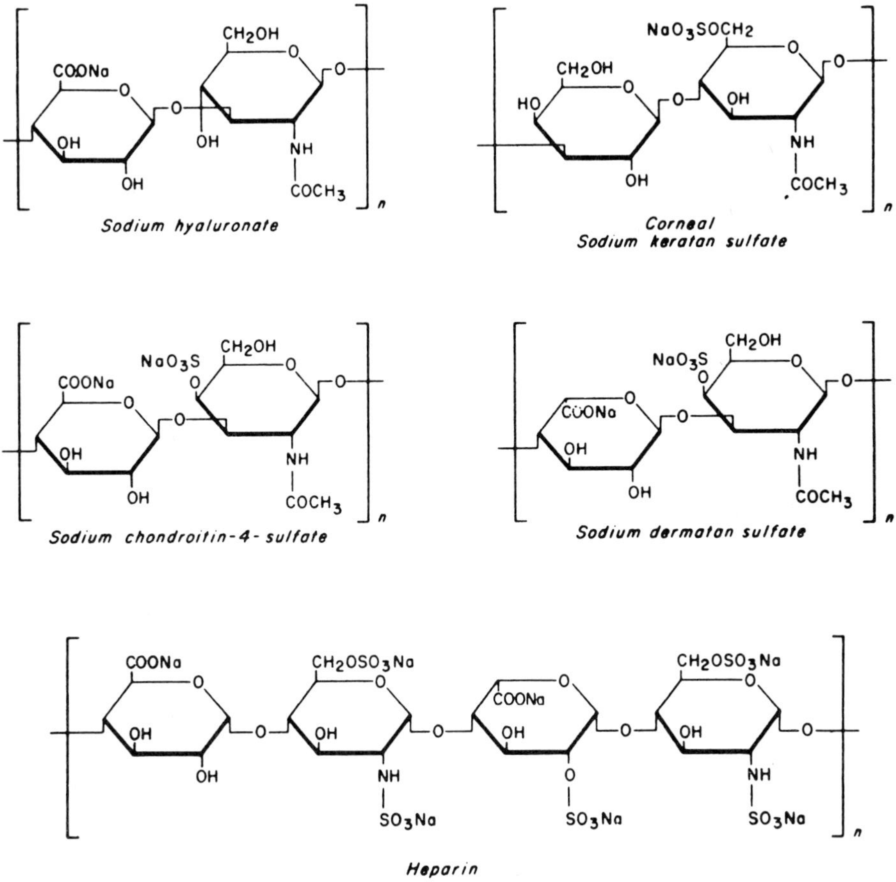

Sodium hyaluronate

Corneal Sodium keratan sulfate

Sodium chondroitin-4-sulfate

Sodium dermatan sulfate

Heparin

FIGURE 5.1 Repeating constituents of representative glycosaminoglycans. Specific components for hyaluronic acid are: glucuronic acid and N-acetylglucosamine; for keratan sulfate: galactose and N-acetylglucosamine-6-sulfate; for chondroitin sulfate: glucuronic acid and N-acetylgalactosamine-4- or -6-sulfate; for dermatan sulfate: iduronic acid (or small quantities of glucuronic acid) and N-acetylgalactosamine-4-sulfate; for heparin: glucuronic acid or iduronic acid-2-sulfate and N- and O-sulfated glucosamine. For heparan sulfate, glucuronic acid is the predominant uronic acid and the glucosamine moieties are N-sulfated and N-acetylated.
Source: Toole, BP. 1976. Morphogenetic role of glycosaminoglycans. In Neuronal Recognition, S. H. Barondes (ed.), p. 275. Plenum Press, New York. Reprinted with permission.

TABLE 5.1

Glycosaminoglycan Composition

Glycosaminoglycan	Approximate Molecular Weight	Major Component Sugars	Location of Sulfate	Linkage
Hyaluronic acid	$5 - 50 \times 10^5$	N-acetylglucosamine	—	β-(1→4)
		glucuronic acid		β-(1→3)
Chondroitin-4-sulfate	$2 - 5 \times 10^4$	N-acetylgalactosamine	4	β-(1→4)
		glucuronic acid		β-(1→3)
Chondroitin-6-sulfate	$2 - 5 \times 10^4$	N-acetylgalactosamine	6	β-(1→4)
		glucuronic acid		β-(1→3)
Dermatan sulfate	$2 - 5 \times 10^4$	N-acetylgalactosamine	4	β-(1→4)
		iduronic acid	2	α-(1→3)[a]
		glucuronic acid		β-(1→3)
Heparin	$0.5 - 4 \times 10^4$	glucosamine	6,N	α-(1→4)
		glucuronic acid		β-(1→4)
		iduronic acid	2	α-(1→4)[a]
Heparan sulfate	$1 - 5 \times 10^4$	glucosamine	6,N	α-(1→4)
		N-acetylglucosamine		α-(1→4)
		glucuronic acid		β-(1→4)
		iduronic acid	2	α-(1→4)[a]
Keratan sulfate	$5 - 20 \times 10^3$	N-acetylglucosamine	6	β-(1→3)
		galactose	6	β-(1→4)

[a] The linkage of L-iduronic acid is identical to the β-linkage of D-glucuronic acid, but iduronic acid possesses an L rather than a D configuration so this bond is designated α rather than β.

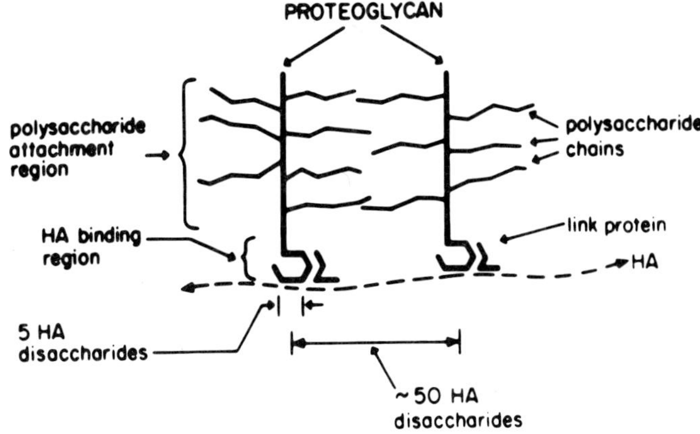

FIGURE 5.2 Diagram of multimolecular proteoglycan aggregate. Polysaccharide chains represent individual glycosaminoglycan molecules covalently linked to protein core. In collaboration with a link protein, proteoglycan protein cores interact non-covalently with hyaluronic acid. Multiple different glycosaminoglycans may be bound to a single protein core. Source: Heinegard, D and Hascall, V. 1974. Aggregation of cartilage proteoglycans. J Biol. Chem. 249: 4250-4256. Reprinted with permission.

the other molecules in the group in not being covalently bound to a protein core, in being unsulfated, and in having a substantially higher molecular weight (Toole 1976; Jeanloz 1970; Silbert 1982; Meyer 1938).

Hyaluronate does interact in a highly specific fashion with proteoglycan protein cores to form multimolecular aggregates or "megacomplexes" (Toole 1976; Heinegard and Hascall 1974) (Figure 5.2) but the interaction is non-covalent (Nieduszynski et al. 1980). A strongly hydrated hyaluronate decasaccharide unit is involved and the linkage is stabilized by a link protein (molecular weight = 44,000) (Perkins et al. 1981).

Study of the physical and chemical behavior of hyaluronic acid has been extensive (Meyer and Palmer 1934; Schoenberg and Moore 1964; Ogston 1970; Laurent 1966) and has led to theories proposing a significant role for hyaluronate in directing events at a cellular level. Because of its negative charge and large size, hyaluronate forms an extended random coil in dilute solution and occupies an enormous molecular domain (Toole 1976). At concentrations found in tissues, hyaluronate has been envisaged as a dense mesh work capable of restricting the flow of water, hindering diffusion and/or transport of solutes, excluding macromolecules, and exerting an osmotic pressure (Toole 1976). These physical capacities may have important operational consequences in tissue morphogenesis.

Chondroitin and the Chondroitin Sulfates

Chondroitin and the chondroitin sulfates are composed of D-glucuronic acid and 2-acetamido-2-deoxy-D-galactose; the sulfated and unsulfated forms differ from one another only in the content and location of sulfate ester groups (Jeanloz 1970). The individual polysaccharide chains possess 30-50 disaccharide units and have molecular weights of $2\text{-}5 \times 10^4$ daltons (Table 5.1) (Sharon 1975). Microheterogeneity in the proportion of sulfate esters present accounts for some disaccharide units being unsulfated, while others are 4-sulfated or 6-sulfated. Oversulfation of either the glucuronic acid or the galactosamine moieties and hybrid molecules possessing both 4-sulfated and 6-sulfated galactosamine residues have been described (Sharon 1975).

Dermatan Sulfate

First isolated from pig skin (Meyer and Chaffee 1941), dermatan sulfate was originally known as chondroitin sulfate B. It resembles chondroitin sulfate except that iduronic acid replaces most of the glucuronic acid moieties. Previously, the molecule was considered to consist entirely of repeating L-iduronic acid-N-acetylgalactosamine units (Jeanloz 1970; Sharon 1975); but, it is now clear that dermatan sulfate is a hybrid possessing both iduronic acid and glucuronic acid.

Keratan Sulfate

Keratan sulfate contains no uronic acids (Figure 5.1); instead, its repeating disaccharide is composed of galactose alternating with N-acetylglucosamine. Varying degrees of sulfation are observed at the C6 position of both components and additional heterogeneity is explained by the presence of other sugars such as fucose, mannose, sialic acid, and N-acetylgalactosamine (Sharon 1975).

Heparin and Heparan Sulfate

Heparin and heparan sulfate have a more complicated structure than the other glycosaminoglycans and cannot be portrayed as simple repeating disaccharide units (Figure 5.1) (Silbert 1982). Heparin's major component sugars include glucosamine, glucuronic acid, and iduronic acid. Heparan sulfate contains these sugars and N-acetylglucosamine. Variations in the content of uronic acid and sulfate occur throughout the chains; heparan sulfate also exhibits variations in amounts of N-sulfate and N-acetyl (Silbert 1982).

INITIAL STUDIES OF GLYCOSAMINOGLYCANS DURING WOUND REPAIR

Histochemical Characteristics of Wound Granulation Tissue

Experiments by Balazs and Holmgren (1949; 1950) were among the first to study wound granulation tissue carbohydrates that might be involved in regulating cellular behavior. Growing tissues had been observed to undergo a characteristic metachromatic change when stained with the basic dye, toluidine blue (Balazs and Holmgren 1949; 1950; Penny and Balfour 1949). Onset of metachromasia was attributed to increased levels of high molecular weight, extracellular polysaccharides, that is, sulfated glycosaminoglycans. When granulation tissues from skin wounds in rats were studied over a period of 30 days, dye uptake was initially low, it subsequently increased, peaking on days 6-9 and then decreasing to values seen in normal skin by day 15. The functional consequences of such changes were evaluated by exposing fibroblasts in culture to aqueous extracts of granulation tissues derived from the same series of wounds. Growth was markedly suppressed when fibroblasts were cultured in extracts of 6-9 day tissue but was significantly promoted when cultured in extracts from younger tissues. The inhibitory influence of the older tissue extracts was considered to be related to the presence of metachromatic glycosaminoglycans.

Dunphy and Udupa (1955) subsequently extended these histochemical techniques for monitoring rat granulation tissue glycosaminoglycans. They relied upon toluidine blue metachromasia, a glycosaminoglycan-specific colloidal iron stain, and a periodic acid-Shiff reagent, to qualitatively assess glycosaminoglycans and overall carbohydrate content. A regular sequence of events leading to complete wound closure was observed. An amorphous extracellular matrix was identified after early proliferation of fibroblasts. Toluidine blue metachromasia of the matrix peaked on days 5-6 and subsequently declined. When wound tissues were assayed chemically for hexosamine, maximal levels were found immediately after wounding (Dunphy and Udupa 1955; Edwards, Pernokas and Dunphy 1957; Grillo, Watts and Gross 1958). These observations were attributed to an accumulation of non-sulfated glycosaminoglycans during the first few days of healing; a transition to sulfated glycosaminoglycans was presumed to occur before the end of the first post-wound week. Glycosaminoglycans appeared to be present in abundance during early wound repair, but when the totally nonspecific nature of hexosamine as a measure of tissue glycosaminoglycan was recognized, the initially elevated hexosamine levels were explained on the basis of simple serum exudation (Jackson, Flickinger and Dunphy 1960).

Cetyl Pyridinium Chloride (CPC)-Precipitable Polysaccharides

Clearly, initial investigations were impeded by lack of adequate methods for glycosaminoglycan isolation and identification. As a result, Scott's (1956) observation that the quarternary ammonium detergent, cetyl pyridinium chloride (CPC), formed water-insoluble complexes with glycosaminoglycans represented a significant technical advance. Depending upon charge density, the resulting complexes were soluble to varying degrees in salt solutions. Jackson, Flickinger and Dunphy (1960) employed this characteristic of the CPC-complexes to successfully isolate glycosaminoglycans from open rat skin wound granulation tissue. The CPC fraction precipitating between 0.5 M and 0.9 M Na_2SO_4 was presumed to be a mixture of chondroitin sulfate, dermatan sulfate, and keratan sulfate. In this manner, concentrations of granulation tissue glycosaminoglycans were found to be relatively constant between days 6 and 15 and were invariably lower than normal skin. Because of the small quantities of material available for analysis, the exact identity of individual glycosaminoglycans was not determined.

Further modifications and improvements in CPC-precipitation techniques reported by Antonopoulos and coworkers (1965) were applied to analysis of wound granulation tissue glycosaminoglycans by Bentley (1967). Based upon their differential solubility in various salt-CPC solvents, glycosaminoglycan mixtures could be precipitated on the surface of cellulose columns previously treated with CPC. Subsequent elution would allow glycosaminoglycans to be separated from each other and from other hexosamine-containing substances. After homogenization and digestion with papain, tissue samples were centrifuged, dialyzed, ethanol-precipitated, redissolved, and precipitated with CPC. Samples were then dissolved in the different solvents and run through cellulose microcolumns. All solvents included at least 0.5% CPC. The material isolated from a column run with 1% CPC was treated with HCl at 105°C and hexosamine determination performed on the resulting hydrolysate. Hexosamine measured from this column reflected keratan sulfate content. The hexosamine measured from a column run with 0.3 M NaCl, and 0.05% CPC represented hyaluronate. Chondroitin sulfate was identified by running the column with 0.75 M NaCl, 0.1% acetic acid, 0.05% CPC, followed by acid hydrolysis and measurement of hexosamine. Exclusion of acetic acid from the solvent allowed recovery of dermatan sulfate.

Bentley's experiments showed that progressive increases in chondroitin sulfate and dermatan sulfate occurred from day 5 through 17 for open wounds in rats (Figure 5.3). This pattern resembled that seen for wound collagen (Dunphy and Udupa 1955; Hosoda 1960) and suggested that massive early production of chondroitin sulfate and dermatan sulfate was not a prerequisite for collagen synthesis.

Of particular interest was the analysis of the 0.3 M NaCl (hyaluronate) fraction. Initially elevated hyaluronate levels declined near the end of the first postwound week and then remained constant (Figure 5.4). A decline in hyaluronate content coupled with a concomitant rise in sulfated glycosaminoglycans was consistent with earlier work (Balazs and Holmgren 1949; Campani, Zonta and Ugazio 1959). The predominance of non-sulfated glycosaminoglycans in early wounds was felt to promote fibroblastic proliferation in some way, but the role of the sulfated glycosaminoglycans during later repair was unclear. Increased sulfated glycosaminoglycan might stimulate collagen production (Balazs and Holmgren 1949; Campani, Zonta and Ugazio 1959) but, more likely, both collagen and sulfated glycosaminoglycans were the common products of a single differentiative event.

Healing in a variety of specialized systems was subsequently studied (Dorner 1967; Anseth 1961; Cintron and Kublin 1977). Dorner (1967) investigated repair of surgical incisions in rabbit tendons and found that the most pronounced changes in connective tissue composition occurred during the first three weeks: hyaluronate decreased from approximately 50% of total CPC-precipitable glycosaminoglycan at 4 days to about 20% at the end of the study. The content of dermatan sulfate increased from 10% to over 40% during the same period. Further, but less rapid, decreases in hyaluronate and increases in dermatan sulfate occurred during the next 100 days. Variable levels of chondroitin-4-sulfate and low but constant quantities of chondroitin-6-sulfate were also identified. By four months, the composition of the healing tissue closely resembled that of mature uninjured tendon (Dorner 1967).

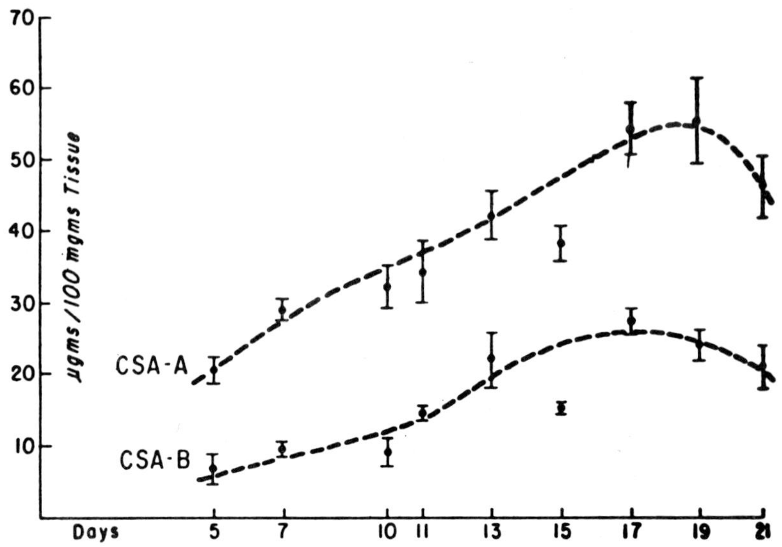

FIGURE 5.3 Changes in content of chondroitin-4-sulfate (CSA-A) and dermatan sulfate (CSA-B) for skin wound granulation tissue as a function of time (data points expressed as mean ± 1 S.D.). Separations and identifications were based on the differential solubility of glycosaminoglycan-CPC complexes in various solvents.
Source: Bentley, JP. 1967. Rate of chondroitin sulfate formation in wound healing. Annals of Surgery 165:186-191. Reprinted with permission.

FIGURE 5.4 Profile of hyaluronic acid content (0.3M NaCl fraction) of skin wound granulation tissue as a function of time. (Data points expressed as mean ± 1 S.D.)
Source: Bentley, JP. 1967. Rate of chondroitin sulfate formation in wound healing. Annals of Surgery 165:186-191. Reprinted with permission.

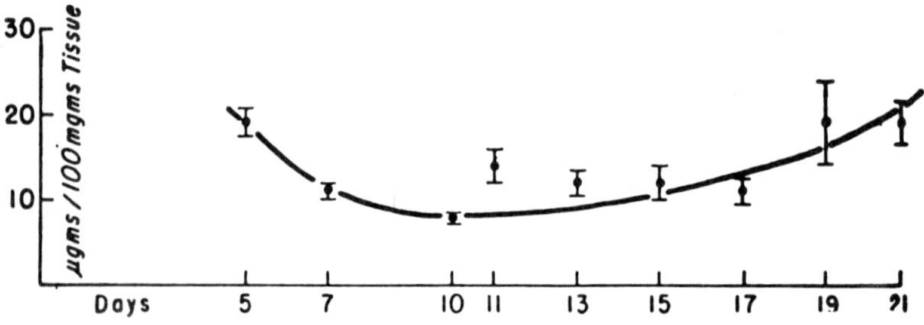

Anseth (1961) studied corneal wound healing in rabbits and found that the glycosaminoglycans normally present in the corneal stroma decreased significantly following wounding both in samples from the wound area and from the surrounding corneal tissue. Chondroitin sulfate and/or dermatan sulfate were synthesized or deposited in the wound during the entire period of study whereas fully-sulfated keratan sulfate, normally present in high concentrations in cornea, was not replenished even in 90-day old wounds. Increased hyaluronate during early corneal healing was considered a distinct possibility, but was not directly evaluated.

Subsequently, Cintron and Kublin (1977) detected hyaluronate, heparan sulfate, and an under-sulfated keratan sulfate in corneal wound tissue and proposed a recapitulation of corneal ontogenetic processes by comparing glycosaminoglycan and collagen content during repair and development.

Consistent with these reports, Campani and collaborators (1959) studied [^{35}S]-sulfate uptake into granulation tissue surrounding cotton pledgets and found no synthesis of sulfated polysaccharides during early stages of tissue formation. The obvious implication of such work was that hyaluronate predominated during early repair but was replaced with sulfated glycosaminoglycans as wounds matured.

Use of Polysaccharidases for Identifying Glycosaminoglycans

Even with development of CPC-precipitation techniques for isolating glycosaminoglycans, wound healing studies continued to be hindered by inadequate specificity. The lack of a convincing and unifying theory on the role of glycosaminoglycans in embryonic tissues was also an impediment. A structural role for glycosaminoglycans based upon their physical and chemical properties was almost certain; indeed, specific physical characteristics of connective tissues were attributed to the molecular properties of various glycosaminoglycans. The high water content, low serum protein content, turgidity, viscosity and other mechanical features seemed entirely consistent with the perceived properties of glycosaminoglycans or associated proteoglycans (Toole 1976). Real advances, however, toward understanding glycosaminoglycans in healing tissues did not occur until a more specific method emerged for identifying such molecules and until developmental biologists proposed potential functions beyond strictly structural ones.

Toole and Gross (1971) described an improved method for identifying glycosaminoglycans based upon a differential susceptibility to various polysaccharidases. By this technique,

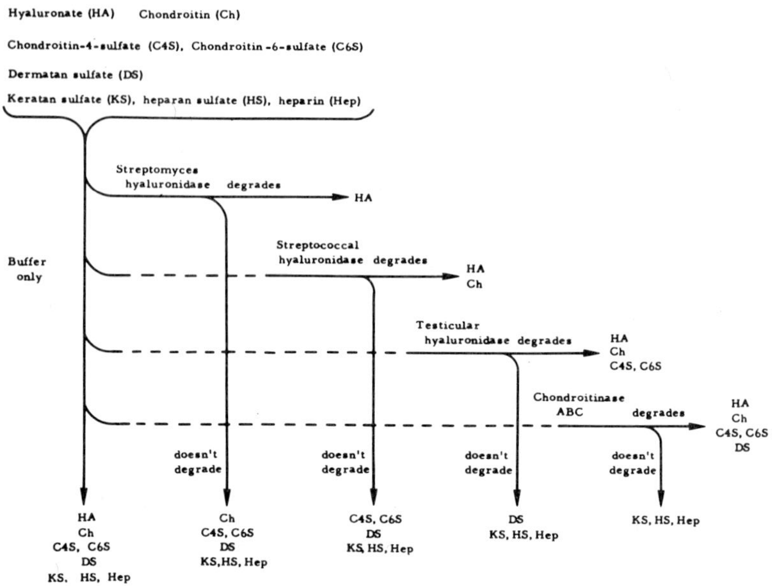

FIGURE 5.5 Technique for identifying glycosaminoglycans on the basis of their differential susceptibility to highly specific polysaccharidases. See text for explanation.
Source: Toole, BP. Morphogenetic role of glycosaminoglycans. Neuronal Recognition, p 275. S. H. Barondes (ed.). Plenum Press, New York. Reprinted with permission.

aliquots of radioactively labeled glycosaminoglycans were degraded with substrate-specific polysaccharidases Figure 5.5); Streptomyces hyaluronidase was used to degrade hyaluronic acid; streptococcal hyaluronidase degraded hyaluronic acid and chondroitin; testicular hyaluronidase degraded hyaluronate, chondroitin, chondroitin-4-sulfate, and chondroitin-6-sulfate; chondroitinase ABC degraded hyaluronate, chondroitin, chondroitin-4-sulfate, chondroitin-6-sulfate, and dermatan sulfate. After precipitation of reaction mixtures with cetyl trimethylammonium bromide (CTAB), solubilized radioactivity was indicative of glycosaminoglycans susceptible to the polysaccharidase employed; radioactivity contained within the pellet material was used to quantitate resistant glycosaminoglycans. Although only Streptomyces hyaluronidase was monospecific for hyaluronic acid, the overlapping substrate specificities of the enzymes permitted precise measurement of several individual glycosaminoglycans. For example, the difference in solubilized radioactivity after treatment with streptococcal hyaluronidase and after *Streptomyces* hyaluronidase would be directly attributable to labelled chondroitin in the sample. Differences in radioactivity between testicular hyaluronidase degradation products and streptococcal hyaluronidase products would be attributable to chondroitin-4-sulfate and chondroitin-6-sulfate. The difference between testicular hyaluronidase and chondroitinase ABC would be a reflection of labelled dermatan sulfate. The only limitation of the method was its inability to distinguish between chondroitin-4-sulfate and chondroitin-6-sulfate, nor between keratan sulfate, heparan sulfate, and heparin. Naturally, this assay required radioactively labeled glycosaminoglycans and, as such, was really a measure of the rate of glycosaminoglycan synthesis. After the initial description by Toole and Gross (1971), a colorimetric assay was devised by Hatae and Makita (1975) based upon a technique reported by Reissig and coworkers (1955). By monitoring supernatant solutions after enzymatic degradation, the amount of terminal reducing N-acetylhexosamine could be used as a very direct indication of the amount of glycosaminoglycan present. Using the carbazole method of Bitter and Muir (1962), uronic acid levels of reaction products could also be measured.

WOUND HEALING AS A DEVELOPMENTAL PHENOMENON

Glycosaminoglycan Regulatory Functions During Development

The first major application of polysaccharidase degradation as a means for measuring glycosaminoglycan content and synthetic rate was in developmental systems (Toole 1976; 1972; Toole and Gross 1971; Toole and Trelstad 1971; Toole, Jackson and Gross 1972; Orkin and Toole 1978; 1980a; 1980b; Polansky, Toole and Gross 1974). In this context, a regulatory role for glycosaminoglycans was proposed that went beyond merely structural functions. Among the various developmental systems that have been studied, extensive work has been performed with regenerating newt limbs (Toole and Gross 1971), developing chick embryo corneas (Toole and Trelstad 1971), limb bud and axial chondrogenesis (Toole 1972), and chick heart, brain, and skin development (Orkin and Toole 1978; 1980a; 1980b; Polansky, Toole and Gross 1974). These studies correlated the synthesis of hyaluronate and its enzymatic removal in developmental sequences *in vivo* with the accumulation and differentiation of mesenchymal cells. Specifically, Toole and Trelstad (1971) examined endogenous tissue hyaluronidase activity as the mechanism by which changes in tissue hyaluronate content were produced. Corneal extracts of various developmental stages were exposed to exogenous hyaluronate substrates and the release of terminal reducing N-acetylglucosamine was determined. A unit of hyaluronidase activity was defined as one microgram of N-acetylhexosamine released per milligram protein per 37°C, 8-hour incubation. At developmental Stage 34, hyaluronidase activity increased from undetectable levels to approximately 25 units (Figure 5.6); after Stage 39, hyaluronidase activity diminished sharply. In a complementary study, [^{3}H]-acetate uptake that could be attributed specifically to incorporation into hyaluronate or into chondroitin sulfate was determined and expressed as a percentage of incorporation into total glycosaminoglycan. From Stage 34 to Stage 38, hyaluronate incorporation dropped from 60% to less than 10%. Hyaluronidase activity remained maximal during this period (Figure 5.6). The data implied that synthesis of new hyaluronate decreased as existing hyaluronate was degraded under the influence of a corneal hyaluronidase. Importantly, uptake of radioactive acetate into hyaluronate expressed as a percentage of total glycosaminoglycan incorporation could decrease while the actual amount of hyaluronic acid might be constant or increasing. Without demonstrating a drop in the actual amount of hyaluronate, it is difficult to confirm that hyaluronidase functions by removal of extant hyaluronate. When Toole and Gross (1971) expressed incorporation of [^{3}H]-acetate as CPM per milligram protein for the regenerating newt limb, they found that over the first ten days, hyaluronate incorporation peaked and then diminished during the next 25 days. Removal of hyaluronic acid began on the tenth day of regeneration and was associated with increased levels of hyaluronidase activity. As hyaluronate content decreased, levels of chondroitin sulfate rose. It appeared that glycosaminoglycans in regenerating newt limb changed in accord with the trends seen in developing cornea; however, since both the corneal and limb regeneration studies relied upon radioisotopes, each was really a measure of the amount of incorporation during the time of isotope administration (i.e., rate of glycosaminoglycan synthesis). How indicative such information is of the actual quantity of glycosaminoglycan present would need to be evaluated in the context of the time and duration of isotope administration. Certainly, previously synthesized glycosaminoglycans would remain unlabeled and undetected. When the question involves extant hyaluronate rather than rate of synthesis, the Hatae-Makita (1975) determina-

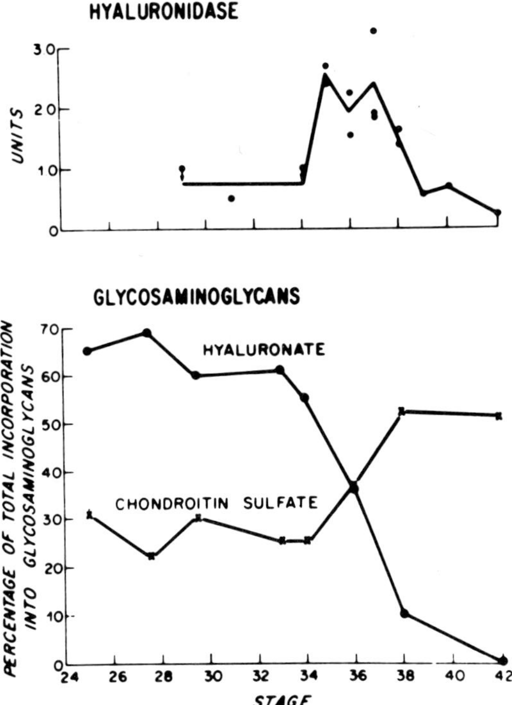

FIGURE 5.6 Metabolism of glycosaminoglycans in embryonic chick cornea. Hyaluronate synthesis predominates during early corneal development. Onset of hyaluronidase activity is temporally correlated to cessation of hyaluronate synthesis and to increased levels of chondroitin sulfate production.
Source: Toole, BP and Trelstad, RL. 1971. Hyaluronate production and removal during corneal development in the chick. Dev. Biol. 26:28-35. Reprinted with permission.

tion described earlier would be appropriate. In this way, a measure of total hyaluronate at the time of assay is obtained; in addition, the amount of other glycosaminoglycans can be determined by using other polysaccharidases with different substrate specificities.

In addition to studies describing changes in the quantity and nature of specific glycosaminoglycans in developmental systems, Toole, Jackson, and Gross (1972) determined the direct effects of hyaluronate on developing cells in vitro. Despite the fact that primary and passaged cultures of chick embryo cells synthesize and secrete substantial levels of hyaluronidase (Orkin and Toole 1980a), cell cultures of embryonic chondroblasts, which normally aggregate to produce metachromatic nodules, failed to form either colonies or metachromatic nodules when exposed to nanogram per milliliter quantities of exogenous hyaluronate. Based on these studies (Toole and Gross 1971; Toole and Trelstad 1971; Toole 1972; Toole, Jackson and Gross 1972; Orkin and Toole 1978; 1980a; 1980b; Polansky, Toole and Gross 1974), the hypothesis was advanced that: 1) hyaluronate prevents aggregation of mesenchymal cells and consequently facilitates their migration, 2) removal of hyaluronate by hyaluronidase permits aggregation and subsequent differentiation to proceed in the proper sequence for tissue organization, and 3) the effect of hyaluronate on cell aggregation could possibly lead to alterations in the rates of synthesis of specific differentiation products (that is, chondroitin sulfate, keratan sulfate, and collagen). In the developmental systems studied for changing levels of glycosaminoglycans, a similar sequence has been observed, so the contention that hyaluronic acid and its removal under the influence of hyaluronidase play important parts in normal sequences of tissue morphogenesis has gained popularity.

The specific mechanism of hyaluronate function remains unknown. Since the hyaluronate molecule possesses a high density of negative charges and occupies a large molecular domain, it can associate with enormous quantities of water. This hydrating property has been proposed as the mechanism for facilitating cellular migration (Toole and Trelstad 1971). In the embryonic chick cornea, for example, a massive swelling of the primary corneal stroma begins on the fifth day of development in response to the secretion of hyaluronate by the corneal epithelium. Primary mesenchymal cells derived from the neural crest wait along the periphery of the cornea until such swelling takes place; only then do they migrate into the primary corneal stroma (Toole and Trelstad 1971). Even the pattern of cellular migration into the stroma seems to be dictated by a hyaluronate gradient since the leading edge of cells is immediately adjacent to the corneal endothelium where hyaluronate concentration is highest (Hay and Revel 1969). Corroborating this view, Morris (1979) showed that glycosaminoglycan influence on cell behavior might be explained by steric factors related to polymer configuration, viscosity, molecular weight, and concentration. Such macromolecules might therefore affect cell migration and reorganization during morphogenesis in an entirely non-specific fashion.

As a highly anionic molecule, hyaluronate might also function in the capacity of an extracellular calcium depot (Spooner 1975). In this way, hyaluronate's ability to facilitate cellular migration might be related to the calcium-dependence of the cytoplasmic microfibrillar contractile apparatus implicated in cellular locomotion (Spooner 1975).

Turley and Roth (1979) proposed a different, more specific mechanism when they found that migratory activity was high for fibroblasts cultured on a hyaluronate substrate but low for fibroblasts cultured on chondroitin sulfate. Based upon the spontaneous glycosylation of glycosaminoglycan substrates by adherent fibroblasts, they attributed substrate effects to specific interactions between glycosaminoglycans and cell surface glycosyltransferases. The nature of the interaction will be discussed subsequently.

Finally, hyaluronate might function by means of a direct interaction with particular cells. Dahlgren and Björkstein (1982) studied the effect of hyaluronic acid on polymorphonuclear leukocyte cell surface properties and found that exposure to hyaluronate caused a marked increase in hydrophobic and negatively charged groups on the leukocyte surface; it also enhanced leukocyte function and rendered cells more liable to hydrophobic interactions. The role such factors may play in mammalian wound repair is not known, but hyaluronate concentrations are highest during the first week after injury (Bertolami and Donoff 1978; 1982) when leukocytic infiltration is also maximal (Peacock and Van Winkle 1976), so a hyaluronate-mediated influence on leukocyte function certainly appears plausible.

Glycosaminoglycan Regulatory Functions During Wound Repair

Given a specific regulatory role for glycosaminoglycans during development, the similarities long recognized between developmental and wound healing processes justified the expectation that glycosaminoglycans might function similarly in reparative tissues (Bertolami and Donoff 1978; 1979a,b; 1982; Bertolami 1978). Cellular proliferation, migration, differentiation, synthesis/resorption of large quantities of extracellular matrix, and programmed cellular death are events shared by both systems. Since the signal for removal of hyaluronate in development was a discrete peak in hyaluronidase activity with subsequent hyaluronate degradation and onset of differentiation (Toole and Gross 1971; Toole and Trelstad 1971; Toole 1972; Toole, Jackson and Gross 1972; Orkin and Toole 1978; 1980a; 1980b; Polansky, Toole and Gross 1974), the granulation tissues from open skin wounds in rabbits were studied to determine if a specific, wound-associated hyaluronidase existed (Bertolami and Donoff 1978; 1979a,b; 1982; Bertolami 1978).

As predicted, a hyaluronidase-like enzyme was found in healing granulation tissues on and after the seventh postwound day (Bertolami and Donoff 1978). The complete absence of hyaluronidase activity before this time presumably favored accumulation of unsulfated glycosaminoglycans in the manner described for developmental systems. The fact that the amount of hyaluronate measured in central wound granulation tissue was 50% higher on postwound day 7 than on day 14 suggests a functioning degradative system during the second postwound week analogous to that observed during embryonic development. Since the observed changes in hyaluronate are in agreement with those described by Bentley (1967), it appears that *Streptomyces* hyaluronidase provides a simple yet specific method for measuring hyaluronate content that can be correlated to endogenous hyaluronidase activity. The early presence of hyaluronate should not be confused with the initially high levels of non-metachromatic hexosamine-containing substances characteristic of incipient wound repair. As mentioned, initial increases in hexosamine are secondary to serum exudation during inflammation (Jackson, Flickinger and Dunphy 1960) and are maximal immediately after wounding.

In the peripheral regions of the open wound, a distinctly different tissue topography was noted which consisted of an overlying sheet of migrating epithelium and a deep layer of granulation tissue. The characteristics of this "whole edge" tissue were determined separately. In whole edge tissue, enzyme activity was not present until relatively late (14 days). During the absence of enzyme, hyaluronic acid levels were quite high, at nine days the hyaluronate content of hyaluronidase-negative whole edge tissue was 3-fold greater than that of the corresponding hyaluronidase-positive central granulation tissue. Tissue subjacent to edge epithelium was distinguished easily from presumably more mature granulations in that it resembled hyaluronate-rich embryonic tissue with characteristically large intercellular spaces (Bertolami and Donoff 1978; 1982). The prolonged elevation of hyaluronic acid levels in edge tissues and associated effects on mesenchymal cell migration in this region could be important relative to the phenomenon of wound contraction (Bertolami 1978).

In developmental systems (Toole and Gross 1971; Toole and Trelstad 1971; Toole 1972; Toole, Jackson and Gross 1972; Orkin and Toole 1978; 1980a; 1980b; Polansky, Toole and Gross 1974), the level of sulfated glycosaminoglycan increased as the amount of hyaluronate decreased. A similar phenomenon was suggested for the healing wound by a more than 5-fold increase in central granulation tissue uronic acid between days 7 and 14 accompanied by a marked drop in hyaluronate. The increasing level of uronic acid could not be attributed to hyaluronate since hyaluronate levels were declining; the apparent cause for such uronic acid increases was the synthesis of sulfated glycosaminoglycans; for example, dermatan sulfate and/or chondroitin-4-sulfate and chondroitin-6-sulfate (Bertolami and Donoff 1978; 1982). Onset of toluidine blue metachromasia during this period confirms this interpretation (Dunphy and Udupa 1955). Since such sulfated substances are characteristically the products of differentiated cells, it appeared that hyaluronate degradation by hyaluronidase was contemporary with cellular differentiation. Whether hyaluronidase resorption of hyaluronic acid initiates the process of differentiation remains speculative, but the sequence of events operative in healing wounds certainly appears similar to that described for developmental systems.

Characterization of Mammalian Skin Wound Hyaluronidase

Characterization of the crude wound enzyme revealed a pH optimum of 4.5, a value well within the range of optima described for other mammalian hyaluronidases (DeSalequi, Plonska and Pigman 1967; Yang and Srivastava 1975). Although the cell responsible for the manufacture and secretion of wound hyaluronidase is not known, the pH optimum suggested that neither acute nor chronic inflammatory cells are involved since leukocytic hyaluronidase has a markedly lower pH optimum (Tynelius-Bratthall and Attström 1972). Macrophages as a potential source of the enzyme were similarly excluded since Goggins and associates (1968) observed a pH optimum of 3.9 for rabbit macrophage hyaluronidase. Others (Tsuda et al. 1974) have failed to find any hyaluronidase activity whatsoever in macrophages. Although periods of maximal enzyme activity did not correspond to periods of maximal inflammatory cell infiltration (Bertolami 1978), recent evidence (Castor et al. 1981) suggesting that lymphocyte and platelet growth factors may be involved in glycosaminoglycan metabolism indicates the need for further study. A bacterial origin for the enzyme must also be considered, but this possibility seems remote due to the complete absence of the unsaturated cleavage products characteristic of bacterial hyaluronidase action (Bertolami and Donoff 1982).

In general, hyaluronidase-type enzymes range from being extremely narrow in their spectrum of activity to being rather broad. Streptomyces hyaluronidase is very specific and degrades only hyaluronic acid (Hatae and Makita 1975; Ohya and Kaneko 1970). Streptococcal hyaluronidase acts not only upon hyaluronate, but also upon the non-sulfated glycosaminoglycan, chondroitin (Toole and Gross 1971). Testicular hyaluronidase has the broadest spectrum of activity and catalyzes the cleavage of chondroitin-4-sulfate and chondroitin-6-sulfate in addition to hyaluronic acid and chondroitin (Toole and Gross 1971). Crude and subsequently purified wound enzyme were shown to be active against hyaluronic acid and chondroitin-4-sulfate, but not against chondroitin-6-sulfate or dermatan sulfate (Toole and Gross 1971). Apparently, a desulfation occurred during the course of the reaction against chondroitin-4-sulfate since substitution in the C4 position would normally interfere with the formation of the intermediate required for color development (presumably a glucoxazoline) (Reissig, Strominger and LeLoir 1955). The possibility that the wound enzyme was actually active against chondroitin-6-sulfate as well but that the sulfated cleavage products were simply not detectable was excluded since substitution in the C6 position is known not to exert an effect comparable to position 4 substitution (Reissig, Strominger and LeLoir 1955). The ability to differentiate chondroitin-4-sulfate and chondroitin-6-sulfate is a property shared by a tadpole tail skin hyaluronidase described by Silbert and DeLuca (1970); however, the tadpole enzyme does not involve an associated desulfation.

Like other hyaluronidases, the wound enzyme functioned in a strictly endoglycosidic manner. This fact was established by incubating wound enzyme with a formate buffer and with saccharo-1,4-lactone monohydrate (Polansky, Toole and Gross 1974; Levvy and Marsh 1959); both have been shown to inhibit β-N-acetyl-glucosaminidase and β-glucuronidase, the exoglycosidases likely to be present.

The hyaluronidase contained within wound granulation tissue was unaffected by skin grafting (Bertolami and Donoff 1979a). In both open and grafted wounds, collagen concentrations are known to increase during healing despite marked collagenase activity and resultant net collagen loss (Donoff and Grillo 1975). Since concentration depends not only upon the deposition and resorption of collagen, but also upon the turnover of non-collagenous wound substances, hyaluronidase in open and grafted wounds may contribute to resorption of hyaluronate and hence to an increase in collagen concentration concomitant with net collagen loss (Bertolami and Donoff 1979a).

Relationship Between Glycosaminoglycans and Collagen Synthesis

In healing wounds, several explanations for a relationship between glycosaminoglycan production and collagen synthesis have been offered (Dunphy and Udupa 1955; Layton et al. 1958; Meyer 1947; Green and Hamerman 1964; Green and Goldberg 1963; 1965) but none have been completely satisfactory. Several investigators (Dunphy and Udupa 1955; Layton et al. 1958; Meyer 1947) believed that the glycosaminoglycan component of the extracellular matrix was physically and chemically necessary for deposition of collagen; but, Jackson, Flickinger, and Dunphy (1960) observed that constant, low levels of sulfated glycosaminoglycans were present throughout the course of healing, so high concentrations of sulfated glycosaminoglycans could not be essential for normal collagen formation.

A similar conclusion was reached by Bentley (1967). Although fibroblasts were known to synthesize both collagen and glycosaminoglycans, distinctly different mechanisms for controlling production of each substance became apparent when Green and Hamerman (1964) found that clonal isolates of 3T6 fibroblasts grown to saturation density made both substances in the same culture while 3T3 fibroblasts, possessing a decreased capacity for collagen synthesis, elaborated hyaluronate at the same rate as line 3T6 (Green and Goldberg 1965). Interestingly, the synthesis of collagen by established fibroblast lines followed a course remarkably similar to that of collagen in open wound granulation tissues (Green and Goldberg 1963).

In contrast, other work (Rokosová-Čmuchalová and Bentley 1968; Flint 1971; LeRoy 1972; Uitto et al. 1971; Fleischmajer and Perlish 1972; Toole and Lowther 1968; Linares and Larson 1978) has suggested that glycosaminoglycans might participate in controlling the rate of collagen synthesis. Evidence for a relationship between the biosynthesis of collagen and glycosaminoglycans has been based on a concomitant inhibition of both chondroitin sulfate synthesis and collagen production in epiphyseal cartilage by sodium salicylate; non-collagen protein remained unaffected (Rokosová-Čmuckalová and Bentley 1968). Collagen formed in the salicylate-treated series aggregated into more mature fibrils faster than in controls. Similarly, Flint (1971) observed a temporal and spatial correlation between the disaggregation of collagen fibers and the appearance of increased quantities of glycosaminoglycans in the repair of split thickness skin graft donor sites.

In addition, increased hexosamine and sialic acid concentrations (suggesting increased glycoprotein content) have been demonstrated in tissue culture studies of scleroderma skin (LeRoy 1972). Two studies of glycosaminoglycan concentration in scleroderma skin using CPC precipitation and resolution in buffers of increasing ionic strength reported an increase in total glycosaminoglycan concentration. One study found chondroitin-4,6-sulfate (Uitto et al. 1971) and the other found dermatan sulfate (Fleischmajer and Perlish 1972) to be the fractions responsible for the increase.

A specific role for dermatan sulfate in the formation and orientation of collagen was suggested (Toole and Lowther 1968) when covalently bound dermatan sulfate-protein complexes were found to instantaneously precipitate tropocollagen in the form of "native type" fibrils. In healing wounds, a further postsynthetic/postsecretion function for sulfated glycosaminoglycans was proposed when Linares and Larson (1978) attributed to chondroitin sulfate the ability to protect collagen against collagenolysis. Aberrations in wound proteoglycan content might thus relate to the excessive collagen deposition characteristic of hypertrophic scars and keloids. Whether these _in vitro_ studies actually reflect the situation _in vivo_ has not been established; in fact, Shoshan (1981) has suggested that it may be the collagen that reduces glycosaminoglycan degradation (David and Bernfield 1979) rather than the reverse.

A complete resolution to the conflicting evidence for a direct relationship between the collagen and sulfated glycosaminoglycan content of wound tissues has not been achieved. Certainly, some of the parallels may result from the fact that both substances are the products of differentiated cells; any factor that influences cellular differentiation might generate coincident but otherwise unrelated effects.

Specific Interactions Between Cells and Glycosaminoglycans

Turley and Roth (1979) proposed a specific interaction between cells and matrix glycosaminoglycans when they observed a spontaneous glycosylation of glycosaminoglycan substrates by adherent fibroblasts. The presence of cell surface glycosyltransferases (Shur and Roth 1975) that can interact with extracellular saccharide acceptors provides a means by which cellular adhesive recognition (Bossmann 1972; Shur and Roth 1975), migration (Shur 1977a; 1977b), and matrix-mediated cellular induction (Shur 1977a; 1977b) might occur. The role discussed earlier for hyaluronate in cell movement (Toole 1976; Pratt, Larsen and Johnston 1975) makes the possibility of an interaction between a glycosaminoglycan-containing matrix and surface transferases particularly attractive. Shur (1977b) suggested that such interaction could be responsible for the recognition and adhesive forces required for directed cellular migration.

In a slightly different context, glycosaminoglycans that are present on cell surfaces may also be involved in other cell-matrix interactions (Stamatoglou and Keller 1982). Using Swiss mouse 3T3 and SV3T3 cells, cell surface heparan sulfate has been shown to bind to native calf skin collagen and to fibronectin (Stamatoglou and Keller 1982). Such binding is reversed by heparin and dermatan sulfate but not by chondroitin-4-sulfate or chondroitin-6-sulfate. Cell surface chondroitin sulfate binds to collagen but not to fibronectin; cell surface hyaluronate binds to neither. Specific glycosaminoglycan-mediated binding between cell surfaces and extracellular matrix constituents may also provide insight into cellular adhesion in wound healing, tissue organization, and metastatic invasion (Stamatoglou and Keller 1982).

Glycosaminoglycans and the Phenomenon of Wound Contraction

In evaluating the analogy between embryonic development and wound healing, it may be instructive to consider the phenomenon of wound contraction as a type of morphogenetic movement. Embryonic organ morphogenesis is, in part, a product of the local motor activity of individual cells (Spooner 1975). Wound contraction could be the result of a similar mechanism. The wound periphery appears to be important in the generation of forces necessary for wound contraction (Grillo, Watts and Gross 1958); this region also possesses the highest concentrations of hyaluronate (Bertolami and Donoff 1978; 1982). Given hyaluronate's ability to promote cellular migration and proliferation (Toole 1972; 1976; Toole and Gross 1971; Toole and Trelstad 1971; Toole, Jackson and Gross 1972; Orkin and Toole 1978; 1980a; 1980b; Polansky, Toole and Gross 1974; Pratt, Larsen and Johnston 1975), forces arising in the wound edge could be entirely comparable to those responsible for true embryonic morphogenetic movements. The cells giving rise to such forces are not known, but the most widely accepted theory of wound contraction assigns an important role to a specialized muscle-like cell, the myofibroblast (Gabbiani, Chaponnier and Hüttner 1978; Bertolami and Donoff 1979a,b). How the glycosaminoglycan composition of wound granulation tissue influences myofibroblasts has not been adequately explored.

REFERENCES

Anseth, A. 1961. Glycosaminoglycans in corneal regeneration. Exp. Eye Res. 1:122-127.

Antonopoulos, CA, Gardell, S and Hamnström, S. 1965. Separation of the glycosaminoglycans (mucopolysaccharides) from aorta by a column procedure using quarternary ammonium compounds. J. Athero. Res. 5:9-15.

Balazs, A, and Holmgren, HJ. 1950. The basic dye-uptake and the presence of a growth-inhibiting substance in the healing tissue of skin wounds. Exp. Cell Res. 1:206-216.

Balazs, A, and Holmgren, HJ. 1949. Wound extracts and their effects on the growth of hen fibroblasts. Nature 163:488-489.

Bentley, JP. 1967. Rate of chondroitin sulfate formation in wound healing. Ann. Surg. 165:186-191.

Bertolami, CN. 1978. A Study of Wound Healing as a Developmental Phenomenon. D. Med. Sc. thesis, Harvard University.

Bertolami, CN, and Donoff, RB. 1982. Identification, characterization, and partial purification of mammalian skin wound hyaluronidase. J. Invest. Derm. 79:417-421.

Bertolami, CN, and Donoff, RB. 1979a. The effect of skin grafting upon prolyl hydroxylase and hyaluronidase activities in mammalian wound repair. J. Surg. Res. 27:359-366.

Bertolami, CN, and Donoff, RB. 1979b. The effect of full thickness skin grafts on the actomyosin content of contracting wounds. J. Oral Surg. 37:471-476.

Bertolami, CN, and Donoff, RB. 1978. Hyaluronidase activity during open wound healing in rabbits: A preliminary report. J. Surg. Res. 25:256-259.

Bitter, T, and Muir, HM. 1962. A modified uronic acid carbazole reaction. Anal. Biochem. 4:330-334.

Bossmann, HB. 1972. Platelet adhesiveness and aggregation. II. Surface sialic acid, glycoprotein: N-acetylneuraminic acid transferase and neuraminidase of human blood platelets. Biochim. Biophys. Acta. 279:456-474.

Campani, M, Zonta, A and Ugazio, G. 1959. Ricerche sul tessuto di riparazione della ferite cutanee. Proc. Simposio Della Societa Italiana E Della Societa Tedesca Di Patologia. Milano 6-7.

Castor, CW, Bignall, MC, Hossler, PA, and Roberts, DJ. 1981. Connective tissue activation. XXI. Regulation of glycosaminoglycan metabolism by lymphocyte (CTAP-I) and platelet (CTAP-III) growth factors. In Vitro 17:777-785.

Cintron, C, and Kublin, CL. 1977. Regeneration of corneal tissue. Dev. Biol. 61:346-357.

Dahlgren, C, and Björkstén, B. 1982. Effect of hyaluronic acid on polymorphonuclear leukocyte cell surface properties. Scand. J. Hematol. 28:376-380.

David, G, and Bernfield, MR. 1979. Collagen reduces glycosaminoglycan degradation by cultured mammary epithelial cells: Possible mechanism for basal lamina formation. Proc. Natl. Acad. Sci. USA 76:786-790.

DeSalequi, M, Plonska, H, and Pigman, W. 1967. A comparison for serum and testicular hyaluronidase. Arch. Biochem. Biophys. 121:548-554.

Donoff, RB, and Grillo, HC. 1975. The effects of skin grafting on healing open wounds in rabbits. J. Surg. Res. 19:163-167.

Dorner, RW. 1967. Glycosaminoglycans of regenerating tendon. Arth. Rheum. 10:275-276.

Dunphy, JE, and Udupa, KN. 1955. Chemical and histochemical sequences in the normal healing of wounds. New England J. Med. 253:847-851.

Edwards, LC, Pernokas, LN, and Dunphy, JE. 1957. The use of plastic sponge to sample regenerating tissue in healing wounds. Surg. Gyn. Obstet. 105:303-309.

Fleishmajer, R, and Perlish, JS. 1972. Glycosaminoglycans in scleroderma and scleredema. J. Invest. Derm. 58:129-132.

Flint, MH. 1971. The role of mucopolysaccharides in the healing and remodelling of split skin donor sites. In Trans. Fifth Internat. Cong. Plast. Reconstr. Surg., edited J. T. Hueston, p. 730. Melbourne: Butterworths.

Gabbiani, G, Chaponnier, C, and Hüttner, I. 1978. Cytoplasmic filaments and gap junctions in epithelial cells and myofibroblasts during wound healing. J. Cell Biol. 76:561-568.

Goggins, JF, Lazarus, GS, and Fullmer, HM. 1968. Hyaluronidase activity of alveolar macrophages. J. Histochem. Cytochem. 16:688-692.

Green, H, and Goldberg, B. 1965. Collagen synthesis by cultured cells. In Structure and Function of Connective and Skeletal Tissue, edited by S. F. Jackson, pp. 288-296. London: Butterworths.

Green, H, and Goldberg, B. 1963. Kinetics of collagen synthesis by established mammalian cell lines. Nature 200:1097-1098.

Green, H, and Hamerman, D. 1964. Production of hyaluronate and collagen by fibroblast clones in culture. Nature 201:710.

Grillo, HC, Watts, GT, and Gross, J. 1958. Studies in wound healing: I. Contraction and the wound contents. Ann. Surg. 148:145-152.

Hatae, Y, and Makita, A. 1975. Colorimetric determination of hyaluronate degraded by Streptomyces hyaluronidase. Anal. Biochem. 64:30-36.

Hay, EE, and Revel, JP. 1969. Fine structure of the developing avian cornea. In Vol. I of Monographs in Developmental Biology, edited by A. Wolsky and P. S. Chem, pp. 78-118. Basel: Karger.

Heinegard, D, and Hascall, VC. 1974. Aggregation of cartilage proteoglycans. III. Characteristics of the proteins isolated from trypsin digests of aggregates. J. Biol. Chem. 249:4250-4256.

Hosoda, Y. 1960. Studies on granulation tissue. I. Soluble collagen in wound healing. II. Fibrogenesis and nucleic acids. Keio J. Med. 9:261-286.

Jackson, DS, Flickinger, DB, and Dunphy, JE. 1960. Biochemical studies of connective tissue repair. Ann. N.Y. Acad. Sci. 86:943-947.

Jeanloz, R. 1970. Mucopolysaccharides in higher animals. In The Carbohydrates: Chemistry and Biochemistry, second edition IIB, edited by W. Pigman and D. Horton, p. 590. New York: Academic Press.

Laurent, TC. 1966. In vitro studies on the transport of macromolecules through the connective tissue. Fed. Proc. 25: 1128.

LeRoy, EC. 1972. Connective tissue synthesis by scleroderma skin fibroblasts in cell culture. J. Exp. Med. 135:1351-1362.

Levvy, GA, and Marsh, CA. 1959. Preparation and properties of β-glucuronidase. Adv. Carbohydr. Chem. 14:381-428.

Layton, LL, Frankel, DR, Sher, IH, Scapa, S, and Friedler, G. 1958. Importance of the synthesis of acidic polysaccharide for wound healing. Nature 181:1543-1544.

Linares, HA, and Larson, DL. 1978. Proteoglycans and collagenase in hypertrophic scar formation. Plast. Reconstr. Surg. 62:589-593.

Meyer, K. 1947. Biological significance of hyaluronic acid and hyaluronidase. Physiol Rev. 27:335-359.

Meyer, K. 1938. The chemistry and biology of mucopolysaccharides and glycoproteins. Cold Spring Harbor Symp. Quant. Biol. 6:91-102.

Meyer, K, and Chaffee, E. 1941. The mucopolysaccharides of skin. J. Biol. Chem. 138:491-499.

Meyer, K, and Palmer, JW. 1934. The polysaccharide of vitreous humor. J. Biol. Chem. 107:629-634.

Morris, JE. 1979. Steric exclusion of cells: A mechanism of glycosaminoglycan-induced cell aggregation. Exp. Cell Res. 129:141-153.

Nieduszynski, IA, Sheehan, JK, Phelps, CF, Hardingham, TE, and Muir, II. 1980. Equilibrium-binding studies of pig laryngeal cartilage proteoglycans with hyaluronate oligosaccharide fractions. Biochem. J. 185:107-114.

Ogston, AG. 1970. The biological functions of glycosaminoglycans. In Chemistry and Molecular Biology of the Intercellular Matrix, Vol. 3, edited by E. A. Balazs, pp. 1231-1240. New York: Academic Press.

Ohya, T, and Kaneko, Y. 1970. Novel hyaluronidase from streptomyces. Biochim. Biophys. Acta. 198:607-609.

Orkin, RW, and Toole, BP. 1980a. Isolation and characterization of hyaluronidase from cultures of chick embryo skin- and muscle-derived fibroblasts. J. Biol. Chem. 255:1036-1042.

Ordin, RW, and Toole, BP. 1980b. Chick embryo fibroblasts produce two forms of hyaluronidase. J. Cell Biol. 85:248-257.

Orkin, RW, and Toole, BP. 1978. Hyaluronidase activity and hyaluronate content of the developing chick embryo heart. Dev. Biol. 66:308-320.

Peacock, EE, and Van Winkle, W. 1976. Wound Repair, second edition, pp. 1-21, Philadelphia: Saunders.

Penny, JR, and Balfour, BM. 1949. Effect of vitamin C on mucopolysaccharide production in wound healing. J. Pathol. Bacteriol. 61:171-178.

Perkins, SJ, Miller, A, Hardingham, TE, and Muir, H. 1981. Physical properties of the hyaluronate binding region of proteoglycan from pig laryngeal cartilage. J. Mol. Biol. 150: 69-95.

Polansky, JR, Toole, BP, and Gross, J. 1974. Brain hyaluronidase: Changes in activity during chick development. Science 183:862-864.

Pratt, RM, Larsen, MA, and Johnston, MC. 1975. Migration of cranial neural crest cells in a cell-free hyaluronate-rich matrix. Dev. Biol. 44:298-305.

Reissig, JL, Strominger, JL, and LeLoir, LF. 1955. A modified colorimetric method for the estimation of N-acetylamino sugars. J. Biol. Chem. 217:959-966.

Rokosová-Čmuchalová, B, and Bentley, JP. 1968. Relation of collagen synthesis to chondroitin sulfate synthesis in cartilage. Biochem. Pharmacol. Suppl. 17:315-327.

Schoenberg, MD, and Moore, RD. 1964. The conformation of hyaluronic acid and chondroitin sulfate C: Metachromatic reaction. Biochim. Biophys. Acta. 83:42-51.

Scott, JE. 1956. The preparation and fractionation of acid polysaccharides using long-chain quarternary ammonium compounds. Biochem. J. 62:31P.

Sharon, N. 1975. Complex Carbohydrates. Their Chemistry, Biosynthesis, and Functions. pp. 258-281, Massachusetts: Addison-Wesley.

Shoshan, S. 1981. Wound healing. Int. Rev. Connect. Tiss. Res. 9:1-26.

Shur, BD. 1977a. Cell-surface glycosyltransferases in gastrulating chick embryos I. Dev. Biol. 58:23-39.

Shur, BD. 1977b. Cell surface glycosyltransferases in gastrulating chick embryos II. Dev. Biol. 58:40-55.

Shur, BD, and Roth, S. 1975. Cell surface glycosyltransferases. Biochim. Biophys. Acta 415:473-512.

Silbert, JE. 1982. Structure and metabolism of proteoglycans and glycosaminoglycans. J. Invest. Derm. 79 Suppl. 1: 31s-37s.

Silbert, JE, and DeLuca, S. 1970. Degradation of glycosaminoglycans by tadpole tissue: Difference in activity toward chondroitin-4-sulfate and chrondroitin-6-sulfate. J. Biol. Chem. 245:1506-1508.

Spooner, BS. 1975. Microfilaments, microtubules and extracellular materials in morphogenesis. BioScience 25:440-451.

Stamatoglou, SC, and Keller, JM. 1982. Interactions of cellular glycosaminoglycans with plasma fibronectin and collagen. Biochim. Biophys. Acta 719:90-97.

Toole, BP. 1976. Morphogenetic role of glycosaminoglycans (acid mucopolysaccharides) in brain and other tissues. In Neuronal Recognition, edited by S. H. Barondes, pp. 275-329. New York: Plenum Press.

Toole, BP. 1972. Hyaluronate turnover during chondrogenesis in the developing chick limb and axial skeleton. Dev. Biol. 29:321-329.

Toole, BP, and Gross, J. 1971. The extracellular matrix of the regenerating newt limb: synthesis and removal of hyaluronate prior to differentiation. Dev. Biol. 25:57-77.

Toole, BP, Jackson, G, and Gross, J. 1972. Hyaluronate in morphogenesis: Inhibition of chondrogenesis in vitro. Proc. Natl. Acad. Sci. USA 69:1384-1386.

Toole, BP, and Lowther, DA. 1968. Dermatan sulfate-protein: Isolation from and interaction with collagen. Arch. Biochem. Biophys. 128:567-578.

Toole, BP, and Trelstad, RL. 1971. Hyaluronate production and removal during corneal development in the chick. Dev. Biol. 26:28-35.

Tsuda, T, Dannenberg, AM, Ando, M, Rojas-Espinosa, O, and Shima, K. 1974. Enzymes in tuberculous lesions hydrolyzing protein, hyaluronic acid, and chondroitin sulfate. J. Retic. Soc. 16:220-231.

Turley, EA, and Roth, S. 1979. Spontaneous glycosylation of glycosaminoglycan substrates by adherent fibroblasts. Cell 17:109-115.

Tynelius-Bratthall, G, and Attström, R. 1972. Acid phosphatase, hyaluronidase, and protease in crevices of healthy and inflammed gingiva in dogs. J. Dent. Res. 51:279-283.

Uitto, J, Helin, G, Helin, P, Lorenzen, I. 1971. Connective tissue in scleroderma. Acta Derm. Venerol. 51:401-406.

Yang, C, and Srivastava, PN. 1975. Purification of bull sperm hyaluronidase by concanavalin-A affinity chromatography. Biochim. Biophys. Acta 391:382-387.

PART II
Cellular Response to Fracture

6
Fracture Healing

R. Bruce Heppenstall

BONE FUNCTION

The two primary functions of bone are to support the human frame and to provide a source of calcium. Bone also serves as an anchor for the origin and insertion of the surrounding musculature and protects several vital soft tissue structures. Since bone makes up the human skeleton, it is essential to locomotion. Despite its active role in these body functions, bone is a light structure, when one considers that it represents only one tenth of the entire body weight. Bone has a breaking strength comparable to that of medium steel, yet it is a flexible and elastic structure. This elasticity allows bone to be bent or twisted and still return to its original state following removal of the deforming force, provided that force has not exceeded the limits of elasticity. Bone is able to resist axial stresses but is limited in its ability to resist rotational forces. One important point to bear in mind with regard to bone is that, like the liver, it is one of the few organs able to undergo spontaneous regeneration rather than just simple repair with restoration of structure. This property is more of a regenerative phenomenon, as the entire anatomical structure is restored to the state that existed prior to injury.

Fracture healing has many similarities to soft tissue healing, but also has some unique features owing to the anatomical struc-

---

ture and characteristics of bone. There has been a lag in investigative studies on the healing of osseous tissue compared with that of soft tissue, because many of the techniques applied to soft tissue studies are not applicable to the anatomical structure of bone. A simple example is the difficulty of isolating intact mitochondria from osseous tissue as opposed to the relative ease of obtaining mitochondria from soft tissue.

BONE STRUCTURE

The gross structure of bone has been divided into two specific types--tubular and flat. Tubular bone provides normal weight-bearing functions and locomotion. Flat bone, such as the skull, serves to protect vital soft tissue structures. Anatomically, tubular bones are formed with a diaphysis and an epiphysis, or secondary ossification center. Diaphyseal bone is made up of a lamellar structure, indicative of mature bone, with collagen fibril bundles which are arranged in layers, strata, or lamellae. Primitive nonlamellar bone is known as fibrous bone, and it occurs in embryonic life, at fracture sites, and at the metaphysis during active new bone formation. The epiphyseal plate is located at the junction of the diaphysis and epiphysis in the area where normal longitudinal growth occurs in tubular bone. In flat bone there is no epiphyseal plate.

The periosteum is a fibrous sheet that surrounds bone. This important anatomical structure plays an active role in the fracture healing process. It is subdivided into an outer fibrous layer and an inner layer known as the cambium layer (Fig. 6.1). Active new bone cell proliferation occurs from the cambium layer during fracture repair. The periosteum has a much greater osteogenic potential in the child than in the adult. This is important to the fracture healing process since nonunion is very rare in childhood. The inner portion of bone, known as the marrow cavity, is lined with a fibrous sheet called the endosteum, which also is actively involved in the fracture healing process.

The functioning unit of mature bone is known as the haversian system or osteon. This structure consists of a haversian canal in the center, containing one or more blood vessels (capillaries and venules), which is surrounded by lamellae (Fig. 6.2). The surrounding lamellae have lacunae, each of which contains an osteocyte with a cytoplasmic process extending through canaliculi to communicate with the haversian vessels. The size of the osteon is limited by the fact that the

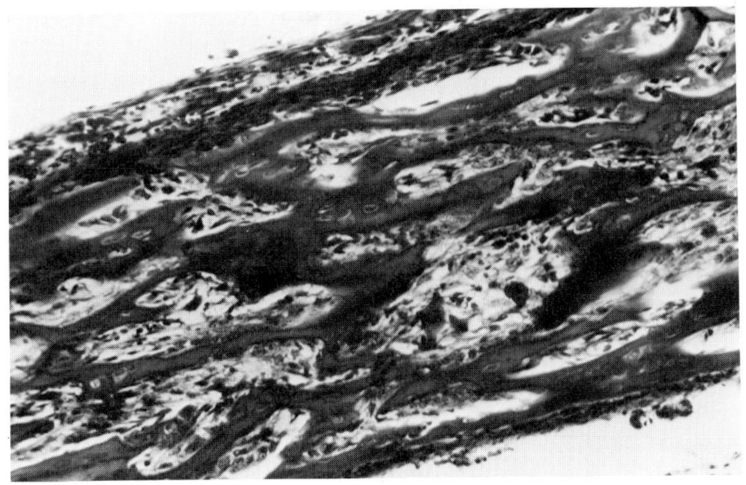

FIGURE 6.1 Longitudinal section of bone demonstrating the periosteum as an outer fibrous layer and an inner cambrium layer.

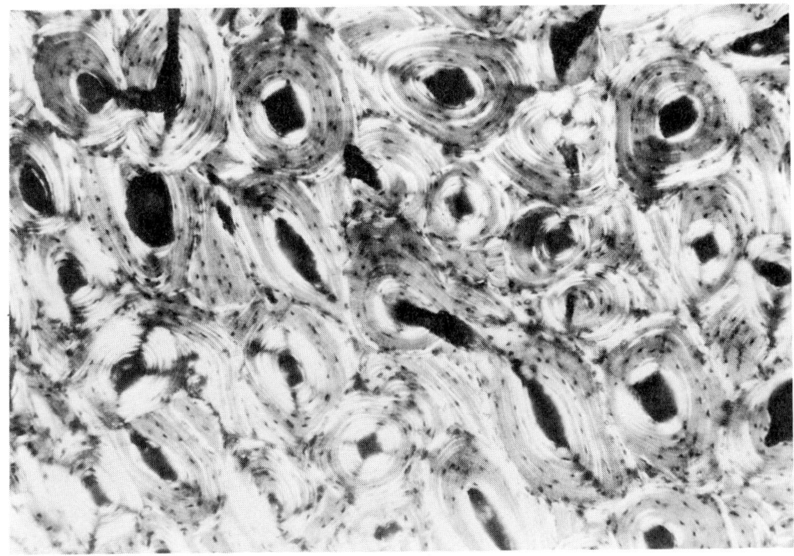

FIGURE 6.2 Polarized light demonstration of the osteonal structure of bone. Note the surrounding lamellae.

haversian canal supplies the nutrition, and Ham has demonstrated that bone cells in general cannot survive farther than 0.1 mm away from a capillary.[16,17]

Bone Formation

Bone formation occurs through two distinct mechanisms, endochondral and membranous. Endochondral bone formation occurs at the epiphyseal plate in long bones and accounts for growth and length (growth in width of bone develops by subperiosteal appositional bone formation). Endochondral bone requires the laying down of a pre-formed cartilage model. This cartilage is gradually resorbed and replaced by new bone. It is important to have a thorough knowledge of endochondral bone formation as this sequence of events has been described in fracture healing. An organizational structure, such as the epiphyseal plate, does not develop during fracture healing. However, several of the events, such as the formation of a cartilage model, do occur, and many investigators feel that the fracture healing process is similar to events that occur in the epiphyseal plate. In fact, several recent studies have pointed out the similarities in the physiological events that take place at a fracture site and those that take place at the epiphyseal plate.[22] Therefore, it is possible that bone growth and bone repair are governed essentially by the same mechanisms.

Membranous bone formation does not involve a cartilage model. This type of bone forms when mesenchymal cells differentiate directly into osteoblasts, which then lay down osteoid. This is followed by mineralization to form new bone. This type of bone is seen in the calvarium, most facial bones, the clavicle and mandible (both mixed), and subperiosteal bone. The specific type of bone formation has a direct bearing on fracture repair, as skull, for example, generally heals by fibrous union and not by new bone formation.

Bone Composition

A typical mature lamellar bone has a composition of approximately 8 percent water and 92 percent solid material. The solid material portion can be divided into an organic phase of 21 percent and an inorganic phase of 71 percent.

Organic Constituents

The organic material, also known as the matrix, supplies form and supporting structure for the deposition and crystallization of inorganic salts. The matrix is composed of approximately 98 percent collagen, with the remaining 2 percent or less consisting of ground substance. Bone collagen is made up of type 1, which consists of two alpha-1 chains and an alpha-2 chain. Type 1 collagen is very similar to skin and tendon collagen. The hydroxylation of proline and lysine requires oxygen, iron, and ascorbic acid. It is important to bear in mind that very little oxygen is required to hydroxylate all available proline and lysine. Therefore, the hydroxylation process can occur under conditions of relative hypoxia. It is interesting that the number of hydroxylysine residues in humans is the same in both bone and skin collagen. This does not apply to the glycosylation of the hydroxylysine residues, as this process is less frequent in bone collagen than in other types of collagen.

Lane recently demonstrated that in the rat 40 to 60 percent of collagen synthesis in the callus and pericallus tissues during the second and fourth week postfracture was type 2 collagen. The presence in the fracture callus of type 2 collagen, which had previously been identified in the epiphyseal plate, provided strong biochemical evidence that endochondral bone formation occurs during the fracture healing process.[24] However, if compression plating is employed for the fixation of fractures, very little callus develops, and the collagen formed is then type 1.

Several investigators have felt that the cross-linking pattern in bone collagen may differ from that of other types of collagen. It is true that bone collagen is extremely insoluble compared with other collagens. It has also been demonstrated that animals administered β-aminopropionitrile and made lathyritic have 40 percent of their bone collagens soluble in neutral salt solution, which consists primarily of the alpha components. Lathyrogens have been demonstrated in the past to prevent covalent cross-linking in collagen. Therefore, it is reasonable to conclude that the insolubility of bone collagen may be due to a high degree of cross-linking, or that the cross-linking is of a different type than that in other collagens. It has also been suggested that the insolubility of bone collagen may be due to keto-aldimine cross-linking as well as other aldimine cross-links which may be reduced during maturation. Collagen degradation occurs by action of the enzyme collagenase. The enzyme cleaves the collagen molecules at a specific site to yield two peptides, which are then susceptible to other proteases under normal physiological conditions. Although the exact regulation of collagenase activity is a very complex subject, it is known that collagenase activity is partially controlled by parathyroid hormone, thyroxin, and steroid metabolism.

The matrix also includes a group of substances that make up less than 2 percent of its composition and are known as ground substance. They include the glycosaminoglycans (previously known as acid mucopolysaccharides) and proteoglycans. The glycosaminoglycans (GAG) are highly-charged polyanions composed of repeating disaccharide units. These units include a carboxyl or a sulfate group or both, consisting of uronic acid and hexosamine moieties, except for keratan sulfate, which is an exception to this rule.

The GAG structure, which has been evaluated in several studies, includes hyaluronate, chondroitin-4-sulfate, chondroitin-6-sulfate, keratan sulfate, dermatan sulfate, heparan sulfate, and heparin. The difference between these structures is essentially a different repeating disaccharide structure. The GAG structures as a rule do not exist as isolated polysaccharide chains in vivo but are linked covalently to protein and are known as proteoglycans. It has recently been proposed that hyaluronate may not exist as the proteoglycan, in contrast to sulfated GAG, but as individual GAG chains occurring in the extra-cellular matrix. Interestingly, the molecular weight of hyaluronate is several times that of the sulfated GAG chains. Some investigators believe that the glycosaminoglycans and proteoglycans may be involved in the calcification mechanism, although their exact role has not been delineated. It is probable that the interaction of collagen and cartilage proteoglycan plays an important part in cartilage matrix deposition.

Inorganic Constituents

The principle inorganic salt is crystalline in the form of hydroxyapatite, $Ca_{10}(PO_4)_6(OH)_2$. The role played by bone carbonate in relation to calcium carbonate has been extensively debated in the past.[7] Recent theories have focused on the inclusion of carbonate $CO_3^=$ in the interior volume of the apatite structural model. The difficulty of this theory lies in how carbonate is incorporated into the hydroxyapatite structure. It is possible that it may be substituted for phosphate ion, or trapped interstitially, or substituted for the hydroxyl radical. It is also possible that $CO_3^=$ interferes with the formation of hydroxyapatite by replacing $PO_4^=$ or $HPO_4^=$ at the surface of the developing crystallite. Further studies will be required before the exact role of the carbonate ion is definitely established.

The mineral crystals are extremely small, being approximately 25 to 75 Å in diameter and approximately 200 Å in length. This provides a very large surface area. In fact, the surface area of bone mineral is enormous and has been estimated to be approximately 100 square meters per gram. There is a shell of water surrounding the surface crystals (hydration shell), and ions may move freely between the hydration shell and the crystalline surface. Glimcher has demonstrated a definite relationship between bone crystal and collagen structure.[14,15] The bone crystals appear to align in a specific pattern within the collagen molecule, with the long axis of the crystal aligned parallel to the longitudinal axis of the collagen fiber in a band pattern with the collagen fibril. In other words, bone crystals appear in the hole zone of the collagen fibril, increasing the surface area.[21] As an example, the skeleton of a 150-pound man would equal approximately 100 acres of surface area. Two theories have been advanced regarding the relation of bone crystal and collagen fiber. The first is that a direct physical bond exists between the collagen fibers and the initial apatite crystallites. This theory is based on the results of electron paramagnetic resonance studies. The second theory is that a specific charge exists on the collagen fiber, initiating the formation of crystals, which are held in this position by electrostatic forces.

Cellular Components

Three principal bone cells are identified during bone formation and remodeling. These are the osteoblast, osteocyte, and osteoclast. A similar series of cells has been demonstrated in cartilage formation, and these are known as the chondroblast, chondrocyte, and chondroclast. In bone, the osteoblast is the cell primarily involved in the formation of the matrix. The osteocyte acts in a dual capacity as a bone-forming and bone-destroying cell. The osteoclast is involved with bone destruction and resorption and also plays a part in the remodeling process.

In an excellent series of investigative studies[1] Belanger described bone resorption as being mediated by the osteocyte and termed this process osteocytic osteolysis.[6] He felt that the normal day-to-day resorption occurring in bone remodeling was mediated by the osteocyte, whereas pathological resorption was mediated by the osteoclast. The osteocyte produces collagen and is believed to elaborate the proteoglycans and the protein polysaccharides. The osteocyte is found within the haversian system in lamellar bones and in a lacuna communicating with a haversian canal from which it obtains nourishment and oxygen supply. As described by Ham, osteocytes generally occur in compact bone no more than 0.1 mm away from a functioning capillary.[16] The blood supply of compact bone is derived from one or two capillaries or slightly larger vessels that are present in each haversian canal. The haversian canal and the enclosed capillaries lie more or less parallel to the shaft of a long bone.

During fracture repair, osteoblasts appear to originate from cells of the cambium layer of the periosteum and endosteum. Several names have been attached to these cells in the past, including fibroblast, osteoprogenitor, and undifferentiated mesenchymal cell. Many investigators believe that the periosteum contains osteogenic cells and participates in the formation of the external callus (Fig. 6.3).[38,39] Therefore, it should be preserved, if at all possible, during the surgical management of fractures. However, as will be discussed, the endosteum is ultimately the most important portion of the bone involved in fracture healing.

The osteoclast is a multinuclear cell, which generally is located along the peripheral aspect of the bone substance. Its primary function is bone resorption. The peripheral aspect of an osteoclast presents a ruffled border in association with resorption of the adjacent bone.

It is probable that mesenchymal cells subjected to appropriate mechanical and biophysical stimuli may transform directly into osteoblasts and produce bone. Bassett demonstrated that cells subjected to a combination of compression and low oxygen tensions transformed directly into chondroblasts and formed cartilage.[4] If the cells were then administered an adequate amount of oxygen and placed under tension rather than compression, they differentiated into fibroblasts and produced dense fibrous tissue. One problem in interpreting these results is separating the effects of compression and tension from the effects of varying oxygen tensions on the stimulation of cells to form various linkages. It is a clinical axiom that bone forms in compression and fails in tension

FRACTURE HEALING

Primary type bone healing is somewhat artificial in that it is possible only with rigid internal fixation and excellent anatomical position. This is not usually the case in the nonoperative treatment of fractures. The goal of primary bone healing is therefore obtained only by primary operative internal fixation. It has been adequately demonstrated by Perren and the Associa-

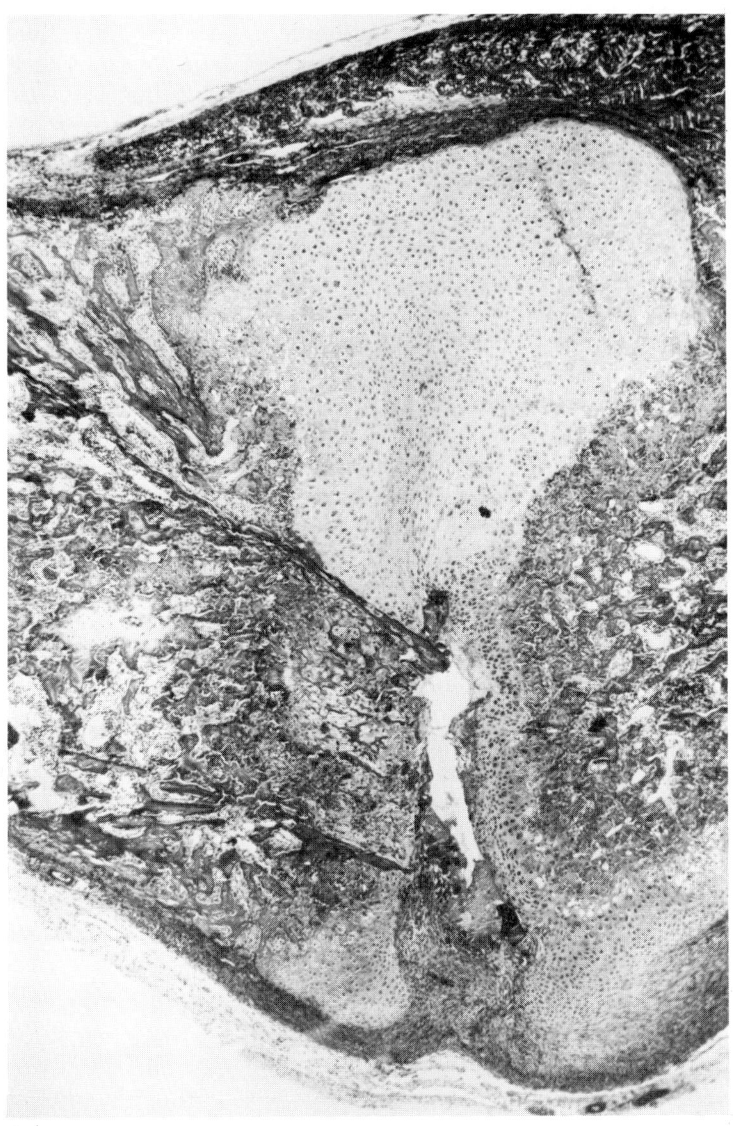

FIGURE 6.3 The extent of the periosteal collar may be viewed in this fracture at the top of this low power photomicrograph demonstrating the osteogenic potential of the periosteum at the proximal and distal aspects of the fracture and the cartilage cells in the center of the periosteal collar. Development of the abundant periosteal collar is secondary to gross motion at the fracture site.

tion for the Study of Internal Fixation (AO Group) that fractures treated in this manner reveal evidence of primary bone healing without any sign of fibrous tissue or cartilage during the healing process.[29] There is no evidence of external callus formation with this type of treatment. The destruction of osteons close to the fracture site, initiated by the destruction of local blood supply, stimulates an intensive regeneration of new haversian systems in the area. Osteoclasts form spearheads at the ends of the haversian canals close to the fracture site, and these become enlarged in preparation for the formation of a new system. The osteoclast spearhead (cutting cone) can advance at a rate of 50 to 80 μ per 24 hours up to and through the fracture surface, with the production of enlarged haversian canals, which cross from one fragment to the opposite fragment. Osteoblasts follow immediately to form new osteons which traverse the fracture site. If rigid internal fixation is employed, it will take approximately five to six weeks for new osteons to be constructed. Therefore, the repair is produced by new osteons developing and crossing the fracture site to replace the old osteons that had been deprived of their local blood supply. If a gap exists between the fracture fragments, or if there is not rigid immobilization, this type of healing does not occur. It is replaced by healing that is normally observed in the nonoperative management of fractures, which will be discussed further on. A great deal of credit must be given to the Association for the Study of Internal Fixation for thoroughly evaluating this type of fracture repair.

Stages of Repair

Impact

Bone will absorb energy until a failure occurs. The greater the rate of application of force or load, the greater the energy bone may absorb. The amount of energy that can be absorbed by bone is inversely proportional to the modulus of rigidity. Also, the amount of energy absorbed by osseous tissue is directly proportional to the volume of bone. A fracture line will follow the path of least resistance. If drill holes have been placed in bone prior to impact, the fracture line will pass through the drill holes because they produce areas of stress concentration. This is extremely important to remember when large compression plates are removed following internal fixation and during fracture healing. The limb must be protected until the osseous tissues around the drill holes have a chance to react to the new stresses and abolish the stress concentration. It usually requires at least four to six weeks for the bone to adapt to the new stress. If compression plates are left on for a prolonged period, osteoporosis may develop beneath them, and this of course will weaken the resistance of bone to impact.

Induction

At the present time, the exact duration of the stage of induction is unknown. This stage may occur at any time from impact to the completion of the stage of inflammation. Cells in the area of the fracture are induced to form new bone. Although the exact origin of new osteoblasts is still a matter of controversy, it is fair to state that two separate mechanisms appear to operate. In the first mechanism, the periosteal cell, endosteal cell, and osteocyte undergo modulation in order to produce new osteoblasts. The second mechanism involves differentiation of fibroblasts, endothelial cells, muscle cells, and undifferentiated mesenchymal cells. The exact stimulus of modulation and differentiation is unknown at the present time. It is possible that the initial disruption of the blood supply and the production of a state of relative hypoxia with a large oxygen gradient may stimulate formation of an osteoblast linkage, as previously proposed by the author.[18,19] An acidic pH rapidly develops in the local area, and this may also be a stimulus. Lysosomal enzymes are released following cell disruption. Although each is a possible initial stimulant, it is probable that the stimulation is multifactorial.

Inflammation

This stage begins immediately after the fracture occurs and persists until cartilage or bone formation is initiated. Clinically, the end of this stage is usually associated with a decrease in pain and swelling. This interval varies but usually lasts for three to four days. There is a gross disruption of the vascular supply with attendant hemorrhage and hematoma formation (Fig. 6.4). A state of hypoxia exists with an acidic environment. The bone at the edge of the fracture site, both the periosteal and endosteal surfaces, becomes necrotic. There is a gross disruption of the osteons and the lacunae with the release of lysosomal enzymes. Mast cells, containing vasoactive substances as well as heparin, may be identified now and are thought to play an active role at this stage. As in other areas of inflammation, the macrophage removes metabolic by-products and dead tissue. Recent work suggests that the macrophage

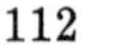

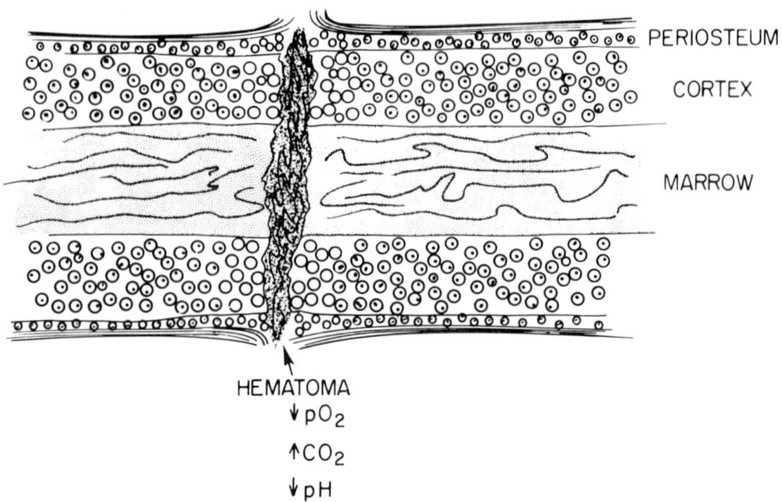

FIGURE 6.4 A hematoma develops at the fracture site as a result of disruption of the osseous structure and attending vascular supply. The bone at the edges of the fracture site becomes necrotic. This produces empty lacunae at the fracture margins.

may be the activator of fibroblasts in soft tissue repair, and it is conceivable that the same mechanism operates in fracture repair. Osteoclasts begin to mobilize, and osteolytic activity may be seen along the ruffled border of the cell.

Soft Callus

This is a very active phase in which both an external and an internal soft callus are formed (Fig. 6.5). The external callus plays an important role by helping to immobilize the fracture fragments. Urist and Johnson[41] likened the callus cuff to a bridge span, because it makes it possible to stabilize the fracture and to load the bone long before the process of union is complete. The external callus is achieved by an active proliferation of osteoblasts in the cambium layer of the periosteum. This is evident not only at the fracture site but also along the undersurface of the periosteum away from the fracture site. In effect, this produces a collar of soft tissue callus, with each end approaching the other from each fragment. The fibrous layer of the periosteum is elevated proximal to the fracture site for some distance by the proliferation of the underlying osteoblasts. In the proximal portion of the periosteum the

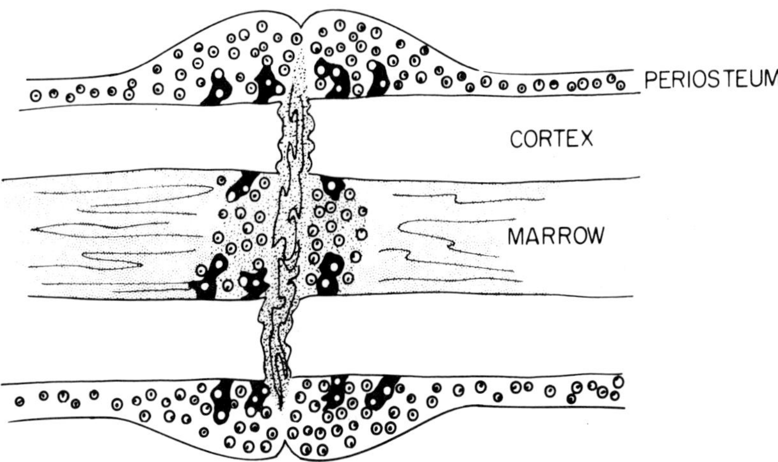

FIGURE 6.5 The stage of soft callus with a periosteal collar forming to bridge the fracture surface. Note the periosteal reaction that occurs both proximal and distal to the fracture site proper.

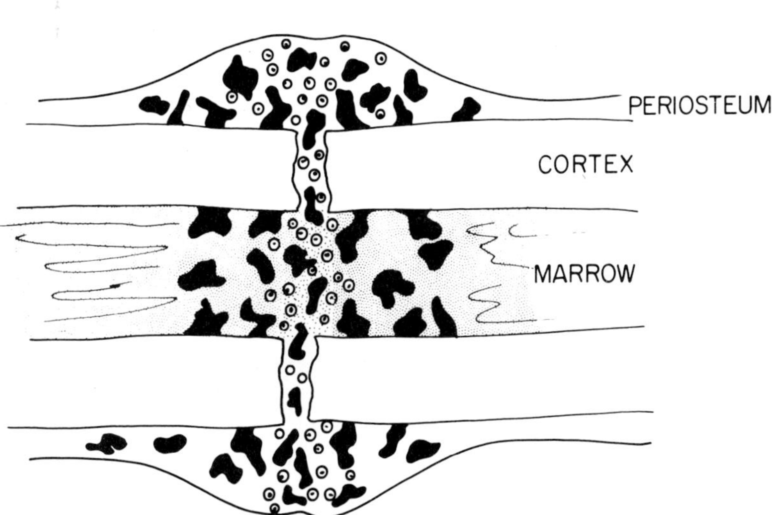

FIGURE 6.6 The stage of hard-callus formation with the conversion of the internal and external callus to fiber bone. Studies have revealed hypertrophic cells within the callus similar to those seen in the epiphyseal plate prior to calcification.

osteoblasts form new bone directly. However, as the fracture site is approached, cartilage cells as well as active osteoblasts are evident. Tonna demonstrated in a series of experiments that cartilage cell formation at the fracture site occurs by means of osteogenic cell progeny transformation.[39] He labeled the cells at the fracture site and found that newly formed cartilage cells were labeled with the same frequency as osteogenic cell progeny. He concluded that osteogenic cells were osteochondrogenic cells which were equally capable of giving rise to osteoblasts, or chondrocytes. Therefore, these cells can form cartilag or bone, depending on the local environment. As the fracture site is approached, there is an associated gradual ingrowth of new vascularity. However, new cells are increasing at a more rapid rate, and the cellularity outstrips the vascular supply, producing a state of relative hypoxia. This was initially demonstrated by Wray[42,43] and has been further documented by the author.[18] The importance of the endosteal blood supply has been thoroughly evaluated in several excellent studies by Rhinelander.[30-35] Suffice it to state that the periosteal circulation initially provides blood supply to the fracture site, but the endosteal circulation eventually plays a major role in the fracture healing process. The surface of the soft callus is electronegative and remains so throughout this stage, which usually lasts three to four weeks, or until the bony fragments are united by fibrous and/or collagenous tissue. The end of this stage is clinically evident when the osseous fragments are no longer grossly mobile and are at least in a "sticky" phase.

Hard Callus

At this stage the external and internal callus gradually convert to fiber bone (Fig. 6.6). If internal fixation has not been employed in the treatment of these fractures, endochondral bone formation dominates. If the fragments have been well immobilized with a compression plate, however, membranous bone formation will predominate. In this state there is a definite increase in vascularity but also an abundant increase in cellularity. Therefore, the cellular structure is still operating under conditions of relative hypoxia. The pH of the matrix now reverts to neutral, but the external and internal surfaces of the callus remain electronegative. There is continued development of the endosteal blood supply throughout this stage, and the osteoclasts are still active in removing the remaining dead bone. This stage begins at three to four weeks and continues until the fragments are firmly united with new bone. The fracture site is now clinically and roentgenographically healed (Figs. 6.7

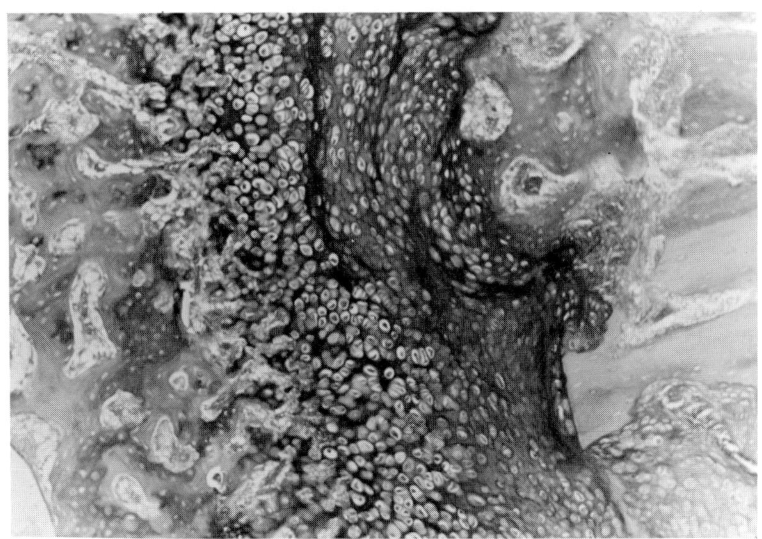

FIGURE 6.7 A high-power view of the advanced periosteal and endosteal reaction. Note the fracture surface in the mid-portion on the right. The abundant periosteal new fiber bone and endosteal conversion to fiber bone is evident.

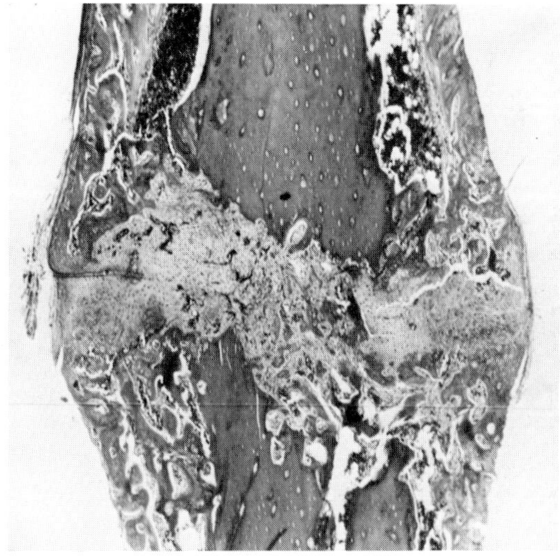

FIGURE 6.8 This is an obvious nonunion for comparison with Figure 6.7. Note that the periosteal and endosteal callus has not progressed to form new fiber bone. Cartilage and fibrous tissue persist.

and 6.8). The average elapsed time in an adult is three to four months for major long bones. This time is significantly decreased in the pediatric age group.

Remodeling

In this stage the newly formed fiber bone is gradually converted to lamellar bone. Osteoclasts are active in remodeling the external surface of the bone to decrease the size of callus or "bump." The medullary canal is reconstituted in a similar manner. The local tissue oxygen supply reverts to normal. The surface charge of the fracture site is no longer electronegative. The duration of the remodeling stage is variable: it may last for a few months, but there is evidence in human biopsy studies that it may continue for several years. The capability for remodeling is vastly increased in pediatric patients compared with adults. This effect is believed to be mediated through the epiphyseal plate, but the exact mechanism of its action has not been adequately evaluated. It is not uncommon in pediatric patients to have a bone heal in an angulated state only to be actively remodeled, and in follow-up one year postfracture to find that the angulation has been remodeled and the gross anatomical alignment of the bone has been restored. Adult bone lacks this increased ability to actively remodel angulatory deformities at the fracture site, and therefore adult fractures must be properly reduced if alignment is to be maintained (Figs. 6.9, 6.10, and 6.11).

Role of the Hematoma. The exact function of the hematoma at a fracture site has been actively debated in the past. Lexer[5] believed that the fracture hematoma represented an inactive stuffing material between ends of the fracture, without value for union. If the hematoma was increased, then periosteal cells would organize the hematoma extensively. He concluded that if this occurred, the cells produced fibrous tissue instead of bone. On the other hand, Phemister[5] felt that fibrin in the hematoma may stimulate cell regeneration and aid in immobilizing the fracture ends. Through this mechanism, granulation could advance into the hematoma with resorption and perform the same function as in soft tissue repair.

Most investigators now agree that the active role of the hematoma is not as important in the fracture healing process as was once believed.[43,44] The larger the dead space created by the disruption at the fracture site, then the more extensive the hematoma formation. The real physiological question is the following: does the hematoma function as an initial stimulus for

FIGURE 6.9 A roentgenograph of a healed dog fibula. Note the remodeling that has occurred at the fracture site.

FIGURE 6.10 A longitudinal section of a healed dog fibula demonstrating the remodeling and reconstitution of the endosteal bone.

FIGURE 6.11 Low-power magnification shows that the medullary space has not been reconstituted in this longitudinal section of a dog fibula. Cartilage is still present at the fracture site.

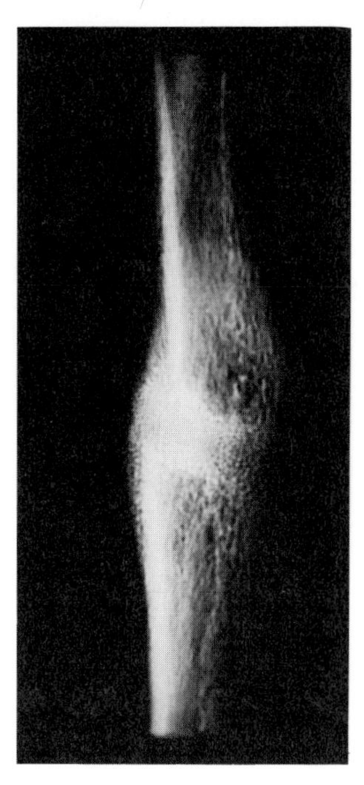

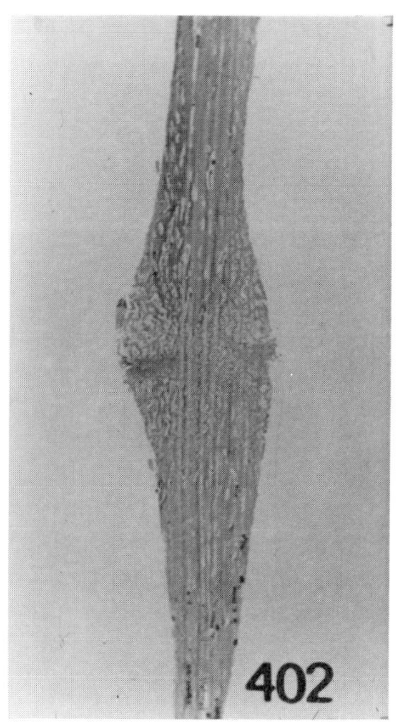

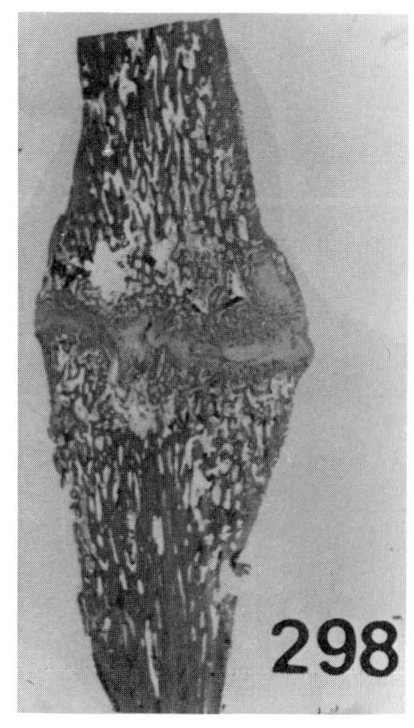

the differentiation of primitive mesenchymal cells for active repair at the fracture site? Considerable debate continues to surround this point, but the general feeling is that the hematoma itself does not play a significant physiological stimulatory role in the repair of fractures. In fact, the studies of the AO Group, demonstrated that the hematoma between the fracture ends is virtually eliminated in rigid anatomical internal fixation, the condition in which primary bone healing occurs.[29]

Blood Supply and Fracture Healing

Our present understanding of the microcirculation in fracture healing was advanced by Trueta's work,[40] but it remained for the classic studies of Rhinelander to outline and document the microcirculatory changes during the fracture healing process.[30-35] These studies represent an excellent example of a scientific approach to the problem, and all personnel involved with skeletal physiology should be thoroughly familiar with Rhinelander's work. A brief summary of his findings follows.

Microangiographic techniques revealed that fracture of a contralateral forelimb of a canine ulna produced a physiological stimulation of the circulation of the uninjured forelimb. Rhinelander believed that the difference between the normal stimulated circulation and the normal resting circulation, shown in Figure 6.12, represented an enormous potential for increased vascular function within bone. A classification of the blood vessels comprising the normal circulation was developed on the basis of function rather than anatomical location. An afferent and an efferent vascular system were described. The three primary components of the afferent vascular system were the principal nutrient artery, the metaphyseal arteries, and the periosteal arterioles. The efferent vascular system included the large emissary veins and *vena comitans* of the nutrient vein, which drain the medullary contents exclusively, the cortical venous channels, and the periosteal capillaries. All these components convey blood toward the exterior. The endosteal circulation supplies the medullary area and the inner two thirds to three quarters of the compactum. The periosteal arterioles supply the outer third or quarter of the compactum only in localized areas that are related to fascial attachments, and these periosteal arterioles become more active when the medullary supply is interrupted.

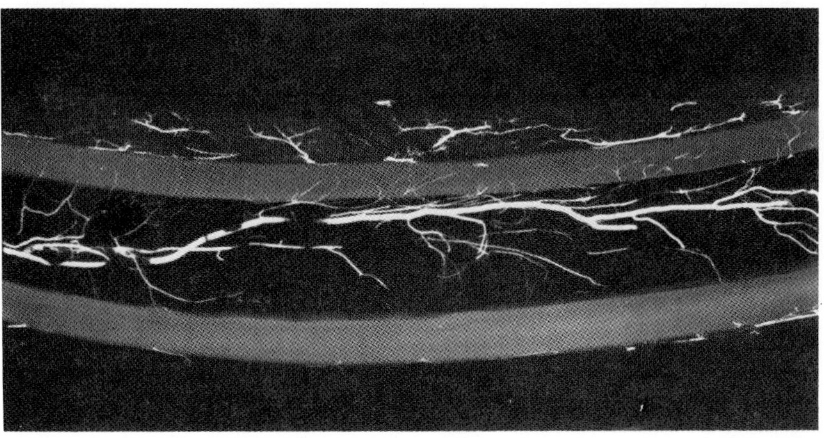

FIGURE 6.12 Microangiogram of the midshaft of a normal dog radius with the circulation in a resting state. Note the prominence of the medullary vessels.
Source: Courtesy of F. W. Rhinelander and Journal of Bone and Joint Surgery. The normal microcirculation of diaphyseal cortex and its response to fracture. J.B.J.S. 50A:784-800, 1968.

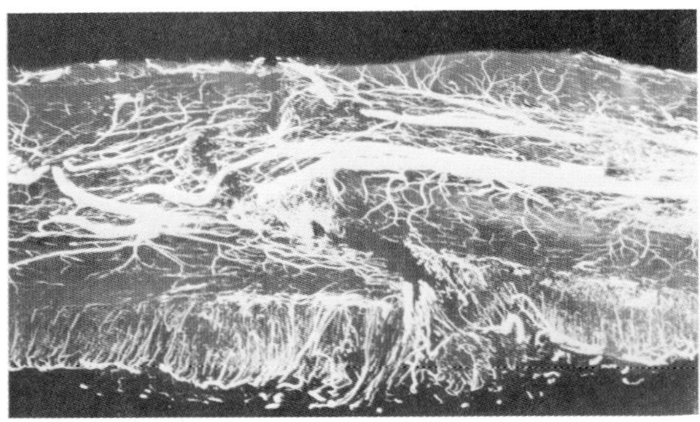

FIGURE 6.13 Microangiogram of three-week-old displaced radial fracture with reestablishment of the medullary circulation. The extensive periosteal callus shows the characteristic arrangement of blood vessels perpendicular to the cortical surface. (x6).
Source: Courtesy of F. W. Rhinelander and Journal of Bone and Joint Surgery. The normal microcirculation of diaphyseal cortex and its response to fracture. J.B.J.S. 50A:784-800, 1968.

Brookes felt that the normal centrifugal blood flow could be reversed with interruption of the nutrient blood system so that the periosteal system could convey blood to the compactum.[33] However, Rhinelander was unable to demonstrate a major reversal in direction of flow of blood supplied by the so-called periosteal circulation when the medullary blood supply was interrupted. It is true that a small supply of new blood develops in relation to the soft tissue attachments at the fracture site, and these temporarily provide blood to the external callus (Fig. 6.13). Following canine fractures that were well reduced and stabilized, he was able to demonstrate that the endosteal osseous callus can bridge the fracture gap within three weeks without the intermediate production of fibrocartilage. Arteries derived from the medulla permeated the cortex of both fracture fragments and rendered these fragments extremely porotic, with the result that by six weeks they traversed it completely to afford the major blood supply even to the external callus. This provided further evidence that blood supply of the cortex was functionally centrifugal in direction of flow.

This sequence of events did not occur when the fracture fragments were widely displaced or comminuted. In displaced fractures the periosteal afferent circulation derived from the overlying soft tissues was initially important in supplying blood to the external callus that attempted to bridge the fracture gap. However, the periosteal bridging callus was never responsible for the primary osseous union. It always contained a zone of fibrocartilage. The medullary circulation was also stimulated following fracture in each main fragment with the production of the endosteal osseous callus. If the fracture fragments were widely displaced or comminuted, then the periosteal afferent circulation persisted for much longer in supplying the chief areas of bone repair. However, Rhinelander was able to demonstrate that the endosteal circulation makes every effort to assume the major function of afferent blood supply as soon as possible. In short, the endosteal blood supply is ultimately the most important blood supply in the fracture healing process (Figs. 6.14 and 6.15).

Special Types of Repair

Small Osseous Defects

This type of repair has been studied in animals by means of a small drill hole in bone. The periosteum is destroyed at the penetrating site. As in a fracture, the surrounding bone

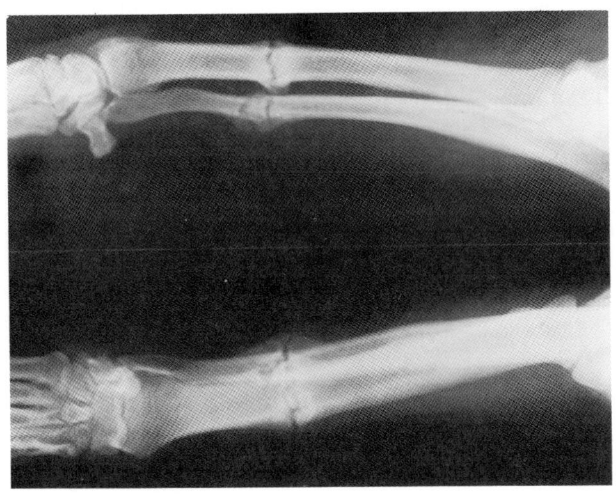

FIGURE 6.14 Roentgenograph revealing delayed union of six-week-old displaced fractures of both forelimb bones in a dog. Source: Courtesy of F. W. Rhinelander and Journal of Bone and Joint Surgery. The normal microcirculation of diaphyseal cortex and its response to fracture, J.B.J.S. 50A:784-800, 1968.

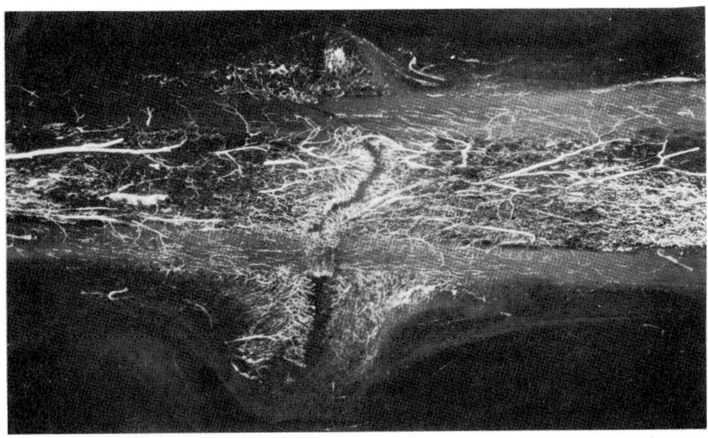

FIGURE 6.15 Microangiogram of radial fracture shown in Figure 6.14. Note the vascular pattern corresponding to the roentgenographic appearance of delayed union. (x6). Source: Courtesy of F. W. Rhinelander and Journal of Bone and Joint Surgery. The normal microcirculation of diaphyseal cortex and its response to fracture. J.B.J.S. 50A:784-800, 1968.

and marrow become necrotic for at least a few millimeters around the hole, and a small hematoma develops in the osseous defect. Polymorphonuclear leukocytes are seen in the hematoma almost immediately, and by 24 hours plasma cells, lymphocytes, and macrophages are evident. Granulation tissue gradually replaces the hematoma. The periosteum reacts as it does to a normal fracture. The cambium layer becomes thickened by the proliferation of new osteoblasts, elevating the fibrous layer. This reaction extends for some distance from the drill site. The osteoblastic cells within the periosteal layer eventually form a bridge across the defect in a peculiar way that resembles the external callus of normal fracture healing. The endosteum responds in a similar manner. The transformation of undifferentiated mesenchymal cells is more rapid with this type of defect. Intramembranous bone formation occurs within the central portion of the defect. In general, the major portion of the trabeculae is oriented at right angles to the osseous shaft. Lamellar bone gradually replaces fiber bone within the osseous defect, and large intertrabecular spaces are gradually abolished. In the early phase of this repair (by three weeks), a mixture of fibrous and lamellar bone bridges the gap. There is no definite evidence of endochondral bone formation in this defect. Cutting cones gradually replace the reactive bone, with new bone oriented in the same direction as the remainder of the shaft. Remodeling of the excess periosteal and endosteal callus is evident.

Intramedullary Fixation

Several types of intramedullary devices are now available for internal fixation. This technique was introduced by Küntscher[23] in 1940 with a report of the results of intramedullary rod fixation of femoral fractures. This device has its most useful application in the femoral region. Several other devices have been described in the literature over the past two decades and are now available, including the Schneider, Hanson-Street, and Fluted Sampson devices. The femoral medullary cavity must be reamed extensively before any of these is inserted; the effect of such reaming has been studied by Rhinelander with microangiographic techniques. The main intramedullary vascular supply is destroyed during the initial reaming prior to insertion of the rod. The periosteal blood supply then increases its function in an attempt to compensate for the lost endosteal circulation. The deficit is compounded if the periosteum is "stripped" during the insertion of the rod.

Rhinelander demonstrated that the best design for an intramedullary device is a fluted one because it permits control of rotation but at the same time allows regeneration of the endosteal vascular blood supply between the flutes.[34,35] If a solid intramedullary rod without flutes is employed, the main medullary circulation is destroyed, and an extensive period is required for its regeneration along the border of the device. However, if a fluted rod has been inserted, the endosteal blood supply may regenerate between the flutes. In other words, besides controlling rotation, the fluted design allows for a rapid reconstitution of the endosteal blood supply compared with the nonfluted one.

If there is good solid fixation of the fracture site by the intramedullary device, a small amount of external callus develops, with a decreased amount of endochondral bone formation. However, if a loose-fitting rod is inserted and there is motion at the fracture site, the major portion of the bone deposited between the fragments will be the result of endochondral bone formation. Clinically, it is difficult to decide when a fracture site is completely healed, as a portion of the fracture is obscured by the intramedullary device. Most authors feel that at least one and one half years should elapse before the device is removed.

An important point to bear in mind is that if there is evidence of comminution at the fracture site, a bone graft from the iliac crest should be used along with the internal fixation device. In fact, we have seen many cases presenting with initial comminution that are bone grafted in this manner and the rod removed at a later date. Following removal of the rod, it is not uncommon to see a fracture line in the intramedullary area that was once occupied by the rod. However, there is usually extensive bone formed around this area, bridging the two main fragments. The author takes this to mean that if the fracture had not been bone grafted initially, it probably would not have healed primarily, even with the internal fixation device. Therefore, it is a good rule of thumb to employ a bone graft as well as internal fixation for open reduction of comminuted femoral fractures.

Compression Plating

As described earlier, the role of a compression plate is to provide rigid internal fixation, reducing motion at the fracture site and allowing excellent apposition of the osseous fragments (Fig. 6.16). Several outstanding studies performed by the Association for the Study of Internal Fixation have documented

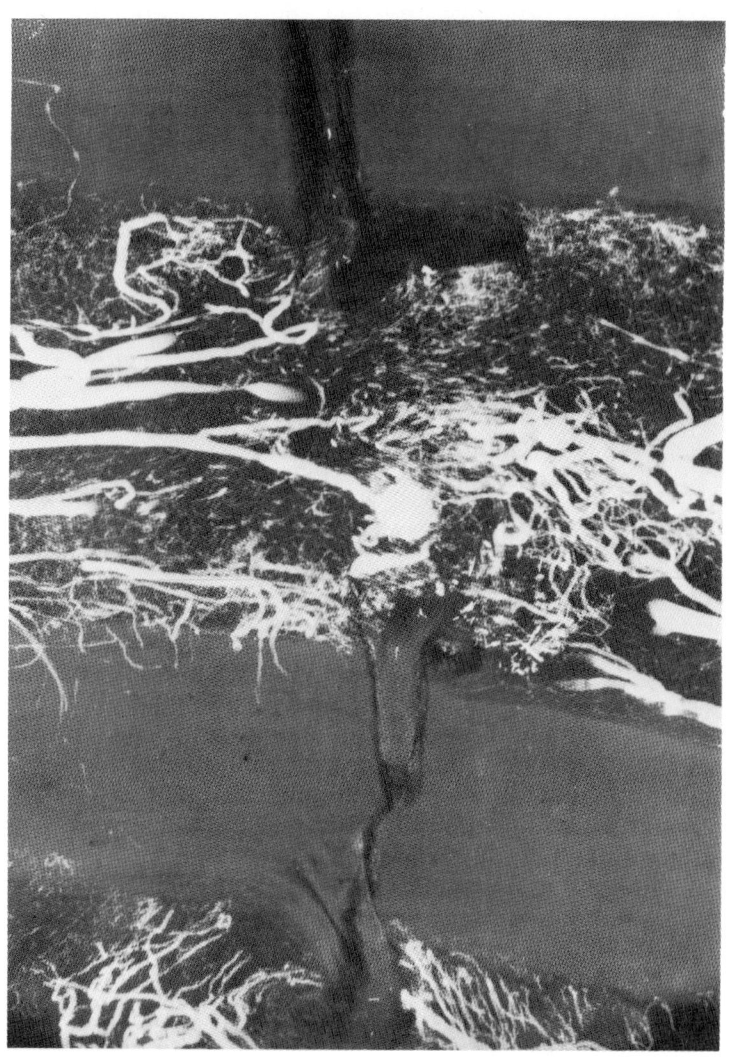

FIGURE 6.16 Microangiogram of a dog radius one week after transverse osteotomy and secure plate fixation showing reconstitution of the medullary vessels (x25).
Source: Courtesy of F. W. Rhinelander and Journal of Bone and Joint Surgery. The normal microcirculation of diaphyseal cortex and its response to fracture. J.B.J.S. 50A:784-800, 1968.

the beneficial effect of compression plates.[29] Primary bone healing is common in this type of repair. The osseous fragments unite with new bone that is osteonal, without endochondral bone formation, and of normal orientation. The bone fragments under the compression plate should be approximated as closely to anatomical as possible. However, the cortices opposite the plate are often poorly approximated owing to the differing configurations of the bone and the compression plate. Every effort should be made to reconcile the two by bending the plate if this is to be prevented. In this connection, it is important to recall that bone heals under compression and fails under tension. Therefore, it is not only theoretically sound to obtain good apposition of both cortices, but it is also very practical. A hematoma does not form between the bone fragments if apposition is satisfactory with a compression plate. There is a mild inflammatory reaction in the soft tissues adjacent to the periosteum and in the marrow. New cutting cones originate at the junction of live and dead bone. Osteoclasts lead the cutting cones and migrate directly across the fracture site along an empty haversian canal, resorbing the matrix. They cross the fracture site and enter another apposing empty haversian canal or begin to cut into necrotic bone on the other fragment. This means that a new living osteon is produced immediately behind the cutting cone. The obvious question that arises is, what is the significance of the finding of an external callus? The finding of an external callus means by inference that there has been motion at the fracture site. If motion at the fracture site can be eliminated, an external callus is not formed, and primary bone healing takes place. With an external callus, endochondral bone formation is present, whereas with compression plating and the consequent absence of an external callus, primary bone healing without intervening cartilage occurs. It is important to remember that a compression plate, if left in place, will continue to absorb the major portion of the stress instead of the stress being absorbed by the osseous tissue underneath the plate. When this occurs, osteoporosis underneath the plate is the ultimate result. If flexible compression plates are employed instead of rigid fixation plates, the severe osteoporosis underneath the plate is not as significant. The design of improved plates and the timing of their removal are the subjects of extensive investigation.

Physiological Effects of Oxygen on Growth and Repair

In the past, it was felt that adequate blood supply with a high oxygen tension stimulated growth in the epiphyseal plate. Brighton and Heppenstall documented the oxygen tensions in various zones of the epiphyseal plate.[8] The result of this study indicates that active bone growth in the metaphyseal area of the epiphyseal plate occurs under conditions of relative hypoxia. It was further noted that a large oxygen gradient existed between the zone of cell columns, the zone of hypertrophic cells, and the metaphyseal area. The oxygen tension in the zone of cell columns averaged 57 mm Hg. In the zone of hypertrophic cells it measured 24.3 mm Hg. In the metaphyseal area where active new bone formation occurs the oxygen tension measured 19.8 mm Hg. It was postulated that the relative hypoxia in the metaphyseal area might be a stimulus for new bone formation. These studies were then expanded to include fracture repair. Brighton and Krebs, utilizing the same oxygen microelectrode technique, measured the oxygen tensions at a fracture and nonunion site.[9] Once again, the oxygen tensions were noted to be relatively low during active new bone formation in the course of repair. In a separate study utilizing a different oxygen-measuring technique, the author was able to demonstrate that active new bone formation at the site of an osseous defect occurred under conditions of relative hypoxia (Fig. 6.17).[18] An additional finding in the same study was that the oxygen consumption during rapid active new bone formation was not elevated above that of normal bone. This provided evidence that the low oxygen tension was not due to rapid consumption but rather to an increase in cellularity above that of vascularity. In other words, the cells were outstripping their blood supply, in a sequence of events similar to that in soft tissue repair. Kelly and his associates have measured the blood flow to fractures in animals with the use of radioisotope techniques.[25,28] They were able to demonstrate that the blood flow to a canine fractured tibia reached a maximum on the tenth day and decreased thereafter but did not return to normal values until 112 days postfracture. Rhinelander has also demonstrated through microangiographic techniques a gradual increase in the vascular supply. If these studies are correlated, it appears that the blood supply is increased at a fracture site, but that cellularity is also increased above vascularity, producing a state of relative hypoxia during active new bone formation.

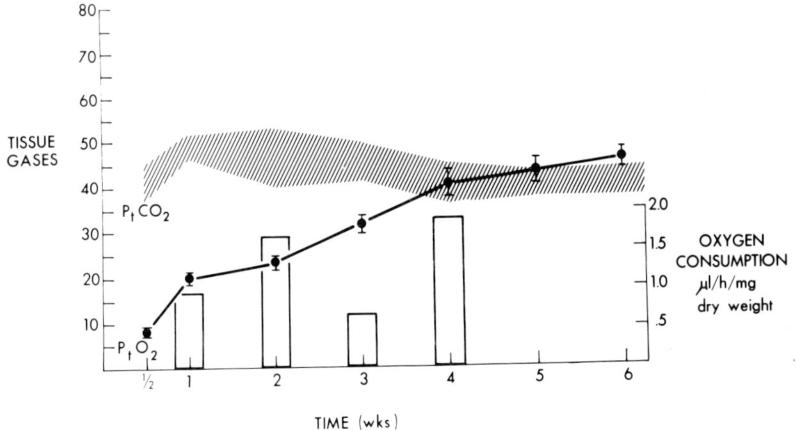

FIGURE 6.17 The tissue oxygen, carbon dioxide, and oxygen consumption values obtained in healing dog rib defects as a function of time. Of interest was the fact that at three to four weeks, when bone was actively being formed, the oxygen tension remained low and was associated with a slightly elevated carbon dioxide tension and no evidence of an increase in oxygen consumption above that of normal bone.
Source: Courtesy of R. B. Heppenstall et al. and Clinical Orthopedics and Related Research. Tissue gas tensions and oxygen consumption in healing bone defects. Clin. Orthop. 106:357-365, 1975.

A further study was performed by the author in an attempt to evaluate the effect of chronic systemic hypoxia on the fracture healing process (Fig. 6.18).[19] It was noted that a sustained chronic systemic hypoxia produced a delay in fracture healing. The author proposed that one cause of delay in fracture healing might be the fact that systemic hypoxia abolished the normally large oxygen gradient at the fracture site, as had been previously demonstrated.

Hyperbaric oxygen studies have produced conflicting results. Some studies have indicated that the fracture healing process may be stimulated by the addition of hyperbaric oxygen treatments.[27] However, a recent study on bone turnover with the use of hyperbaric oxygen reveals that this technique increases the amount of bone resorption above that of bone formation, with a negative net effect.[12] It is also known that a high concentration of oxygen over a prolonged period is detrimental to cell function.

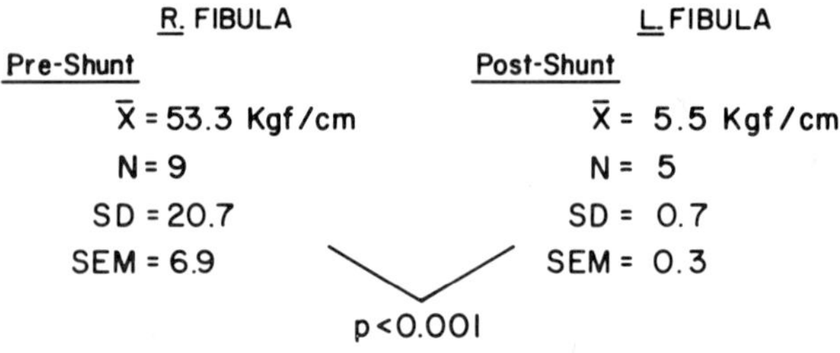

FIGURE 6.18 Modulus of bending of a healing fiber fracture in the dog. The pre-shunt measurements were taken prior to the production of chronic systemic hypoxia. The post-shunt measurements were in dogs with central arteriovenous shunts producing a state of chronic systemic hypoxia. Note the deficit in breaking strength in the post-shunt or chronically hypoxic dogs compared with that in the normal dogs.
Source: Courtesy of R. B. Heppenstall et al. and Journal of Bone and Joint Surgery. Fracture healing in the presence of chronic hypoxia. J.B.J.S. 58A:1153-1156, 1976.

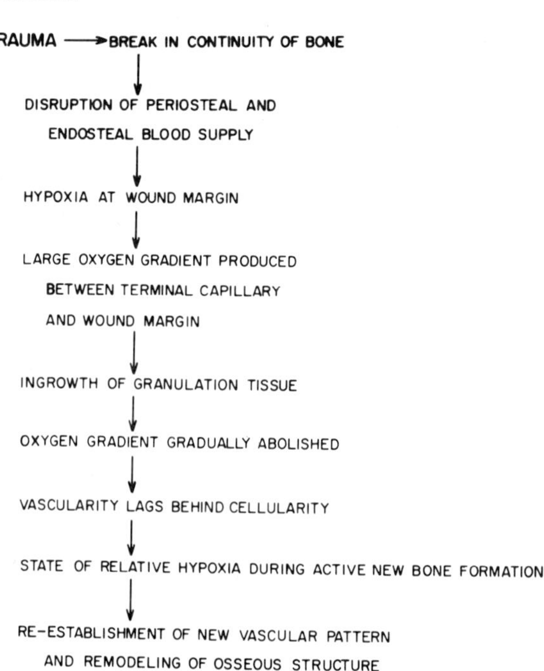

FIGURE 6.19 A hypothetical sequence of events in relation to oxygen and fracture healing.

What then can we accurately state regarding the effect of oxygen on the fracture healing process? Seven facts appear to emerge:

1. All the available proline and lysine that is hydroxylated in tissues can be hydroxylated by a small amount of oxygen, well below the levels measured for normal fracture repair.
2. Fractures normally heal under a state of relative hypoxia by mechanisms similar to those of soft tissue repair.
3. A large oxygen gradient across the reparative surface is probably the initial stimulus for healing.
4. A state of chronic systemic hypoxia definitely delays the fracture healing process.
5. Studies of hyperbaric oxygen have produced conflicting results, but hyperbaric oxygen has been shown to have a detrimental effect on bone turnover by producing increased resorption compared to formation. It is also well documented that a high oxygen concentration for a prolonged period of time is detrimental to cell function.
6. The blood supply to a fracture increases well above normal during the early phases of repair, but a concomitant increase in cellularity produces a state of relative hypoxia during active new bone formation.
7. Bone cells have been demonstrated to follow predominantly an anaerobic pathway (Fig. 6.19).

The unanswered question at present concerns the effect of a mild elevation in local oxygen tension above that normally seen during active repair. Studies are currently in progress.

Anemia and Fracture Healing

A review of the literature concerning the effects of anemia on soft tissue healing has produced conflicting opinions. A recent study has provided well-documented evidence that an uncomplicated normovolemic anemia does not alter soft tissue healing. A similar study was performed by the author to evaluate the effect of anemia on fracture healing (Fig. 6.20).[20] Rothman had earlier demonstrated that an iron deficiency anemia definitely delays the healing process.[37] However, iron deficiency anemia is not the usual clinical situation in fracture healing. The author was able to demonstrate that an uncomplicated normovolemic anemia does not delay fracture healing. If, however, hypovolemia is associated with the anemia, the fracture healing process is definitely delayed. Normally, a hypovolemic anemia is rarely encountered in the course of fracture healing in humans. There-

RESULTS

	Hct	Modulus of elasticity	Roentgenogram
Group A	38±2	45 ± 5.2 Kgf/cm	Normal Healing
Group B	30±1	43 ± 4.4 Kgf/cm	Normal Healing
Group C	32±1	16 ± 6.5 Kgf/cm	Delayed Healing

FIGURE 6.20 Effect of anemia on fracture healing. Group A included fractures of the rabbit fibula at three weeks, blood withdrawn and reinfused. Group B, Normovolemic rabbits. Group C, Hypovolemic Anemia. Note the decreased breaking strength in the hypovolemic state.
Source: Courtesy of R. B. Heppenstall and C. T. Brighton and Clinical Orthopedics and Related Research. Fracture healing in the presence of anemia. Clin. Orthop. 123:253-258, 1977.

fore, it is not acceptable today to administer blood transfusions when the hemoglobin drops below an arbitrarily selected level (in the past, 8 to 10) in anticipation of stimulating the fracture healing process. Oxygen delivery to the fracture surface will be normal in the presence of a normovolemic anemia. Since fracture healing is not stimulated by blood transfusion, exposing the patient to the known risks of blood transfusion is not warranted. This rule is probably not valid in managing debilitated patients who have anemia and a fracture. Blood transfusions in this clinical situation may stimulate fracture healing because of the various components present in blood and not because of oxygen delivery.

Theories of Calcification

A complete discussion of this subject is beyond the scope of this book. A summary of several proposed theories will be outlined.

A significant amount of investigation has been done on the exact mechanism of calcification, and several theories have been formulated on the basis of these experiments. It is fair to state that the exact mechanism of calcification in bone is still unknown. One of the stumbling blocks to developing a theory of calcification is overcoming the fact that calcification can occur in cartilage and osseous tissues without occurring in soft tissue at the same time. This leads the observer to suspect that a specific mechanism must exist for the calcification of bone. In the past, significant emphasis was placed on hard tissue collagen as a nucleation catalyst. However, recent research has directed attention to the function of mitochondria and matrix vesicles in calcification.[1,2,10,22,26] It is now recognized that the main inorganic constituent of bone is minute crystals of hydroxyapatite.

One of the earliest theories of calcification was put forth by Robison and revolved around the idea that a local increase in concentration of phosphate ions could be produced by hydrolysis of ester phosphates by a phosphatase.[36] The popularity of this theory has waxed and waned over the past three decades. Some authors have suggested that the protein polysaccharides may play an important role in the calcification process. Chondroitin sulfate may inhibit calcification through a mechanism that limits ion diffusion and binds calcium. It has also been proposed that chondroitin sulfate acts in conjunction with collagen to initiate calcification through the formation of specific nucleation centers.

The theory of crystal nucleation followed by crystal growth has received recent attention and enthusiasm. Glimcher has proposed that hydroxyapatite crystals form within the fibers of the collagen matrix, oriented in a specific way relative to the fiber axis.[14,15] They appear to be associated with a particular portion of the collagen band pattern (hole zone), which suggests that the collagen matrix may in fact be the nucleation site. It has been demonstrated that fibers with 640 Å periodicity are capable of being calcified.[21] It appears that the other forms of collagen aggregation cannot be calcified, suggesting that the spatial arrangement of a quarter-stagger found in the native form of collagen is required for nucleation to occur.

Another possible mechanism in calcification involves adenosine triphosphate as an energy source. The adenosine triphosphate (ATP) binds calcium in the formation of an ATP-calcium complex. ATPase then hydrolyzes the complex, producing adenosine, sodium acid phosphate, and calcium acid pyrophosphate. The final step involves hydrolysis to form hydroxyapatite. Orthophosphoric acid is also formed, undergoing in turn a reaction with adenosine to regenerate ATP.

A further suggestion is that the specific nucleation site resides in the monosaccharide or disaccharide attached to the hydroxylysine residue of collagen. To carry this a step further, the glycosylation of the hydroxylysine residues may inhibit mineralization through a mechanism of steric hindrance in the hole zones of the polymerized collagen molecule. It is possible that the hole region within the collagen fibril is the nucleation site and that unglycosylated hydroxylysine could be the specific factor in the nucleation process. However, it has been demonstrated that bone treated with β-aminopropionitrile and made lathyritic (which inhibits the cross-linking mechanism) will still calcify. This observation tends to confuse the issue unless we consider the presence of the hydroxyl group of hydroxylysine in the hole region of the collagen fibril to be an important factor.

Current theory, which the author tends to favor, involves the mitochondria and matrix vesicles as key components in the calcification mechanism. This is particularly true in the epiphyseal plate, and it is likely that fracture healing is just an extension of the physiological mechanisms that occur within the growth plate. Ketenjian and Arsenis[22] were able to separate mitochondria from the hypertrophic zone of the growth plate of the calf scapula and costochondral junction. They observed that calcium phosphate ions may be concentrated and stored inside the mitochondria and through a rate-dependent, membrane-regulated phenomenon become transferred to deposition sites along the collagen fibrils.[22] It is possible that the mitochondrial membranes are degraded by lysosomal enzymes, which then set the granules free to become the seeds for growth of extracellular apatite microcrystallites. Lehninger hypothesized that in calcifying tissues, intramitrochondrial deposits of amorphous calcium phosphate were released from the mitochondria and transported as small stable aggregates to other sites, where they served as precursors for the larger and more stable mineral deposits characteristic of calcified tissues.[26] He believed that in this manner the mitochondria played a vital role in the calcification mechanism.

Brighton and Hunt demonstrated that mitochondria and cell membranes accumulate calcium in the growth plate and concluded that both of these structures may well be involved in the calcification of the growth plate.[10] They noted that the mitochondria and the cell membranes accumulated calcium in the upper zones of the epiphyseal plate, however, at the bottom of the zone of hypertrophic cells the mitochondria tended to lose their calcium as the matrix vesicles began to accumulate calcium (Figs. 6.21 and 6.22). It has previously been shown that glycogen storage occurs in the zone of cell columns where the oxygen tension is high and aerobic metabolism occurs. However, the glycogen is utilized in the zone of hypertrophic cells where the oxygen

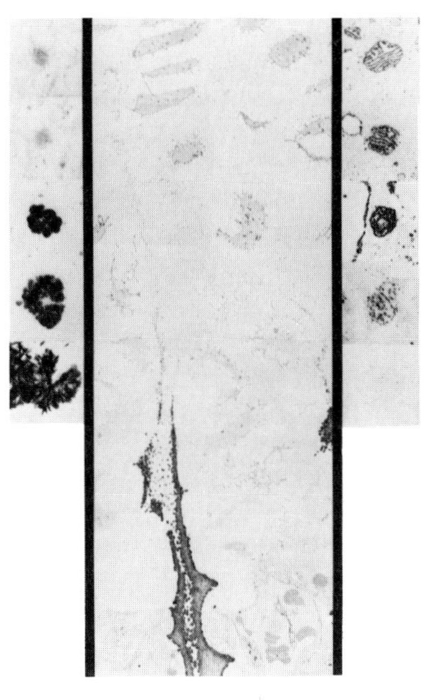

FIGURE 6.21 Composite electron micrograph of hypertrophic zone of epiphyseal plate. Central portion demonstrates relationship of cartilage cells to calcified matrix. Right hand portion depicts mitochondria calcium at the top of the zone of hypertrophic cells and loss of calcium at bottom of the zone. Left hand portion depicts matrix vesicles taking up calcium as they approach the lower portion of the zone. Source: Courtesy C. T. Brighton and R. M. Hunt and Journal of Bone and Joint Surgery, 1978.

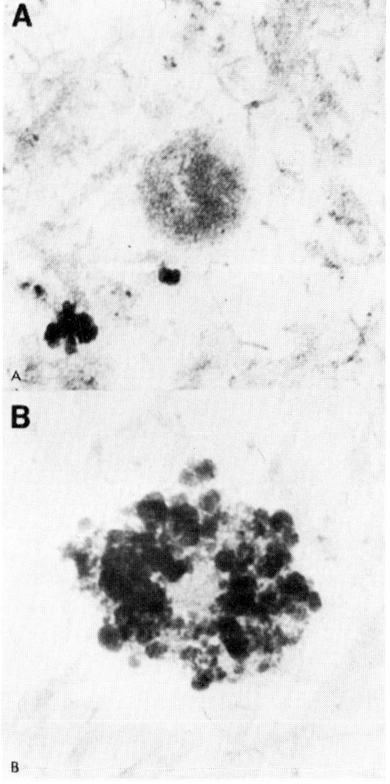

FIGURE 6.22 A. Electron micrograph of matrix vesicle from top portion of hypertrophic zone. Calcium stain fails to reveal calcium within the vesicle. B. Matrix vesicle staining from lower portion of the hypertrophic zone reveals calcium in the vesicles.

tension is known to be low.[8] Lehninger has demonstrated that the uptake and retention of calcium by mitochondria is an active process requiring energy.[26] Studies by Azzi and Chance have revealed that mitochondria release their calcium when exposed to an anoxic environment.[3] Therefore, it is entirely probable that all of these mechanisms may be involved in the calcification process.

The sequence of events would be as follows. At the upper portion of the growth plate, glycogen is accumulated and aerobic metabolism occurs. As the midportion of the growth plate are approached, mitochondria can be seen to accumulate calcium, as demonstrated by Brighton and Hunt.[10] As the lower portion of the epiphyseal plate is approached, particularly the lower half of the zone of hypertrophic cells, the oxygen tension is low (as measured previously by the author), and the glycogen is consumed as a source of energy. Since there is no other energy source available for the uptake and retention of calcium in this region of low oxygen tension, the mitochondria lose their calcium to the extracellular environment. At this level and in the lower portion of the zone of hypertrophic cells, calcium begins to appear in the matrix vesicles. It is true that these studies have been performed in the growth plate, but if we extrapolate these theories to fracture healing, the same physiological mechanism may operate.

The author has demonstrated that the oxygen tension and the oxygen consumption are low during active new bone formation at the site of an osseous defect.[18] Ketenjian and Arsensis have shown that all the components of growth plate cartilage are found in the callus of a healing fracture.[22] They also demonstrated extracellular vesicles in the hypertrophic sections of the fracture callus. Mitochondria tend to accumulate calcium-containing granules in the callus. A shift of oxidative glycolysis with cartilage maturation was seen in the callus, as in the growth plate. Lane has demonstrated a persistence of type 2 cartilage well into the beginning of the calcification process.[24] Therefore, it is entirely possible the same mechanism exists at a fracture site as in the growth plate to initiate calcification. At the present time, this appears to be a very attractive hypothesis. However, there are still several unanswered questions, and a great deal of further investigation into the mechanism of bone formation is required.

Hormones in Bone Metabolism

Parathyroid Hormone

The parathyroid glands play a primary role in calcium metabolism. Parathormone has a direct effect on bone, and its release increases the serum calcium. It also has a direct effect on osteoclasts which are normally present in bone. The action of parathormone is believed to take place within the cell. Osteoclasts contain large quantities of acid phosphatase and citrate, and it is possible that a stimulation of both these substances may be responsible for the mobilization of calcium from bone. Urinary hydroxyproline is formed from insoluble bone collagen and is an indication of collagen catabolism. Parathormone causes an increase in hydroxyproline excretion, which is directly related to the amount of parathormone released.

The hormone has a stimulatory effect both on the number and action of the osteoclasts and on osteocytic osteolysis. Bone resorption occurs not only through a mechanism of osteoclast stimulation but also through osteocyte function within the haversian system. Therefore, it may be seen that parathyroid hormone has a direct effect on calcium metabolism. In general it has nine basic functions:

1. It increases plasma calcium concentration and decreases plasma PO_4 concentration.
2. It increases urinary excretion of PO_4 and hydroxyproline-containing peptides and decreases urinary excretion of calcium.
3. It increases the rate of skeletal remodeling and the net rate of bone resorption.
4. It increases the extent of osteocytic osteolysis in bone and increases the number of osteoclasts and osteoblasts.
5. It increases the conversion of 25-hydroxycholicalciferol to 1,25-dihydroxycholicalciferol in the kidney.
6. It activates adenylcyclase in target cells.
7. It causes an initial increase in calcium entry in target cells.
8. It alters the acid-base balance of the body.
9. It increases gastrointestinal absorption of calcium.

Calcitonin. Copp originally discovered calcitonin and thought it was derived from the thyroid gland.[11] Therefore, it was originally called thyrocalcitonin. It became apparent that calcitonin originates from the C cells of the thyroid, derived embryonically from ultimobranchial origins. This hormone has a direct regulatory function in calcium metabolism. It is believed to act in concert with parathormone to maintain calcium balance.

Its primary function is to decrease the calcium and phosphate plasma concentrations. The effects of calcitonin in bone include the following: (1) it decreases resorptive activity of osteoclasts and osteocytes; (2) it decreases the rate of activation of osteoprogenitor cells to preosteoclasts and osteoclasts; and (3) it increases modulation of osteoclasts to osteoblasts. When calcitonin is given prior to parathormone, it initially blocks the effect of parathormone on hydroxyproline excretion, osteocytic osteolysis, and activation of new metabolic units, with the result that eventually parathormone escapes. It does not act at a cellular level as an antiparathormone.

Calcitonin increases the production of both cancellous and compact bone. Although there is still a great deal to learn about the exact mechanism of calcitonin action, we are all indebted to Copp's initial investigative work in isolating and identifying this substance.

Growth Hormone. Recent research has revealed that growth hormone circulates through the liver and acquires a sulfation factor; this metabolite is the growth-stimulating factor and not growth hormone per se. Growth hormone has been demonstrated to increase collagen synthesis in bone and also to increase the ability of tissue to mineralize, as measured by calcium accretion rates. Autoradiographic studies have failed to demonstrate a target cell for growth hormone, and this tends to support the theory that growth hormone operates through its intermediary, known as somatomedin. Animal studies have revealed a decrease in the healing time of fractures with administration of growth hormone. It also may be that its effect on the fracture healing process is due to its direct influence on protein metabolism. Somatomedin increases periosteal bone formation and endosteal bone resorption. It also increases calcium and phosphate absorption in the intestine and renal tubular reabsorption.

Insulin. Insulin appears to increase bone collagen synthesis and may increase excretion of urinary hydroxyproline. The effects of insulin seem to be mediated by protein synthesis. It has been demonstrated that isolated bone cell preparations will increase RNA synthesis after exposure to insulin. A generalized systemic osteoporosis has been noted both in diabetic humans and in alloxan diabetic rats. In humans, the osseous structures of diabetics have reduced numbers of osteoid seams, slower rates of normal osteons, closure, and slower development of resorptive centers. It is also possible that the effect of insulin on bone is related to its effect on carbohydrate metabolism.

Thyroxine. Hypothyroidism leads to a state of generalized growth retardation, and the administration of thyroid hormones produces an acceleration of skeletal and somatic growth. Thyroid hormone itself may have a permissive effect on growth hormone. This is suggested by the fact that growth hormone by itself cannot reverse the linear growth deficit in hypophysectomized-thyroidectomized rats. However, if thyroxin and growth hormone are administered together to hypophysectomized animals, normal linear bone growth will be restored.

Increased bone resorption in humans has been noted in a state of thyrotoxicosis. Another interesting finding is a decrease in the radiodensity in the skeletons of hyperthyroid children. Both triliodothyronine (T_3) and thyroxine (T_4) will increase the differentiation and resorption of cartilage, leading to new bone formation within a fracture callus.

ACTH and Cortical Steroids. It has been demonstrated that low doses of cortisol (0.5 to 2.5 mg per kg) produce direct inhibition of the modulation of osteoclast to osteoblast. If they are administered in higher doses (greater than 5 mg per kg), the rate of osteoprogenitor cell activation falls, so that in spite of secondary increase in parathormone there is a decreased formation of new osteoclasts. The skeleton remodeling rate declines, but net resorption persists. At all doses of administration there is a direct inhibition of osteoblasts.

Soft tissue studies have also shown that administration of steroids will decrease wound healing and may increase susceptibility to infection. This is also true of fracture healing. The net effect is to produce a state of protein catabolism, which definitely retards healing. Steroids have been demonstrated to impair the mobilization rate of osteogenic precursor cells during fracture healing. It has also been noted that very large doses of cortisone are required to inhibit the initial process of callus formation.

Vitamins and Bone Metabolism

Vitamin A

This vitamin has a direct effect on cartilage cells of the growth plate. Decreased growth may result if it is deficient in the diet, although this is rarely seen today. Severe vitamin A deficiency will produce an apparent overgrowth or thickening of bone. Severe hypervitaminosis A will result in the thinning of cortical bone secondary to the direct effect of lysis. It has been suggested that low doses of vitamin A decrease the fracture healing time and increase cellular proliferation and matrix formation. However, the precise action of vitamin A on bone is poorly documented.

Vitamin C

Collagen formation is dependent upon vitamin C, which is necessary for the hydroxylation of proline. If vitamin C is not plentiful, bone and cartilage matrix will be deficient. Therefore, fracture healing requires the presence of vitamin C for normal collagen formation. If it is not present, normal matrix synthesis will not occur. Vitamin C deficiency is not seen today, and therefore vitamin C supplementation is not necessary to stimulate fracture healing.

Vitamin D

In vitamin D deficiency there is a failure of normal mineralization, a decreased osteoclast count, and diminished bone resorption for the parathormone level. Administration of vitamin D reestablishes the normal calcification front on osteoid surfaces, possibly accounting for the initial decrease in calcium, which requires the presence of parathormone. There is then an increase in the osteoclast count. Vitamin D deficiency also affects the epiphyseal plate. Mitochondrial concentration of calcium is reduced, with fewer matrix calcification vesicles, decreased calcification of cartilaginous matrix, and an absence of chondroclasts to remove calcified cartilage. All of these effects are reversed with vitamin D administration.

The mode of action of vitamin D on bone is as follows: vitamin D deficiency will cause a decreased rate of entry of calcium into the cells or mitochondria, resulting in a diminished mitochondrial calcium pool and the extracellular calcium pool. It is now known that the active agent of vitamin D is D_3 or cholecalciferol, which was originally thought to be a vitamin but is now considered a hormone. D_3 is converted to 25-hydroxycholecalciferol in the liver and to 1,25-dihydroxycholecalciferol in the kidney. An increase in parathormone level will stimulate the conversion of 25-hydroxycholecalciferol to 1,25-dihydroxycholecalciferol. This hormone accelerates the active transcellular transport of calcium and increases the growth and maturation of intestinal mucosal cells.

Vitamin D has been demonstrated to increase citrate production in bone cells by stimulating the conversion of pyruvate first to oxaloacetate and then to citrate in the Krebs cycle. Citrate promotes mobilization of calcium ion from bone by chelating calcium and removing ionized calcium. Many investigators believe that this action of vitamin D plays an important role in the remodeling phase of fracture healing.

It is readily apparent that a great deal is still to be learned in regard to fracture healing in general and to new procedures that may stimulate repair, so that morbidity and recuperation time may be decreased.

NOTES

1. Anderson, HC. Matrix vesicles of cartilage and bone. In Bourne, G (ed), The Biochemistry and Physiology of Bone—Calcification and Physiology. Vol. IV, pp. 135-157. New York: Academic Press, 1976.

2. Ali, SY, Sajdera, SW, and Anderson, HC. Isolation and characterization of calcifying matrix vesicles from epiphyseal cartilage. Proc. Natl. Acad. Sci. USA 67:1513-1520, 1970.

3. Azzi, A, and Chance, B. The "energized state" of mitochondria; lifetime and ATP equivalence. Biochim. Biophys. Acta 189:141-151, 1969.

4. Bassett, CAL, and Herrmann, I. Influence of oxygen concentration and mechanical factors on differentiation of connective tissue in vitro. Nature 190:460-461, 1961.

5. Bassett, CAL. Current concepts in bone formation. J. Bone Joint Surg. 44A:1217-1244, 1962.

6. Bélanger, LF. In Bourne, G (ed), Biochemistry and Physiology of Bone. Vol. III, 2nd Ed., pp. 239-270. New York, Academic Press, 1971.

7. Blitz, RM, and Pellegrino, ED. The nature of bone carbonate. Clin. Orthop. 129:279-292, 1977.

8. Brighton, CT, and Heppenstall, RB. Oxygen tension in zones of the epiphyseal plate, the metaphysis and diaphysis. J. Bone Joint Surg. 53A:719-728, 1971.

9. Brighton, CT, and Krebs, AG. Oxygen tension of healing fractures in the rabbit. J. Bone Joint Surg. 54A: 323-332, 1972.

10. Brighton, CT, and Hunt, RM. Mitochondrial calcium and its role in calcification. Histochemical localization of calcium in electron micrographs of the epiphyseal growth plate with K-pyroantimonate. Clin. Orthop. 100:406-416, 1974.

11. Copp, DH. Parathyroid Hormone, Calcitonin and Calcium Homeostasis. Summary. In Talmage, RV, and Bélanger, LF (eds). Parathyroid Hormone and Thyrocalcitonin (calcitonin). New York: Excerpta Medica Foundation, 1968.

12. Edwards, CC. The effect of hyperbaric oxygen and DCAF fluorescein on the rate of bone formation in rabbits. Transactions of The Orthopaedic Research Society Meeting. New Orleans, 1976, p. 18.

13. Ehrlich, HP, Grislis, G, and Hunt, TK. Metabolic and circulatory contributions to oxygen gradients in wounds. Surgery 72:578-583, 1972.

14. Glimcher, MJ. Molecular biology of mineralized tissues with particular reference to bone. Rev. Mod. Physics 31:359-393, 1959.

15. Glimcher, MJ. Specificity of molecular structure of of organic matrices in mineralization. In Sognnaes, RF (ed). Calcification in Biological Systems, pp. 421-487. Washington, D.C.: The American Association for the Advancement of Science, 1960.

16. Ham, AW. Some histophysiological problems peculiar to calcified tissues. J. Bone Joint Surg. 34A:701-728, 1952.

17. Ham, AW, and Harris, WR. Repair and transplantation of bone. In Bourne, G (ed), Biochemistry and Physiology of Bone. Vol. III, 2nd Ed., pp. 337-397. New York: Academic Press, 1972.

18. Heppenstall, RB, Grislis, G, and Hunt, TK. Tissue gas tensions and oxygen consumption in healing bone defects. Clin. Orthop. 106:357-365, 1975.

19. Heppenstall, RB, Goodwin, CW, and Brighton, CT. Fracture healing in the presence of chronic hypoxia. J. Bone Joint Surg. 58A:1153-1156, 1976.

20. Heppenstall, RB, and Brighton, CT. Fracture healing in the presence of anemia. Clin. Orthop. 123:253-258, 1977.

21. Katz, EP, and Li, ST. Structure and function of bone collagen fibrils. J. Mol. Biol. 80:1-15, 1973.

22. Ketenjian, AY, and Arsenis, C. Morphological and biochemical studies during differentiation and calcification of fracture callus cartilage. Clin. Orthop. 107:266-273, 1975.

23. Kuntscher, G. Intramedullary surgical techniques and its place in orthopaedic surgery. J. Bone Joint Surg. 47A: 809-813, 1965.

24. Lane, J, Murphy, L, Irwin, J, and Beller, P. Collagen and proteoglycan structure and metabolism during fracture repair. Transactions of the Orthopaedic Research Society Meeting. Las Vegas, 1977, p. 94.

25. Laurnen, EI, and Kelly, PJ. Blood flow, oxygen consumption, carbon dioxide production and blood-calcium and pH changes in tibial fractures in dogs. J. Bone Joint Surg. 51A:298-308, 1969.

26. Lehninger, AL. Mitochondria and calcium ion transport. Biochem. J. 119:129-138, 1970.

27. Makley, JT, Heiple, KG, Chase, SW, and Herndon, CH. The effect of reduced barometric pressure on fracture healing in rats. J. Bone Joint Surg. 49A:903-914, 1967.

28. Paradis, GR, and Kelly, PJ. Blood flow and mineral deposition in canine tibial fractures. J. Bone Joint Surg. 57A: 220-226, 1975.

29. Perren, SM, Huggler, A, Russenberger, M, et al. The reaction of cortical bone to compression. Acta Orthop. Scand. (Suppl. 125) (1969b).

30. Rhinelander, FW. Some aspects of the microcirculation of healing bone. Clin. Orthop. 40:12-16, 1965.

31. Rhinelander, FW. The normal microcirculation of diaphyseal cortex and its response to fracture. J. Bone Joint Surg. 50A:784-800, 1968.

32. Rhinelander, FW, Phillips, RS, Steel, WM, and Beer, JC. Microangiography in bone healing. II. Displaced closed fractures. J. Bone Joint Surg. 50A:643-662, 1968.

33. Rhinelander, FW. Circulation in bone. In Bonine, G (ed), The Biochemistry and Physiology of Bone. Vol. II, 2nd Ed., pp. 2-76. New York: Academic Press, 1972.

34. Rhinelander, FW. Effects of medullary nailing on the normal blood supply of diaphyseal cortex. AAOS Instructional Course Lectures, pp. 161-187. St. Louis: C. V. Mosby, 1973.

35. Rhinelander, FW. Tibial blood supply in relation to fracture healing. Clin. Orthop. 105:81, 1974.

36. Robison, R. Possible significance of hexosephosphoric esters in ossification. Biochem. J. 17:286-293, 1923.

37. Rothman, RH, Klemek, JS, and Toton, JJ. The effect of iron deficiency anemia on fracture healing. Clin. Orthop. 77: 276-283, 1971.

38. Tonna, EA, and Cronkite, EP. Cellular response to fracture studied with tritiated thymidine. J. Bone Joint Surg. 43A:352-362, 1961.

39. Tonna, EA, and Pentel, L. Chondrogenic cell formation via osteogenic cell progeny transformation. Lab. Invest. 27: 418-426, 1972.

40. Trueta, J, and Caladias, AX. A study of the blood supply of the long bones. Surg. Gynecol. Obstet. 118:485-498, 1964.

41. Urist, MR, Wallace, TH, and Adams, T. The function of fibrocartilaginous fracture callus. Observations on transplants labelled with tritiated thymidine. J. Bone Joint Surg. 47B:304-318, 1965.

42. Wray, JB. Vascular regeneration in the healing fracture. Angiology 14:134-138, 1963.

43. Wray, JB, and Goodman, HO. Post fracture vascular changes and healing process. Arch. Surg. 87:801-804, 1963.

44. Wray, JB. The biochemical characteristics of the fracture hematoma in man. Surg. Gynecol. Obstet. 130:847, 1970.

7
Biological Basis for the Imperfect Repair of Articular Cartilage Following Injury

Lawrence Rosenberg

PROPERTIES OF ARTICULAR CARTILAGE

Articular cartilage is a highly specialized connective tissue which consists of relatively few cells distributed throughout an abundant extracellular matrix. Articular cartilage is a hard yet elastic tissue which provides smooth gliding surfaces in diarthrodial joints. Articular cartilage transmits load, absorbs impact, and sustains shearing forces, yet resists wear to a surprising degree.

These remarkable mechanical properties of articular cartilage are directly related to the structure and properties of the extracellular matrix. The extracellular matrix of normal articular cartilage consists mainly of type II collagen, cartilage-specific proteoglycans, a variety of matrix proteins, and water. The cartilage-specific proteoglycans exist mainly in the form of huge aggregates with potent elastic properties, formed by the non-covalent association of proteoglycan monomers, link protein and hyaluronic acid. The cartilage-specific proteoglycan monomers consist of chondroitin sulfate and keratan sulfate chains covalently bound to a protein core.

The mechanical properties of normal articular cartilage, which enable it to resist wear, result from the structure and properties of the extracellular matrix formed when cartilage-specific proteoglycan aggregates at high concentration are entangled and constrained in a dense network of type II collagen fibers.

This work was supported by United States Public Health Service Grants CA AM 23945 and HL 16387 from the National Institutes of Health.

In the imperfect repair of articular cartilage lesions which result from injury penetrating into subchondral bone, type II collagen is partially replaced by type I collagen, cartilage-specific proteoglycan aggregates of huge size with potent elastic properties are probably replaced by dermatan sulfate-containing proteoglycans of much smaller size with feeble elastic properties, and a normal cartilage extracellular matrix is not restored. These abnormalities in the extracellular matrix of the reparative tissue are probably related to the imperfect repair of articular cartilage following injury penetrating into subchondral bone.

RESPONSE OF ARTICULAR CARTILAGE TO INJURY

Mature articular cartilage does not contain blood vessels and it is walled off from cell types which participate in the inflammatory response to injury by the zone of calcified cartilage and the synovial fluid. There are two fundamentally different types of injury to articular cartilage, based on the capacity of the defect created by the injury to undergo repair.

The first type of injury produces a defect (Type I defect) restricted to the substance of articular cartilage, which does not involve subchondral bone, its blood vessels or the cellular elements of marrow (Meachim 1963; Mankin 1974; Moskowitz et al. 1973; 1979). Since the Type I defect is restricted to articular cartilage and is walled off from the blood vessels and cellular elements in marrow by the zone of calcified cartilage, cell types in the marrow and vessels of subchondral bone which participate in an inflammatory response do not have access to the defect. Therefore Type I lesions restricted to the substance of articular cartilage do not elicit an inflammatory response and do not heal.

The second type of injury is an injury which penetrates and extends into subchondral bone, its blood vessels and marrow (Meachim and Roberts 1971; Mankin 1974; Mitchell and Shepard 1976; 1980; Furukawa et al. 1980; Salter et al. 1980). A defect (Type II defect) is created in which cells from marrow and vessels capable of participating in an inflammatory response and repair have access to the defect. The Type II defect undergoes repair which appears to be satisfactory during the first two months following injury. However, the structure of the reparative tissue is imperfect, and the integrity of the reparative tissue is not maintained. In the discussion that follows, we will focus on the histologic and biochemical characteristics of the reparative tissue which fills Type II defects involving subchondral bone, and we will attempt to provide a partial explanation for the imperfect repair of these lesions.

HISTOLOGY OF REPAIR IN TYPE II DEFECTS

To study the evolution of the healing process in Type II defects, Type II defects were created in the articular cartilage of the distal femur in mature white New Zealand rabbits. Defects which were 2 mm in diameter were created by drilling through the articular cartilage surface into bleeding subchondral bone using a 2 mm drill bit in an orthopedic hand drill. The healing defects were then examined at 24 hrs, 48 hrs, 1 week, 2 weeks, 3 weeks, 1 month, 2 months, 6 months, and 1 year following injury. Serial sections were prepared throughout the defects and the microscopic sections were stained with H&E, or with safranin O and fast green (Rosenberg 1971).

At 24 and 48 hours following injury, fibrin clot containing mononuclear cells filled the defect. At one week, fibroblasts and collagen fibers filled the defect, which were oriented parallel to the articular cartilage surface. At one month post-injury, fibroblasts had differentiated into chondrocytes separated by broad areas of extracellular matrix which stained heavily with safranin O. Figure 7.1a shows the appearance of normal articular cartilage from the distal femur of a rabbit stained with safranin O and fast green. The darker staining of the articular cartilage is the result of the heavy staining of proteoglycans in the articular cartilage with safranin O. The bone, and the cartilage surface which contains bundles of collagen fibers but very little proteoglycan, stains much lighter with fast green.

Figs. 7.1b and 1c show the reparative tissue from one rabbit at two months post-injury stained with H&E (1b) and with safranin O and fast green (1c). The morphology of the reparative tissue resembles that of cartilage and the extracellular matrix stains heavily with safranin O. Fig. 7.1d shows the healing cartilage from another rabbit at two months post-injury. At two months, repair seems to be satisfactory, in that the morphology of the reparative tissue resembles that of cartilage, and a proteoglycan rich extracellular matrix has been formed.

Figs. 7.1e and 1f show the reparative tissue in a defect at 6 months post-injury stained with H&E (Fig. 7.1e), and with safranin O and fast green (Fig. 7.1f). Except for the surface, the integrity of the reparative tissue has been preserved.

FIGURE 7.1 Response of articular cartilage to injury which penetrates and extends into subchondral bone, its blood vessels and marrow.

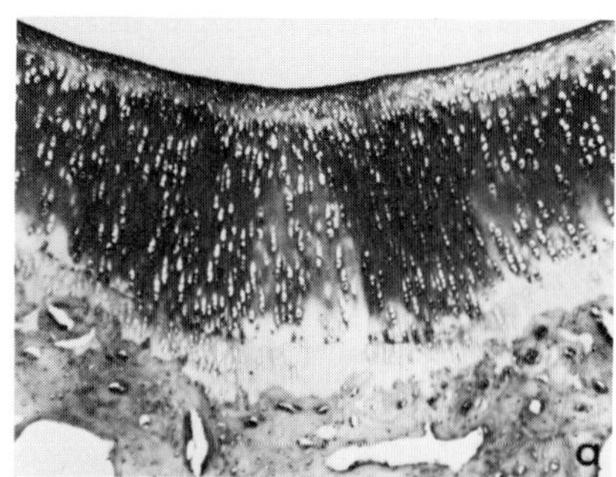

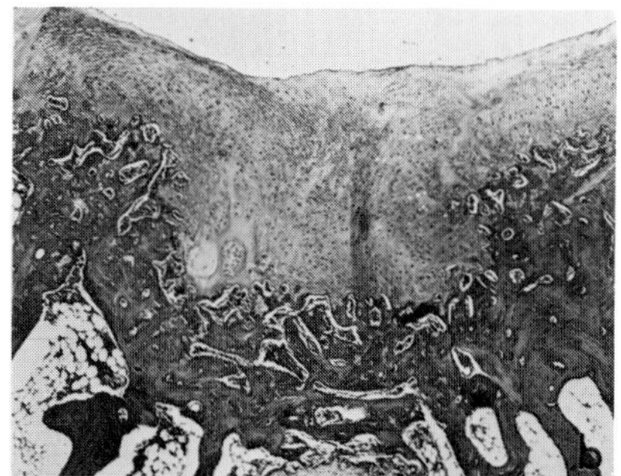

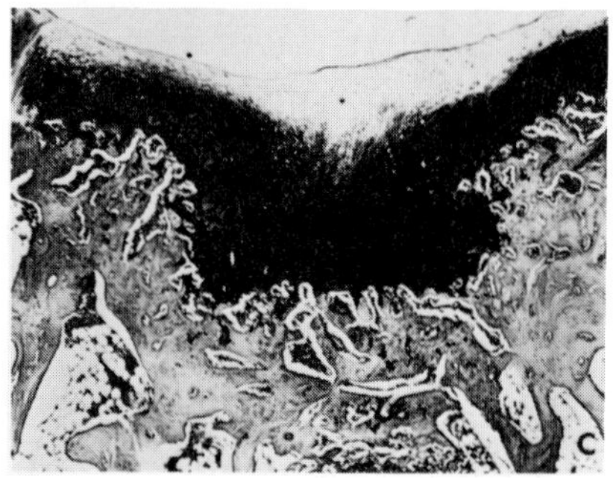

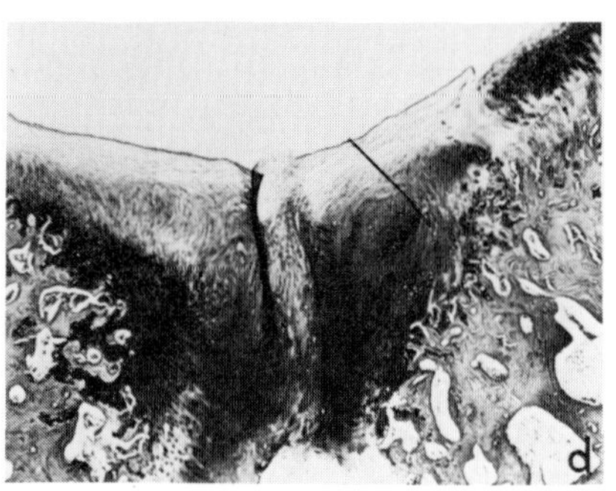

Fig. 1a shows the appearance of normal articular cartilage from the distal femur of a mature rabbit stained with safranin O and fast green. Safranin O is a cationic dye that binds to the anionic groups of glycosaminoglycans. The dark staining throughout most of the articular cartilage is the result of the heavy staining of proteoglycans in the articular cartilage with safranin O. The cartilage surface which consists mainly of bundles of collagen fibers and very little proteoglycan, does not stain with safranin O, but stains much lighter with fast green.

Fig. 1b shows the reparative tissue from a 2 mm defect at 2 months postinjury, stained with H&E.

Fig. 1c shows a serial section through the same defect, stained with safranin O and fast green. At two months, the morphology of the reparative tissue resembles that of cartilage, and the extracellular matrix stains heavily with safranin O.

<u>Fig. 1d</u> shows another defect at 2 months, stained with safranin O and fast green.

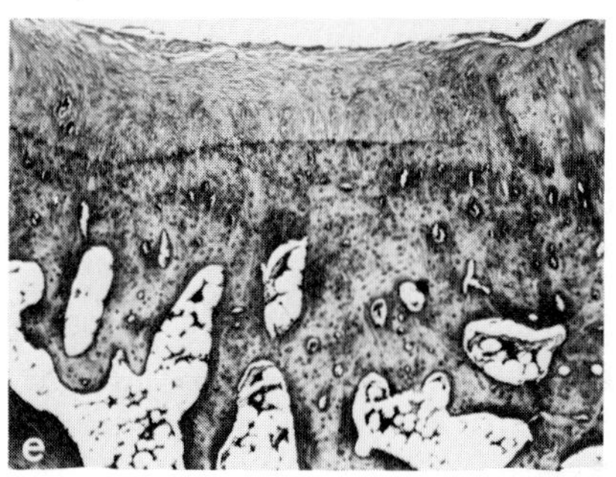

<u>Fig. 1e</u> shows the reparative tissue in a defect at six months post-injury stained with H&E.

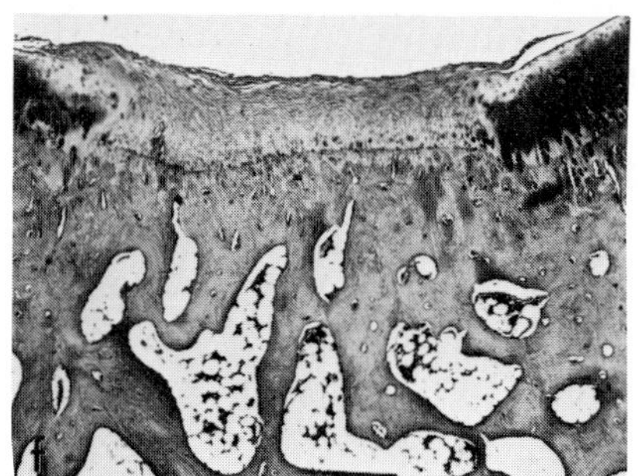

<u>Fig. 1f</u> shows a serial section through the same defect stained with safranin O and fast green. At six months post-injury, little or no safranin O staining was present in the reparative tissue of any of the defects created in 20 rabbits.

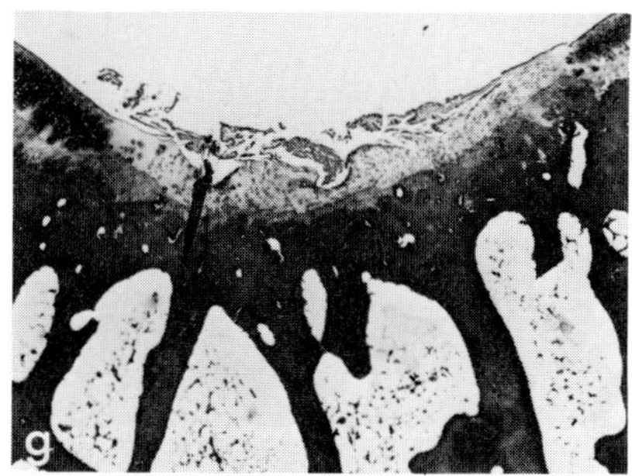

<u>Fig. 1g</u> and <u>1h</u> show the appearance of defects in two animals at six months post-injury, in which the reparative tissue has undergone extensive degenerative changes.

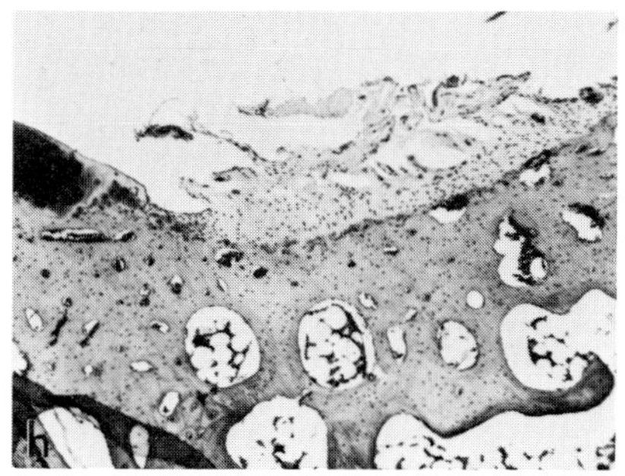

However, little or no safranin O staining is present in the reparative tissue, indicating that proteoglycan which was present throughout the extracellular matrix at two months post-injury is not demonstrable by safranin O staining in the extracellular matrix at six months post-injury. Of twenty mature rabbits studied at six months post-injury, none had proteoglycan demonstrable in the extracellular matrix of the reparative tissue at six months post-injury. Moreover, in 50% of these animals, the reparative tissue did not maintain its integrity, underwent fibrillation, and decreased in thickness, as shown in Figs. 1g and 1h.

Similar changes were noted in defects examined at one year post-injury. Based on these histologic studies, lesions of articular cartilage which penetrate into subchondral bone appear to undergo satisfactory healing initially at two months post-injury, but subsequently degenerate into erosive lesions which resemble human chondromalacia and the early stages of human osteoarthritis.

BIOCHEMICAL BASIS FOR THE IMPERFECT REPAIR OF TYPE II ARTICULAR CARTILAGE LESIONS

What is the biochemical basis for the imperfect repair of type II lesions of articular cartilage? What is wrong with the chemical composition and structure of the reparative tissue, so that the properties of normal cartilage are not restored? Why does the reparative cartilage lose its capacity to resist wear and undergo fibrillation and degeneration? Few studies have focused on these questions and there has been little work in this area.

One important abnormality in the reparative tissue is that an extracellular matrix is formed whose chemical composition, structure and properties are different from those of normal articular cartilage. The extracellular matrix of normal articular cartilage consists mainly of type II collagen, cartilage-specific proteoglycan aggregates and noncollagenous matrix proteins. In the imperfect repair of type II articular cartilage lesions type I collagen is substituted for type II collagen.

David Eyre and his co-workers have determined the amounts of type I and II collagen which are present in healing cartilage (Furukawa et al. 1980). Defects, which were 3 mm in diameter and extended into subchondral bone were created in the patellar groove of the femora of two groups of New Zealand white rabbits. One group consisted of 10- to 12-month-old rabbits, with closed epiphyses, which were skeletally mature. The other group of 6- to 7-month-old rabbits were almost mature, but had open epiphyses. Biochemical studies on the reparative tissue were carried out at 3, 4, 6, 12, 24, and 48 weeks following the creation of the defects. Samples of normal articular cartilage from the femoral condyles of the same joint were taken for controls. To determine the amounts of type I and type II collagen, CNBr peptides of the cartilage collagens were prepared and separated by SDS-PAGE on 10% polyacrylamide slab gels. The gels were stained with Coomassie blue and scanned at 550 nm. The amounts of type I and type II collagens were then determined from the amounts of the peptides α1(II)CB 10 and α2CB 3,5. Fig. 7.2 shows the results obtained by SDS-PAGE of the CNBr peptides from control type I collagen from bone, control type II collagen from normal rabbit articular cartilage, and from the reparative tissue at 3 weeks to 48 weeks post-injury.

Table 7.1 shows the relative amounts of type I and type II collagen in the reparative tissue calculated from the scans of the gels. At 3 to 4 weeks, when the reparative tissue is differentiating into hyaline cartilage, less than 40% of the collagen is type II collagen. At 8 weeks, more than 40% of the collagen in the reparative tissue is type I collagen. It should be emphasized that at 8 weeks (Figs. 7.1b, 1c, and 1d) the reparative tissue appears to have differentiated into a satisfactory hyaline cartilage, based on its histologic appearance and the high concentration of proteoglycans in its extracellular matrix as indicated by safranin O staining. Between 2 months and 6 months, the reparative tissue contains 25% to 33% type I collagen. This is the period during which proteoglycan seems to disappear from the reparative tissue, and during which it undergoes fibrillation and degenerates. Even at 1 year post-injury, approximately 20% of the collagen in the reparative tissue is type I collagen. Thus repair is imperfect in the sense that type I collagen is substituted for type II collagen.

Connective tissues which synthesize and secrete type I collagen usually simultaneously synthesize and secrete dermatan sulfate-containing proteoglycans into the extracellular matrix. Type I collagen and dermatan sulfate-containing proteoglycans are the characteristic extracellular products of undifferentiated mesenchymal cells and many types of fibroblasts. Compared with the cartilage-specific proteoglycan, the dermatan sulfate-containing proteoglycan is a much smaller proteoglycan, with feeble elastic properties. I would like to advance the hypothesis that in the imperfect repair of type II lesions of articular carti-

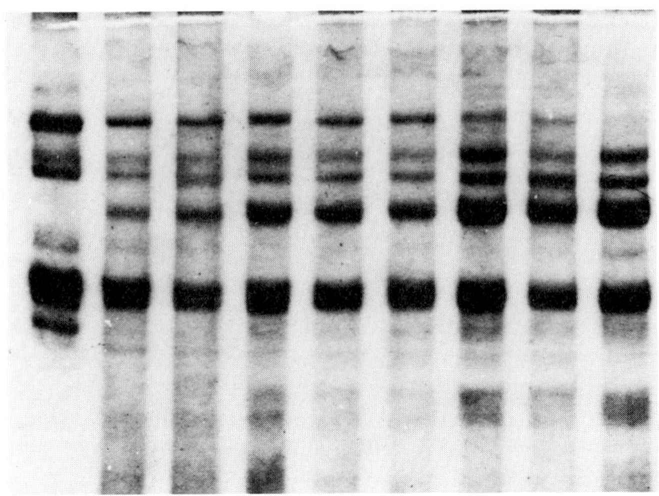

FIGURE 7.2 Cyanogen bromide peptides from control type I bone collagen, control type II collagen from normal rabbit articular cartilage, and of the collagens from reparative tissue from the cartilage defects. The cyanogen bromide peptides have been stained with Coomassie Blue following SDS-PAGE on a 10% polyacrylamide slab gel.
Source: Furukawa et al. 1980.

lage, cartilage-specific proteoglycan aggregates with potent elastic properties are partially replaced by dermatan sulfate-containing proteoglycans of much smaller size with weak elastic properties; also, that the substitution of the dermatan sulfate containing proteoglycan for the cartilage-specific proteoglycan contributes to the decreased capacity of the reparative cartilage to resist wear, and to its degeneration.

It should be emphasized that this is a hypothesis. There have been no studies which show that in the repair of type II lesions of articular cartilage, cartilage-specific proteoglycans of huge size with potent elastic properties are partially replaced by dermatan sulfate-containing proteoglycans of small size with feeble elastic properties. Proof of this concept requires that microanalytical methods be developed to demonstrate the presence of dermatan sulfate proteoglycans in the reparative tissue as a function of time. The presence of the dermatan sulfate proteoglycan in the reparative tissue and healing cartilage might also be demonstrated by immunofluorescent localization or immunoelectron microscopy, using antisera to the isolated dermatan sulfate proteoglycan.

The time is ripe for such studies. In the last two years, dermatan sulfate proteoglycans have been isolated from a variety of tissues and characterized. The methods which have been developed can now be applied to isolate and quantitate the dermatan sulfate proteoglycan in healing cartilage. The dermatan sulfate proteoglycans have properties which are strikingly different from those of the cartilage-specific proteoglycans, and explain why the properties of normal articular cartilage will not be restored if dermatan sulfate proteoglycans are substituted for cartilage-specific proteoglycans during the imperfect healing of articular cartilage. To study the role of dermatan sulfate proteoglycan in the imperfect repair of type II lesions of articular cartilage, it is useful to first examine what has been learned about the dermatan sulfate proteoglycans from other tissues, the methods developed for their isolation, and their special properties. It is particularly informative to compare the properties of the dermatan sulfate proteoglycans to those of the cartilage-specific proteoglycans.

PROPERTIES OF CARTILAGE-SPECIFIC PROTEOGLYCANS

In normal young articular cartilages, most of the proteoglycan exists as proteoglycan aggregates of large size, formed by the non-covalent association of proteoglycan monomers, hyaluronic acid and link proteins (Rosenberg et al. 1975; 1976; Hascall and Kimura 1982; Buckwalter and Rosenberg 1982). A diagrammatic model of the structure of the cartilage-specific proteoglycan aggregate is shown in Fig. 7.3. The cartilage proteoglycan monomer consists of a core protein from which arise many chondroitin sulfate and keratan sulfate chains. The chondroitin sulfate and keratan sulfate chains are covalently attached to serine and threonine residues within the protein core. Chondroitin sulfate, keratan sulfate, dermatan sulfate and hyaluronate are linear polymers composed of sugar residues. They are members of the group of polysaccharides called <u>glycosaminoglycans</u> or <u>mucopolysaccharides</u>, found in the ground substance of a variety of connective tissues.

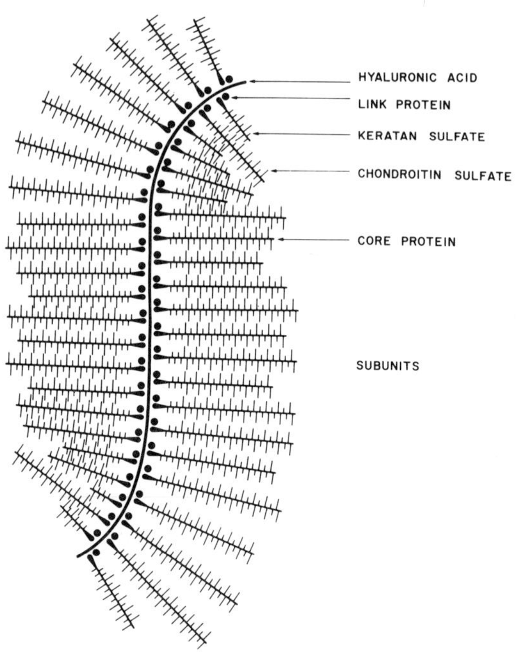

FIGURE 7.3 Diagrammatic model of the molecular architecture of a cartilage proteoglycan aggregate.
Source: Rosenberg 1975.

Glycosaminoglycans are made up of two different sugar residues which alternate regularly in the polysaccharide chain. One sugar residue is an amino sugar, formed when the hydroxyl group of the number two carbon of glucose or galactose is replaced by an amino group, which is acetylated. Therefore, in the glycosaminoglycans, one sugar residue is the amino sugar N-acetylglucosamine or N-acetylgalactosamine. The other sugar residue is usually glucuronic acid, in which the number six carbon of glucose carries a carboxyl group. The structures of the glycosaminoglycans and of their linkage regions to protein are shown in Fig. 7.4. In hyaluronic acid, glucuronic acid and N-acetylglucosamine alternate regularly in the polymer chain. Chondroitin 4-sulfate contains glucuronic acid alternating with N-acetylgalactosamine. Each glycosaminoglycan is described

```
                                   GLYCOSAMINOGLYCAN
SO4                         SO4
 ↓                           ↓
 4                           4
GalNAC(β1→4)GlcUA(β1→3)GalNAc(β1→4)GlcUA(β1→3) Gal (β1→3)Gal(β1→4)Xyl→Ser
                                   CHONDROITIN 4-SULFATE

                         SO4
                          ↓
                          6
Gal(β1→4)GlcNAc(β1→3)Gal(β1→4)GlcNAc(β1→3)Gal(β1→4)GlcNAc(β1→6)GalNAc→Thr
                                                                      3
                                                                   β  ↑
                                                                      1
                                    KERATAN SULFATE     NeuAc(α2→3)Gal

GlcNAc(β1→4)GlcUA(β1→3)GlcNAc(β1→4)GlcUA(β1→3) Gal (β1→3)Gal(β1→4)Xyl→Ser
                                   HYALURONATE

SO4                        SO4
 ↓                          ↓
 4                          4
GalNAc(β1→4)IdUA(α1→3)GalNAc(β1→4)GlcUA(β1→3) Gal (β1→3)Gal(β1→4)Xyl→Ser
                                   DERMATAN SULFATE

 SO4                        SO4
  ↓                          ↓
  6                          6
GlcNAc(α1→4)IdUA(α1→4)GlcNAc(α1→4)GlcUA(β1→3)  Gal (β1→3)Gal(β1→4)Xyl→Ser
                                   HEPARAN SULFATE

 SO4          SO4          SO4
  ↓            ↓            ↓
  6            2            6
GlcNSO3⁻(α1→4)IdUA(α1→4)GlcNAc(α1→4)GlcUAc(β1→3)Gal(β1→3)Gal(β1→4)Xyl→Ser
                                        HEPARIN
```

FIGURE 7.4 Structures of the glycosaminoglycans and their linkage regions to protein.

in terms of the sugar residues which comprise its disaccharide repeating unit.

The disaccharide-repeating unit of dermatan sulfate consists of L-iduronic acid and N-acetylgalactosamine. L-iduronic acid is the C-5 epimer of D-glucuronic acid, in which the carboxyl group is in an axial rather than an equatorial position. As indicated in Fig. 7.4, dermatan sulfate chains also carry disaccharide-repeating units composed of glucuronic acid and N-acetylgalactosamine, like those present in chondroitin sulfate (Fransson 1968; Coster et al. 1975; Malmstrom et al. 1975). Thus, dermatan sulfate is a hybrid, in which the glycosamino-glycan chain is a copolymer of dermatan sulfate and chondroitin sulfate-repeating units. The different classes of proteoglycan monomers are distinguished from one another by the different kinds of glycosaminoglycan chains attached to the proteoglycan monomer core protein, and by the fact that they possess different core proteins as demonstrated by immunologic analyses or peptide mapping.

An important feature of the chemical structure of the glycosaminoglycans is that the sugar residues carry closely spaced negatively charged carboxyl and sulfate groups. Because of the repelling forces of the closely spaced negatively charged groups, the glycosaminoglycan chains arising from the proteoglycan monomer core protein assume a stiffly extended conformation. In the cartilage-specific proteoglycan monomer, the chondroitin sulfate and keratan sulfate chains stick out from the core protein like the bristles on a brush. The extended conformation causes the proteoglycan monomer molecule to spread out in a relatively large volume of solution. The stiffness of the chains makes the molecule resistant to compression into a smaller volume of solution. This property is partially responsible for the elasticity of cartilage.

Cartilage specific proteoglycan monomers from articular cartilage are polydisperse and vary in size and chemical composition. However, an average representative proteoglycan monomer would have a protein core of approximately 200,000 in molecular weight, measuring about 2000 Å long. To this protein core would be attached approximately 100 condroitin sulfate side chains, each 20,000 to 30,000 in molecular weight, and around 500 to 600 Å long. Keratan sulfate chains 5000 to 10,000 in molecular weight, 100 to 200 Å in length, would also be attached to the protein core. The entire proteoglycan monomer would be approximately two million in molecular weight.

In native cartilage, most of the proteoglycan exists in the form of aggregates of high molecular weight (Rosenberg et al. 1975; Buckwalter and Rosenberg 1982; Hascall and Kimura 1982). A representative cartilage-specific proteoglycan aggregate from bovine articular cartilage would consist of 100 proteoglycan monomers non-covalently bound together with link protein to a hyaluronic acid chain 4000 nm in length. Such an aggregate would be approximately 200 million in molecular weight. As shown in Fig. 7.3, the aggregate is formed by the non-covalent association of many proteoglycan monomers with hyaluronic acid and link protein. Hyaluronic acid forms the central filamentous backbone of the proteoglycan aggregate. Fig. 7.5 shows the molecular architecture of a proteoglycan aggregate from calf nasal cartilage as demonstrated by electron microscopy (Buckwalter and Rosenberg 1982). A detailed description of the

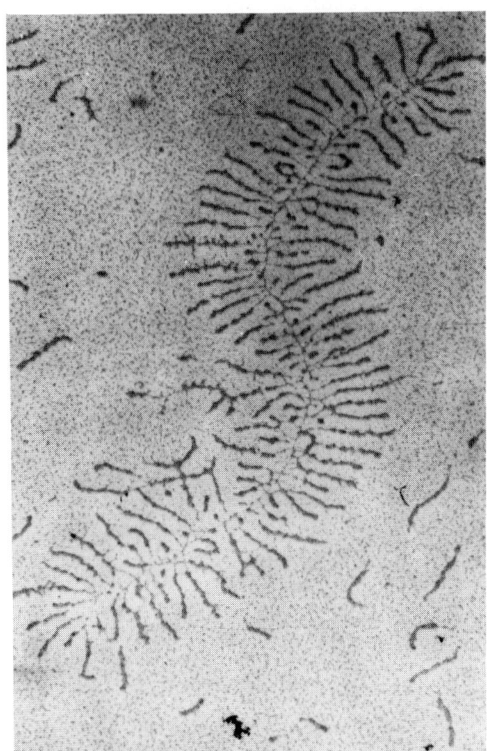

FIGURE 7.5 Electron micrograph showing the molecular architecture of a proteoglycan aggregate from calf nasal cartilage. Source: Buckwalter and Rosenberg 1982.

dimensions of proteoglycan aggregates determined by electron microscopy has been reported recently (Buckwalter and Rosenberg 1982). The formation of such huge aggregates depends upon the capacity of the cartilage-specific proteoglycan monomer to non-covalently bind to hyaluronic acid (Hardingham and Muir 1972; 1973; 1974; Hascall and Heinegard 1974; Hascall 1977). This, in turn, depends upon the presence of a hyaluronic acid binding region in the core protein of the cartilage-specific proteoglycan monomer.

As shown in Fig. 7.3, proteoglycan monomer core protein consists of three distinct regions which differ in structure and function. One end of proteoglycan monomer core protein contains little or no chondroitin sulfate or keratan sulfate, and consists of a region of core protein approximately 70,000 in molecular weight with a globular conformation. This region contains the binding region of core protein for hyaluronic acid. Another region, which comprises most of the length of the core protein and extends toward the other end of the proteoglycan monomer molecule, contains all of the chondroitin sulfate chains and some of the keratan sulfate chains, and is called the chondroitin sulfate-rich region. Between the chondroitin sulfate-rich region and the hyaluronic acid binding region is located a third region consisting of a short peptide to which are attached mainly keratan sulfate chains. This region is called the keratan sulfate-rich region (Heinegard and Axelsson 1977).

In the cartilage-specific proteoglycan aggregate, link proteins are centrally located in the region where proteoglycan monomer binds to hyaluronate. The link proteins bind simultaneously to the hyaluronic acid binding region of proteoglycan monomer core protein, and to hyaluronate, and stabilize the binding of proteoglycan monomer to hyaluronate (Hardingham 1979; Tang et al. 1979). Once the link proteins have been incorporated into the cartilage-specific proteoglycan aggregate, the aggregate will not dissociate unless exposed to agents like 4 M GdmCl, which break non-covalent bonds. However, the aggregates formed by the self-association of dermatan sulfate-containing proteoglycan monomers appear to reversibly dissociate when exposed to shearing forces or increased pressure, as discussed below.

Because of the repelling forces of the thousands of closely spaced negatively charged groups on their chondroitin sulfate and keratan sulfate chains, these huge proteoglycan aggregates tend to spread out into a relatively large domain of solution. The volume of solution occupied by proteoglycan aggregates in solution in vitro is far greater than that available to them in native cartilage. In native cartilage, the aggregates expand until they are constrained by the surrounding network of collagen fibers. The aggregates in native cartilage exhibit elastic forces (Mow et al. 1983) which are balanced by the tensile forces of collagen fibers. When articular cartilage is subjected to a compressive force, the aggregates are temporarily compressed into a smaller domain, and water is simultaneously extruded from the cartilage. When the compressive force is relieved, the aggregates expand, the articular cartilage simultaneously imbibes water, and the volume of the cartilage increases until further increases in volume are prevented by the collagen fibers. These are the properties of the huge, stable cartilage-specific proteoglycan aggregates which are responsible in part for the elastic properties of normal articular cartilage.

PROPERTIES OF THE DERMATAN SULFATE-CONTAINING PROTEOGLYCAN

As noted above, thus far there have been no studies of the dermatan sulfate proteoglycan from healing cartilage defects.

Methods are now available to demonstrate the presence, and to determine the concentration of the dermatan sulfate proteoglycan in healing cartilage defects. The amounts of dermatan sulfate proteoglycan which can be isolated from reparative tissue may be too small for its detailed characterization and an extensive study of its properties. However, much useful information about the properties of this species can be obtained from the study of similar species from tissues other than reparative tissue.

For example, the series of events which occurs during cartilage repair (Figs. 7.1b to 1d) is somewhat analogous to the series of events which occurs during limb development. Goetinck and his co-workers have extensively studied the biosynthesis of the dermatan sulfate proteoglycan and the cartilage-specific proteoglycan during the chondrogenesis which occurs in limb bud development (Goetinck et al. 1974; Pennypacker and Goetinck 1976; Goetinck and Pennypacker 1977; Royal and Goetinck 1977; McKeown and Goetinck 1979; Royal et al. 1980).

Prior to the advent of chondrogenesis, the developing limb bud consists of a core of mesenchyme covered by ectoderm. The mesenchymal cells are closely spaced and separated by relatively small amounts of extracellular matrix. Before chondrogenesis begins, the extracellular matrix of the mesenchyme contains mainly type I collagen and a dermatan sulfate-containing proteoglycan, and much smaller amounts of cartilage-specific proteoglycan. With the advent of chondrogenesis, synthesis of the cartilage-specific proteoglycan suddenly increases and synthesis of the dermatan sulfate proteoglycan greatly decreases. Goetinck's studies have shown that the dermatan sulfate proteoglycan is much smaller in size than the cartilage-specific proteoglycan monomer, and it does not bind to hyaluronic acid to form large aggregates.

To obtain dermatan sulfate proteoglycans in amounts sufficient for their detailed characterization, we isolated dermatan sulfate proteoglycans from bovine fetal epiphyseal cartilage (Rosenberg et al. 1983). The isolation procedure which we developed is summarized in Table 7.1. The isolated species showed a single band on agarose acrylamide gels and appeared as a single component with a sedimentation coefficient (s^0_{20}) of 5S in sedimentation velocity studies.

The chemical composition of the cartilage-specific proteoglycan monomer from bovine fetal epiphyseal cartilage is shown in Table 7.3. In the purified monomer, dermatan sulfate represents 39.9% of the total glycosaminoglycan. The dermatan sulfate-containing proteoglycan monomer has a much higher

TABLE 7.1

Isolation of Dermatan Sulfate-Containing Proteoglycan Monomers

1. Extract fresh wet cartilage in 4 M GdmCl, 0.05 M EDTA, 0.15 M sodium acetate, at pH 7 containing protease inhibitors at 5° for 24 h.
2. Dialyze extract against 20 volumes of 0.15 M sodium acetate, 0.05 M EDTA, at pH 7 containing protease inhibitors, for 16 h at 5°.
3. Equilibrium density gradient centrifugation under associative conditions at 3.5 M CsCl at 40,000 rpm for 50 h at 5°. Cut fractions A1 to A6.
4. Determine dermatan sulfate content of fractions A1 to A6 using chondroitinases AC and ABC. Pool the dermatan sulfate-containing fractions.
5. Equilibrium density gradient centrifugation under dissociative conditions of dermatan sulfate-containing fractions in 3M CsCl, 4M GdmCl, at 40,000 rpm for 65 h at 5°. Cut fractions D1 to D6.
6. Determine dermatan sulfate content of fractions D1 to D6 using chondroitinases AC and ABC.
7. Chromatography on DEAE-Sephacel in 6 M urea, 0.025 M Tris, at pH 6.5.
8. Chromatography on Sephacel S-200 in 4 M GdmCl. Dialyze against water. Lyophilize.
9. Dissolve in 0.15 M sodium acetate, pH 6.3, precipitate with three volumes of ethanol, wash in ethanol and ether and dry.

protein content than the cartilage-specific proteoglycan monomer, and appears to contain a substantial number of mannose-rich oligosaccharides.

Antisera were raised against the isolated dermatan sulfate-containing proteoglycan monomer, and against the cartilage-specific proteoglycan monomer from bovine epiphyseal cartilage (Rosenberg et al. 1983) and the reactivity of antibodies from the two antisera with each proteoglycan monomer was studied by ELISA. The antibodies to dermatan sulfate proteoglycan monomer reacted strongly with this monomer but showed <u>no</u> reaction with cartilage-specific proteoglycan monomer. Antibodies to cartilage-specific proteoglycan monomer did not cross react with dermatan sulfate proteoglycan monomer. Thus the two proteoglycan monomers possess different protein cores. These observations are directly applicable to the study of the imperfect repair of articular cartilage. Using the procedure shown in Table 7.1, dermatan sulfate proteoglycan might be isolated from the fetal cartilage of a particular species. Antibodies to the dermatan sulfate proteoglycan might then be used to demonstrate the presence of the dermatan sulfate proteoglycan in the reparative tissue of healing cartilage defects.

DERMATAN SULFATE-CONTAINING PROTEOGLYCANS FROM BOVINE SCLERA

Bovine sclera is a rich source of dermatan sulfate proteoglycans from which this species may be isolated in amounts sufficient for its detailed characterization, and for studies of its unusual properties. Dermatan sulfate proteoglycans have been extensively studied by Fransson, Coster and their coworkers (Fransson 1976; Fransson and Coster 1979; Fransson

TABLE 7.2

Relative Amounts of Types I and II Collagens in Reparative Tissue at Various Times After Injury

Time After Injury	Type II Collagen as % of Type I and Type II
3 weeks	30
4 weeks	39
6 weeks	53
8 weeks	59
12 weeks	57
24 weeks	76
48 weeks	81

Note: Calculated from scans of Coomassie Blue stained CNBr peptides following SDS-PAGE.
Source: Furukawa, T, Eyre, D, Koide, S, and Glimcher, M. Biochemical studies on repair cartilage resurfacing experimental defects in the rabbit knee. *J. Bone and Joint Surg.* 62A:79-89, 1980.

TABLE 7.3

Chemical Composition of the Dermatan Sulfate-Containing Proteoglycan Monomer from Bovine Fetal Epiphyseal Cartilage. Values Shown as Percent of Dry Weight

Protein	35.50%
Hexuronate	11.51
Galactosamine	13.25
Glucosamine	4.13
Mannose	1.03
Galactose	0.88
Xylose	0.45
Fucose	0.21
Glucose	0.16
Sialate	1.00
Chondroitin sulfate	15.8
Dermatan sulfate	10.5
(DS/CS+DS) × 100	39.9

Source: Rosenberg, L, et al. 1983. Isolation, characterization and immunohistochemical localization of a dermatan sulfate-containing proteoglycan from bovine fetal epiphyseal cartilage. In Kelley, RO, Goetinck, PF, and MacCabe, JA (eds), Limb Development and Regeneration, Part B. New York: Alan R. Liss. With the permission of the publishers.

et al. 1979; Carlstedt et al. 1981; Coster and Fransson 1981; Coster et al. 1981). The dermatan sulfate proteoglycans were extracted from bovine sclera with 4 M guanidine hydrochloride (GdmCl) in the presence of protease inhibitors and purified by ion exchange chromatography on DEAE-cellulose in 6 M urea, equilibrium density gradient centrifugation, and by gel chromatography on Sepharose CL-2B in 4 M GdmCl. Two proteoglycan monomers of different size, called proteoglycans I and II, were separated by gel chromatography on Sepharose CL-2B in 4 M GdmCl. Under associative conditions on gel chromatography, the larger proteoglycan monomer (I) tended to self-associate into aggregates, while the smaller proteoglycan monomer (II) did not. The sizes of proteoglycans I and II under associative conditions were not increased by the addition of hyaluronic acid, indicating that the dermatan sulfate proteoglycan monomers did not react with, or bind to hyaluronate to form proteoglycan aggregates of the kind formed by cartilage specific proteoglycans (Fig. 7.2).

The molecular weights of the scleral proteoglycan monomers were determined by sedimentation velocity, diffusion and sedimentation equilibrium experiments in 6 M GdmCl. In 6 M GdmCl, the molecular weights of proteoglycan monomers I and II were 160,000 to 220,000 and 70,000 to 100,000 respectively.

The average molecular weight of the dermatan sulfate side chain was 24,000. Proteoglycan monomer I contained 45% protein and proteoglycan monomer II contained 60% protein. Thus, the molecular weights of the protein cores of monomers I and II are approximately 85,000 and 46,000 respectively. This indicates that proteoglycan monomer II contains one or two dermatan sulfate chains bound to a core protein approximately 46,000 in molecular weight, while proteoglycan monomer I contains 4 or 5 dermatan sulfate chains bound to a core protein approximately 85,000 in molecular weight.

SELF-ASSOCIATION OF DERMATAN SULFATE-CONTAINING PROTEOGLYCAN MONOMERS

Sedimentation equilibrium and light scattering studies under associative conditions in 0.15 M NaCl, pH 7.4, revealed that proteoglycan monomers I and II self-associated to form aggregates of higher molecular weights. Moreover, the propensity to form aggregates and the size of the aggregates formed varied under different conditions and was dramatically increased under the conditions prevailing in the light scattering experiments. Proteoglycan monomer I self-associated into aggregates with molecular weights of 500,000 to 800,000 in sedimentation equilibrium experiments in 0.15 M NaCl, while proteoglycan monomer II showed little tendency to self-associate and gave molecular weights of 90,000 to 110,000.

In light-scattering experiments, both proteoglycan monomers I and II exhibited an enhanced propensity for self-association. Under associative conditions in 0.15 M NaCl, proteoglycan monomers I and II showed molecular weights of 3.1×10^6 and 3.4×10^6 respectively. Thus dermatan sulfate proteoglycans, even in a maximally aggregated state, have molecular weights which are approximately the same as cartilage-specific proteoglycan monomers, and which are 20 to 100 times less than those of cartilage-specific proteoglycan aggregates.

The properties of the dermatan sulfate proteoglycans from bovine sclera are summarized in Table 7.4. One of the most interesting properties is the capacity of the dermatan sulfate proteoglycans to undergo different degrees of self-association depending upon the experimental conditions. Thus, under the conditions of light-scattering experiments, where the macromolecules are not subjected to shearing forces or pressure, the highest degree of self-association into aggregates of large size readily occurs.

In sedimentation equilibrium experiments, where the macromolecules are subjected to pressure, the degree of self-association is somewhat less. In gel chromatography experiments, the larger dermatan sulfate-containing proteoglycan (proteoglycan I) self-associates slightly to form small aggregates, while the smaller dermatan sulfate-containing proteoglycan (proteoglycan II) does not. The possibility exists that the proteoglycan aggregates formed by the self-association of dermatan sulfate-containing proteoglycans are reversibly dissociated by shearing forces and/or pressure.

This phenomenon would have important implications for the biomechanical properties of reparative tissues filling cartilage defects, in which dermatan sulfate-containing proteoglycans were substituted for cartilage-specific proteoglycans. Cartilage-specific proteoglycan aggregates, which are formed by the non-covalent association of proteoglycan monomers, link protein and hyaluronate, are stabilized against dissociation by link protein, and there is no indication that they dissociate when subjected to shearing forces or pressure. The proteoglycan aggregates formed from dermatan sulfate-containing proteoglycans are much smaller in size than the cartilage-specific proteoglycan aggregates. The dermatan sulfate-containing proteoglycan aggregates may dissociate into small dermatan sulfate-containing proteoglycan monomers, with molecular weights of 70,000 to 220,000 when subjected to the shearing forces or pressure to which articular cartilage is usually exposed.

The small dermatan sulfate-containing proteoglycans would be less effectively enmeshed with, and constrained by the surrounding network of collagen fibers. Because of their relatively small size, the dermatan sulfate proteoglycans might not be retained in the extracellular matrix of the tissue, and might gradually be lost from the reparative tissue. This phenomenon might explain the sequence of changes shown in Figs. 7.1c, 1d, 1e, and 1f.

The dermatan sulfate proteoglycans would not possess the strong elastic properties of the huge cartilage-specific proteo-

TABLE 7.4

Properties of Dermatan Sulfate Proteoglycans from Bovine Sclera

Numbers of monomers	I	II
Monomer molecular weight	160K to 220K	70K to 100K
Core protein molecular weight	85K	46K
Glycosaminoglycan molecular weight	24K	24K
Numbers of glycosaminoglycan chains	4 to 5	1 or 2
Mannose oligosaccharides	yes	yes
Binds to hyaluronate	no	no
Self-associates	yes	yes
Light scattering	3.1×10^6	3.4×10^6
Sedimentation equilibrium	500K to 800K	90K to 110K
Gel chromatography	slight	none
Mechanism of self-association:	Interactions between dermatan sulfate chains	

glycan aggregates. The dermatan sulfate proteoglycan would be incapable of forming together with collagen a fibrous composite similar to that present in normal articular cartilage. The biomechanical properties of the reparative tissue would be different from those of normal articular cartilage. These biochemical changes might contribute to the imperfect repair of articular cartilage following injury, whose histologic characteristics are shown in Fig. 7.2.

REFERENCES

Buckwalter, JA, and Rosenberg, LC. 1982. Electron microscopic studies of cartilage proteoglycans. Direct evidence for the variable length of the chondroitin sulfate-rich region of proteoglycan subunit core protein. J. Biol. Chem. 257, 9830-9839.

Carlstedt, I, Coster, L, and Malmstrom, A. 1981. Isolation and characterization of dermatan sulphate and heparan sulphate proteoglycans from fibroblast cultures. Biochem. J 197, 217-225.

Coster, L, and Fransson, LA. 1981. Isolation and characterization of dermatan sulphate proteoglycans from bovine sclera. Biochem. J. 193, 143-153.

Coster, L, Fransson, LA, Sheehan, J, Nieduszynski, IA, and Phelps, CF. 1981. Self-association of dermatan sulphate proteoglycans from bovine sclera. Biochem. J. 197, 483-490.

Coster, L, Malmstrom, A, Sjobert, I, and Fransson, LA. 1975. The copolymeric structure of pig skin dermatan sulphate. Distribution of L-iduronic acid sulphate residues in copolymeric chains. Biochem. J. 145, 379-389.

Fransson, LA. 1976. Interaction between dermatan sulphate chains. I. Affinity chromatography of copolymeric galactosaminoglycans on dermatan sulphate-substituted agarose. Biochim. Biophys. Acta 437, 106-115.

____ 1968. Structure of dermatan sulfate. III. The hybrid structure of dermatan sulfate from umbilical cord. J. Biol. Chem. 243, 1504-1510.

Fransson, LA, and Coster, L. 1979. Interaction between dermatan sulphate chains. II. Structural studies on aggregating glycan chains and oligosaccharides with affinity for dermatan sulphate-substituted agarose. Biochim. Biophys. Acta 528, 132-144.

Fransson, LA, Coster, L, Malmstrom, A, and Sheehan, JK. 1982. Self-association of scleral proteodermatan sulfate. Evidence for interaction via the dermatan sulfate side chains. J. Biol. Chem. 257, 6333-6338.

Fransson, LA, Nieduszynski, IA, Phelps, CF, and Sheehan, JK. 1979. Interactions between dermatan sulfate chains. III. Light-scattering and viscometry studies of self-association. Biochim. Biophys. Acta 586, 179-188.

Furukawa, T, Eyre, DR, Koide, S, and Glimcher, M. 1980. Biochemical studies on repair cartilage resurfacing experimental defects in the rabbit knee. J. Bone and Joint Surg. 62-A, 79-89.

Goetinck, PF, and Pennypacker, JP. 1977. Controls in the acquisition and maintenance of chondrogenic expression. In Vertebrate Limb and Somite Morphogenesis, edited by D. A. Ede, J. R. Hinchliffe, and M. Balls, Cambridge: Cambridge University Press.

Goetinck, PF, Pennypacker, JP, and Royal, PD. 1974. Proteochondroitin sulfate synthesis and chondrogenic expression. Exptl. Cell Res. 87, 241-248.

Hardingham, TE. 1979. The role of link-protein in the structure of cartilage proteoglycan aggregates. Biochem. J. 177, 237-247.

Hardingham, TE, and Muir, H. 1974. Hyaluronic acid in cartilage and proteoglycan aggregation. Biochem. J. 139, 565-581.

____, 1973. Hyaluronic acid in cartilage. Biochem. Soc. Trans. (DUBLIN) 1, 282-284.

____, 1972. The specific interaction of hyaluronic acid with cartilage proteoglycans. Biochim. Biophys. Acta 279, 401-405.

Hascall, VC. 1977. Interaction of cartilage proteoglycans with hyaluronic acid. J. Supramolecular Struc. 7, 101-120.

Hascall, VC, and Heinegard, D. 1974. Aggregation of cartilage proteoglycans. I. The role of hyaluronic acid. J. Biol. Chem. 249, 4232-4241.

Hascall, VC, and Kimura, JH. 1982. Proteoglycans: Isolation and characterization. In Methods in Enzymology edited by L. W. Cunningham and D. W. Frederiksen. Vol. 82, pp. 769-800. New York: Academic Press.

Heinegard, D, and Axelsson, I. 1977. Distribution of keratan sulfate in cartilage proteoglycans. J. Biol. Chem. 252, 1971-1979.

Malmstrom, A, Carlstedt, I, Aberg, L, and Fransson, LA. 1975. The copolymeric structure of dermatan sulphate produced by cultured human fibroblasts. Different distribution of iduronic acid- and glucuronic acid-containing units in soluble and cell-associated glycans. Biochem. J. 151, 477-489.

Mankin, HJ. 1974. The reaction of articular cartilage to injury and osteoarthritis. New England J. Med. 291, 1285-1292.

McKeown, PJ, and Goetinck, PF. 1979. A comparison of the proteoglycans synthesized in Meckel's and sternal cartilage from normal and nanomelic chick embryos. Develop. Biol. 71, 203-215.

Meachim, G. 1963. The effects of scarification on articular cartilage of the rabbit. J. Bone and Joint Surg. 45B, 150-161.

Meachim, G, and Roberts, C. 1971. Repair of the joint surface from subarticular tissue in the rabbit knee. J. Anat. 109, 317-327.

Mitchell, N, and Shepard, N. 1980. Healing of articular cartilage in intra-articular fractures in rabbits. J. Bone and Joint Surg. 62A, 628-634.

____, 1976. The resurfacing of adult rabbit articular cartilage by multiple perforations through the subchondral bone. J. Bone and Joint Surg. 58A, 230-233.

Moskowitz, RW, Howell, DS, Goldberg, VM, Muniz, O, and Pita, JC. 1979. Cartilage proteoglycan alterations in an experimentally induced model of rabbit osteoarthritis. Arth. and Rheum. 22, 155-163.

Moskowitz, RW, Davis, W, Sammarco, J, Martens, M, Baker, J, Mayor, M, Burstein, AH, and Frankel, VH. 1973. Experimentally induced degenerative joint lesions following partial meniscectomy in the rabbit. Arth. and Rheum. 16, 397-405.

Mow, VC, Mak, AF, Lai, WM, Rosenberg, LC, and Tang, LH. 1983. Viscoelastic properties of proteoglycan subunits and aggregates in varying solution concentration. Submitted to J. Biomechan.

Pennypacker, JP, and Goetinck, PF. 1976. Biochemical and ultrastructural studies of collagen and proteochondroitin sulfate in normal and nanomelic cartilage. Develop. Biol. 50, 35-47.

Rosenberg, L. 1975. Structure of cartilage proteoglycans. In Dynamics of Connective Tissue Macromolecules, edited by P. M. C. Burleigh and A. R. Poole, pp. 105-128. Amsterdam: North-Holland Publishing Company.

Rosenberg, L. 1971. Chemical basis for the histological use of safranin O in the study of articular cartilage. J. Bone and Joint Surg. 53A, 69-82.

Rosenberg, L, Hellmann, W, and Kleinschmidt, AK. 1975. Electron microscopic studies of proteoglycan aggregates from bovine articular cartilage. J. Biol. Chem. 250, 1877-1883.

Rosenberg, L, Tang, L, Choi, H, Pal, S, Johnson, T, Poole, AR, Roughley, P, Reiner, A, and Pidoux, I. 1983. Isolation, characterization and immunofluorescent localization of a dermatan sulfate-containing proteoglycan from bovine fetal epiphyseal cartilage. In Limb Development and Regeneration. Part B, edited by R. O. Kelley, P. F. Goetinck, and J. A. MacCabe. New York: Alan R. Liss.

Rosenberg, L, Wolfenstein-Todel, C, Margolis, R, Pal, S, and Strider, W. 1976. Proteoglycans from bovine proximal humeral articular cartilage. Structural basis for the polydispersity of proteoglycan subunit. J. Biol. Chem. 251, 6439-6444.

Royal, PD, and Goetinck, PF. 1977. In vitro chondrogenesis in mouse limb mesenchymal cells: Changes in ultrastructure and proteoglycan. J. Embryol. Exp. Morph. 39, 79-95.

Royal, PD, Sparks, KJ, and Goetinck, PF. 1980. Physical and immunochemical characterization of proteoglycans synthesized during chondrogenesis in the chick embryo. J. Biol. Chem. 255, 9870-9878.

Salter, RB, Simmonds, DF, Malcolm, BW, Rumble, EJ, MacMichael, D, and Clements, N. 1980. The biological effect of continuous passive motion on the healing of full-thickness defects in articular cartilage. An experimental investigation in the rabbit. J. Bone and Joint Surg. 62A, 1232-1251.

Tang, LH, Rosenberg, L, Reiner, A, and Poole, AR. 1979. Proteoglycans from bovine nasal cartilage. Properties of a soluble form of link protein. J. Biol. Chem. 254, 10523-10531.

PART III
Induction of Repair

8
Clinical and Immunobiological Studies of Human Extra-Embryonic Membranes in Wound Healing

Jiri T. Beranek, W. Page Faulk, J.P. Ortonne and B.L. Hsi

INTRODUCTION

A successful treatment of chronic venous leg ulcers with amniotic epithelium [1,2] has prompted us to explore further the immunobiological role of this extra-embryonic membrane in the metabolism of tissue cells known to be involved in wound healing. Matthews, Fault & Bennett have recently reviewed the beneficial effects of amnion in surgical practice.[3] These promising clinical results now require a larger and more randomized investigation. Such a study would be difficult to realize on a large scale with the use of human amnion epithelium, due to technical reasons of amnion supply, culture and application. However, if amnion conditioned medium (ACM) could enhance wound repair, it could provide a novel, convenient and easily available approach to the problem of non-healing wounds.[4] We wish to herewith present basic and clinical results from such a study in which ACM was used in the treatment of non-healing ulcers of the leg.

METHODS AND MATERIALS

Laboratory Studies

Human amnions were collected aseptically from elective Caesarean sections in otherwise healthy women at term. The

---

Note: Magnification numbers given within figure legends in this chapter pertain to original magnification. The photographs have been reduced to fit house specifications.

membranes were immediately immersed in ice-cold Dulbecco's phosphate buffered saline (PBS), and transported to the laboratory where they were cleaned of blood clots and decidual tissue and washed in two changes of ice-cold PBS.

The culture method of Burgos and Faulk[5] was initially used, but this was modified as follows: Whole amniochorion was cut into pieces approximately 5 × 5 cm which were separated in halves and cultured in separate 245 × 245 × 20 mm polystyrene dishes in 400 ml of the Dutch modification of RPMI 1640 to which were added: 10% heat-inactivated newborn calf serum (NCS), 10 mM sodium bicarbonate, 2 mM L-glutamine, gentamycin 80 mg/l, and fungizon 2 mg/l. The membrane culture was maintained at 37° in a humid atmosphere containing 2% CO_2 as long as the buffering capacity of the medium permitted, which was usually about 10 days. After culture, the medium was collected and lyophilized for storage. Control medium was treated in the same way, but without amniochorion.

The viability of cultured amniotic epithelium was monitored by the DNA-binding assay with propidium iodide according to Yeh et al.[6] as well as by using a modification of the dye-exclusion technique with trypan-blue as described by Hudson and Hay.[7] Pieces of amniotic epithelium were dissected from the underlying connective tissue, and chorion and amnion were placed in Petri dishes filled with 0.05% trypan-blue in saline for 5 minutes at room temperature followed by two rinses in PBS to remove excess dye. The tissue was then observed through a microscope equipped with phase-contrast illumination in order to obtain an overall estimation of dead and living cells.

In order to produce whole amnion conditioned medium (WACM) amnion epithelium conditioned medium (AECM), and chorion conditioned medium (CHCM), 5 × 5 cm pieces of the corresponding tissues were placed in 100 mm tissue culture dishes filled with the Dutch modification of RPMI 1640 medium with 2 mM L-glutamine and enriched either with 10% heat inactivated fetal calf serum (FCS) or 10% NCS, or no serum, and cultured for 3 days under the same conditions as described above.

The influence of ACM on the growth of different cell types was studied by experiments _in vitro_ with the use of mouse bone marrow (MBM) cells. The cells were obtained from mouse femurs[8] and suspended in RPMI 1640 medium (Dutch modification) supplemented with 10% FCS, 2 mM L-glutamine and gentamycin, 80 mg/l. The cells at different densities were seeded into 35 mm culture dishes filled with 3 ml of the same medium. All cultures were incubated at 37°C in a humid atmosphere with 2% CO_2.

Media were changed at weekly intervals and subcultures were done when the bottom of the experimental dish was covered by large confluent cell colonies, that is, approximately every 10-14 days. Human bone marrow cells were obtained from marrow samples collected in vials containing 100 I.U. preservative-free heparin. The samples were diluted by adding alpha medium, transferred into narrow tubes and centrifuged for ten minutes at 1800 RPM in a clinical centrifuge, resuspended and separated on a Ficoll gradient.

Quantitative experiments were carried out by means of a colony forming unit (CFU) culture assay in methyl cellulose semi-solid medium as described by Iscove et al.[9] In this assay, 100,000 human or mouse bone marrow cells contained in 1 ml of semi-solid medium were plated in 35 mm tissue culture dishes. The medium contained 20% FCS, 20% ACM providing stimulating activity, 20% alpha medium, and 40% methyl cellulose stock solution. The stock solution contained 2% methylcellulose in alpha medium and was enriched with 2% essential amino acids solution, 1% non-essential amino acids solution, and 0.4% L-asparagine (10 mg/l). The plates were incubated at 37° in a humid atmosphere with 6% CO_2 for 7 days for mouse cells or 14 days for human cells, and the number of colonies (more than 50 cells) was counted.

To assay phagocytosis, a suspension of charcoal particles in complete culture medium (1:20, vol/vol.) was prepared. Three drops of charcoal suspension were mixed with the medium in a cell culture dish, and the dish was incubated at 37°C for four hours. After incubation, the cultures were washed and evaluated with the use of a phase-contrast microscope.

To liberate cells for subcultures, they were trypsinized for 10 minutes at 37°C in a solution of Trypsin-Versen, and a cell scraper was used to detach the cells from the bottoms of their dishes.

Clinical Studies

Selection of Patients

For the randomized study, patients with long lasting, unhealing and relapsing ulcers accompanying venous insufficiency were selected. After a period of preparatory treatment which did not exceed 14 days, the initial debridement and cleaning of ulcers as well as the treatment of peri-ulcerative dermatitis were accomplished. During this period of time, the patients were randomized into experimental or control groups by the flip of a coin. Non-healing ulcers accompanying other diseases such as arteriosclerosis were accepted for treatment, but these patients were not considered as being part of the randomized study. All patients in this investigation were hospitalized.

Experimental Treatment

Following randomization, all ulcers were photographed and their outlines were traced onto transparent film. A pretreatment biopsy was taken from the center of the ulcer. Reconstituted ACM (designated Medium A) was applied twice a day by means of a saturated gauze dressing covered by an impermeable membrane for 14 days. Patients in the control group received culture medium without amniochorion (designated, Medium B) under the same conditions. After the first week of treatment, the ulcers were photographed. At the end of treatment, the ulcers were again photographed and their outlines were traced onto a transparent film, and a follow-up biopsy was done. During the treatment, the patients did not receive medical treatment (such as steroids) which could alter wound healing.

Biopsy

Punch biopsies 8 mm in diameter were obtained from the center of the ulcer bed. The obtained tissue was divided in half. One half was placed in 10% buffered formalin for histological examination (H-E), Masson's trichrome stain, PAS, and Wilder's reticulin stain), and the other half was frozen in liquid nitrogen and processed for Factor VIII by immunohistology according to Matter and Faulk.[10] Second biopsies were sufficiently removed from the first so as to avoid errors in interpretation.

RESULTS

Laboratory Studies

In the first experiment, 3,250,000 MBM cells in 16 ml medium were seeded into 25 cm^2 Falcon flasks, and 25% ACM was added to experimental dishes. After 5 days, a proliferation of adherent MBM cells in colonies was observed in the experimental dishes while cells in the control flasks did not manifest any growth. Dose-response experiments were then done employing 1,000,000 MBM cells in 5 ml of medium seeded into 35 mm culture dishes supplemented with ACM ranging from 1 to 80%. The most intense cellular proliferation appeared in the experimental dishes containing 20% ACM. This concentration was therefore used in the following experiments.

750,000 MBM cells in 5 ml of media were seeded into 35 mm culture dishes. The cells in experimental dishes were stimulated by the addition of 20% WACM, CHCM, or AECM, all produced by the cultivation of the corresponding tissues in the media with FCS, NCS, or without serum. The proliferation of MBM cells was observed with all of these conditioned media, but growth was definitely more vigorous in the conditioned media produced in the presence of FCS or NCS, prompting us to culture all future amniotic membrane in medium containing serum.

The next experiment was done to study what type of cell was stimulated by ACM. MBM cells (500,000) were seeded into 35 mm culture dishes in 3 ml of medium, and the experimental dishes received 20% ACM. Two populations of cells were visible in both the experimental and control dishes after 24 hours. These consisted of large attached cells and smaller ones which were either unattached or loosely attached. After 48 hours, the attached cells in the experimental dishes appeared noticeably enlarged in comparison with their counterparts in the control dishes, and by 72 hours small colonies of large, round or spreading cells appeared in experimental dishes. By the sixth day there was a vigorous growth of colonies in the experimental dishes (Fig. 8.1), and in the control dishes there were no colonies at all. By 10 days, 1-2 small colonies could however, be noticed in the control dishes, but at this time the experimental dishes contained colonies of spread cells which were often covered by masses of loosely attached cells. It was possible to detach these round cells by pipetting and to subculture them. If they were subcultured in sufficiently high density, they began to form new colonies of large, spread cells in about 4 days. When cells from both the experimental and control dishes were harvested by trypsinization, growth was obtained only from the experimental dishes.

When charcoal particles were added into the dishes which contained proliferating MBM cells, more than 90% of the cells were observed to phagocytose these particles (Fig. 8.2), suggesting that the proliferating cells were macrophages.

Finally, we used the colony forming unit assay to quantitate the biological activity of each preparation of ACM. Table 8.1 shows our results with the use of both human bone marrow (BM) and MBM cells.

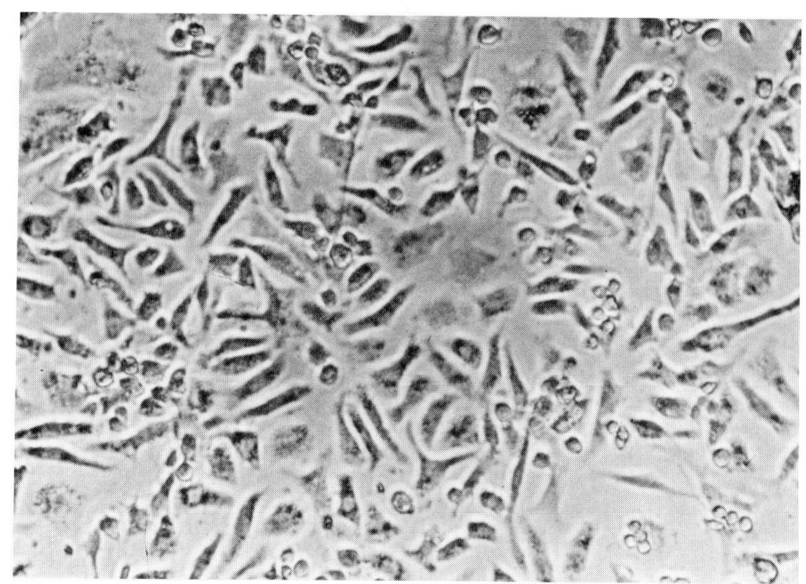

FIGURE 8.1 Colony of MBM cells on the 6th day of culture. (180x)

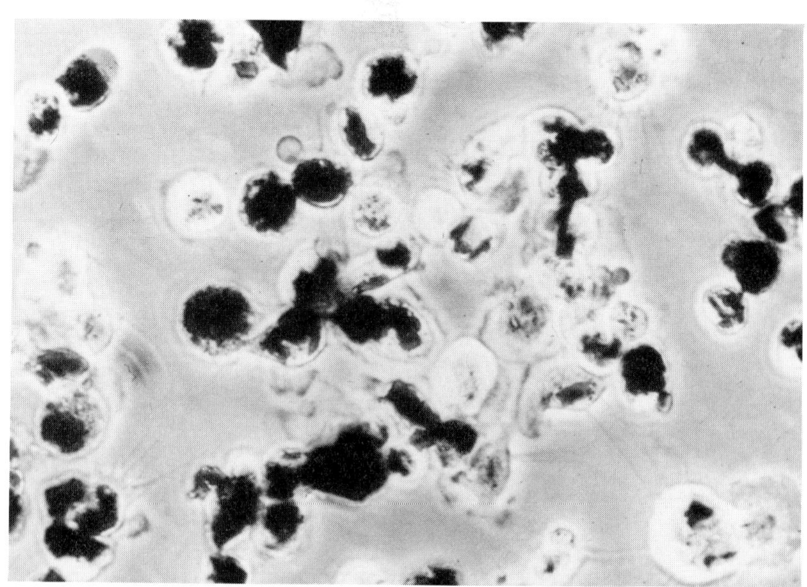

FIGURE 8.2 Phagocytosis of charcoal particles. (360x)

TABLE 8.1

Colony Stimulating Activity of ACM*

Number	Human BMC† Colonies	Mouse BMC Colonies	Day of Culture
1	31 ± 5	52 ± 3	1 - 3
2	34 ± 4		1, 2, 3 - 4
3	23 ± 9		1, 2, 3 - 4
4	80 ± 12		1, 2, 3 - 5
5	88 ± 18		1, 2, 3 - 6
6	104 ± 11		1, 3, 3 - 6
7_A**	80 ± 7		1 - 3
7_B	87 ± 6		4 - 6
8_1**		122 ± 7	1 - 10
8_2		93 ± 14	1 - 10
9_1		88 ± 4	1 - 10
9_2		213 ± 9	1 - 10
10_1		223 ± 23	1 - 10

* ACM is amnion conditioned medium.
† BMC is bone marrow cells.
**Lettered subscripts are ACM from different times, numbered subscripts are from different halves of same amniochorion.

Clinical Studies

To date, we have successfully treated six patients with venous leg ulcers with the use of intact amniotic epithelium according to Bennett et al.[2] and Faulk et al.,[1] and the results of that preliminary study confirmed in every detail the findings of previous investigators who have used intact extra-embryonic membranes in the treatment of stasis ulcers (for a review, see Matthews, Bennett & Faulk).[11] In the present randomized study, we have treated 9 patients with the use of ACM, the details of which are given in Table 8.2. As can be seen in the table, the application of ACM improved healing of leg ulcers in the majority of cases, and control medium had a minimum and largely negligible effect. Such healing could be correlated not only with the quality of granulation tissue, but also with epithelization (Figs. 8.3 and 8.4).

TABLE 8.2

Clinical Studies of Human Amniochorion: Leg Ulcers Treated with ACM or Control Medium (9 patients with less than 2 year follow-up)

Age/Sex	Duration (years)	Diagnosis	Treatment* With Medium	Clinical/Biopsy Results
75/F	2	Venous	A	Improved 3+
64/M	2/12	Venous	B	Deteriorated
60/M	6	Venous	A	Improved 1+
61/M	10	Venous	B	Stable
86/F	20	Venous	B	Stable
73/F	40	Venous	B	Improved 2+
80/F	20	Arteriosclerosis	A	Stable
75/M	4/12	Arteriosclerosis	A	Improved 3+
64/M	2/12	Venous	A	Improved 2+

* Medium A is ACM, medium B is control.

Histological pictures of biopsies obtained from leg ulcers before treatment were characterized by the presence of thick-walled capillaries with narrow lumina which were very similar to those reported by Faulk and co-workers.[1] These were rarely filled with blood and were delimited by a layer of flat endothelial cells (Fig. 8.5). Besides these capillaries, non-canalized young vessels vaguely similar to sweat ducts (Fig. 8.6) and necrotic capillaries were also seen. Reticulin stains revealed that the basement membranes possessed a honey-combed appearance (Fig. 8.7). Immunohistological reactions for Factor VIII-related antigen, a marker of endothelial cells,[10] have shown that most cells of the thick-walled capillaries are of endothelial origin (Fig. 8.8). Some endothelial cells even detached from the capillary walls, suggesting that they may exceptionally migrate into the extra-vascular spaces.

Application of control medium did not change the character of the vessels in any of the cases we have treated. This is true even in patient no. 6 who manifested a clinical improvement on medium B. (See Table 8.2.) In contrast, the application of ACM has been followed in all cases by an appearance of thin-walled capillaries filled with blood. Reticulin stains on biopsies of ulcers after treatment with ACM have revealed thin-walled capillaries with well-formed basement membranes (Fig. 8.9), and these observations of an improvement in vascularity have been corroborated by immunohistological reactions for Factor VIII showing well-formed intracytoplasmic granules of Factor VIII reactive endothelial cells (Fig. 8.10).

DISCUSSION

The discovery of angiogenic factors in tumor[12] and normal tissues[13] was followed by attempts to use these factors in the therapy of diseases with insufficient vascularization. This approach was impeded by ethical considerations which prevented the use of tumor tissues for the production of such factors. However, the use of amniochorions poses no ethical, medical or legal problems, and they are easily available for culture. Thus, when it became apparent that amnion epithelium exerted a beneficial effect on the healing of leg ulcers[1,2] and many other types of non-healing wounds,[3,14] we decided to explore further the possibility of making a more universally-available preparation of amnion for treatment, and we were attracted to the idea that ACM was both easily accessible and inexpensive.

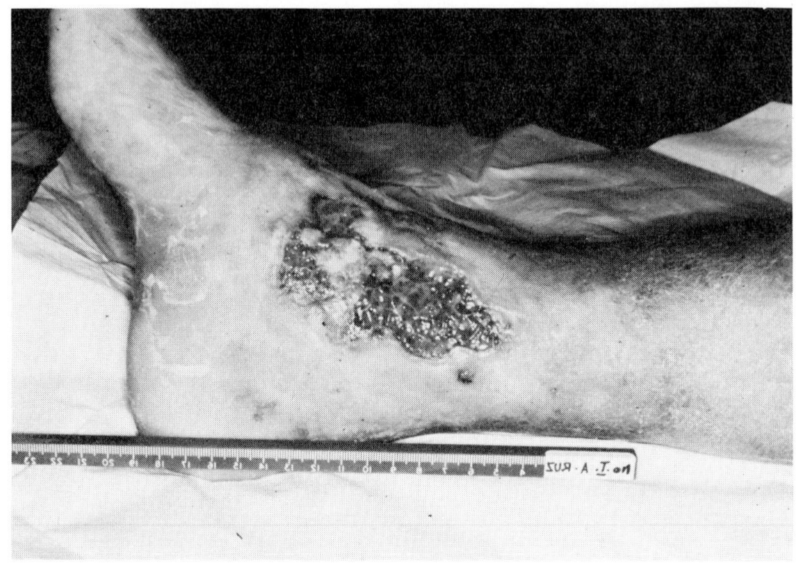

FIGURE 8.3 Typical leg ulcer before treatment with ACM.

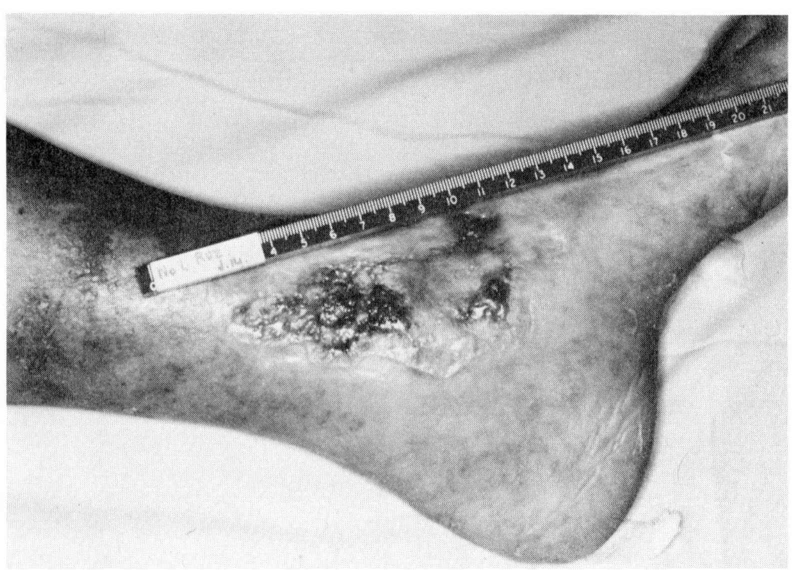

FIGURE 8.4 The same leg ulcer as in Fig. 8.3, but after 14 days of treatment with ACM.

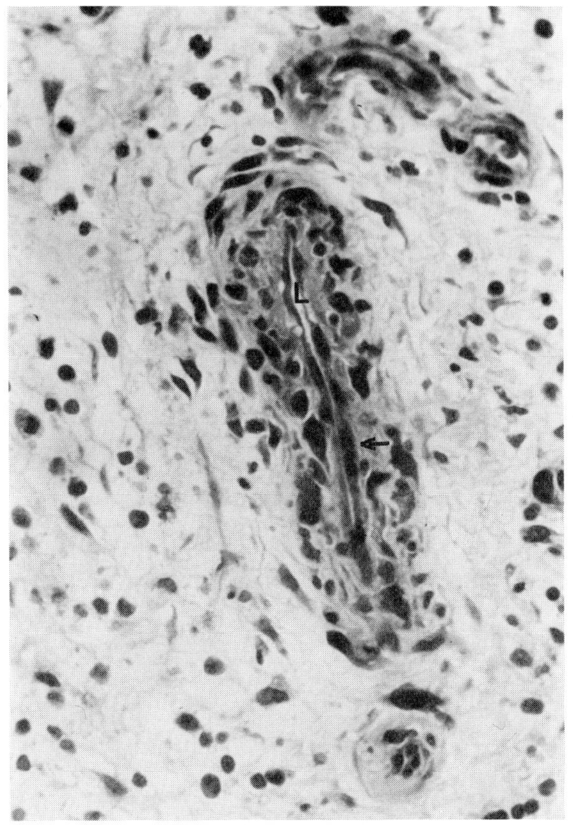

FIGURE 8.5 (right) Parasagittal section of a hyperplastic capillary before ACM treatment. Note narrow slit-like lumen. (446x)

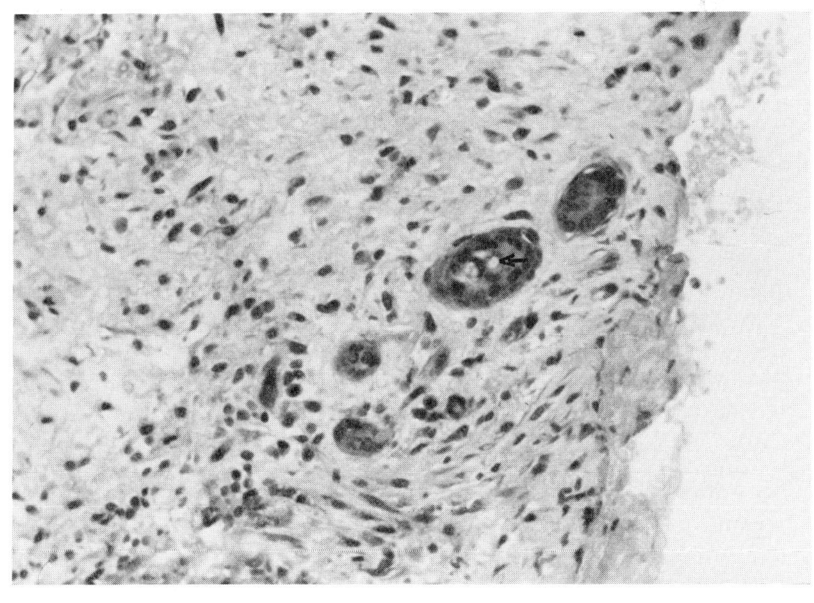

FIGURE 8.6 (below) Hyperplastic capillary sprouts without lumina. H&E stain of leg ulcer biopsy taken before application of ACM. (446x)

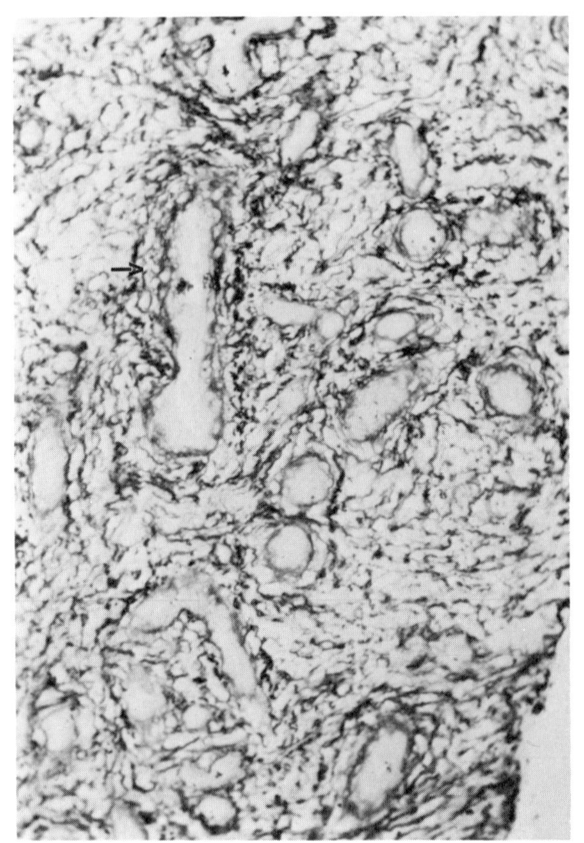

FIGURE 8.7 (left) Honey-combed appearance in reticulin stain of basement membranes of hyperplastic capillaries in leg ulcer biopsy before treatment with ACM. (176x)

FIGURE 8.8 (below) Hyperplastic capillaries in leg ulcer biopsy taken before ACM treatment showing immunoreactivity for Factor VIII in most cells. Note some cells appear to be entirely detached from capillary wall. (446x)

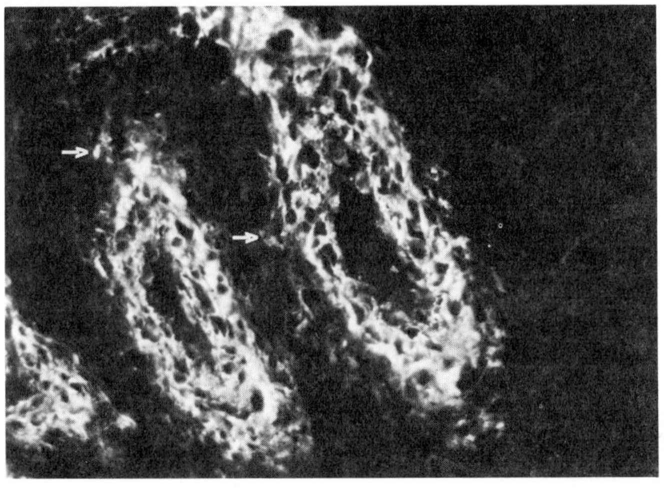

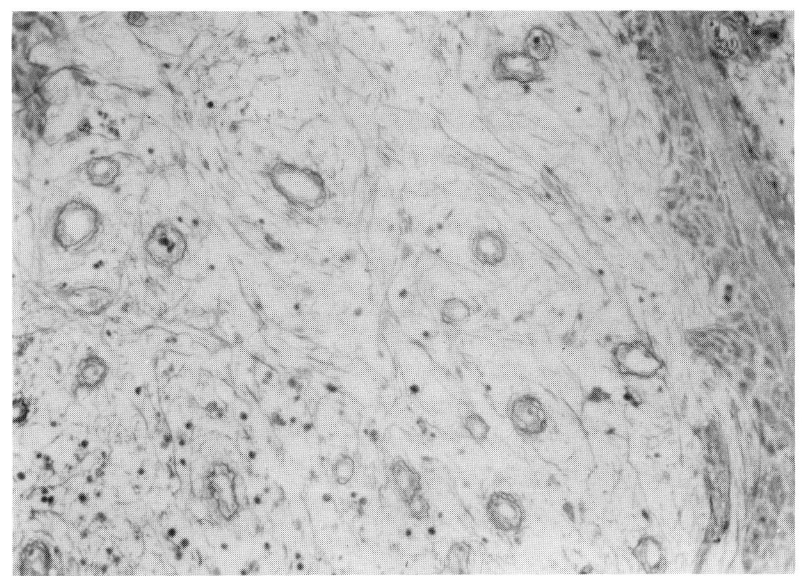

FIGURE 8.9 Post-ACM treatment. Leg ulcer biopsy stained for reticulin showing basement membranes of thin-walled capillaries. (176x)

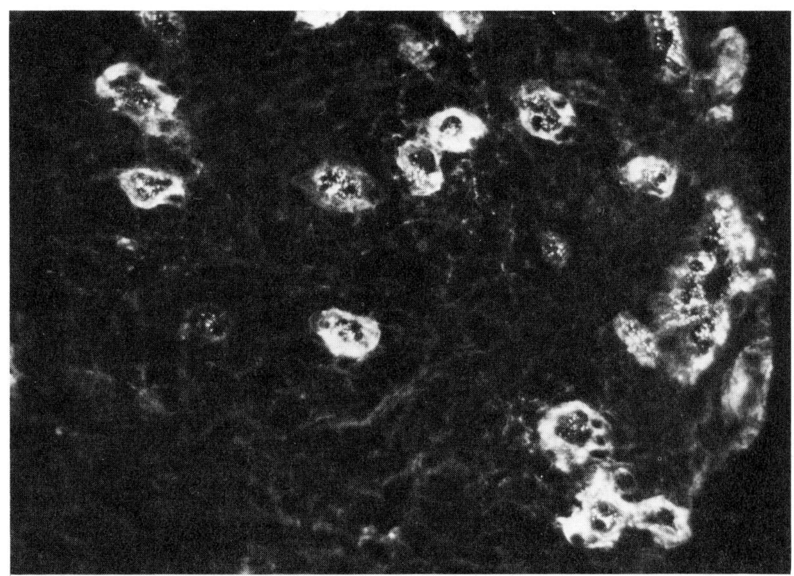

FIGURE 8.10 Post-ACM treatment. Leg ulcer biopsy showing immunoreactivity of Factor VIII related antigen in thin-walled capillaries. (176x)

In order to learn how ACM works, we turned our attention to bone marrow, as this contains many progenitor cells, and we were curious to learn which of these were stimulated by ACM. Following a good deal of experimentation, it seems fairly clear that the principal cell type to be stimulated in marrow is the macrophage. This observation does not, however, exclude a direct action of ACM on endothelial cells or capillaries. The macrophage has a well-known role in wound healing, including supposed angiogenic functions, thus putting forward the possibility that the role of ACM in wound healing is mediated by macrophages which stimulate the formation of new capillaries. There are, unfortunately, no quantitative in vivo or in vitro methods to measure angiogenesis, causing us to turn to the use of the colony forming unit (CFU) assay as a possible technique to measure the activity of our preparations. Our decision to use this assay was based on the idea of a common origin for endothelial and hematopoietic cells,[15] and the possibility that these cells might have retained sensitivities to the same growth-promoting factors.

There is a general consensus that the main reason for the development of venous ulcers is venous hypertension which damages cutaneous capillaries, and that capillaries react to venous hypertension by endothelial hyperplasia and inflammation.[16] Indeed, when we had an opportunity to study the ulcer bed biopsies obtained before treatment with ACM, we were impressed by the intensity of endothelial proliferation which in some sections was reminiscent of capillary hemangiomas. We also took careful note of the relative absence of inflammatory changes in capillaries, even necrotic ones.

The presence of noncanalized hyperplastic capillary sprouts suggests that capillaries in the nonhealing wounds may not have become hyperplastic because of the venous hypertension, but that they might have grown in such a way from the beginning. The narrow lumina and thick walls of these hyperplastic capillaries which are rarely filled with blood indicate that they function inefficiently, and this impression is supported by the observation that the pattern of Factor VIII reactivity in these vessels is not at all like that which one might expect to find in normal endothelium. The presence of human Factor VIII in the cells situated on the outer side of hyperplastic capillaries or even in the cells detached from the capillary suggests their possible migration into the extravascular space, as has been described for some vascular tumors.[17]

The use of ACM as an adjunct in wound healing for venous ulcers undoubtedly increases the amount of vascular tissue.

Nevertheless, it seems that the most important action of ACM is its capacity to induce the formation of normal thin-walled capillaries filled with blood, thus it is possible that ACM acts more as a differentiating factor than as a growth factor. The question of whether this is a differentiating factor produced secondarily by macrophages or primarily by ACM remains to be answered by future research.

SUMMARY

After a successful treatment of chronic venous ulcers with human amnion epithelium, the possibility of using amnion conditioned medium (ACM) in their therapy was explored. ACM was produced by culturing human amniochorions with 10% new-born calf serum. The medium was collected, lyophilized and used after reconstitution. The growth-promoting property of this material was studied in cultures of mouse bone marrow cells with 20% ACM. This stimulated proliferation of adherent cells in colonies. These cells phagocytized charcoal particles, suggesting that they were macrophages. The macrophage growth promoting factor was quantified with a colony forming culture assay by using human or mouse bone marrow cells. The clinical usefulness of ACM on wound healing was studied with the cooperation of nine patients with chronic leg ulcers, mostly of venous origin. These were treated with ACM or control medium.

The application of ACM clinically improved healing of ulcers and control medium had a negligible effect. Histological pictures of biopsies from leg ulcers before treatment were dominated by the presence of thick-walled capillaries with narrow lumina. Their endothelial cells possessed Factor VIII-related antigen. They were often only loosely separated from extra-vascular spaces by honey-combed basement membranes. The use of control medium did not change the character of these capillaries, but the application of ACM was followed by an appearance of thin-walled capillaries filled with blood and having more normal basement membranes. These results suggest that ACM might have a positive influence on both the growth and differentiation of capillaries.

NOTES

1. Faulk, WP, Matthews, RN, Stevens, PJ, Bennett, JP, Burgos, H, Hsi, BL. Human amnion as an adjunct in wound healing. Lancet 1 (1980):1156-1158.

2. Bennett, JP, Matthews, R, Faulk, WP. Treatment of chronic ulceration of the legs with human amnion. Lancet 1 (1980):1153-1156.

3. Matthews, RN, Faulk, WP, Bennett, JP. A review of the role of amniotic membranes in surgical practice. Obstet. Gynec. Annl. 11 (1982):31-58.

4. Faulk, WP, Hsi, BL, McIntyre, JA, Yeh, GCJ, Mucchielli, A. Antigens of human extra-embryonic membranes. J. Reprod. Fert. In press.

5. Burgos, H, Faulk, WP. The maintenance of human amniotic membranes in culture. Brit. J. Obstet. Gynaecol. 88 (1981):294-300.

6. Yeh, GCJ, Hsi, BL, Faulk, WP. Propidium iodide as a nuclear marker in immunofluorescence. II. Use with cellular identification and viability studies. J. Immunol. Meth. 43 (1981):269-275.

7. Hudson, L, Hay, FC. In Practical Immunology. Oxford, London, Edinburgh, Melbourne, Blackwell Publications (1976), p. 115.

8. Metcalf, D. Hemopoietic Colonies. New York: Springer Verlag (1977), p. 12.

9. Iscove, NN, Seiber, F, Winterhalter, KH. Erythroid colony formation in cultures of mouse and human bone marrow: Analysis of the requirement for erythropoietin by gel filtration and affinity chromatography on agarose-concanavalin A. J. Cell. Physiol. 83 (1974):309-320.

10. Matter, L, Faulk, WP. Fibrinogen degration products and Factor VIII. Consumption in normal pregnancy and pre-eclamsia: Role of placenta. In Hypertension in Pregnancy, Bonnar, J, McGillivray, I, Symonds, M (eds.). Lancaster: M.T.P. Press (1980), pp. 357-369.

11. Matthews, RN, Bennett, J, Faulk, WP. Amnion on wounds: A perspective. In Reproductive Immunology, Gleicher, N (ed.). New York: Liss Publications (1981), pp. 269-280.

12. Greenblatt, M, Shubik, P. Tumor angiogenesis. Transfilter diffusion studies in the hamster by the transparent chamber technique. J. Natl. Cancer Institute 41 (1968):111-124.

13. Nismioka, K, Ryan, TJ. The influence of the epidermis and other tissues on blood vessels growth in hamster cheek pouch. J. Invest. Dermatol. 58 (1972):33-45.

14. Matthews, RN, Bennett, J, Faulk, WP. Wound healing using amniotic membranes. Brit. J. Plastic Surg. 34 (1981): 76-78.

15. Smith, RA, Glomski, CA. Hemogenic endothelium of the embryonic aorta: Does it exist? Developm. Comp. Immunol. 6 (1982):359-368.

16. De Graciansky, P, Boulle, M, Boulle, S, Guilaine, J. Ulcere de jambe. In Atlas de Dermatologie, Vol. X (Texte). Paris: Maloine (1973).

17. Beranek, J. Activities enzymatiques des hemangiomes cutanes. Etude histologique et histoenzymologique. Memoire pour le Titre d'Assistant Etranger. Faculté de Medecine de Paris (1970), 128 pp.

9
Effect of Angiogenic Factors on the Vascularization of IVALON™ Sponge Implants

David S. Jackson, Lola Kamp,
W. Douglas Sheffield and Barbara Matlaga

INTRODUCTION

A key feature of the wound healing process is neovascularization. This occurs by angiogenesis which involves the budding off of new capillaries from existing blood vessels in neighboring tissues. The new capillaries are formed by the migration and proliferation of endothelial cells into the dead space of the wound. To achieve this neovascularization apparently requires locally produced factors which are chemotactic and/or mitogenic and which are probably secreted by macrophages (see Polverini et al. 1977, Knighton et al., Chapter 3 of this volume) and platelets (Michaeli et al., Chapter 21 of this volume).

In some circumstances, poor vascularization is the underlying cause of poor healing and it may therefore be possible to stimulate neovascularization by the application of angiogenic factors to such wounds. The experiments we report were designed to test this idea, using implanted IVALON™ Sponges as a wound model.

MATERIALS AND METHODS

The isolation and characterization of a number of putative angiogenic factors has been described (see Folkman 1982 for review). In our study the angiogenic factor was derived from

---

The angiogenic factors were kindly provided by Dr. J. B. Weiss, University of Manchester, England. We also thank Linell Griffin for typing the manuscript.

bovine retina or from mouse lymphoma cell conditioned media. In both cases the factor has a molecular weight of 300-400 and was highly active in the standard chorioallantoic membrane (CAM) bioassay.

IVALON™ Sponge Implantation

Discs of IVALON™ Sponges 2 cm in diameter and 2 mm thick were prepared. The discs were boiled in distilled water for 3 hours to remove residual formaldehyde, dried at 60°C, weighed and sterilized by autoclaving. Immediately before implantation, the sponges were impregnated with the test material dissolved in phosphate buffer saline (PBS). Control sponges were impregnated with PBS alone. The dilution of the angiogenic factor was based on the results of the CAM assay.

The sponges were implanted subcutaneously in Sprague-Dawley rats weighing approximately 300 gms. Two sponges were implanted in each rat and 3 rats were used for each time point.

Analysis of Sponges

In the first experiment, the sponges and the surrounding capsule were removed intact and placed in neutral formalin for histological examination with H&E staining. Sponges were removed 7, 13 and 21 days after implantation.

In the second experiment, at each time point, two sponges with capsule were prepared for histological examination with azure eosin staining. Four sponges from which the capsule had been removed, were analyzed for collagen by hydroxyproline determination using the method of Woessner (1961). Sponges were removed 4, 7, 9 and 14 days after implantation.

Morphometric analysis of neovascularization was performed on control and treated sponges removed on Day 14 following implantation.

RESULTS

Retinal Factor

There was some vascularization of the control sponges at Day 7, but the vascular response of the treated wound is con-

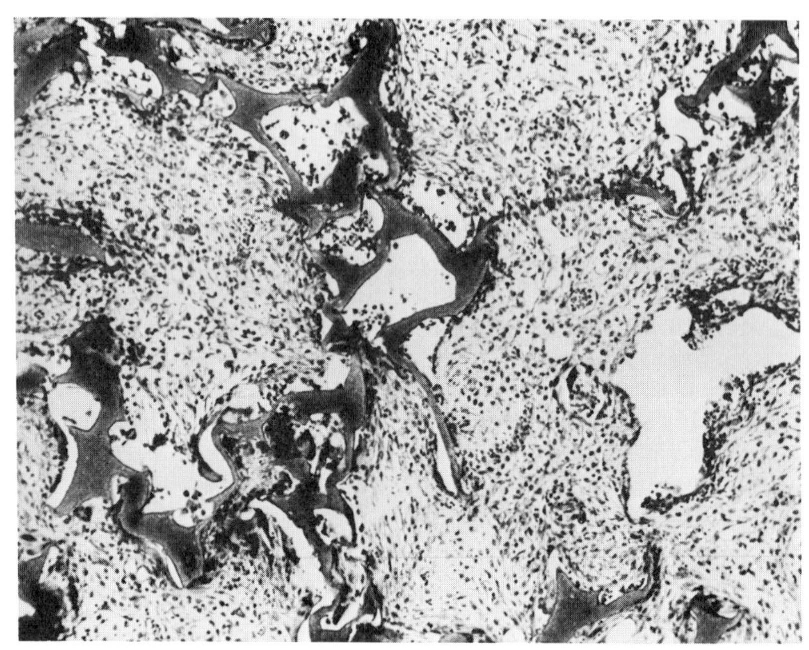

FIGURE 9.1 (a) (above) Center of control sponge. (b) (below) Center of sponge impregnated with bovine retinal angiogenic factor. 7 day implantation H&E. Mag X 25.

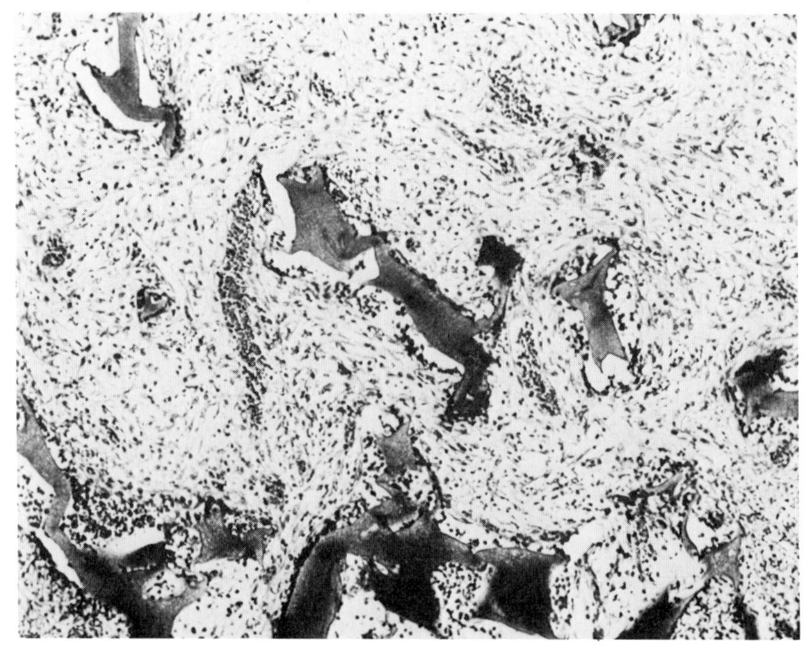

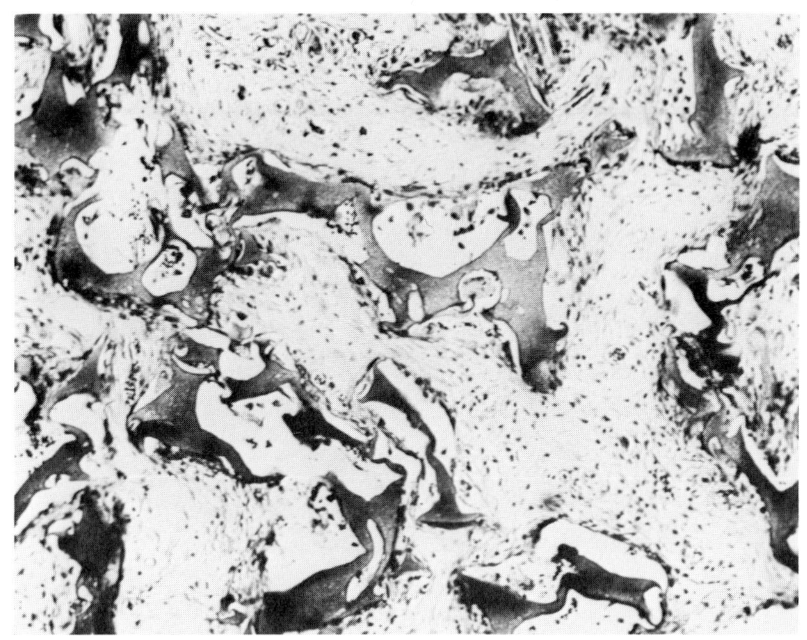

FIGURE 9.2 (a) (above) Control sponge. (b) (below) Sponge impregnated with bovine retinal angiogenic factor. 13 day implantation H&E. Mag X 25.

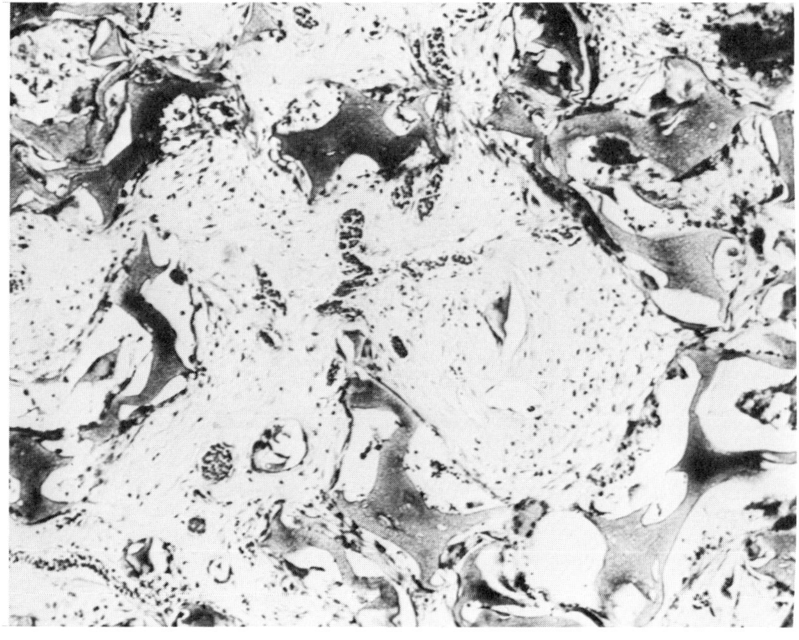

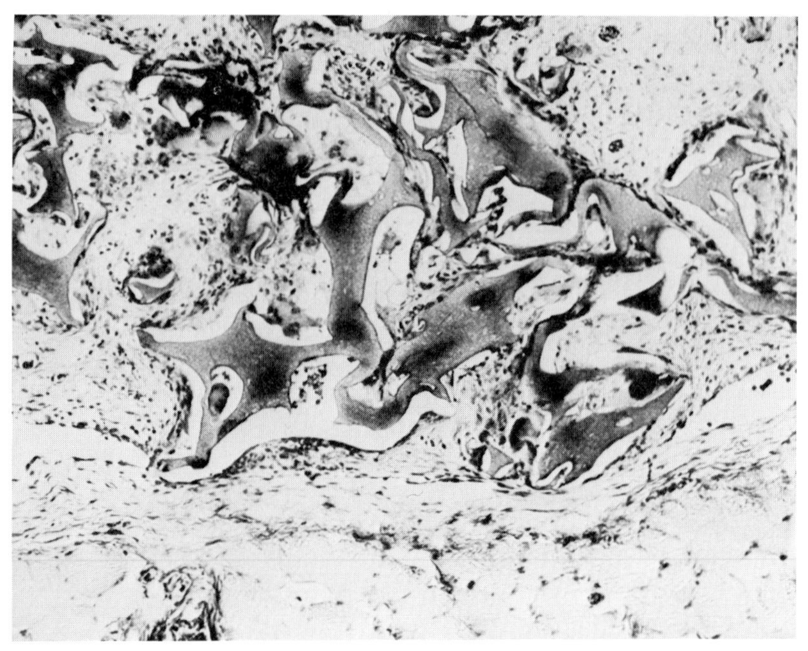

FIGURE 9.3 (a) (above) Capsule region control. (b) (below) Capsule region of sponge impregnated with bovine retinal angiogenic factor. 13 day implantation H&E. Mag X 25.

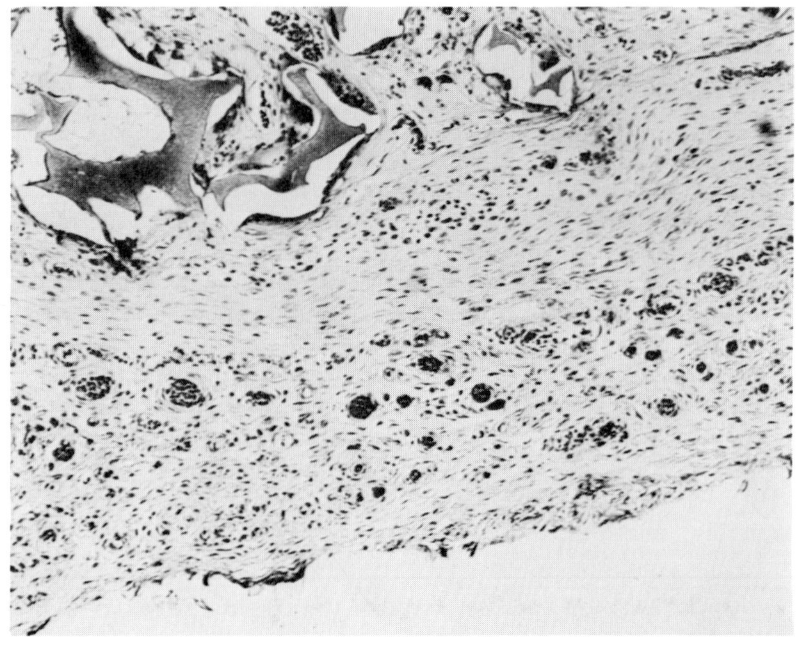

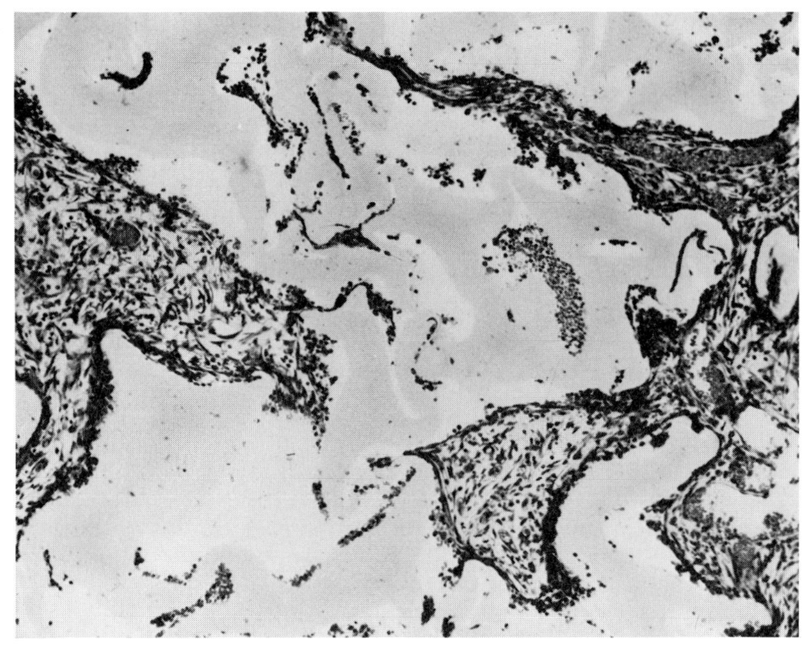

FIGURE 9.4 (a) (above) Control sponge. (b) (below) Sponge impregnated with mouse lymphoma angiogenic factor. 7 day implantation azure eosin. Mag X 25.

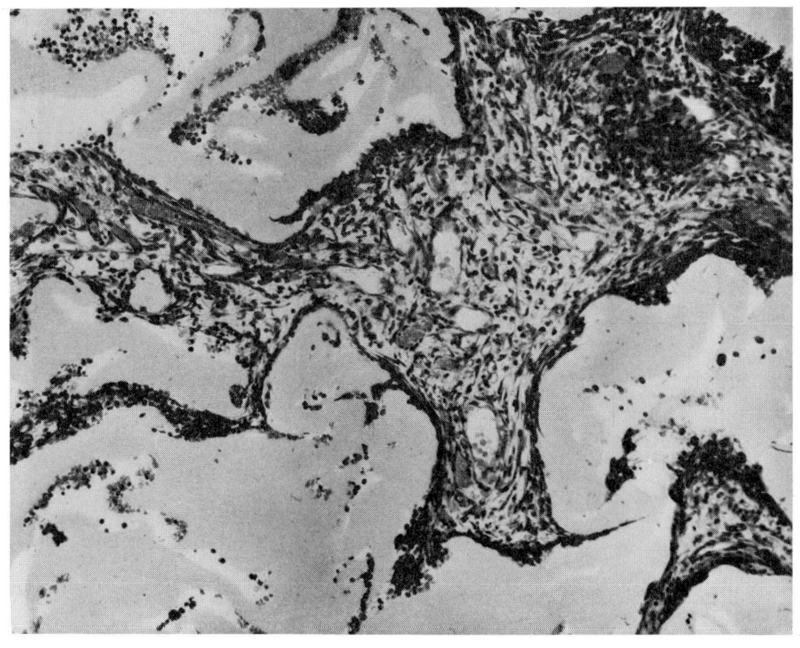

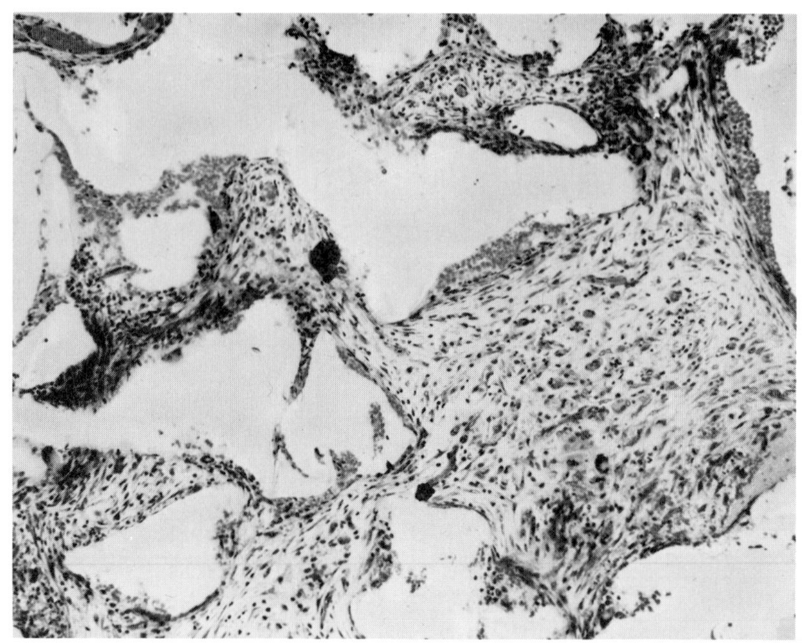

FIGURE 9.5 (a) (above) Control sponge. (b) (below) Sponge impregnated with mouse lymphoma angiogenic factor. 9 day implantation azure eosin. Mag X 25.

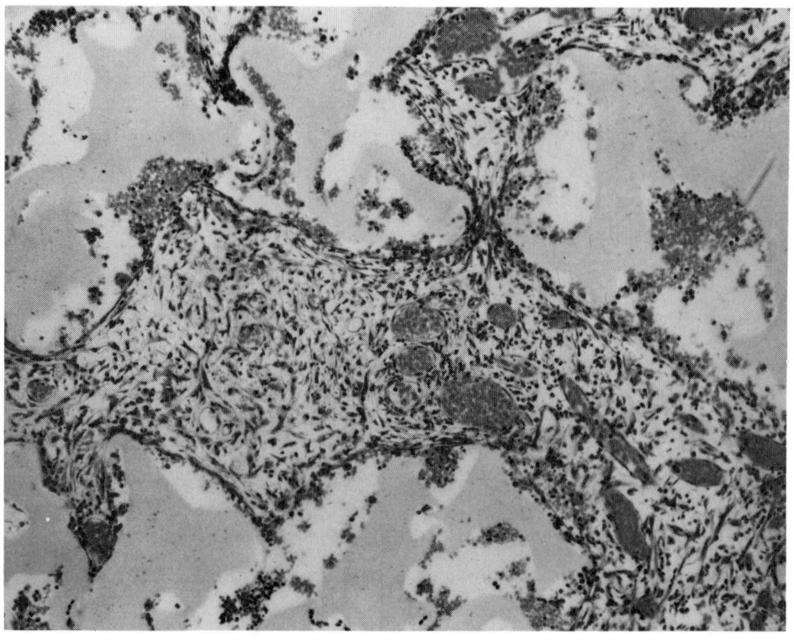

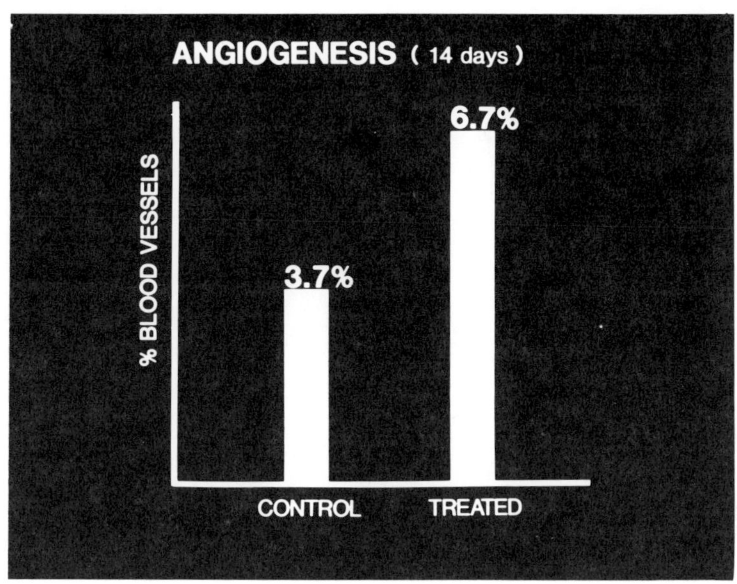

FIGURE 9.6 (above) Morphometric analysis of vascularization of sponges at 14 days. 5 randomly chosen sites from two samples each of control and treated sponges were evaluated.

FIGURE 9.7 (below) (a) Control sponge. (b) Sponge impregnated with mouse lymphoma angiogenic factor. 14 day implantation. Van Gieson Mag X 63.

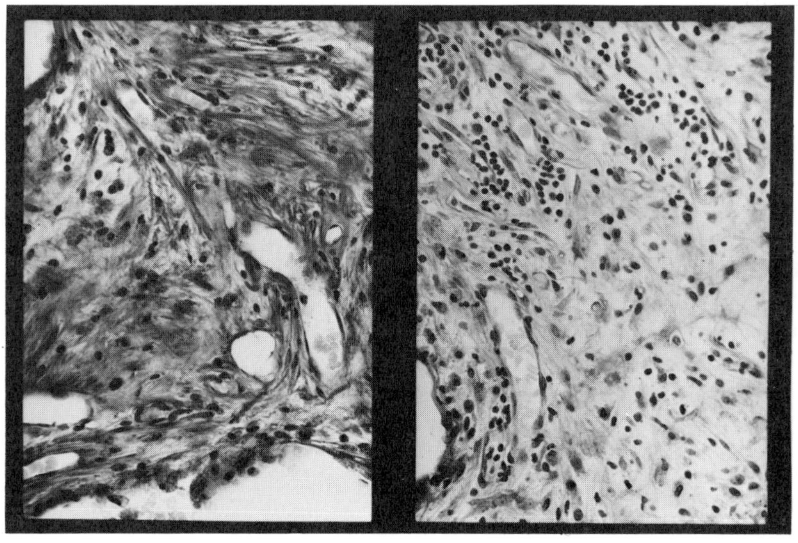

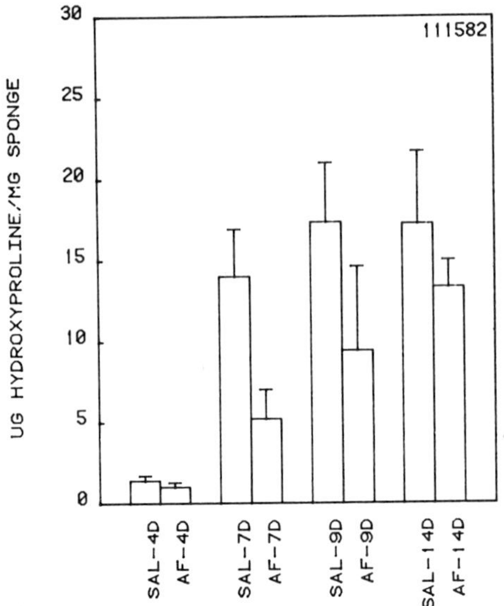

* SAL–Saline; AF–Angiogenic Factor.

FIGURE 9.8 Collagen content of control and treated sponges measured as hydroxyproline.

siderably greater (Fig. 9.1). There are more capillaries and the diameters of the capillaries are greater. By Day 13 the difference between the control and treated sponges is even more obvious (Fig. 9.2). In the treated sponges, branching blood vessels are frequently seen but occur rarely in the controls.

Figure 9.3 shows the vascularization of the capsule which forms around the sponges. Here again the vascularization of the treated sponge is much richer. Also noteworthy is the fact that all the vessels appear to be running in parallel across the surface since virtually all the vessels in the capsule are seen in transverse cross-section. The fibrous tissue formed in the treated sponges appeared to be denser and more mature.

Mouse Lymphoma Factor

In contrast to the first experiment, at 7 days the vascularization of the treated sponges was much more sparse then in the controls (Fig. 9.4). By the 9th and 14th day, however, the treated sponges were more richly vascularized (Fig. 9.5). This is confirmed by the morphometric analysis carried out on the 14 day sponges (Fig. 9.6): the average blood vessel area of the treated sponge being almost twice that of the controls.

In the treated sponges there was a general tendency for the granulation tissue to maintain an immature appearance, with numerous hypertrophic, basophilic fibroblasts and endothelial cells remaining at the later time periods. There was also a corresponding paucity of collagen deposition, an extreme example being seen in Figure 9.7. The delay in collagen formation is also seen in the analyses of the collagen content of the sponges (Fig. 9.8).

DISCUSSION

The results with the retinal factor show that neovascularization is stimulated by angiogenic factor applied locally. There is an increase in both number and size of the capillaries invading both the sponge and the capsule surrounding it. Similar results are seen with a factor derived from platelets (see Michaeli et al., Chap. 21 of this volume).

However, the events observed with mouse lymphoma factor follow a different time course in that both vascularization and granulation tissue formation are delayed. Increased vascularity is eventually obtained as can be seen in Figure 9.6 and by Day 14 collagen formation is approaching that of the control (Fig. 9.8). A possible explanation for the different time course of events between the two angiogenic preparations may be in the nature of angiogenic factors and the difficulty of quantifying their potency. The factors used in this study are extremely potent, possibly at picogram and certainly at nanogram levels (Dr. J. B. Weiss, personal communication). They are available only in minute amounts and in the absence of a chemical identity the actual amount applied to each sponge is not known. Further, the CAM assay is not quantitative so that the actual angiogenic activity applied to the sponge is not known. To compound the issue further, it is now known that above a certain level the angiogenic factor is inhibitory rather than stimulatory, both of neovascularization and of endothelial cell proliferation *in vitro* (Dr. J. B. Weiss, personal communication).

A possible explanation for this result observed with the mouse lymphoma factor is that the initial concentration was high enough to be inhibitory. As the factor diffused out of the sponge the concentration would fall until it reached a level at which neovascularization was stimulated. This might account for the delay in neovascularization to the 9th day following implantation. This delay could also account for the delay in the maturation of the granulation tissue since this will depend on the availability of a good blood supply.

The rate of maturation of granulation tissue in sponges treated with retinal factor correlated with the increased vascularity. This is also seen with platelet derived angiogenesis, as reported by Michaeli et al., in Chapter 21 of this volume.

Recently we have used lower concentrations of mouse lymphoma angiogenic factor with results similar to those obtained with the retinal factor. Thus both, this study and that of Michaeli et al., suggest that, at least in the IVALON™ Sponge model, the rate and degree of vascularization of granulation tissue can be increased with locally applied angiogenic factor and that this can result in increased connective tissue formation.

REFERENCES

Folkman, J. Angiogenesis: Initiation and control. In Annals. N.Y. Acad. Sci. 401:212-227 (1982).

Polverini, PJ, Coltran, RS, Gimbrone, MA, and Unanue, ER. Activated macrophages induce vascular proliferation. Nature 269:804-805 (1977).

Woessner, J. The determination of hydroxyproline in tissue and protein samples containing small proportions of this amino acid. Arch. Biochem. Biophys. 93:440-448 (1961).

10
Biophysics of Fracture Repair and Bone Regeneration

Carl T. Brighton

INTRODUCTION

Biophysics is the study of the physical forces acting upon or within living cells. Of the various physical forces that one might expect to pertain to bone or cartilage cells, i.e. mechanical, heat, electricity, only electricity has been studied in depth. This chapter will review the electrical signals present in bone (endogenous signals), the effects of applying electricity to bone (exogenous signals), the clinical application of the use of electricity in treating nonunions of fractured bones, and it will review the possible mechanisms of electrically induced osteogenesis.

Endogenous Electrical Signals in Bone

Two types of electrical potentials have been described in bone: 1) stress generated potentials and 2) bioelectric potentials.

Stress generated potentials were originally described by Yasuda in 1953.[127] They originate from the organic component of bone when it is mechanically stressed, are not dependent upon cell viability, occur in both wet and dry bone, are electronegative on the side of compression and electropositive on the side of tension, occur in bone, cartilage, and tendon, and are thought to be caused by streaming potentials and/or piezoelectricity.[5,52,54,85,89,103,112,116] Studies with microelec-

---

Supported in part by USPHS grant AM 18033.

trodes (Figure 10.1) have shown that, as the haversian canal is approached in an osteon under tension, the electrical potential becomes more positive (or less negative); and as the haversian canal is approached in an osteon under compression, the potential becomes more negative.[105] Since the area immediately adjacent to the haversian canal is the most reactive region in the osteon, a region where bone is formed or resorbed, the following associations become tenable:

(a) Compression → Electronegativity → Bone Formation
and
(b) Tension → Electropositivity → Bone Resorption

As will be shown later, experiments with exogenously applied electrical signals to bone support (a) the bone formation side of the association, but no evidence as yet is present supporting (b) the bone resorption side of the association. It should be noted here that the microelectrode studies described above are the best evidence to date linking stress generated potentials to a physiological function, that is, bone formation.

Bioelectric potentials were originally described by Friedenberg and Brighton in 1966.[45] Such potentials are static, in contradistinction to the dynamic stress generated potential. Bioelectric potentials are dependent on cell viability, are not dependent on mechanical stress, are electronegative in areas of active growth and repair, and are neutral or electropositive in less active areas.[46,48] When a fracture is present in bone, a strong peak of electronegativity appears over the healing area (see Figure 10.2). This peak of electronegativity is present throughout the entire healing process although, as the fracture heals, the amplitude of the peak gradually declines. Whether or not this peak of electronegativity has physiological significance is not known, for the peak could be present either as a cause or as an effect.

A secondary peak of electronegativity occurs over the growth plate at the proximal end of a long bone in which a fracture is present in the shaft (as shown in Figure 10.2). This secondary peak may have physiological significance when one considers that a fractured long bone in a child frequently overgrows. Such overgrowth or increase in longitudinal growth occurs in the growth plates. The signal that instructs the growth plate to increase linear growth is unknown. The secondary peak of electronegativity does not appear to be present as an effect, since the original trauma and its attendant cellular activity and response are far removed from the growth plate.

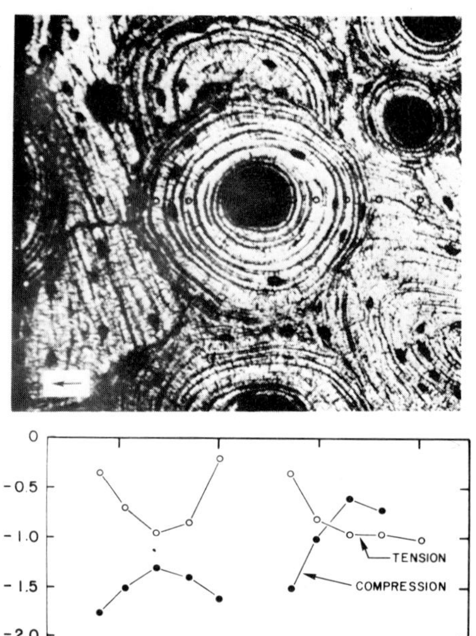

FIGURE 10.1 Composite picture showing (top) transverse section of bone with a Halversian osteon in the center and (bottom) graph of the stress generated potentials at various loci in relationship to the Haversian canal with the bone in tension versus compression.
Source: Electrical Properties of Bone and Cartilage, Brighton, CT, Black, J, and Pollack, SR (eds), p. 75. New York: Grune and Stratton, 1979. Reprinted with permission.

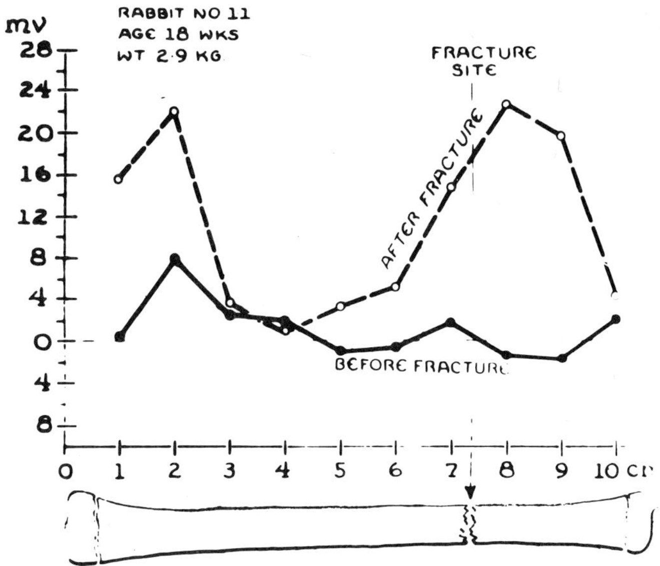

FIGURE 10.2 Graph showing bioelectric potentials from the surface of the in situ rabbit tibia before and after fracture.

Hence, it is possible that the signal that turns on the growth plate in such circumstances is the secondary peak of electronegativity.

It is postulated that stress generated potentials play a physiological role in bone remodeling and bone maintenance, whereas bioelectric potentials play a role in bone growth and repair. Whether or not this hypothesis is correct awaits further experimentation.

Exogenous Electrical Signals Applied to Bone

There are several methods of applying electricity to bone. The great majority of the studies investigating the effects of electricity on bone have employed direct current (Figure 10.3). Many investigators have confirmed and considerably expanded upon the original observation of Yasuda that bone forms in the vicinity of the cathode given the proper current and voltage.[9, 36,49,50,51,55,57,58,64,65,66,68,69,75,80,82,88,92,95,96,107, 114,115,118,121,122,123,126,128]

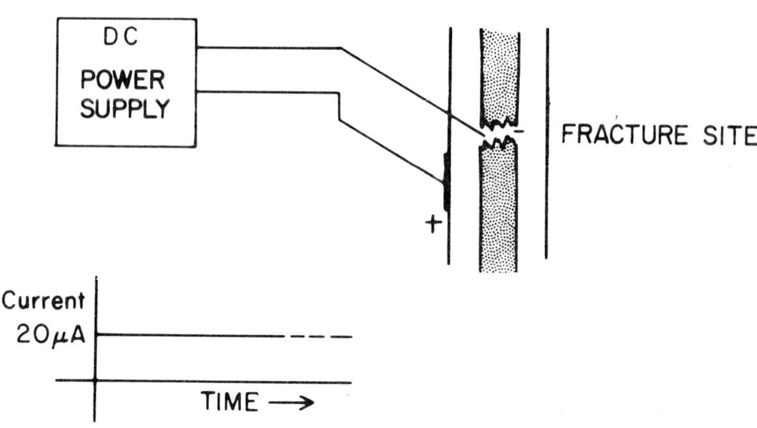

FIGURE 10.3 Drawing depicting apparatus used for direct current stimulation of osteogenesis. Note that the cathode must be in the area to be stimulated; the anode may be placed on the skin even at sites remote from the cathode. Using stainless steel cathodes, 20 μamps constant direct current has been found to be optimal for osteogenesis.

Using various in vitro and in vivo models in our laboratory, we have developed the following principles as they apply to osteogenesis induced by direct current: (1) given the proper parameters of current and voltage, and using stainless steel electrodes, bone forms only in the vicinity of the cathode, whereas cell necrosis occurs around the anode[51]; (2) resistance rapidly increases between the electrodes, leading to a concomitant decrease in current; if a constant current is to be maintained, an active power supply utilizing a transistorized control circuit must be provided[51]; (3) electrically induced osteogenesis exhibits a dose-response curve in which current levels of less than five microamperes delivered through a stainless steel cathode do not produce osteogenesis, current levels of five to 20 microamperes produce progressively increasing amounts of bone formation, and current levels greater than 20 microamperes show bone formation giving way to cellular necrosis[50,51]; (4) electricity can favorably influence fracture-healing in laboratory animals, but to do so, the cathode must be directly in the fracture site[49]; (5) given the proper parameters of current and voltage, electricity can induce bone formation in the absence of trauma and in areas where bone formation is not presently active, as for example in the medullary canal of an adult animal[50]; (6) the reaction at the cathode results in oxygen consumption and hydroxyl radical production[20]: $2H_2O + 4e^- + O_2 \rightarrow 4\,OH^-$; (7) pulsed direct current is not as effective in producing osteogenesis as is constant direct current[33,118]; and (8) the electrically "active" area of the cathode is at the junction of the insulation and bare wire and measures approximately 0.02 square millimeter; thus, the actual current density utilizing stainless steel as the cathode is 1×10^{-3} amperes per square millimeter.[16,33]

Alternating current has not been shown to date to be able to stimulate significant amounts of new bone formation.

Electricity can also be induced in bone by means of inductive coupling (Figure 10.4). A time-varying electrical signal is applied to a pair of Helmholtz coils, and a time-varying magnetic field is produced. This time-varying magnetic field, in turn, induces a time-varying electrical field in the tissues situated between the coils. Bassett et al.[10] were the first to apply inductive coupling for stimulating osteogenesis. An alternating current applied to coils placed external to the skin on either side of a dog's osteotomized fibula produced a time-varying magnetic field which, in turn, induced a time-varying electrical field in the bone centered between the coils. The signal used had a pulse duration of 150 microseconds repeated at sixty-five Hertz (cycles per second), and a peak amplitude of 20 millivolts per centimeter in bone. At the end of 28 days, the fibulae were mechanically tested to determine stiffness. Results indicated that the osteotomized fibulae subjected to the electrical field were significantly stiffer than control fractured fibulae not subjected to the electrical field.

Bassett[5,13] and his group have studied various pulse shapes and patterns and have refined the signal several times. At present they use a bipolar, quasirectangular-base pulse pattern which is asymmetrical in timing and amplitude. The main polarity portion of each pulse is 200 microseconds in duration and the opposite polarity portion of each pulse is 20 microseconds. This allows the pulses to be grouped in a burst configuration, the duration of which is five milliseconds. Each burst of pulses repeats at a rate of 15 Hertz. The peak amplitude of each individual pulse induces in bone a peak current density of 10 microamperes per square centimeter.

A third method used to apply electricity to bone is termed capacitive coupling. In capacitive coupling, an electrical field is induced in bone by an external capacity; that is, two charged metal plates are placed on either side of an animal's limb and

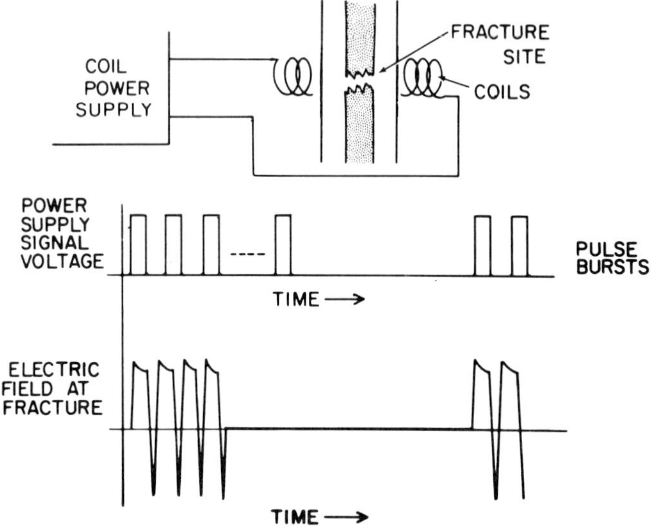

FIGURE 10.4 Drawing depicting apparatus used for stimulation of osteogenesis with inducative coupling. A time varying electrical field (power supply signal voltage) is applied to the pair of coils, producing a time varying magnetic field, which, in turn, induces a time varying electrical field in the bone and tissue located between the coils.

are attached to an appropriate voltage source (Figure 10.5). Several studies have shown that both constant and pulsed capacitively-coupled electrical fields can favorably influence fracture repair in rabbits[6] and in vitro epiphyseal plate growth.[27,101] The voltages employed in these early studies, however, were too high for clinical use. Recently, capacitively-coupled fields of much lower voltages (output signal 5 volts peak-to-peak sinusoidal wave form, and a frequency of 60 KHz) have been found to be stimulating to the rabbit proximal tibial growth plate.[24]

Clinical Application of Electrically Induced Osteogenesis

Based on the laboratory studies just summarized, the clinical usefulness of electrically induced osteogenesis began to be explored in the early 1970s. To date, the vast majority of all this clinical investigation has been with nonunions, or fractures that failed to unite. Since all of the early laboratory studies employed direct current, it follows that the early clinical studies also used direct current. The first patient treated for nonunion showed solid bone-healing of the medial malleolus after nine weeks of constant direct current of 10 microamperes.[47] This was the first recorded instance of healing of a nonunion with electricity in modern times (although there were isolated reports of the use of electricity in treating nonunion and congenital pseudarthrosis during the last century.[56,86] Further

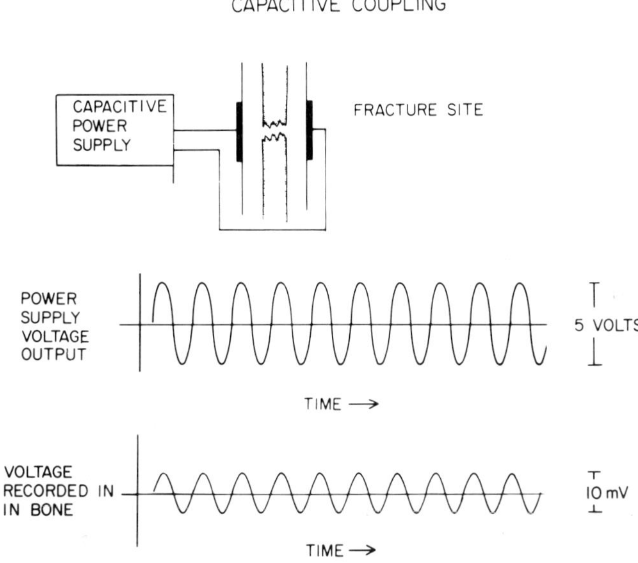

FIGURE 10.5 Drawing depicting apparatus used for stimulation of osteogenesis with capacitive coupling. A time varying electrical signal (power supply voltage output) is applied to capacitor plates located on the limb surface. This produces a time varying electrical field in the bone and tissue placed between the capacitor plates.

experience with the use of direct current in treating nonunion, demonstrated that solid bone-healing was achieved in 84% of the patients when proper electrical parameters were employed.[21,28-30]

In 1977 the study was expanded to include 12 participating investigators throughout the United States. The results indicate that, given proper electrical parameters and proper cast immobilization, a rate of bone union comparable to that seen with bone-graft surgery was achieved.[26]

Experience dictated that four cathodes, each delivering 20 microamperes of constant direct current for 12 weeks, were required to heal a nonunion of a long bone. Of 178 nonunions in 175 patients treated with adequate electricity in the University of Pennsylvania series, 149 (83.7%) achieved solid bone union. Patients with a history of osteomyelitis had a healing rate of 74.4%. The presence of previously inserted metallic fixation devices did not affect the end-result healing rate. Of eighty nonunions in 79 patients treated with electricity in the participating investigators' series, 58 (72.5%) achieved solid bone union.

Review of the nonunions treated unsuccessfully with constant direct current suggested that inadequate electricity, the presence of synovial pseudarthrosis or infection, and dislodgment of the electrodes are causes for failure with the procedure. Complications of the electrical treatment were minor and there was no deep infection resulting from this procedure in patients without previous osteomyelitis. It was concluded that the practicing orthopaedic surgeon utilizing constant direct current to treat nonunion should be adhering to proper fracture management, and by applying the proper current and voltage, be able to achieve a rate of union comparable to that of bone graft surgery at a lower associated risk.

Many other investigators have verified the above clinical studies that constant direct current can, indeed, be employed successfully to heal nonunions[14,15,27,38,67,83,91,117,124,129] or congenital pseudarthrosis of the tibia.[81] A few investigators have also utilized pulsed direct current to heal nonunion.[62,72,73]

Direct current may be applied to nonunion through percutaneously inserted electrodes (Figure 10.6), a semi-invasive technique in which the cathodes are inserted through the skin down into the nonunion site, the anode is placed on the skin, and the power supply is incorporated in plaster. Direct current may also be applied to nonunion through a totally invasive system (Figure 10.7) in which the cathode is placed in the nonunion site and the anode and power supply are buried in the sub-

Methods of Applying Electricity to Bone

Semi-Invasive: Direct Current

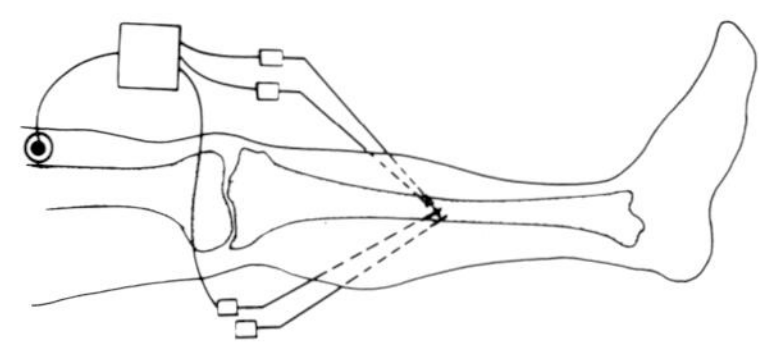

Advantages:	Disadvantages:
Portable	Cathode Irritation/Infection
No Open Procedure	Requires Patient Co-operation

FIGURE 10.6 Drawing showing a semi-invasive method of applying direct current in the treatment of nonunion. Some of the advantages and disadvantages of this method of treatment are given. Four cathodes are inserted percutaneously into the nonunion site. The anode is placed on the skin, and the power pack is incorporated in plaster

Methods of Applying Electricity to Bone

Invasive: Direct Current

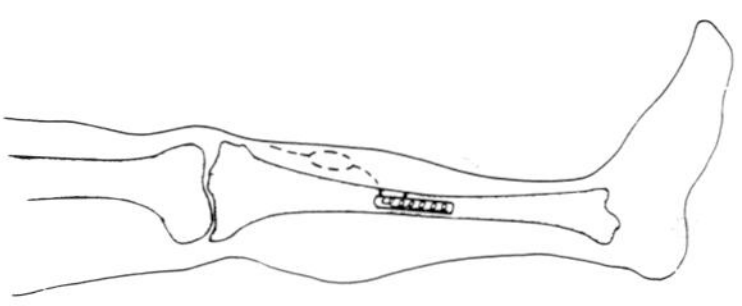

Advantages:	Disadvantages:
Portable	Two Open Surgical Procedures
Independent of Patient Cooperation	Infection Risk × 2
	Cathode Left Behind
Spine Pseudarthrosis	Cannot Be Monitored

FIGURE 10.7 Drawing showing a totally invasive method of applying direct current in the treatment of nonunion. The cathode is wound into a helical configuration and is inserted into a slot made in the bone at the nonunion site. The power pack and anode are buried in the subcutaneous tissue. Advantages and disadvantages of this method are given.

cutaneous tissue. Both methods are reported to give the same rate of healing (80-85%); and this is the same rate of healing reported for bone graft surgery in treating nonunion.[19,20,76,130] Some of the advantages and disadvantages of the two methods are depicted in Figures 10.6 and 10.7.

Bassett et al.[10] in 1974, were the first to employ the principles of inductive coupling in treating nonunion. The signal that eventually evolved has been described previously in this article. In the several series reported by Bassett on the treatment of nonunion with pulsing electromagnetic fields (PEMFs), he found a healing rate of 80-87%.[8,11,12] The advantages and disadvantages of this noninvasive form of treating nonunions with electricity are depicted in Figure 10.8.

Several other investigators have employed various forms of inductive coupling in treating nonunion, and success rates have varied from 64-85%.[49,74,120] In addition, inductive coupling has been employed by Bassett[13] and others[25] in treating congenital pseudarthrosis. The series reported so far are too small to draw any conclusions, but the success rates are apparently not as high as in acquired nonunions.

Methods of Applying Electricity to Bone

Non-Invasive: Inductive Coupling

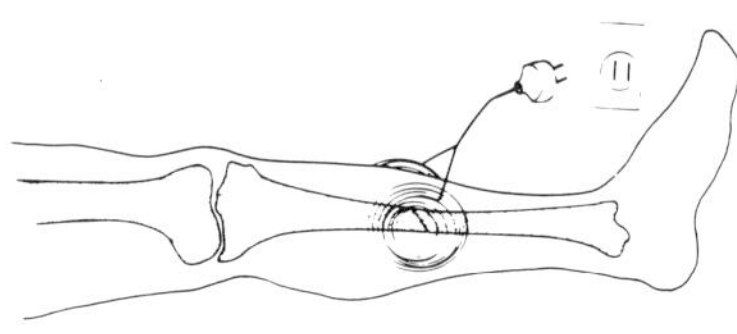

Advantages:	Disadvantages:
No Operative Procedure	Not Portable
No Infection Risk	Requires Patient Co-operation

FIGURE 10.8 Drawing showing a noninvasive inductive coupling method of applying electricity to bone in the treatment of nonunion. A pair of Helmholtz coils is centered over the nonunion site. Advantages and disadvantages of this method are given.

To date only one patient has been treated for nonunion with a capacitively coupled electrical field.[25] A 29-year-old male with nonunion of the tibia of two years' duration, in whom previous bone graft surgery had failed, was treated for 24 weeks with signal output of five volts peak-to-peak, symmetrical sine wave, of frequency 60 KHz (see Figure 10.9). At the end of that time, roentgenograms out of plaster revealed the nonunion to be healed (see Figure 10.10). The theoretical advantages and disadvantages of a capacitively-coupled electrical field in treating nonunion are depicted in Figure 10.11. A large multicenter study to evaluate this method of treating is now underway.

Electricity in various forms is also being studied for possible use in the treatment of delayed union, failed fusions, aseptic necrosis, and osteoporosis. However, none of these studies has been reported in the literature as yet.

Direct current has been used in augmenting spinal fusions, but the series is too small to be meaningful.[41,74]

The subject of treating fresh fractures in patients with electricity is controversial at this time. Studies in laboratory animals have indicated an increased stiffness to mechanical testing of callus fractures exposed to various forms of electricity as compared to that of the controls.[49] However, this increased stiffness is only present during the middle phase of fracture healing. Early and late in the course of fracture healing, there were no differences in stiffness between control and experimental calluses. The net result was that the time to solidify bony union was the same in control and experimental animals. Jørgenson, on the other hand, reported a slight decrease in healing time in patients with fresh fractures of the tibia treated with a slowly pulsed, asymmetrical direct current.[72,73] Most investigators in this field at the present time believe that only those fresh fractures prone to delayed or nonunion, as for example an open fracture accompanied by extensive soft tissue damage, should be treated with electricity.

Possible Mechanisms of Electrically Induced Osteogenesis

The mechanisms by which electricity induces osteogenesis are largely unknown. However, in considering possible mechanisms, it is convenient to consider changes in the microenvironment, which are indirect effects, and direct cellular effects.

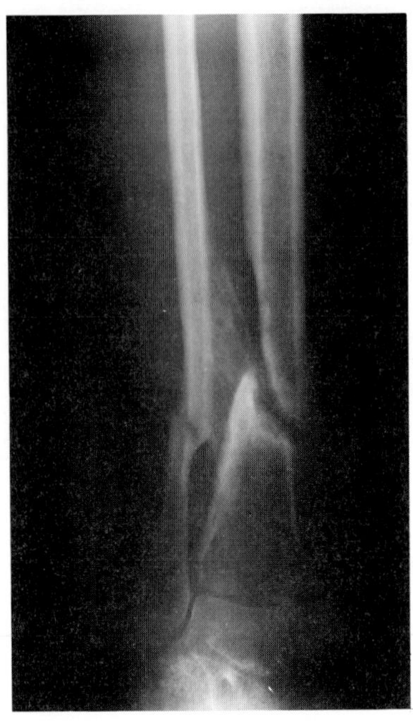

FIGURE 10.9 (left) Antero-posterior roentgenographic view of the nonunion of the left tibia. A previous posterior bone graft procedure has resulted in a cross union between the distal fragment of the tibia and the fibula. A previous fibular osteotomy has healed. (With permission from J. Trauma, 1983.)

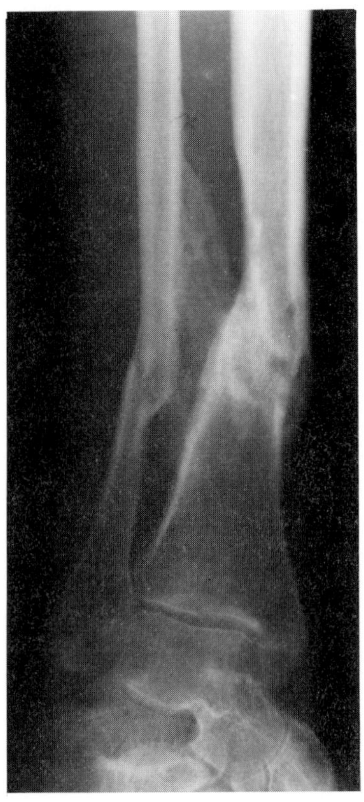

FIGURE 10.10 (right) Antero-posterior roentgenographic view of the left tibia after twelve weeks of continuous treatment with a capacitively coupled electrical field and a second twelve-week period during which time the patient utilized a weight-bearing short leg cast. The nonunion is healed. (With permission from J. Trauma, 1983.)

Methods of Applying Electricity to Bone

Non-Invasive: Capacitive Coupling

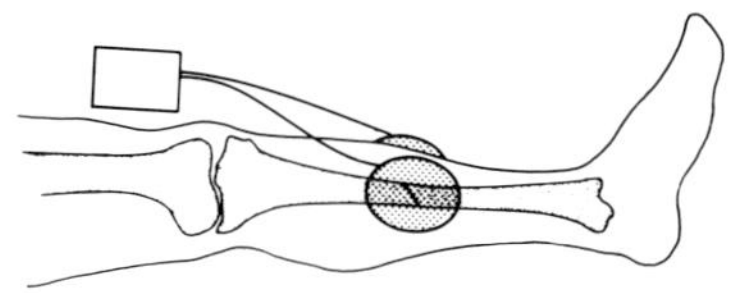

Advantages:	Disadvantages:
Portable	Requires Patient Co-operation
No Operative Procedure	
No Infection Risk	

FIGURE 10.11 Drawing showing a non-invasive, capacitive coupling method of applying electricity to bone in the treatment of non-union. Capacitor plates are placed on the opposite sides of the extremity at the site of nonunion. Some of the advantages and disadvantages of this method are given.

Changes in the microenvironment occur when direct current is used, at least in the vicinity of the cathode. It is known that the cathode consumes oxygen and produces hydroxyl radicals according to the following equation:[16,32]

$$2HO_2 + O_2 + 4e^- \rightarrow 4\ OH^-$$

Thus, according to the above equation, the local pO_2 in the vicinity of the cathode should decrease and the local pH should increase. That this actually occurs *in vivo* in the medullary canal of the tibia was recently shown by Baranowski et al.[4] At 20 microamps direct current, the optimum current for osteogenesis when using stainless steel cathodes, there was a significant ($p < 0.05$) reduction in pO_2 in the medullary canal of the rabbit tibia in the vicinity of the cathode as measured by implanted oxygen needle microelectrodes. At the same time, there was a significant ($p < 0.05$) increase in the pH. At current levels less than optimal, these changes in the microenvironment did not occur.

That low tissue oxygen tension is favorable to bone formation has been demonstrated by a number of studies: (1) low pO_2 values have been measured at the bone-cartilage junction in the growth plate[22] and in newly formed bone and cartilage in fracture calluses[23,61]; (2) optimum in vitro bone growth occurs in a low (5%) oxygen environment[31]; and (3) growth-plate cartilage cells[78] as well as bone cells[17,40,119] follow a predominantly anaerobic metabolic pathway. That an alkaline environment is favorable to calcification has been suggested by the rather high pH (7.70 ± 0.05) found in the growth plate at the calcification front by Howell et al.[63]

Other microenvironmental changes include changes in calcium concentration at the cathode due either to hydrolysis of ATP, in which case calcium phosphate precipitates at the cathode,[87] or to ionic electrophoresis leading to calcium ion accumulation at the cathode.[125]

The noninvasive forms of electrically induced osteogenesis may also bring about changes in the microenvironment by alternating enzyme activity such that changes occur in the extracellular matrix. Thus, pulsing electromagnetic fields have been shown to lead to an increase in lysozyme activity which, in turn, may lead to proteoglycan disaggregation.[97] In the growth plates, proteoglycan disaggregation must occur before the cartilage matrix can calcify. Both alkaline phosphatase[110] and acid phosphatase[111] have been reported to decrease in various pulsing electromagnetic fields, whereas acid mucopolysaccharides, indicating disaggregated proteoglycan and a calcifiable matrix, reportedly increased when exposed to pulsing electromagnetic fields.[111]

The changes in the microenvironment cited above lead indirectly to cellular changes which ultimately result in osteogenesis. Electricity may also act directly on the bone cell. Many authors have studied cellular cyclic AMP in bone and cartilage cells in response to inductively- and capacitively-coupled electrical fields.[18,42,60,71,90,100,101,113] In general, these studies indicated an increase in intracellular cAMP when exposed to an electrical field. However, some authors have suggested that cAMP increased in bone cells whereas it decreased in cartilage cells when subjected to pulsing electromagnetic fields.[60,71,100,101] Lubin et al.[90] demonstrated that mouse calvarial bone cells show a significant decrease in the cAMP response to parathyroid hormone after being exposed to pulsing electromagnetic fields.[90] This suggests that one action of the electrical field is to desensitize the bone cell membrane receptor to parathyroid hormone. If this, indeed, does happen, then PTH-induced bone resorption would be decreased. Somjen et al.[113] found that, at low field strengths, cAMP activity decreased, whereas at higher field strengths cAMP activity increased. They also found that bone cells primarily responded to the higher electrical field.

Intracellular calcium has been shown to increase when bone cells were exposed to pulsing electromagnetic fields by several authors.[7,44,77,93,104,109] Johnson and Rodan[70] showed that a pulsing electromagnetic field led to increased release of arachidonate and increased production of prostaglandin E in rat osteosarcoma-derived osteoblastic cells grown in monolayer.

Other studies have shown an increase in ^{3}H-thymidine,[2,3,34,35,39,77,99,102,108,109] ^{35}S,[1,34,43,44,97,106] ^{3}H- and ^{14}C-proline,[1,7,44,54,90,94] as well as ^{3}H-uridine[7] incorporation in bone and cartilage cells under the influence of pulsing electromagnetic fields or capacitively-coupled fields. Finally, Norton et al.[98] demonstrated increased cellular adherence to glass tubes of bone cells subjected to a capacitively-coupled field and Laub and Korenstein[79] showed increased induction of actin polymerization in bone cells stimulated by a pulsing electromagnetic field.

It is quite obvious from these many studies that electricity of various forms can have profound effects on all bone and cartilage cells. The actual mechanism(s) of action, however, of electrically-induced osteochondrogenesis is certainly not obvious from these studies. More definitive studies linking electrical field to cellular event at the membrane level to cellular response must be performed before mechanisms are understood. In the meantime, biophysics has provided the clinician with an apparently powerful tool for mediating bone and cartilage cell activity exogenously from outside the body.

NOTES

1. Archer, CW, and Ratcliff, NA. The effects of pulsed magnetic fields on bone and cartilage in vitro. Trans. of the Bioelectrical Repair and Growth Soc. 1:1, 1981.

2. Ashihara, T, Kagawa, K, Kamachi, M, Inoue, S, Ohashi, T, and Takeoka, O. ^{3}H-thymidine autoradiographic studies of the cell proliferation and differentiation in the electrically stimulated osteogenesis. In Electrical Properties of Bone and Cartilage, pp. 401-426. Edited by C. T. Brighton, J. Black, and S. R. Pollack. New York: Grune and Stratton, 1979.

3. Assailly, J, Monet, JD, Dautigny, N, and Corvol, MT. Increase of ^{3}H-thymidine uptake in cultured chondrocyte DNA by weak electromagnetically induced pulsating currents. Trans. Bioelectrical Repair and Growth Soc. 1:31, 1981.

4. Baranowski, TJ, Jr, Black, J, and Brighton, CT. Microenvironmental changes associated with electrical stimulation of osteogenesis by direct current. Trans. Bioelectrical Repair and Growth Soc. 2:47, 1982.

5. Bassett, CAL, and Becker, RO. Generation of electrical potentials by bone in response to mechanical stress. Science 137:1063-1064, 1962.

6. Bassett, CAL, and Pawluk, RJ. Noninvasive method for stimulating osteogenesis. J. Biomed. Mater. Res. 9:371-374, 1975.

7. Bassett, CAL, Choski, HR, Hernandex, E, Pawluk, RJ, and Strop, M. The effect of pulsing electromagnetic fields on cellular calcium and calcification of nonunions. In Electrical Properties of Bone and Cartilage, pp. 427-441. Edited by C. T. Brighton, J. Black, and S. R. Pollack. New York: Grune and Stratton, 1979.

8. Bassett, CAL, Mitchell, SN, and Gatson, SR. Treatment of ununited tibial diaphysial fractures with pulsing electromagnetic fields. J. Bone and Joint Surg. 63A:511-523, 1981.

9. Bassett, CAL, Pawluk, RJ, and Becker, RO. Effects of electrical current on bone in vivo. Nature 204:652-655, 1964.

10. Bassett, CAL, Pawluk, RJ, and Pilla, AA. Augmentation of bone repair by inductively coupled electromagnetic fields. Science 184:575-577, 1974.

11. Bassett, CAL, Pilla, AA, and Pawluk, RJ. A non-operative salvage of surgically-resistant pseudarthrosis and non-unions by pulsating electromagnetic fields. A preliminary report. Clin. Orthop. 124:128-143, 1977.

12. Bassett, CAL, Mitchell, SN, Norton, L, and Pilla, AA. Repair of non-unions by pulsing electromagnetic fields. Acta Orthop. Belgica 44:706-724, 1978.

13. Bassett, CAL, Mitchell, SN, Norton, L, Caulo, N, and Gaston, SR. Electromagnetic repairs of nonunion. In Electrical Properties of Bone and Cartilage, pp. 605-630. Edited by C. T. Brighton, J. Black, and S. R. Pollack. New York: Grune and Stratton, 1979.

14. Becker, RO, and Spadaro, JA. Experience with low-current/silver electrode treatment of nonunion. In Electrical Properties of Bone and Cartilage, pp. 631-638. Edited by C. T. Brighton, J. Black, and S. R. Pollack. New York: Grune and Stratton, 1979.

15. Becker, RO, Spadaro, JA, and Marino, AA. Clinical experience with low intensity direct current stimulation of bone growth. Clin. Orthop. 124:75-83, 1977.

16. Black, J, and Brighton, CT. Mechanisms of stimulation of osteogenesis by direct current. In Electrical Properties of Bone and Cartilage, pp. 215-224. Edited by C. T. Brighton, J. Black, and S. R. Pollack. New York: Grune and Stratton, 1979.

17. Borle, AB, Nichols, N, and Nichols, G, Jr. Metabolic studies of bone in vitro. I. Normal bone. J. Biol. Chem. 235: 1206-1210, 1960.

18. Bourret, LA, and Rodan, GA. The role of calcium in the inhibition of cAMP accumulation in epiphyseal cartilage cells exposed to physiologic pressure. J. Cell Physiology 88:353-362, 1976.

19. Boyd, HB, and Lipinski, SW. Causes and treatment of nonunion of the shafts of long bones, with a review of 741 patients (Instructional course lecture). Am. Acad. Orthop. Surg. 17:165-183, 1960.

20. Boyd, HB, Lipinski, SW, and Wiley, JH. Observations on non-union of the shafts of the long bones, with a statistical analysis of 842 patients. J. Bone and Joint Surg. 43A:159-168, 1961.

21. Brighton, CT. Treatment of nonunion of the tibia with constant direct current. J. Trauma 21:189-195, 1981.

22. Brighton, CT, and Heppenstall, RB. Oxygen tension in zones of the epiphyseal plate, the metaphysis, and diaphysis. An in vitro and in vivo study in rats and rabbits. J. Bone and Joint Surg. 53A:719-728, 1971.

23. Brighton, CT, and Krebs, AG. Oxygen tension of healing fractures in the rabbit. J. Bone and Joint Surg. 54A: 323-332, 1972.

24. Brighton, CT, and Pfeffer, GB. _In vivo_ growth plate stimulation in various capacitively coupled electrical fields. _J. Orthop. Res._ 1, 1983.

25. Brighton, CT, and Pollack, SR. Treatment of nonunion of the tibia with a capacitively coupled electrical field: A case report. _J. Trauma_, accepted for publication, 1983.

26. Brighton, CT, Black, J, Friedenberg, ZB, Esterhai, JL, Jr, Day, LJ, and Connolly, JF. A multicenter study of the treatment of nonunion with constant direct current. _J. Bone and Joint Surg._ 63A:2-13, 1981.

27. Brighton, CT, Cronkey, JE, and Osterman, AL. _In vitro_ epiphyseal plate growth in various constant electrical fields. _J. Bone and Joint Surg._ 58A:971-978, 1976.

28. Brighton, CT, Friedenberg, ZB, and Black, J. Evaluation of the use of constant direct current in the treatment of nonunion. In _Electrical Properties of Bone and Cartilage_, pp. 519-546. Edited by C. T. Brighton, J. Black, and S. R. Pollack. New York: Grune and Stratton, 1979.

29. Brighton, CT, Friedenberg, ZB, Mitchell, EI, and Booth, RE. Treatment of nonunion with constant direct current. _Clin. Orthop._ 124:106-123, 1977.

30. Brighton, CT, Friedenberg, ZB, Zemsky, LM, and Pollis, RP. Direct current stimulation of non-union and congenital pseudarthrosis. Exploration of its clinical application. _J. Bone and Joint Surg._ 57A:368-377, 1975.

31. Brighton, CT, Ray, RD, Soble, LW, and Kuettner, KE. _In vitro_ epiphyseal plate growth in various oxygen tensions. _J. Bone and Joint Surg._ 51-A:1383-1396, 1969.

32. Brighton, CT, Adler, S, Black, J, Itada, N, and Friedenberg, ZB. Cathodic oxygen consumption and electrically induced osteogenesis. _Clin. Orthop._ 107:277-282, 1975.

33. Brighton, CT, Friedenberg, ZB, Black, J, Esterhai, JL, Jr, Mitchell, EI, and Montique, F, Jr. Electrically induced osteogenesis: Relationship between charge, current density, and the amount of bone formed. Introduction of a new cathode concept. _Clin. Orthop._ 161:122-132, 1981.

34. Brighton, CT, Unger, A, and Stambough, JA. _In vitro_ capacitively coupled electrical stimulation of bovine articular chondrocyte pellets in varying serum concentrations. _Trans Bioelectrical Repair and Growth Soc._ 2:8, 1982.

35. Brighton, CT, and Wisneski, R. Electrical enhancement of growth plate DNA synthesis _in vitro_ with low voltage capacitive coupling. _Trans. Ortho. Res. Soc._ 27:230, 1981.

36. Cieszynski, T. Studies on the regeneration of ossal tissue. II. Treatment of bone fractures in experimental animals

with electric energy. Arch. Immunol. Ther. Exp. 11:199-217, 1963.

37. Connolly, JF. Healing curve of fractures and the effect of bone growth stimulation. In Electrical Properties of Bone and Cartilage, pp. 547-562. Edited by C. T. Brighton, J. Black, and S. R. Pollack. New York: Grune and Stratton, 1979.

38. Connolly, JF, Hahn, H, and Jardon, JO. The electrical enhancement of periosteal proliferation in normal and delayed fracture healing. Clin. Orthop. 124:97-105, 1977.

39. Corvol, MT, Monet, JD, Dautigny, N, and Assailly, J. Effect of electromagnetically induced pulsating currents on the growth cycle of chick embryo chondrocytes in culture. Trans. Bioelectrical Repair and Growth Soc. 2:41, 1982.

40. Deiss, WP, Jr, Holmes, LB, and Johnson, CC. Bone matrix biosynthesis in vitro. I. Labeling of hexosamine and collagen of normal bone. J. Biol. Chem. 247:3555-3559, 1962.

41. Dwyer, AF, and Wickham, GG. Direct current stimulation in spine fusion. Med. J. Australia 1:73-75, 1974.

42. Facklam, TJ, and Hassler, CR. Electrical stimulation of osteogenic activity in vitro. Trans. Bioelectrical Repair and Growth Soc. 1:5, 1981.

43. Farndale, RW. Stimulation of matrix production by pulsed magnetic fields. Trans. Bioelectrical Repair and Growth Soc. 2:45, 1982.

44. Fitton-Jackson, S, Jones, DB, Murray, JC, and Farndale, RW. The response of connective and skeletal tissues to pulsed magnetic fields. Trans. Bioelectrical Repair and Growth Soc. 1:85, 1981.

45. Friedenberg, ZB, and Brighton, CT. Bioelectric potentials in bone. J. Bone and Joint Surg. 48-A:915-923, 1966.

46. Friedenberg, ZB, Dyer, RH, Jr, and Brighton, CT. Electro-osteograms of long bones of immature rabbits. J. Dental Res. 50:635-639, 1971.

47. Friedenberg, AB, Dyer, RH, Jr, and Brighton, CT. Electro-osteograms of long bones of immature rabbits. J. Dental Res. 50:635-639, 1971.

48. Friedenberg, ZB, Harlow, MC, Heppenstall, RB, and Brighton, CT. The cellular origin of bioelectric potentials in bone. Calcif. Tiss. Res. 13:53-62, 1972.

49. Friedenberg, ZB, Roberts, PG, Jr, Didizian, NH, and Brighton, CT. Stimulation of fracture healing by direct current in the rabbit fibula. J. Bone and Joint Surg. 53-A:1400-1408, 1971.

50. Friedenberg, ZB, Zemsky, LM, Pollis, RP, and Brighton, CT. The response of non-traumatized bone to direct current. J. Bone and Joint Surg. 56-A:1023-1030, 1974.

51. Friedenberg, ZB, Andrews, ET, Smolenski, BI, Pearl, BW, and Brighton, CT. Bone reaction to varying amounts of direct current. Surg., Gyn., and Obstet. 131:894-899, 1970.

52. Fukada, E, and Yasuda, I. On the piezoelectric effect of bone. J. Physiol. Soc. Japan 12:1158-1162, 1957.

53. Goodman, R, Bassett, CAL, and Henderson, AS. Selected electromagnetic field effects on cellular regulatory processes. Trans. Bioelectrical Repair and Growth Soc. 2:42, 1982.

54. Gross, D, and Williams, WS. Streaming potential and the electromechanical response of physiologically moist bone. J. Biomech. 15:277-295, 1982.

55. Harris, WW, Moyen, BJ-L, Thrasher, EL, III, Davis, LA, Cobden, RH, MacKenzie, DA, and Cywinski, JK. Differential response to electrical stimulation. A distinction between induced osteogenesis in intact tibiae and the effect on fresh fracture defects in radii. Clin. Orthop. 124:31-40, 1977.

56. Hartshorne, E. On the causes and treatment of pseudoarthrosis, and especially on that form of it sometimes called supernumerary joint. Am. J. Med. Sci. 1:121-156, 1841.

57. Hassler, CR, Rybicki, EF, Diegle, RB, and Clark, LC. Studies of enhanced bone healing via electrical stimuli. Comparative effectiveness of various parameters. Clin. Orthop. 124:9-19, 1977.

58. Hassler, CR, Cummings, KD, Clark, LC, Rybicki, EF, and Diegle, RB. Augmentation of bone healing via electrical stimuli. In Electrical Properties of Bone and Cartilage, pp. 155-168. Edited by C. T. Brighton, J. Black, and S. R. Pollack. New York: Grune and Stratton, 1979.

59. Heckman, JD, Ingram, AJ, Loyd, RD, Luck, JV, Jr, and Mayer, PW. Nonunion treatment with pulsed electromagnetic fields. Clin. Orthop. 161:58-66, 1981.

60. Hekkelman, JW, Herrmann-Erlee, MPM, Heersche, JNM, and Gaillard, PJ. Studies on the mechanism of parathyroid hormone on embryonic bone in vitro. In Calcium Regulating Hormones, pp. 186-194. Edited by R. V. Talmadge, M. Owen, and L. Parsons. Excerpta Medica, International Congress Series 346. New York: American Elsevier Publishing Co., 1975.

61. Heppenstall, RB, Grislis, G, and Hunt, TK. Tissue gas tension and oxygen consumption in healing bone defects. Clin. Orthop. 106:357-365, 1977.

62. Herbst, E, and von Satzger, G. Electrical pulsed current stimulation in five cases of congenital pseudarthrosis of the tibia. In Electrical Properties of Bone and Cartilage, pp. 639-664. Edited by C. T. Brighton, J. Black, and S. R. Pollack. New York: Grune and Stratton, 1979.

63. Howell, DS, Pital, JC, Marquez, JF, and Madruga, JE. Partition of calcium, phosphate, and protein in the fluid phase aspirated at calcifying sites in epiphyseal cartilage. J. Clin. Invest. 47:1121-1132, 1968.

64. Ida, H. Study on dynamic and electric calluses of bone in vitro. J. Japanese Orthop. Surg. Soc. 31:645-664, 1957.

65. Inoue, S, Ohashi, T. Fukada, F, and Ashihara, T. Electrical stimulation of osteogenesis in the rat: Amperage of three different stimulation methods. In Electrical Properties of Bone and Cartilage, pp. 199-214. Edited by C. T. Brighton, J. Black, and S. R. Pollack. New York: Grune and Stratton, 1979.

66. Inoue, S, Ohashi, T, Yasuda, I, and Fukada, E. Electret induced callus formation in the rat. Clin. Orthop. 124:57-58, 1977.

67. Inoue, S, Ohashi, T, Imai, R, Ichida, M, and Yasuda, I. The electrical induction of callus formation and external skeletal fixation using methyl methacrylate for delayed union of open tibial fractures with segmental loss. Clin. Orthop. 124:92-96, 1977.

68. Jacobs, JD, and Norton, LA. Electrical stimulation of osteogenesis in periodontal defects. Clin. Orthop. 124:41-52, 1977.

69. Janssen, LWM, Akkermans, LMA, and Wittebol, P. Effect of electrical stimulation on embryonic rat calvaria in vitro. In Electrical Properties of Bone and Cartilage, pp. 491-517. Edited by C. T. Brighton, J. Black, and S. R. Pollack. New York: Grune and Stratton, 1979.

70. Johnson, DE, and Rodan, GA. The effect of pulsating electromagnetic fields on prostaglandin synthesis in osteoblast-like cells. Trans. Bioelectrical Repair and Growth Soc. 2:7, 1982.

71. Jones, DB. The effect of pulsing magnetic fields on cAMP metabolism in chick embryo tibiae. Trans. Bioelectrical Repair and Growth Soc. 2:29, 1982.

72. Jørgenson, TE. The effect of electric current on the healing time of crural fractures. Acta Orthop. Scand. 43:421-437, 1972.

73. Jørgenson, TE. Electrical stimulation of human fracture healing by means of slow pulsating, asymmetrical direct current. Clin. Orthop. 124:124-127, 1977.

74. Kane, WJ. The use of supplementary electronic bone growth in primary and secondary lumbosacral fusion. In Electrical Properties of Bone and Cartilage, pp. 563-566. Edited by C. T. Brighton, J. Black, and S. R. Pollack. New York: Grune and Stratton, 1979.

75. Kenner, GH, Precup, JW, Gabrielson, EW, Williams, WS, and Park, JB. Electrical modification of disuse osteoporosis using constant and pulsed stimulation. In Electrical Properties of Bone and Cartilage, pp. 181-188. Edited by C. T. Brighton, J. Black, and S. R. Pollack. New York: Grune and Stratton, 1979.

76. Kirk, NT. End results of one hundred fifty-eight consecutive autogenous bone grafts for non-union in long bones (A) in simple fractures; (B) in atrophic bone following war wounds and chronic suppurative osteitis (osteomyelitis). J. Bone and Joint Surg. 6:760-799, 1924.

77. Korenstein, R, Somjen, D, Danon, A, Fischler, H, and Binderman, I. Pulsed capacitive electric induction of cyclic AMP changes, ^{45}Ca uptake and DNA synthesis in bone cells. Trans. Bioelectrical Repair and Growth Soc. 1:34, 1981.

78. Krane, SM, Parson, V, and Kunin, AS. Studies of the metabolism of epiphyseal cartilage. In Cartilage Degradation and Repair, pp. 43-58. Edited by C. A. L. Bassett. Washington, D.C.: National Academy of Science and National Research Council, 1974.

79. Laub, F, and Korenstein, R. Actin polymerization induced by pulsed electric stimulation of bone cells in vitro. Trans. Bioelectrical Repair and Growth Soc. 2:43, 1982.

80. Lavine, LS, Lustrin, I, and Shamos, MH. Experimental model for studying the effect of electric current on bone in vivo. Nature 224:1112-1113, 1969.

81. Lavine, LS, Lustrin, I, and Shamos, MH. Treatment of congenital pseudarthrosis of the tibia with constant direct current. Clin. Orthop. 124:69-74, 1977.

82. Lavine, LS, Lustrin, I, Shamos, MH, and Moss, ML. The influence of electric current on bone regeneration in vivo. Acta Orthop. Scand. 42:305-314, 1971.

83. Lavine, LS, Lustrin, I, Shamos, MH, Rinaldi, RA, and Liboff, AR. Electric enhancement of bone healing. Science 175:1118-1121, 1972.

84. Lechner, F, and Ascherl, R. Experiences and results of the electrodynamic fields treatment in cases of pseudarthrosis and delayed bone repair. Acta Orthop. Belgica 44:699-705, 1978.

85. Lee, RC, Grodzinsky, AJ, and Glimcher, MJ. The electromechanics of normal and chemically modified articular cartilage. In *Electrical Properties of Bone and Cartilage*, pp. 47-56. Edited by C. T. Brighton, J. Black, and S. R. Pollack. New York: Grune and Stratton, 1979.

86. Lente, RW, Cases of un-united fracture treated by electricity. *New York J. Med.* NS:3117-3129, 1850.

87. Leonard, F, and Wade, CWR. Electrically induced hydrolysis of adenosine 5' triphosphate. *J. Bioelect.* 1:231-237, 1982.

88. Levy, DD, and Rubin, B. Inducing bone growth *in vivo* by pulse stimulation. *Clin. Orthop.* 88:218-222, 1971.

89. Lotke, PA, Black, J, and Richardson, S. Electromechanical properties in human articular cartilage. *J. Bone and Joint Surg.* 56-A:1040-1046, 1974.

90. Luben, RA, Cain, CD, Chen, MC-Y, Rosen, D, and Adey, WR. Effects of electromagnetic stimuli on bone and bone cells *in vitro*: Inhibition of responses to parathyroid hormone by low energy low fields. *Proc. Natl. Acad. Sci.* 79:4180-4184, 1982.

91. Masureik, C, and Eriksson, C. Preliminary clinical evaluation of the effect of small electrical currents on the healing of jaw fractures. *Clin. Orthop.* 124:84-91, 1977.

92. Minkin, C, Poulton, BR, and Hoover, WH. The effect of direct current on bone. *Clin. Orthop.* 57:303-309, 1968.

93. Monet, JD, Assailly, J, Weber. Influencing of pulsating electromagnetic fields on ^{45}Ca kinetics in embryonic chick limb rudiments. *J. Electrochem. Soc.* 126:124, 1979.

94. Mooar, PA, Brighton, CT, Wisneski, RJ, and Pollack, SR. Enhancement of *in vitro* epiphyseal growth plate DNA synthesis in response to a capacitively coupled electric field. *Trans. Bioelectrical Repair and Growth Soc.* 1:33, 1981.

95. Moyen, BJL, Lans, DA, Thrasher, EL, and Harris, WH. La stimulation electrique de l'osteogeneses. Etude de la cathode. *Acta Orthop. Belgica* 44:664-670, 1978.

96. Noguchi, K. Study on dynamic callus and electric callus. *J. Japanese Orthop. Surg. Soc.* 31:641-642, 1957.

97. Norton, LA. Effects of a pulsed electromagnetic field on a mixed chondroblastic tissue culture. *Clin. Orthop.* 167:280-290, 1982.

98. Norton, LA, Bourret, LA, Majeska, RJ, and Rodan, GA. Adherence and DNA synthesis changes in hard tissue cell culture produced by electric perturbation. In *Electrical Properties of Bone and Cartilage*, pp. 443-454. Edited by C. T. Brighton, J. Black, and S. R. Pollack. New York: Grune and Stratton, 1979.

99. Norton, LA, Bourret, LA, and Rodan, GAA. Electrical field enhancement of thymidine incorporation in chondrocytes. J. Dental Res. 56A:105 and 56B:98, 1977.

100. Norton, LA, Rodan, GA, and Bourret, LA. Cyclic AMP fluctuations in bones grown in electric fields. J. Dental Res. 55:215 and 615, 1976.

101. Norton, LA, Rodan, GA, and Bourret, LA. Epiphyseal cartilage cAMP changes produced by electrical and mechanical perturbations. Clin. Orthop. 124:59-68, 1977.

102. Ohashi, T. Electrical callus formation and its osteogensis. J. Japanese Ortho. Assoc. 56:615-633, 1982.

103. Pienkowski, D, and Pollack, SR. Origin of stress generated potentials in fluid saturated bone. J. Orthop. Res. 1:1983.

104. Pilla, AA, and Colacicco, G. Nonfaradic electrochemistry at cell surfaces: Modulation of ^{45}Ca uptake by embryonic chick limb rudiments. J. Electrochem. Soc. 127: 129, 1980.

105. Pollack, SR, Korostoff, E, Starkebaum, W, and Iannacone, W. Microelectrode studies of stress generated potentials in bone. In Electrical Properties of Bone and Cartilage, pp. 69-81. Edited by C. T. Brighton, J. Black, and S. R. Pollack. New York: Grune and Stratton, 1979.

106. Rich, JB, Lee, RC, and Matthews, MB. In vitro electrical stimulation of chondrocyte synthetic response. Trans. Bioelectrical Repair and Growth Soc. 1:32, 1981.

107. Richez, J, Chamay, A, and Bieler, L. Bone changes due to pulses of direct microenvironment. Virchows Arch. Pathol. Anat. 357:11-18, 1972.

108. Rinaldi, RA, Shamos, MH, and Lavine, LS. Uptake of tritiated thymidine during electrical stimulation of induced cortical bone defects. Annals N.Y. Acad. Sci. 238:307-312, 1974.

109. Rodan, GA, Bourret, LA, and Norton, LA. Electrical field stimulation of DNA synthesis in chondrocytes mediated by membrane ion fluxes. J. Dental Res. 58:898, 1977.

110. Rodan, GA, and Johnson, DE. The effects of electromagnetic phosphatase in osteoblast-like cells in culture. Trans. Bioelectrical Repair and Growth Soc. 1:2, 1981.

111. Rooze, MA, and Hinsenkamp, MG. Histochemical modifications induced in vitro by electromagnetic bone tissues. Acta Orthop. Scand. 53: suppl. 196:51-62, 1982.

112. Shamos, MH, Lavine, LS, and Shamos, MI. Piezoelectric effect in bone. Nature 197:81, 1963.

113. Somjen, D, Korenstein, R, Fischler, H, and Binderman, I. Effects of electric field intensity on the response of cultured bone cells to parathyroid hormone and prostaglandin-E_2. In Current Advances in Skeletogenesis. Edited by M. Silvermann and H. Slavkin. Excerpta Medica, International Congress Series S89, New York: American Elsevier Publishing Co., 1982.

114. Stan, S, Sansen, W, and Mulier, JC. Experimental study on the electrical impedance of bone and the effect of direct current on the healing of fractures. Clin. Orthop. 120: 264-267, 1976.

115. Stan, S, Mulier, JC, Sansen, W, and DeWasele, P. Effect of direct current on the healing of fractures. In Electrical Stimulation of Bone Growth and Repair, pp. 45-53. Edited by F. Burny, E. Herbst, and M. Hinsenkamp. New York: Springer-Verlag, 1978.

116. Steinberg, ME. Effect of collagen modification on stress generated potentials (SGPs). In Electrical Properties of Bone and Cartilage, pp. 107-118. Edited by C. T. Brighton, J. Black, and S. R. Pollack. New York: Grune and Stratton, 1979.

117. Traina, GG, and Gulino, G. Medullary rods as electric conductors for osteogenic stimuli in human bone. In Electrical Properties of Bone and Cartilage, pp. 567-579. Edited by C. T. Brighton, J. Black, and S. R. Pollack. New York: Grune and Stratton, 1979.

118. Treharne, RW, Brighton, CT, Korostoff, E, and Pollack, SR. Application of direct, pulsed and SGP-shaped currents in vitro fetal rat tibiae. In Electrical Properties of Bone and Cartilage, pp. 169-180. Edited by C. T. Brighton, J. Black, and S. R. Pollack. New York: Grune and Stratton, 1979.

119. Vaes, GM, and Nichols, G, Jr. Oxygen tension and the control of bone cell metabolism. Nature 193:379-380, 1962.

120. Von Kraus, W, and Lechner, F. Die Heilung von pseudoarthrosen und spontan-frakturen durch strukturbildende elecktrodynamische potentiale. Muhchen med. Wochenschr. 114: 1814-1819, 1972.

121. Von Satzger, G, and Herbst, E. Electric stimulation of osteogenesis. I. Experimental study of bone healing in the rabbit tibia. II. Clinical study of two cases of congenital pseudarthrosis of the tibia. In Electrical Stimulation of Bone Growth and Repair, pp. 55-60. Edited by F. Burny, E. Herbst, and M. Hinsenkamp. New York: Springer-Verlag, 1978.

122. Weigert, M. Plates, cortices and electric potentials. In Electrical Stimulation of Bone Growth and Repair, pp. 45-46.

Edited by F. Burny, E. Herbst, and M. Hinsenkamp. New York: Springer-Verlag, 1978.

123. Weigert, M, and Werhahn, C. The influence of electric potentials on plate bones. *Clin. Orthop.* 124:20-30, 1977.

124. Wilbur, MC, and Russell, HL. Central bioelectric augmentation in the healing of fractures. In *Electrical Properties of Bone and Cartilage*, pp. 597-604. Edited by C. T. Brighton, J. Black, and S. R. Pollack. New York: Grune and Stratton, 1979.

125. Wollast, R, Hinsenkamp, MG, and Burny, F. Physiochemical effect of an electric potential on bone growth. In *Electrical Stimulation of Bone Growth and Repair*, pp. 29-34. Edited by F. Burny, E. Herbst, and M. Hinsenkamp. New York: Springer-Verlag, 1978.

126. Yarington, CT, Jr, and Jaquiss, GW. Electrical control of bone growth is ossicles. Possible future clinical application of this interesting observation. *Arch. Otolaryngol.* 89: 856-860, 1969.

127. Yasuda, I. Fundamental aspects of fracture treatment. *J. Kyoto Med. Soc.* 4:395-406, 1953.

128. Yasuda, I. Electrical callus and callus formation by electret. *Clin. Orthop.* 124:53-56, 1977.

129. Zichner, L, and Happel, MW. Treatment of congenital and acquired nonunions by means of an invasive device. In *Electrical Properties of Bone and Cartilage*, pp. 581-596. Edited by C. T. Brighton, J. Black, and S. R. Pollack. New York: Grune and Stratton, 1979.

130. ZumBrunner, JL, and Brindley, HH. Nonunion of the shafts of the long bones. A review and analysis of 140 cases. *J. Am. Med. Assn.* 203:637-640, 1968.

11
Electrical Effects on Nerve Ganglia *In Vitro*

Betty F. Sisken, Elsie Barr and R. Scott Estes

INTRODUCTION

Electrical stimulation has been used clinically to stimulate bone healing in long term nonunions. In the early studies, metal electrodes were implanted into the fracture site and subsequent osteogenesis was observed in the region of the cathode (see Brighton, et al. 1979). This continues to be a viable approach. More recently, noninvasive methods have been developed to induce currents via applied pulsed electromagnetic fields (PEMF) to stimulate repair (see Bassett, et al. 1979). Comparable success rates are achieved clinically with either method. Basic research into the mechanism whereby applied current results in healing of the lesion has demonstrated effects on proliferation and differentiation of precursor cells.

Our studies have addressed the question of whether applied electric fields stimulate nerve regeneration. Therefore, we have developed an in vitro system using tantalum electrodes immersed in the culture medium to deliver direct current to embryonic sensory ganglia. PEMF is delivered to the ganglia by placing the culture dishes between vertically-oriented Helmholtz coils. Regenerative processes affected by the electric fields are then assayed. In vitro nerve regeneration is characterized by: (1) neuronal survival, (2) neurite outgrowth, (3) synaptic contact to the end-organ, and (4) production of the specific neurotransmitter associated with the neurons in vivo. Previous studies have shown that direct current significantly stimulated neuronal survival and neurite outgrowth to the

---

Supported by ONR N00014-82-K-0105.

cathode (Sisken and Smith 1975; Sisken, et al. 1981). Additionally, direct current is effective in stimulating neuritic outgrowth of 8-day trigeminal ganglia to 8-day co-cultured cornea; the ganglionic neurons and their processes contain positive Substance P fluorescence (Sisken and Beuerman 1983). To ascertain the mechanisms by which this stimulation occurred, we found that amino acid uptake and incorporation in direct current-treated cultures was stimulated over that of control cultures and approximated the values found in cultures treated with nerve growth factor (Sisken and Lafferty 1978).

In all cases, cultures exposed to either type of electrical stimulus are compared to sister cultures containing nerve growth factor (NGF). The effects of NGF on increasing nerve regeneration in vitro are well established (see Varon and Adler 1980), and maximal responses are obtained with concentrations of 10^{-8} to 10^{-9} M. The NGF cultures are used only as a standard for comparing effectiveness of treatment. Since NGF acts primarily as a hormone, the expectation was that the basic mechanism of action of NGF and applied electric fields might be similar but would not be necessarily identical.

In this study we have performed a series of experiments to follow the sequence of morphological and biochemical events that are associated with neuronal growth and differentiation under NGF or applied electric treatments. In addition, we have tested the effects of a commonly-used inhibitor of DNA synthesis, cytosine arabinoside, on the same properties. This drug reduces the mitotically-active, non-neuronal cell population, thereby dissociating the neuronal from the non-neuronal contribution to the regenerative process. We found that neurite outgrowth is independently regulated within the neuronal cells; it remains to be determined if neuronal survival is also independently regulated. Both of these parameters must be stimulated for regeneration to be continued. Preliminary reports of this work have been published (Sisken and Barr 1982).

MATERIALS AND METHODS

Trigeminal Ganglia

Trigeminal ganglia (TG) consisting of both ophthalmic and maxillo-mandibular lobes were dissected from 8 day chick embryos and placed in 6 ml of complete medium in 60 mm Falcon dishes (3002) with no added substrate. Complete medium consisted of 85% Dulbecco's Modified Eagles's Medium, 10% dialyzed fetal bovine serum, 3% glucose to a final concentration of 600 mg%,

1% glutamine (200 mM final) and 1% penicillin-streptomycin mixture. Each set of experiments consisted of 3 dishes/treatment; all sets of experiments were repeated 2-3 times. For each experiment, a control group (untreated) and a group treated with 2.5s nerve growth factor (NGF) 10^{-8} were run in parallel with the electrically-treated group to account for daily variations in culture conditions. All cultures were incubated for 3 days at 39°C in a 5% CO_2 incubator.

A series of experiments were conducted to test the effects of different levels of current on this system. The direct current was applied by connecting a 1.4 V mercury battery to a two-electrode system configured to maintain a non-uniform field in the dish (Figure 11.1A). The center electrode is always the cathode. Figure 11.1B shows the current vs time relationships; the details of this system have been reported (Sechaud and Sisken 1981). Either tantalum metal electrodes (0.25 mm diameter) or platinum electrodes (0.125 mm diameter) were used. Current/voltage curves for each electrode are presented in Figure 11.2 and were obtained using a three-electrode system (Figure 11.3). To discriminate between current applied and potential imposed, we used this three-electrode system to set the potential in our ganglion preparation, incubating these dishes for 3 days in the same incubator. The voltage range tested was -200 mV to -800 mV/Standard Calomel Electrode. Control cultures for this series consisted of tantalum electrodes insulated with 3 coats of plastic; no current was detected in these dishes.

To eliminate any electrode products that form as a result of direct current applied via either metal electrode, we replaced the center electrode with an agar salt bridge; the current value measured with this system was 10 nA (RCA WV511 picoameter™). Replacing both metal electrodes with agar salt bridges produced a current of 6 nA (Figure 11.4 A-B).

Dorsal Root Ganglia

Dorsal root ganglia (DRG) from 7-8 day chick embryos were dissected in Dulbecco's phosphate buffered saline and 6-8 DRGs were immediately placed in 5 ml culture medium in 60 mm culture dishes containing liners (Falcon 3006). The liners are composed of polyester (polyethylene tetrathallate) and their surfaces have been treated to be hydrophilic, thereby increasing cellular attachment. Two media were utilized in these experiments; complete medium (see above) and ara C medium consisting of complete medium with Cytarabine® (Upjohn, cytosine arabinoside) added at a final concentration of 8 μg/ml.

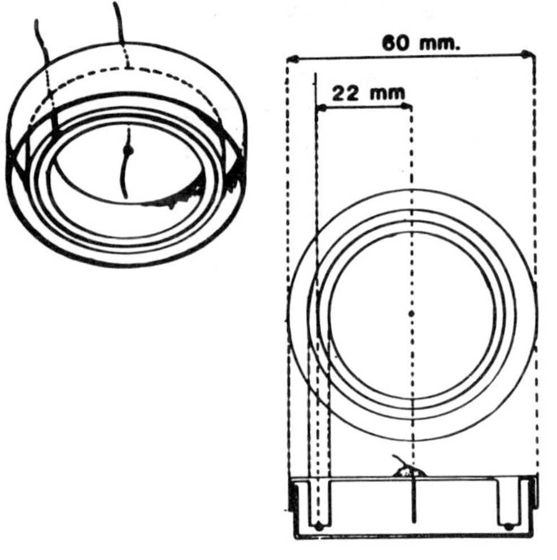

FIGURE 11.1A Diagram of a Falcon culture dish modified to hold wire electrodes. Center cathode and circular anode are connected to a 1.4 V battery.

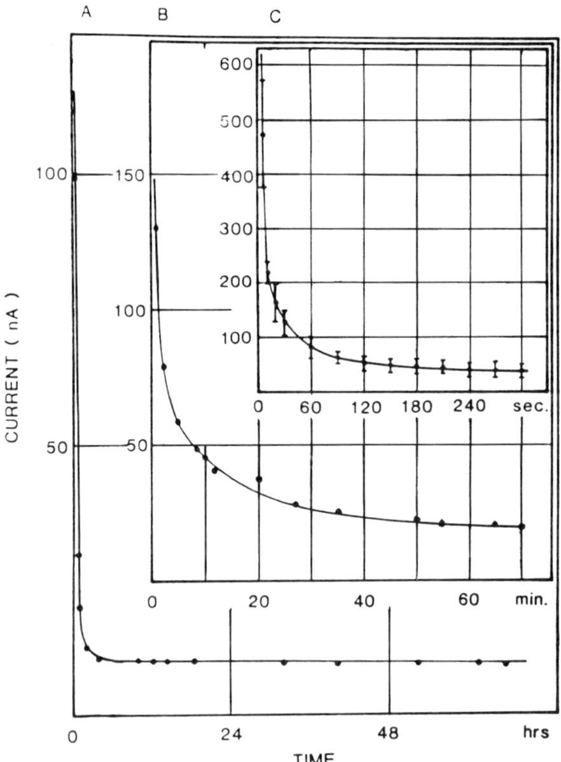

FIGURE 11.1B Current vs. time. Current in 5 dishes was determined for 70 hrs (A) 70 min (B) and 300 secs (C) in culture medium. In (C) the average of 5 dishes is shown; examples of readings are shown in (A) and (B).

FIGURE 11.2 Current vs. potential plots. Tantalum electrodes, right; platinum electrodes, below. The current was determined relative to different potentials fixed with a potentiostat (Tacussel, PRT 20-10). The reference electrode is a saturated calomel electrode separated from the dish by a salt bridge. The readings were made in culture dishes containing culture medium.

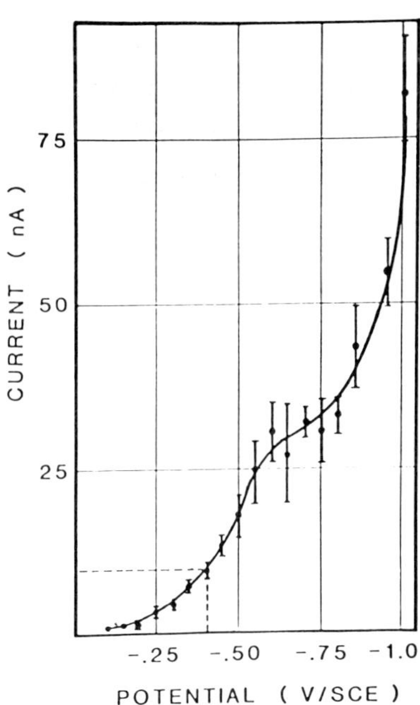

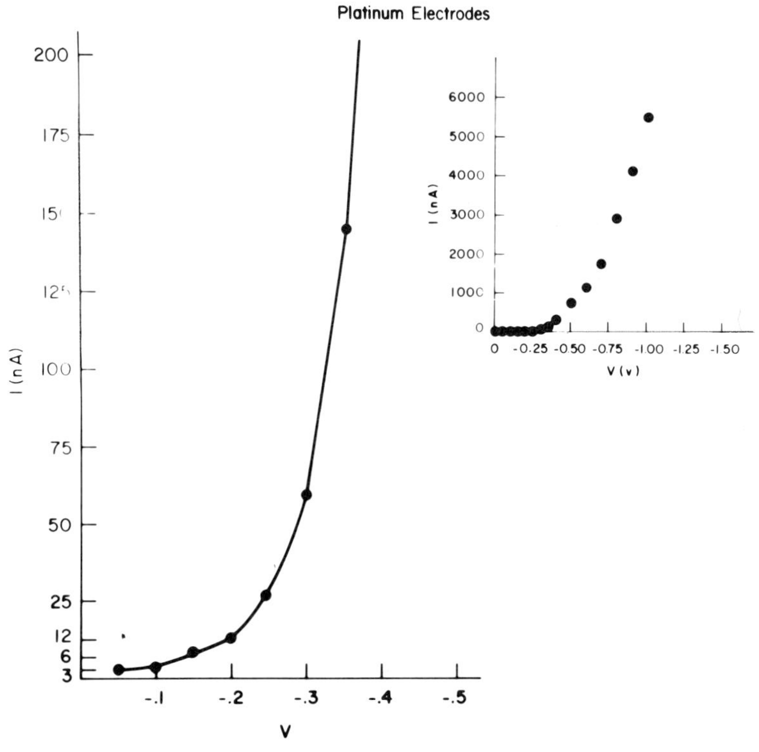

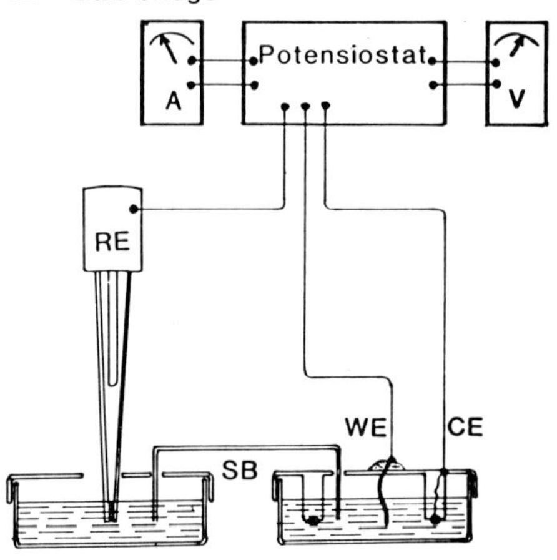

FIGURE 11.3 Three-electrode system for determining current vs. potential curves and for setting the potential.

FIGURE 11.4 Agar salt bridge systems.

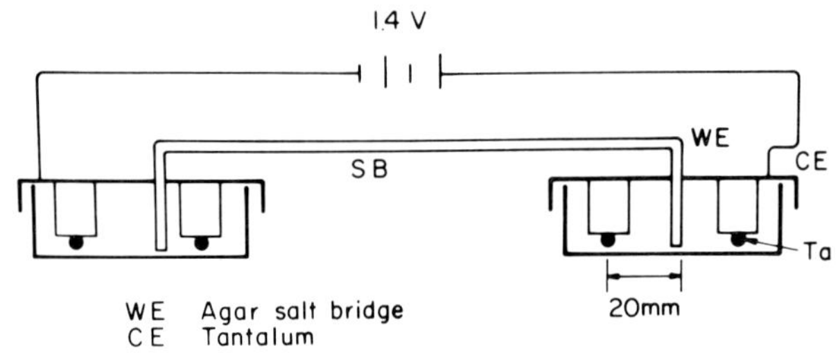

A. Single agar electrode (cathode)

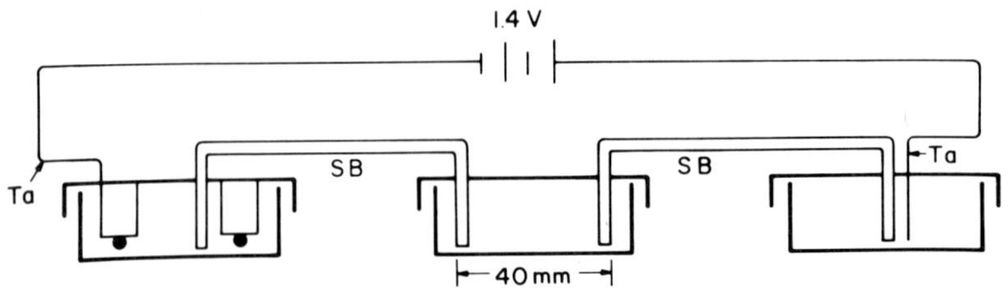

B. Double agar electrode system

Each day's experiment was divided into four treatment groups: a control group which received no treatment; a Nerve Growth Factor (NGF) group which received 2.5s NGF at a final concentration of 10^{-8} M; a group treated with pulsed electromagnetic fields (PEMF); and a group treated with 10nA direct current (DC). Each of the groups had four dishes per experiment; the duration of these experiments was either 3 days or 6 days.

The PEMF dishes were placed vertically between two Helmholtz coils and exposed for two days on a 12 hr. on/12 hr. off schedule (24 hrs total exposure). The characteristics of the PEMF waveform are shown in Figure 11.5 and it consists of a single pulse, repeated at 72 Hz. The current induced in these dishes is maximal in the center and varies non-linearly to zero at the edge (McLeod, et al. 1982). The magnetic component runs parallel to the surface of the dish and is uniform throughout.

Direct current was applied using the tantalum electrode system described above; the total current measured from these dishes was 10 nA (-400mV/SCE). The electric field created in the dish is presented in Figure 11.6.

Neurite Outgrowth

At the end of the incubation, the cultured ganglia were fixed in 3.5% glutaraldehyde in 0.1 M cacodylate buffer at room temperature for 2 hours. Neurite outgrowth was assessed on the fixed cultures using a scoring system reported in previous studies (Sisken, et al. 1981). Representative scores are demonstrated pictorially in Figure 11.7. After scoring, the cultures were refrigerated overnight.

Neuronal Survival

All cultures for these studies were rinsed twice in 4°C cacodylate buffer after glutaraldehyde fixation, post-fixed in 1% osmic acid in 0.1 M cacodylate buffer, dehydrated and processed for Epon embedding. In the TG series, propylene oxide was eliminated and pre-embedding steps consisted of equal parts of absolute alcohol and Epon. Two micron sections cut with a glass knife at 30 µm intervals, were mounted on slides and stained with toluidine blue.

Radioautography

To determine the extent and localization of protein synthesis in these cultures as a result of time and treatment, ^{3}H-proline

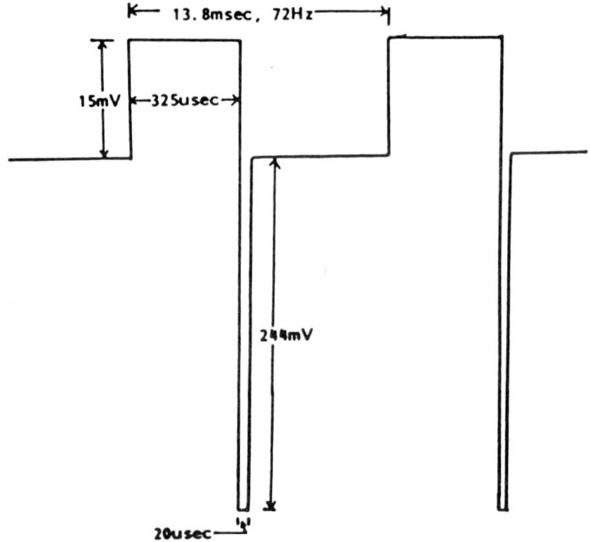

FIGURE 11.5 Single pulse waveform.
Waveform: Pulsed Electromagnetically Induced Current (PEMF)
Magnetic Field Strength: 5.3 Tesla/sec
Maximum Current Density: 0.48 uA/cm^2

FIGURE 11.6 Theoretical distribution of electric field and current density in the culture dish. See Sisken, et al. 1981 for details.

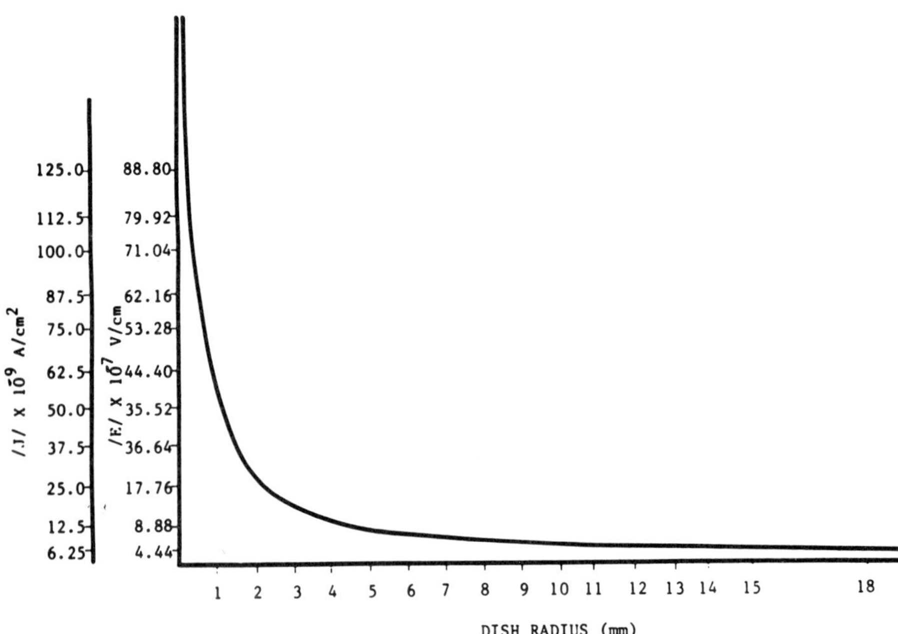

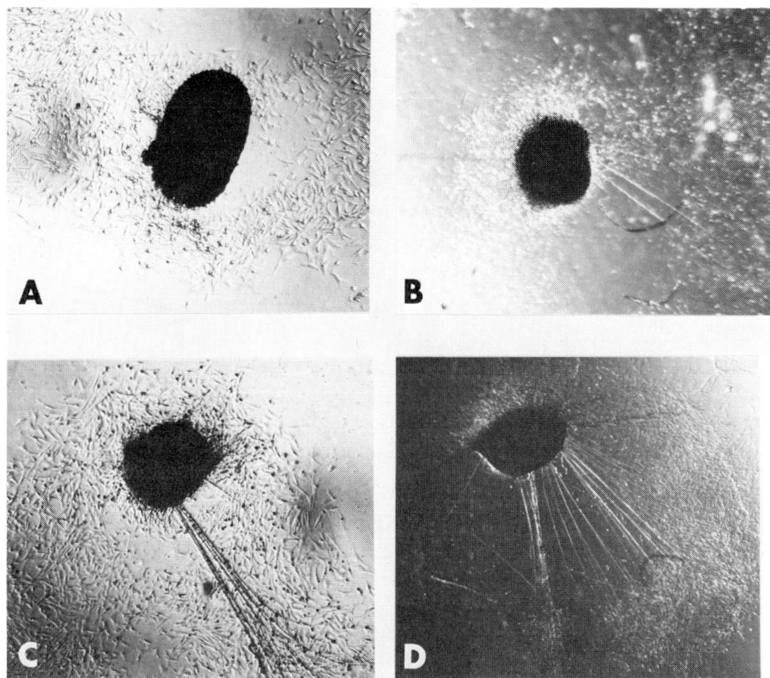

FIGURE 11.7 Neurite scoring system, trigeminal ganglia, 3 DIV. (A), control, score 0; (B) 10nA DC, score 1; (C) 6nA DC (agar electrodes only), score 3; (D) 10 nA DC, score 5. Neurites oriented to the cathode. X 50.

(L-[2,3-^{3}H-proline]), 40 μCi/mM was added 20 hours prior to fixation at a final concentration of 3 μCi/ml. After fixation with glutaradelhyde and 3 washes with 0.1 M cacodylate buffer, the culture dishes were coated with NTB2 liquid emulsion (Kodak) in the dark. The dishes were drained, inverted, and allowed to dry. They were exposed in light-tight boxes at 4°C for 3 weeks. The dishes were then developed at 18°C in Dektol, fixed, washed several times in water and dried. Photographs of the whole explant were taken with a Nikon camera attached to a Nikon inverted microscope.

Statistics

All data were analyzed by R. Kryscio, Dept. of Statistics, using the approximate and exact t-test for comparing the treatment mean effects vs the control mean effects.

RESULTS

The formation of regenerated processes from embryonic sensory ganglia has been well-documented (Yamada, et al. 1971). Growth cone expansions at the end of the elongating axons contain microspikes which aid in attachment to the underlying plastic; in most cultures, these growth cones appear in the first 24 hours of incubation. Continued elongation occurs by assembly of surface material at the growth cone and uptake at the more proximal region (Bray and Bunge 1973). By 48 hours, the neurites have grown considerably, and by 72 hours have reached their maximal length. Previous studies have demonstrated that at 3 DIV, large arrays of microspikes from growth cones of trigeminal ganglia interconnect on the surface of non-neuronal cells after NGF treatment. In contrast, control cultures show limited growth cone formation. DC-treated cultures, however, have well-developed microspikes spreading over underlying cells but these appear to show few connections to microspikes from other cones (Sisken and Lafferty 1978).

Neurite outgrowth (NO) scores in trigeminal ganglia as a function of current and potential are shown graphically in Figure 11.8A. Note that at -400 mV, the total current delivered with tantalum electrodes is 10 nA. This is our standard working level for DC administration. Scores obtained at -200 mV(1 nA) and -600 mV (20 nA) are within the level of significance and fall within a dose response curve; at -800 mV the scores are not different from control values. In contrast, platinum electrodes set at a potential of -400 mV (300 nA) yield scores similar to control cultures. However, setting the potential at -200 mV (12 nA) produces NO scores that are within the range of stimulation found with tantalum electrodes. Substituting either or both wire electrodes with agar salt bridges gave current values of 10 and 6 nA respectively, and the scores overlapped with those in the "current window." In all cases, the NO scores obtained with any of the DC experiments did not reflect maximal stimulation such as that obtained with NGF, as noted in previous studies. The major findings of these experiments are: (1) neurite outgrowth is correlated with the current applied and not the potential imposed, (2) the "current window" encompasses 1-20 nA

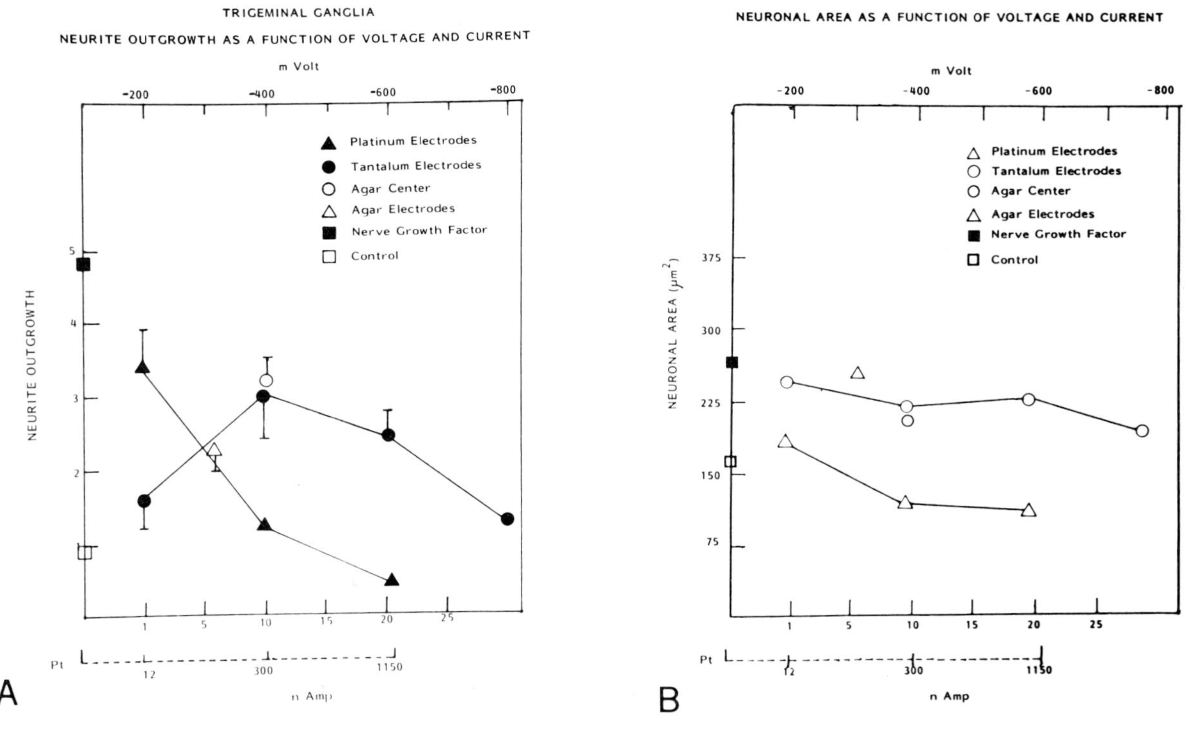

FIGURE 11.8. Neurite outgrowth (A) and neuronal area (B) as a function of current applied and voltage imposed.

and (3) the electrode products produced with metal electrodes do not appear to be involved negatively at these low current levels.

Neuron Survival. Two micrometer sections of ganglia fixed after any of the above treatments are being analyzed for number and area size. Data obtained thus far indicate that the same current values that stimulate neurite outgrowth cause an increase in neuronal cell area comparable to the values obtained with NGF (Figure 11.8B). Representative sections are illustrated in Figure 11.9. With increasing levels of current (20 and 30 nA), the neurons take on a more elongated appearance in contrast to the round shape normally associated with sensory neurons (Figure 9D).

In order to pursue the effects of applied electric fields on nerve regeneration at the molecular level, we turned to a more numerous population of ganglia, the dorsal root sensory ganglia located in the lumbar region. These ganglionic neurons provide sensory innervation to the hindlimbs and contain similar types of neurons as those found in the trigeminal ganglia. With the larger number of ganglia available, we were able to run simultaneous experiments adding a group treated with non-invasively applied pulsed electromagnetically-induced current (PEMF) since previous studies have demonstrated stimulatory effects on nerve regeneration. Our experimental design, therefore, expanded to study four groups; control, NGF, PEMF, and DC. Growth characteristics were assessed as a function of time and treatment in complete medium and in medium containing the DNA synthesis inhibitor, ara C. In our culture system, ara C reduces glia and fibroblasts with no obvious effects on neurite production. Future studies will define quantitatively the extent of the effect of ara C on the numbers and areas of the sensory neurons.

Neurite Outgrowth. Scores for neurite outgrowth in dorsal root ganglia (DRG) as a function of days *in vitro* (DIV) and treatment are presented in Table 11.1. A similar series in the presence of ara C is included. Both are shown graphically in Figure 11.10. At 3 DIV in complete medium, NO is increased with either electric treatment, and significant stimulation is obtained with NGF. All scores decreased with time and although none were significantly different from the control group, NGF, PEMF, and DC remained at a higher level. In the presence of ara C, neurite outgrowth was unaffected at 3 DIV in the treated groups, but the controls showed higher values than those

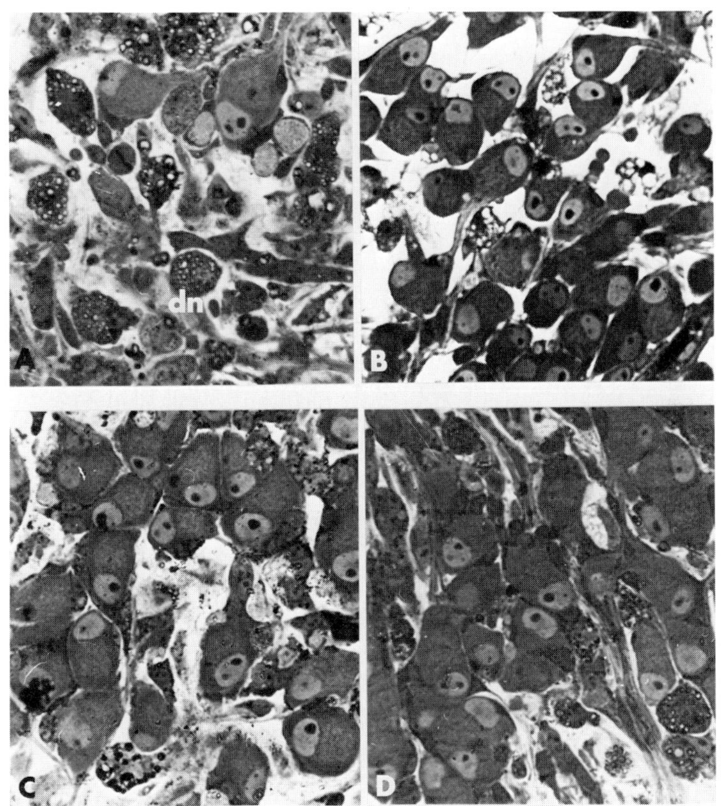

FIGURE 11.9 Two micron Epon sections of trigeminal ganglia after 3 DIV, toluidine blue stain. A, control; B, NGF, C, 10nA DC with agar salt bridge as cathode; D, 20nA DC (-600 mV) tantalum electrodes. Degenerating neurons (dn) are found in all cultures but are most obvious in control cultures. Note elongated neurons with accompanying neurites in 9 D, X 500.

TABLE 11.1

Eight Day Dorsal Root Ganglia Incubated for 3 DIV or 6 DIV

	Complete Medium			Ara-C Medium	
	n Dishes	Neurite Outgrowth*		n Dishes	Neurite Outgrowth*
3 DIV			3 DIV		
Control	12	2.46 ± 0.17	Control	16	3.13 ± 0.18
NGF	12	4.49 ± 0.13	NGF	16	4.32 ± 0.11
PEMF	12	3.22 ± 0.15	PEMF	16	2.92 ± 0.12
D.C.	12	3.33 ± 0.25	D.C.	16	2.97 ± 0.09
6 DIV			6 DIV		
Control	12	1.95 ± 0.23	Control	15	4.25 ± 0.12
NGF	10	3.15 ± 0.40	NGF	14	2.55 ± 0.17
PEMF	10	2.57 ± 0.69	PEMF	13	4.58 ± 0.07
D.C.	13	2.78 ± 0.22	D.C.	13	4.36 ± 0.10

*Mean ± S.E.M.

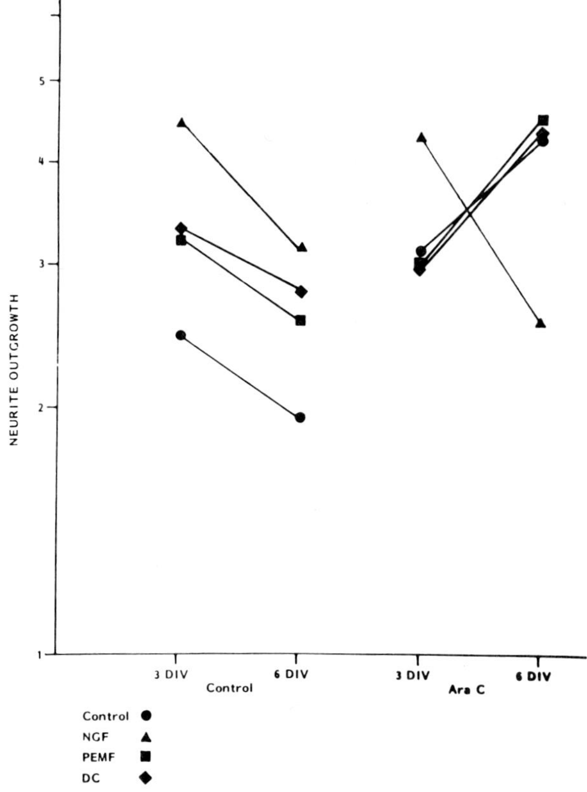

FIGURE 11.10 Neurite outgrowth in dorsal root ganglia at 3 and 6 DIV in complete medium and in medium with ara C.

obtained without the drug, so that C, PEMF and DC values overlap. At 6 DIV all scores significantly increased in these groups while that obtained for NGF significantly decreased. These effects can be seen visually under phase microscopy (Figure 11.13) or in the radioautographs of the ganglia after incubation with ^{3}H-proline.

Radioautography. Localization of protein synthesis as a result of time and treatment in the various cellular types are illustrated in Figures 11.11-11.13. In complete medium at 3 DIV, nerve cells (n) and neurites (nt) stand out as black silhouettes against the more diffusely labeled flattened non-neuronal mat (m).

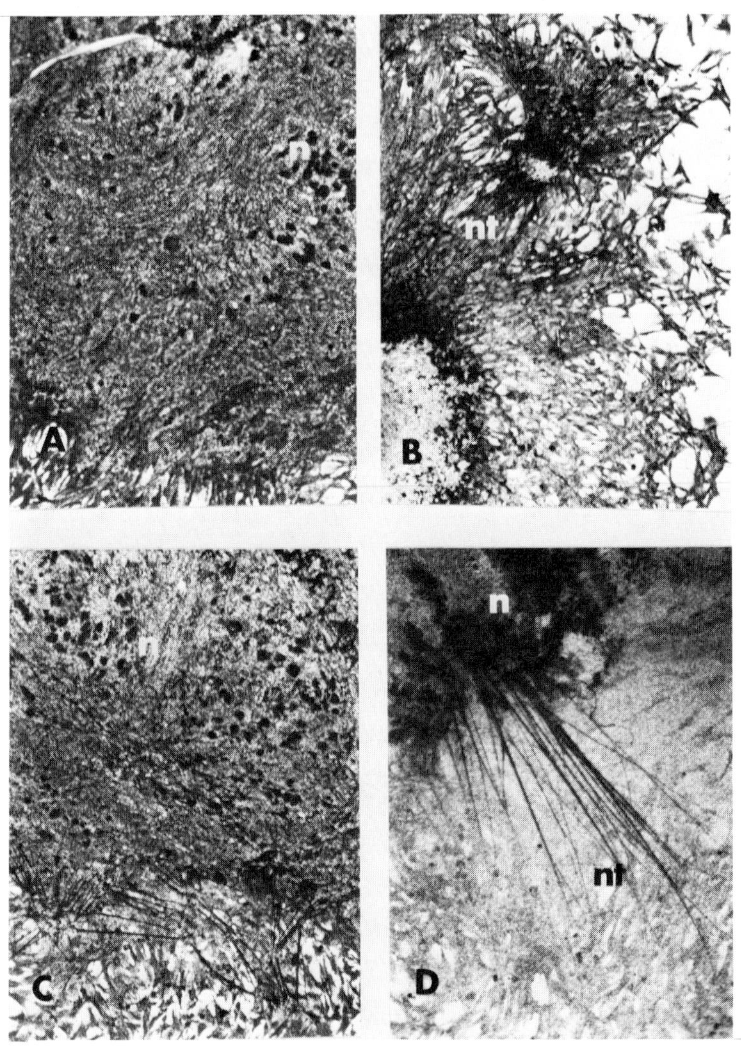

FIGURE 11.11 Radioautographs of dorsal root ganglia after 3 DIV; ^{3}H-proline added for the last 20 hrs. A, control; B, NGF; C, PEMF; D, 10 nA DC. Note black neuronal cells (n) in middle of ganglia in relief against the diffuse grains of the non-neuronal cells. Neurites (nt) contain heavy grain deposits and are prominent especially in NGF (B) and DC (D) cultures. Note black cathodally-oriented neurites in D. X 192.

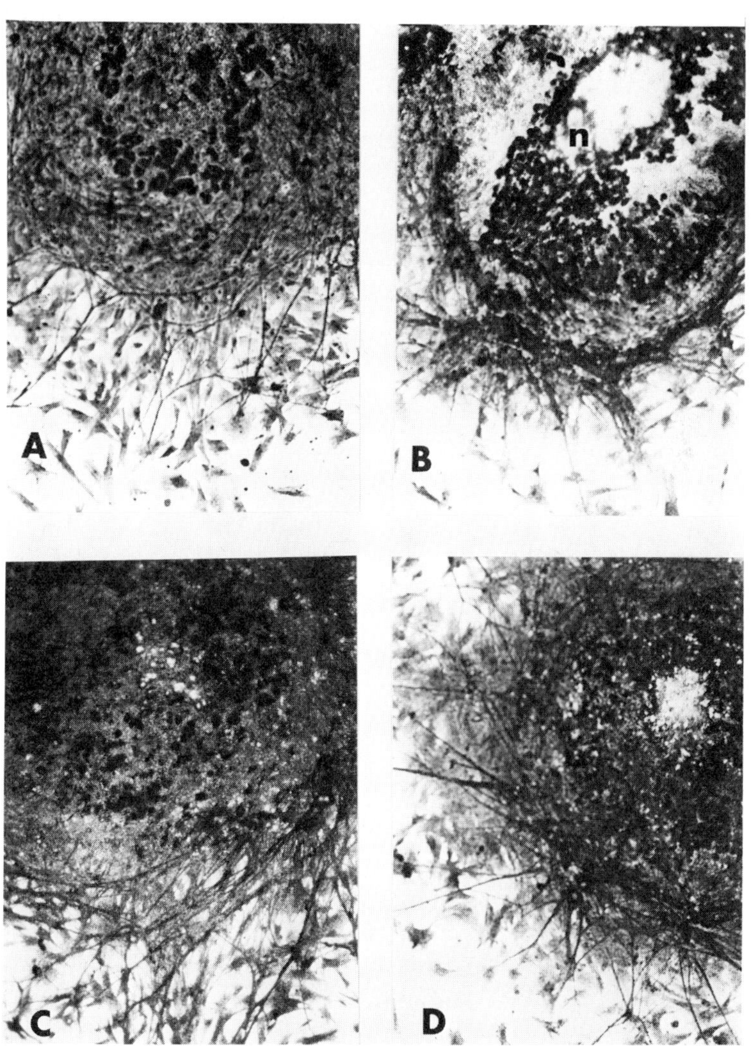

FIGURE 11.12 Radioautographs of dorsal root ganglia after 3 DIV in the presence of 8 μg/ml ara C. A, control; B, NGF; C, PEMF; D, 10nA DC. Note decreased numbers of non-neuronal cells at the periphery of the ganglia. Heavily-stained neurites are present in all four groups. Large numbers of labeled neurons are present in B and D. X 192.

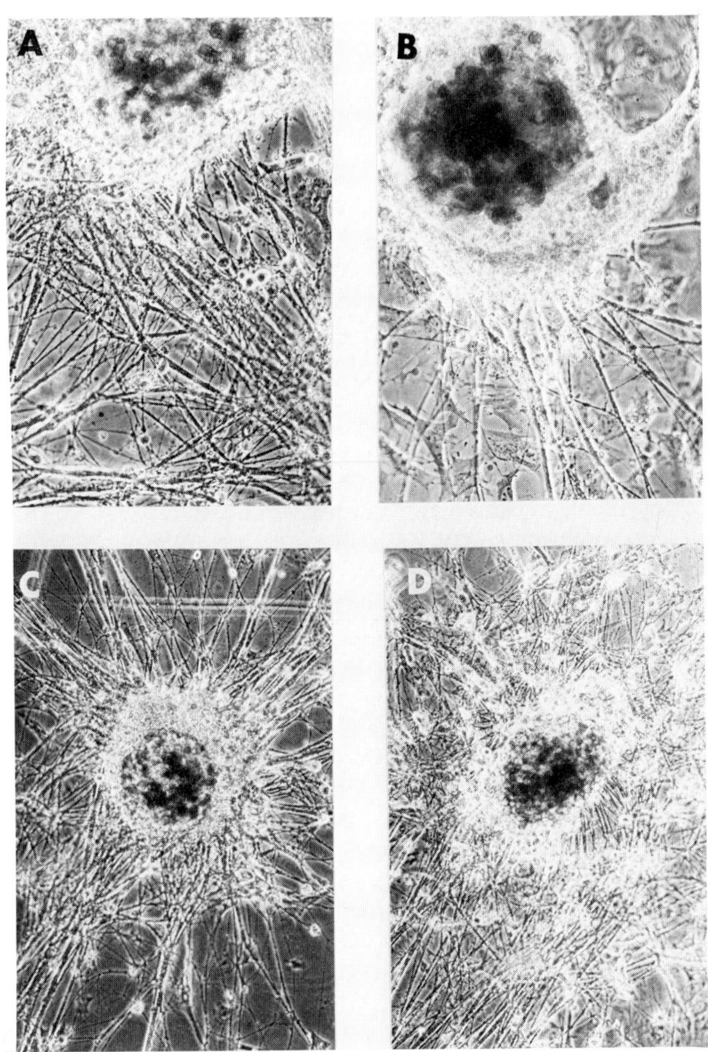

FIGURE 11.13 Phase photomicrographs of dorsal root ganglia after 6 DIV in the presence of 8 μg/ml ara C. A, control; B, NGF; C, PEMF; D, 10 nA DC. Note extensive neurite outgrowth in A, C, D. The neuronal cells in B are grouped centrally and are surrounded by circularly-arranged neurites. X 192.

Heavy label is seen especially in the NGF preparations which contain the greatest number of neurons and neurites (Figure 11.11, B). Long, heavily-labeled neurites are found in DC-treated cultures (Figure 11.11, D). By 6 DIV, non-neuronal cells have taken over and both neurons and their processes are found primarily in the center region of the explant. The neuronal population is diminished in all groups.

In ara C cultures at 3 DIV, the non-neuronal cell population has been considerably diminished and labeled neuritic processes emanate from the centrally-located neurons (Figure 11.12). Few differences between the numbers of processes and neurons are seen in these preparations. In the NGF cultures, heavily-labeled neurons are found centrally and most of the neurite processes are attenuated but still numerous. At 6 DIV (Figure 11.13), a profusion of neurites are seen extending for long distances beyond the explant in C, PEMF and DC groups; the central portion of the ganglia appears reduced in size in all groups. In NGF explants, neurites appear as relatively stubby outgrowths, but the interior of the explant is comparatively larger. Higher magnification of radioautographs of such explants reveal many neurites circling around the center of the ganglia, enclosing closely-packed neurons.

DISCUSSION

Our experiments were designed to investigate the effects of administering electric current using different modes of application to the phenomena of nerve regeneration in vitro. The first series of experiments on trigeminal ganglia assessed the effects of direct current passed through wire electrodes (tantalum or platinum) immersed directly in the culture medium. A dose response curve was obtained wherein current levels of 1-20 nA produced stimulatory effects. Current levels above 20 nA in our culture system were ineffective or deleterious. Substitution of agar salt bridges for the metal electrodes using current levels within the effective "current window" produced comparable stimulatory effects on growth. Increased neurite outgrowth and increased neuronal cell size relative to control values were obtained when direct current was applied with either metal or agar electrodes; these values approached those obtained with a standard nerve growth factor preparation. Since we are engaged in long-term studies of electrical stimulation of nerve regeneration, the metal electrode system remains the system of choice and is preferred due to its ease of handling, minimal contamination problem and the ability to run many cultures concurrently.

We have expanded our studies on the trigeminal ganglia by looking at trophic interactions between the ganglia and co-cultured cornea in the 8 day chick embryo using direct current or NGF to increase outgrowth to this end-organ. Pre-incubation in cyclohexamide (10 μg/ml) was necessary to inhibit corneal epithelial overgrowth leaving the neurite processes unaffected. Synaptic-type contact between trigeminal neurite endings and the corneal stroma were obtained. The neurotransmitter (Substance P) was localized in neurons and neurites in such cultures (Sisken and Beuerman 1983).

The data obtained on cultures of dorsal root ganglia after stimulation with either direct current or pulsed electromagnetically-induced current show less difference relative to control cultures than that obtained in the trigeminal cultures. This may be due to the special liners, but more probably involves the higher growth potential of these ganglia. The scores presented in Figure 11.10 are substantiated by evidence obtained from the radioautographs; this is noted particularly at 6 DIV after ara C treatment. Although the NO scores for controls, PEMF and DC overlap, inspection of the radioautographs find densely-labeled neurons and neurites swirling within the explant prominent in the electrically-stimulated groups. This arrangement of neurites is more dramatic in the NGF-treated ganglia. Further studies to assess numbers and areas of surviving neurons as a function of time in culture and treatment in the presence of ara C, are in progress.

We have preliminary data comparing the numbers of single neurons surviving after 4 DIV in dissociated cultures of DRG; the same degree of stimulation occurred that was found in explant cultures, that is, NGF preserved the maximal number of neurons, while PEMF and DC preserved an intermediate number relative to control cultures. Expanded studies that quantify the numbers of neurons in ara C-treated dissociated cultures are planned. The effect of ara C on neuron survival in dissociated or explant cultures will help to clarify the role that the non-neuronal cells play in maintaining neuronal function. Varon, et al. (1974) have demonstrated that specific proportions of non-neuronal cells are mandatory for neuronal survival in cultures of dissociated DRG. They found that these non-neuronal cells can substitute for NGF.

Application of direct current _in vivo_ with metal electrodes to augment bone repair (cathode in bone) range from 20 μA (in man, Brighton 1979), to 0.5 μA (in rabbits, Spadaro 1979).

Levels of 1-100 nA applied by a bimetallic couple (Pt/Ag) to amputated stumps induced partial limb regeneration in adult frogs (Smith 1967) and young rats (Becker and Spadaro 1972; Sisken, et al. 1979). Such experiments with frogs have been confirmed (Borgens, et al. 1977). Roederer, et al. (1983) applied 10 μA DC to transected spinal cord of the lamprey with wick electrodes; cathodally-directed current significantly reduced the normal "die-back" of cut axons. Marsh and Beams (1946) published the first critical study on the effects of applied direct current to nerve regeneration in vitro. They found that current densities of 120 $\mu A/mm^2$ oriented neurite outgrowth to the cathode. More recent studies (Sisken and Smith 1975; Jaffe and Poo 1979; Sisken, et al. 1981; Hinkle, et al. 1981; and Patel and Poo 1982) on chick ganglia, frog neurons, goldfish retina explants, single Xenopus neurons have demonstrated similar orienting effects of the cathode and stimulation of neurite growth. Reported rates of migration of neurons and their processes to the cathode using time lapse cinemicrography are: 100 μm/hr obtained with trigeminal ganglion explants (Sisken and Smith 1975), and 4.8 μm/hr obtained with single Xenopus neurons (Patel and Poo 1982).

In our second series of experiments, sister cultures of dorsal root ganglia exposed to pulsed electromagnetic fields (PEMF) were added. Although many papers exist in the literature on PEMF effects on organ (bone, cartilage models of long bones) and tissue and cell cultures (chondrocytes, osteoblasts, fibroblasts), few laboratories have developed models to test the effects of PEMF on neuronal cell function. Sisken, et al. (1981) reported on differential stimulation of nerve regeneration with a single pulse waveform in comparison to pulse burst signals. Rein, et al. (1982) noted increased noradrenaline release when phaeochromocytoma (PC12) cells were exposed to low frequency electromagnetic fields in vitro. This release was inhibited by 15 mM magnesium thereby implicating calcium ion fluxes in its effects. These results are consistent with those reported by other investigators studying PEMF effects on bone and cartilage cells. Johnson and Rodan (1982) and Korenstein, et al. (1982) have evidence to suggest that PEMF stimulates calcium fluxes and other second messenger activity, similar to that produced by hormone addition.

Using ara C to eliminate the non-neuronal population of cells in the dorsal root ganglia series demonstrates that the sensory neurons possess the inherent ability to regenerate neurites independently of the surrounding cells. This ability is not restricted to sensory neurons; central nervous system neurons treated with ara C also respond by regenerating their processes (Seil, et al. 1980) as long as they are post-mitotic neurons. Such neurons contain a pool of microtubules necessary for rebuilding the cytoskeleton; new protein synthesis is not mandatory (Yamada and Wessels 1971; Morgan and Seeds 1975; Sisken and Beuerman 1983). The observation that neurite outgrowth begins in ara C medium and continues to lengthen from 3 DIV to 6 DIV in all groups but NGF, suggests that this inherent capability is active for extended lengths of time. The seemingly-paradoxical effects of ara C on NGF neurite outgrowth is clarified by observing radioautographs of such cultures after ^{3}H-proline incorporation. Short, thick processes emerging from the ganglia are heavily-labeled; additionally, layers of labeled processes encircle the centrally-placed neurons. Such a situation was first described by Levi-Montalcini (1966) when excess NGF was present in the culture medium. It is possible that more NGF per neuron is available in the drug-treated cultures since the non-neuronal cells which probably absorb it non-specifically are decreased drastically.

Although neurite production is independently regulated, neuronal survival may ultimately be dependent upon the trophic functions of the non-neuronal cells. Varon, et al. (1974) found that non-neuronal cells can replace the NGF requirement for survival of neurons in dissociated DRG cultures. We have not yet determined neuronal survival in ara C cultures in comparison to those cultures grown in complete medium; it may be that in explant cultures, these accessory cells may also function trophically.

We have shown that application of direct current within limits of 1-20nA stimulates neuronal regeneration of trigeminal ganglia in vitro. Current levels above 20nA are either ineffective or detrimental to the survival of the neurons. By using a mitotic inhibitor, we found that neuronal cells lacking supportive fibroblasts and glia express the inherent ability to regenerate and grow for extended periods of time.

SUMMARY

The effects of various electrical stimuli on nerve regeneration in vitro as defined by neurite outgrowth and neuronal survival, have been documented. A series of experiments were performed on trigeminal ganglia to correlate both parameters of regeneration with different levels of direct current; the current delivered was tested using tantalum or platinum electrodes, or by agar salt bridge electrodes. A dose response curve showed that regeneration was stimulated within a "current window" of 1-20 nA; maximal stimulation occurred with 10 nA. No differences were noted when agar electrodes replaced the metal electrodes, arguing against any involvement of deleterious electrode products. In addition, the growth parameters tested were correlated with current applied rather than voltage imposed. Such trigeminal ganglia stimulated with direct current form "synaptic-type" contacts with the corneal stroma when the ganglia is co-cultured with cornea.

The effects of direct current, pulsed electromagnetic fields or NGF were determined on dorsal root ganglion regeneration as a function of age in culture. In addition, these effects were assessed after treatment with the drug, ara C, to dissociate the electrical or NGF effects on the neuronal cells from those of the non-neuronal cells. Neurite outgrowth was expansive at 3 days *in vitro* in all groups including the controls; this growth continued to 6 days *in vitro* demonstrating the inherent ability of neurons to grow in the absence of supportive cells.

NOTES

1. CAL Bassett, SN Mitchell, L Norton, N Caulo, and SR Gaston. Electromagnetic repairs of nonunions. In Electrical Properties of Bone and Cartilage, ed. CT Brighton, J Black, S Pollack (New York: Grune and Stratton, 1979), p. 605.

2. RO Becker and JA Spadaro, Electrical stimulation of partial limb regeneration in mammals. Bull. N.Y. Acad. Med. 48 (1972):627.

3. RB Borgens, JW Vanable, and LF Jaffe, Bioelectricity and regeneration. I. Initiation of frog limb regeneration by minute currents. J. Exp. Zool. 200 (1977):403.

4. D Bray and MB Bunge. The growth cone in neurite extension. Locomotion of Tissue Cells, Ciba Foundation Symposium (Amsterdam: Elsevier, 1973), p. 195.

5. CT Brighton, ZB Friedenberg, and J Black. Evaluation of the use of constant direct current in the treatment of nonunion. In Electrical Properties of Bone and Cartilage, ed. CT Brighton, J Black, S Pollack (New York: Grune and Stratton, 1979), p. 519.

6. L Hinkle, CD McCaig, and KR Robinson. The direction of growth of differentiating neurones and myoblasts from frog embryos in an applied electric field. J. Physiol. 314 (1981):121.

7. LF Jaffe and MM Poo. Neurites grow faster towards the cathode than the anode in a steady field. J. Exp. Zool. 209 (1979):115.

8. DE Johnson and GA Rodan. The effect of pulsating electromagnetic fields on prostaglandin synthesis in osteoblast-like cells. Trans. Bioelect. Repair and Growth Soc. 2 (1982): 7.

9. R Korenstein, D Somjen, H Fischler and I Binderman. Primary induced cellular changes and cell specificity in pulsed capacitive stimulation of bone cells in vitro. Trans. Bioelect. Repair and Growth Soc. 2 (1982):5.

10. R Levi-Montalcini. The nerve growth factor: Its mode of action on sensory and sympathetic nerve cells. Harvey Lectures 60 (1966):217.

11. G Marsh and HW Beams. In vitro control of growing chick nerve fibers by applied electric currents. J. Cell and Comp. Phys 27 (1946):139.

12. BR McLeod, AA Pilla, and MW Sampsel. Helmholtz coil-cell system spatial relationship and electrical dosage in the electromagnetic modulation of tissue growth and repair. Trans. Bioelect. Repair and Growth Soc. 2 (1982):13.

13. JL Morgan and NW Seeds. Tubulin constancy during morphological differentiation of mouse neuroblastoma cells. J. Cell Biol. 67 (1975):136.

14. N Patel and MM Poo. Orientation of neurite growth by extracellular electric fields. J. Neurosci. 2 (1982):483.

15. G Rein, R Dixey, and B Watson. Electromagnetic induction of neurotransmitter release from a neuronal cell line in tissue culture. Trans. Bioelect. Repair and Growth Soc. 2 (1982):39.

16. E Roederer, N Goldberg, and M Cohen. Modification of retrograde degeneration in transected spinal axons of the lamprey by applied DC current. J. Neurosci. 3 (1983):153.

17. P Sechaud and BF Sisken. Electrochemical characteristics of tantalum electrodes used in culture medium. Bioelectrochem. and Bioenerg. 8 (1981):633.

18. FJ Seil, AL Leiman, and WR Woodward. Cytosine arabinoside effects on developing cerebellum in tissue culture. Brain Res. 186 (1980):393.

19. BF Sisken and E Barr. Nerve regeneration in-vitro: Correlation of current/potential levels with neuroite outgrowth, neurons cell number and area. Trans. Bioelect. Repair and Growth Soc. 2 (1982):38.

20. BF Sisken and R Beuerman. Cellular interaction between co-cultured check trigeminal ganglia and cornea. Submitted (1983).

21. BF Sisken and JF Lafferty. Comparison of the effects of direct current and nerve growth factor on embryonic sensory ganglia. Bioelectrochem. and Bioenerg. 5 (1978):459.

22. BF Sisken, J Lafferty, and D Acree. The effects of direct and inductively coupled current, and the nerve growth factor, on nerve regeneration in vitro. In Mechanisms of Growth Control, ed. RO Becker (ILL: CC Thomas Co., 1981), p. 251.

23. BF Sisken and SD Smith. The effects of minute direct electrical currents on cultured chick embryo trigeminal ganglia. J. Embry. Exp. Morph. 33 (1975):29.

24. BF Sisken, SD Smith and JF Lafferty. A comparison of the effects of direct current, nerve growth factor and direct current plus nerve growth factor on amputated rat limbs. In Electrical Properties of Bone and Cartilage, ed. CT Brighton, J Black, S Pollack (New York: Grune and Stratton, 1979), p. 267.

25. SD Smith. Induction of partial limb regeneration in Rana pipiens by galvanic stimulation. Anat. Rec. 158 (1967): 89.

26. JA Spadaro. Electrical osteogenesis-role of the electrode material. In Electrical Properties of Bone and Cartilage, ed. CT Brighton, J Black, and S Pollack (New York: Grune and Stratton, 1979), p. 189.

27. S Varon and R Adler. Nerve growth factors and control of nerve growth. In Current Topics in Dev. Biology 16 (1980): 207.

28. S Varon, C Raiborn, and P Burnham. Comparative effects of nerve growth factor and ganglionic non neuronal cells on purified mouse ganglionic neurons in culture. J. Neurobiol. 5 (1974):355.

29. KM Yamada and NK Wessels. Effect of nerve growth factor on microtubular protein. Exp. Cell Res. 66 (1971):346.

12
Role of Extracellular Matrix Components in Local Control of Bone Regeneration, Remodeling and Repair

A. Hari Reddi

INTRODUCTION

The major aim of most students of tissue repair is to attain predictable and optimal healing of soft and hard tissues. The factors that regulate initiation, promotion and termination of tissue repair are not well understood. A common feature of most wounds is that the healing process is a local phenomenon. Since wound healing is a focal activity it is logical that factors regulating repair processes are locally released at the site of injury. The aim of this article is to demonstrate local induction of bone formation by demineralized extracellular matrix. The growing experimental evidence in support of the concept that extracellular matrix components carry and convey information to responding cells of the microcosm of tissue repair as a cascade will be presented.

CASCADE OF BONE DEVELOPMENT

The endogenous potential of the hard tissues for repair is well known to students of bone biology. The sequence of events during fracture healing in man is common knowledge to most orthopedic surgeons and traumatologists. However, the cell biology of hard tissue repair and the mechanism of action in the initiation of regeneration of bone is not well understood. A biochemical approach to the problem is inherently complicated by the tissue heterogeneity and the technical difficulty of avoiding adjoining bone and connective tissue. However these deterrents may be circumvented by the use of extracellular matrix-induced bone development system (Urist 1965; Reddi and Huggins 1972; Reddi and Anderson 1976; Reddi 1981; Reddi 1983) in an extraskeletal site. The sequential multistep cellular response to the matrix constitutes a developmental cascade and will be described (Table 12.1).

On implantation of the extracellular bone matrix in subcutaneous sites, a sequential development of endochondral bone is initiated. There was an instantaneous formation of a blood clot at the site of implantation. On day 1, the implant was a button-like, planoconvex plaque consisting of a conglomerate of matrix, fibrin and neutrophils. Then there was chemotaxis for fibroblast-like cells in vivo (Reddi and Huggins 1972). On day 3 the mesenchymal cells proliferated as observed by ^{3}H-thymidine incorporation by biochemical and radioautographic techniques (Rath and Reddi 1979a). Differentiating chondroblasts were seen on day 5. The implant consisted of hyaline cartilage on days 7-8 as observed by histology and $^{35}SO_4$ incorporation into proteoglycans (Reddi et al. 1978). On day 9 vascular invasion into the implant was noted and there was concomitant cartilage calcification. Osteogenic cells and osteoblasts were seen in the vicinity of sprouting capillaries on days 10-11. Bone development was marked by the appearance of Type I collagen (Reddi et al. 1977) and increased ^{45}Ca incorporation (Reddi 1981). The newly formed bone was remodeled on days 12-18 as indicated by the activity of lysosomal enzymes (Rath et al. 1981). Finally, the remodeled ossicle was the site of hematopoietic bone marrow differentiation as monitored by ^{59}Fe incorporation (Reddi and Huggins 1975). This experimental model is a prototype for the study of the role of extracellular matrix in vivo. In view of the biological importance of this phenomenon we have explored the mechanisms underlying the matrix-cell interactions.

REGULATION BY SYSTEMIC FACTORS

The cascade of matrix-induced endochondral bone development is subject to regulation by systemic hormones and nutrition. Bone development and mineralization is pituitary growth hormone dependent (Reddi and Sullivan 1980). There appears to be an additive effect of growth hormone and thyroid stimulating hormone. The influence streptozotocin-induced diabetes on matrix-induced bone formation was studied (Weiss and Reddi 1980b). Mesenchymal cell proliferation was decreased and delayed in diabetes and was corrected by insulin administration. Local administration of corticosteroids such as dexamethasone inhibited cell proliferation of progenitor cells (Rath and Reddi 1979b).

TABLE 12.1

The Cascade of Extracellular Bone Matrix-Induced Bone Development

Time After Implantation	Cellular Events	Molecular Processes
1 min	Blood clot formation. Platelet release.	Fibrin network formation. Release of platelet-derived growth factors.
1 hr	Arrival of polymorphonuclear leukocytes (PMN) by chemotaxis.	Release of proteolytic enzymes such as collagenase, elastase, etc.
3-18 hr	Accumulation of PMN. Adhesion of cells.	Limited proteolysis and release of chemotactic factors for fibroblasts. Binding of plasma fibronectin to implanted matrix.
day 1	Chemotaxis for fibroblasts and cell attachment to the implanted extracellular matrix.	Release of peptides of fibronectin. Increased cell motility. Role of microtubules and microfilaments.
day 2	Continued chemotaxis for fibroblasts. Signal transmission from matrix to cell surface.	Initiation of protein and nucleic acid synthesis. Possible release of growth factors.
day 3	Matrix-cell membrane interactions. Cell proliferation.	^{3}H-thymidine incorporation into DNA. Increase in ornithine decarboxylase activity. Type III collagen synthesis.
day 5	Differentiation of chondroblasts.	Increase in $^{35}SO_4$ incorporation into proteoglycans.

(continued)

(Table 12.1 continued)

Time After Implantation	Cellular Events	Molecular Processes
day 7	Chondrocytes, synthesis and secretion of matrix.	Type II collagen synthesis. Cartilage specific Proteoglycan synthesis.
day 9	Hypertrophy of chondrocytes. Calcification of cartilage matrix. Vascular invasion. Endothelial cell proliferation. Degradation of cartilage.	Increase in ^{45}Ca incorporation and alkaline phosphatase activity. Type IV collagen synthesis. Laminin Factor VIII in blood vessels.
days 10-12	Osteoblasts. Bone formation and mineralization.	Type I collagen synthesis. Bone proteoglycan synthesis. Peak in ^{45}Ca incorporation and alkaline phosphatase activity.
days 12-18	Osteoclasts. Bone remodeling and dissolution of the implanted matrix.	Increase in lysosomal enzymes acid phosphatase, aryl sulfatase and proteases. Upswing in accumulation of γ-carboxyglutamic acid containing protein (Osteocalcin).
day 21	Bone marrow Differentiation.	Increase in ^{59}Fe incorporation into heme. Accumulation of lysozyme. Type III collagen synthesis.

The regulatory role of vitamin D metabolites on skeletal development is well known, and therefore the potential of matrix-induced bone forming system was examined for vitamin D metabolite effects on discrete stages of bone differentiation. $^{35}SO_4$ incorporation into proteoglycans during chondrogenesis was increased by 24,25-$(OH)_2D_3$ as compared to 1,25-$(OH)_2D_3$. Also 24,25-$(OH)_3D_3$ stimulated ^{45}Ca incorporation into bone mineral. On the other hand 1,25$(OH)_2D_3$ appeared to increase bone remodeling (Wientroub and Reddi 1982). These results indicate that a combination of 24,25$(OH)_2D_3$ and 1,25$(OH)_2D_3$ regulates endochondral bone development; the former stimulates chondrogenesis and bone formation, whereas the latter metabolite regulates remodeling.

MECHANISM OF ACTION

The molecular mechanisms underlying the action of extracellular matrix on cells to initiate the developmental cascade are not known. The response to the extracellular matrix is specific and is elicited only by bone and tooth matrix but not by tendon and skin (Reddi 1976). The surface charge on the matrix is crucial (Reddi 1976). Perturbation of the charge characteristics of the matrix by chemical modifications such as N-acetylation, carboxymethylation and modification of the guanidino groups of arginine abolishes the inductive response. Pretreatment of the matrix with heparin, dextran sulfate and the anionic dye Evans blue inhibits bone cell differentiation (Reddi 1976). The physical dimensions of the matrix particles have an important influence on the quantitative response of new bone. The optimal size for bone induction is in the range of 74-850 μm. These observations are consonant with known requirements for the dimensions of substratum in anchorage-dependent cell proliferation (Stoker et al. 1968; Folkman and Moscona 1978; Gospodarowicz et al. 1980; Reddi 1976). The inductive property is acid stable but alkali labile. The biological activity is heat stable (65°C for 8 h), trypsin-sensitive, and appears to be a glycoprotein on the basis of periodate sensitivity. The conformation of disulfides is necessary for biological activity, as reduction with mercaptoethanol abolishes the activity.

In view of the fact the implanted matrix is predominantly collagenous, we have examined the possible role of fibronectin during early matrix-cell interactions (Weiss and Reddi 1980a; 1981). On implantation the matrix binds fibronectin, which may constitute an important initial event for cell attachment to the matrix. The initial orientation of cell surface to matrix is by electrostatic forces. However, this is not sufficient for subsequent changes in the cells. It is likely the collagen-fibronectin interaction helps to bring the putative inductor in contact with focal cell surface receptors. This results in transduction of cell surface information to the genome. Current approaches in our laboratory are directed towards the identification of various factors that might regulate the developmental cascade of matrix-induced bone development.

One of the first events in this cascade is chemotaxis of cells towards the implanted matrix, followed by mitosis and differentiation into cartilage and bone. In view of this we have explored the potential of various dissociative extractants to obtain factors that promote chemotaxis, mitosis and differentiation. Treatment with 4M guanidine hydrochloride (Anastassiades et al. 1978) or 8M urea containing 1 M NaCl or 1% (w/v) sodium dodecylsulfate extracted the bone inductive property from the matrix (Sampath and Reddi 1981). When the lyophilized extract and the residue were tested alone they were devoid of biological activity. However, on reconstitution of the respective residues with extracts by dialysis against water, the bone inductive property was restored. Gel filtration of the 4M guanidine hydrochloride extract on Sepharose CL-4B resulted in a broad heterogeneous peak. Various pooled fractions were tested for bone inductive property by reconstitution and it was found that the fraction consisting of proteins less than 50,000 daltons was active. Current experiments involve further purification of these extracellular matrix components. In view of the fact that chemotaxis and attachment of cells to the matrix is an early step the chemotactic potency of 4M guanidine hydrochloride extracts was examined. Recent experiments (Somerman et al. 1983) demonstrated potent chemotactic activity in proteins eluted from a gel filtration column of Sepharase CL-6B, in the region of 60,000 daltons. Examination of the mitogenic activity in these extracts revealed that osteoinductively active fractions (< 50,000 daltons) were growth-promoting to fibroblasts from rat-embryo and human skin (Sampath et al. 1982) but not bovine aortic endothelial cells.

Taken together, these results imply that there might be a cascade-type mechanism, that governs extracellular matrix-induced bone differentiation. The initial step in this scheme might be the release of chemotactic factors by limited proteolysis. Then the arrival of mesenchymal cells by chemotaxis is followed by attachment to the matrix via fibronectin and related cell adhesive proteins. The release of mitogenic factors from the matrix promotes growth of cells. Finally the cells differentiate into cartilage and bone in response to specific matrix-derived factors. These observations may have important implications for the local control of skeletal differentiation and remodeling in postfetal life. It is likely that extracellular matrix components might specify positional information during embryonic development. It is possible that extracellular matrix functions in the solid state as an affinity matrix to sequester and release in a controlled manner crucial morphogenetic molecules for bone regeneration and hard tissue repair.

PERSPECTIVES

The foregoing consideration of the cell biology of matrix-induced bone development may have important implications for correction of acquired and congenital craniofacial and other skeletal deformities. Indeed, Glowacki et al. (1981) have reported dramatic results with the use of demineralized bone matrix in the correction of craniofacial defects. The growing understanding of bone differentiation may help us undertake a rational therapeutic approach to a variety of orthopedic and periodontal diseases. The future holds much promise for the alleviation of several crippling disorders of hard tissues.

NOTES

Anastassiades T, Puzic O, Puzic R. Effect of solubilized bone matrix components on cultured fibroblasts derived from neonatal rat tissues. Calcif Tiss Res 26:173-179, 1978.

Folkman J, Moscona A. Role of cell shape in growth control. Nature 273:345-348, 1978.

Glowacki J, Kaban LB, Murray JE, Folkman J, Mulliken JB. Application of the biological principle of induced osteogenesis for craniofacial defects. Lancet 1:959-963, 1981.

Gospodarowicz D, Vlodavsky I, Savion N. The extracellular matrix and the control of proliferation of vascular endothelial and smooth muscle cells. J Supramol Structure 13:339-57, 1980.

Rath NC, Reddi AH. Collagenous bone matrix is a local mitogen. Nature 278:855-857, 1979a.

Rath NC, Reddi AH. Influence of adrenalectomy and dexamethasone on matrix-induced endochondral bone differentiation. Endocrinology 104:1698-1704, 1979b.

Rath NC, Hand AR, Reddi AH. Activity and distribution of lysosomal enzymes during collagenous matrix-induced cartilage, bone and bone marrow development. Develop Biol 85:89-98, 1981.

Reddi AH. Collagen and cell differentiation. In Biochemistry of Collagen, Ramachandran GN, and Reddi AH (eds) pp. 449-478. New York: Plenum Press. 1976.

Reddi AH. Cell biology and biochemistry of endochondral bone development. Coll Res 1:209-26, 1981.

Reddi AH. Regulation of local differentiation of cartilage and bone by extracellular matrix: A cascade type mechanism. In Limb Development and Regeneration Part B, Kelley RO, Goetinck PF, and MacCabe JA (eds) pp. 261-268. New York: AR Liss, 1983.

Reddi AH, Anderson WA. Collagenous bone matrix-induced endochondral ossification and hemopoiesis. J Cell Biol 69:557-572, 1976.

Reddi AH, Huggins CB. Biochemical sequences in the transformation of fibroblasts in adolescent rats. Proc Nat Acad Sci USA 69:1601-1605, 1972.

Reddi AH, Huggins CB. Formation of bone marrow in fibroblast transformation ossicles. Proc Nat Acad Sci USA 72:2212-2216, 1975.

Reddi AH, Gay R, Gay S, Miller EJ. Transitions in collagen types during matrix-induced cartilage, bone and bone marrow formation. Proc Nat Acad Sci USA 74:5589-5593, 1977.

Reddi AH, Hascall VC, Hascall GK. Changes in proteoglycan types during matrix-induced cartilage and bone development. J Biol Chem 253:2429-2436, 1978.

Reddi AH and Sullivan NE. Matrix-induced endochondral bone differentiation: Influence of hypophysectomy, growth hormone and thyroid-stimulating hormone. Endrocrinology 107:1291-1299, 1980.

Sampath TK, Reddi AH. Dissociative extraction and reconstitution of extracellular matrix components involved in local bone differentiation. Proc Nat Acad Sci USA 78:7599-7602, 1981.

Sampath TK, DeSimone DP, Reddi AH. Extracellular matrix-derived growth factor. Exp Cell Res 142:460-464, 1982.

Somerman M, Hewitt AT, Varner HH, Schiffman E, Termine J, Reddi AH. Identification of a bone matrix-derived chemotactic factor. Calcif Tiss Int, in press, 1983.

Stoker M, O'Neill C, Berryman S, Waxman V. Anchorage and growth regulation in normal and virus transformed cells. Int J Cancer 3:683-697, 1968.

Urist, MR. Bone: Formation by autoinduction. Science 150: 893-898, 1965.

Weiss RE, Reddi AH. Synthesis and localization of fibronectin during collagenous matrix-mesenchymal cell interaction and differentiation of cartilage and bone in vivo. Proc Nat Acad Sci USA 77:2074-2078, 1980a.

Weiss RE, Reddi AH. Influence of experimental diabetes and insulin on matrix-induced cartilage and bone differentiation. Amer J Physiol 206E:271-279, 1980b.

Weiss RE, Reddi AH. Role of fibronectin in collagenous matrix-induced mesenchymal cell proliferation and differentiation in vivo. Exp Cell Res 133:247-253, 1981.

Wientroub S, Reddi AH. Vitamin D metabolites and endochondral bone development. In Current Advances in Skeletogenesis, Silbermann M, Slavkin HC (eds) pp. 211-217. New York: Elsevier, 1982.

13
Physiological Aspects of Bone Repair Using Demineralized Bone

Julie Glowacki, Leonard B. Kaban, Stephen T. Sonis, Robert K. Rosenthal and John B. Mulliken

CLINICAL BONE GRAFTING

Bone grafting is often necessary to correct craniofacial, orthopedic, and oral skeletal deformities. Bone is routinely transplanted for repair and reconstruction of defects due to congenital malformations, trauma, neoplasia, and infection. The material of choice is fresh cancellous bone chips and marrow from another part of the patient's skeleton termed an autograft. With such a graft, living osteoblasts and preosteoblasts are transplanted to the site where new bone will be synthesized. Cancellous grafts, however, do not provide immediate structural stability nor mass to the recipient site. For segmental defects or contour augmentations, larger grafts of corticocancellous bone may be required. Pieces of ribs, iliac, or tibial bone provide fewer viable cells than cancellous marrow but serve as internal splinting devices.

There are several obvious limitations to the use of fresh autografts. Harvesting of the graft increases operative time and is accompanied by the risk of excessive blood loss, pneumothorax, infection, chronic pain, deformity, and paresthesia (Murray et al. 1979). The amount of donor bone available may be insufficient for correction of a large defect; this is especially so in infants, children, and frail adults. The shape of the donor bone also limits the appropriateness of the transplant. The most serious problem with conventional bone grafts is unpredictable resorption and failure. The failure rate varies with different anatomical sites and can approach 30% in orthopedic surgery (Urist 1980a) and 70% for onlay grafts in nonweight-bearing craniofacial regions (Mulliken et al. 1981).

The development of microsurgical techniques for the transplantation of living bone larger than six centimeters has been successful in craniofacial reconstruction (Taylor et al. 1975) and orthopedic surgery (Weiland and Daniel 1979). Although vascularized tissue transfers would theoretically avoid the complications of graft resorption, they are limited in applicability because of the few anatomically suitable donor sites, the lengthy operative times, and the skill required of the surgical team.

The problem of donor bone availability has received considerable attention. Currently, allogeneic bone implants are prepared for storage in regional or in-hospital bone banks by freezing or freeze-drying cadaver bone (Friedlaender 1982). It is believed that freezing reduces the antigenicity of allogeneic bone to levels that can be tolerated by the patient. Clinical and experimental studies have shown that preserved bone is inferior to fresh autogenous bone (Heiple et al. 1963) and that it is expensive to maintain banks (Doppelt et al. 1981), but it is the only material available.

A variety of synthetic implants have been used to bridge or fill osseous defects, including ceramics, polymers, and metals. Thus far, most of these initiate healing that is too slow or too transitory to withstand the forces exerted upon the skeleton. The search for the perfect replacement for osteoblasts remains intensive, but current clinical reconstructive procedures make use of the skeleton's inherent mechanisms of osseous repair. A review of the physiology of bone healing and of the mechanisms of graft incorporation points out the fundamental differences between the procedures described above and the principle of induced osteogenesis.

MECHANISMS OF BONE HEALING

The physiological mechanisms of bone grafting vary with the different types of implants. New bone can be formed by three basic mechanisms: osteogenesis, osteoconduction, and osteoinduction (Table 13.1).

Osteogenesis

Osteogenesis is the formation of the mineralized matrix of bone by osteoblasts. The transplantation of cancellous chips and marrow from the crest of the ilium, for example, to another part of the body is, in effect, a translocation of osteoblasts and preosteoblasts into a site where they synthesize new bone. Cancellous bone is the most appropriate donor bone because

TABLE 13.1

Mechanisms of Bone Healing

Type	Physiologic Principle	Examples
Osteogenesis	Transplantation of viable osteoblasts and preosteoblasts	Cancellous marrow; periosteum; and vascularized grafts
Osteoconduction	Ingrowth of bone from margins of the defect with gradual resorption of the implant	Cortical segments; banked allogeneic or xenogeneic bone; resorbable materials
Induced Osteogenesis	Phenotypic conversion of mesenchymal cells into skeletal cells	Demineralized bone bone and dentin.

its trabeculae are covered with osteoblasts that survive the transplantation and also because the marrow contains viable osteogenic precursor cells (Ham and Gordon 1952). Thus autogenous cancellous marrow establishes centers of bone formation in sites where new bone is needed. Because the grafted tissue possesses no immediate structural strength, composite implants of cancellous marrow with metallic trays or cortical bone segments have been preferred (Boyne 1969).

Studies on fracture healing demonstrate that the periosteum is a source of osteogenic cells (Ham and Harris 1971). In 1867 Ollier demonstrated the osteogenic potential of transplanted periosteum (Ollier 1867). More recently, Knize has shown that grafts with periosteum undergo less resorption when placed on the skull than grafts bared of periosteum (Knize 1974). Autogenous periosteal grafting, however, is not practical for most osseous reconstructive purposes.

Vascularized bone grafts also involve the translocation of viable tissue to a new site. By maintaining (on a pedicle) or re-establishing (by microanastomoses) the osseous circulation, large segments of cortical bone can survive harvesting. If the transplanted bone maintains approximation to the edges of the defects, healing occurs by a process analogous to primary fracture repair, in which direct union occurs by osteogenic cells.

Osteoconduction

In the transplantation of devitalized bone, direct osteogenesis by the transplant does not take place. Few cells actually survive harvesting of large fresh cortical segments of bone unless they are vascularized. Banked bone, whether frozen, lyophilized, or irradiated, is also devitalized and hence is not a graft but an implant. In these cases, incorporation of the implant occurs by a process quite distinct from osteogenesis. In osteoconduction, dead bone acts as a trellis for the ingrowth of vessels, followed by the resorption of the implant and deposition of new bone derived from the edges of the defect. The cellular mechanisms of implant resorption and bone synthesis are analogous to the process of bony union of an aligned fracture. Trauma to the bone and surrounding tissue is accompanied by disruption of the circulation and death of the osteocytes in the haversian systems for a distance from either side of the fracture line. The surfaces of the dead bone become invaded by capillaries and resorbed by osteoclasts and new bone is formed in a callus of cartilage and woven bone derived from medullary proliferation and periosteum. The callus and adjacent bone are gradually remodeled and creeping repair culminates with consolidation of haversian bone (Simmons 1980). Axhausen is credited for the use of the term "creeping substitution" to describe the process of resorption of an implant that occurs prior to the ingrowth of new bone (Axhausen 1912). With a dense cortical bone transplant, this process is very gradual and may take years before all the dead bone is replaced by new living bone. This same process occurs following the implantation of banked allogeneic bone. Experimental and clinical studies using massive banked osteochondral allo-implants suggest that resorption may not be necessary for the success of these heroic limb-sparing procedures (Mankin et al. 1976). Despite controversial evidence regarding the antigenicity of bone, it appears that the antigenicity of processed banked bone is low enough to be tolerated by patients (Brown and Cruess 1982).

Osteoinduction

Osteoinduction is the phenotypic conversion of connective tissue into bone by an appropriate stimulus. Demineralized bone and dentin are such post-embryonic osteoinductive stimuli (Ray and Holloway 1957; Urist 1965). After implantation into subcutaneous pockets in rats, demineralized bone powders induce the conversion of connective tissue into cartilage, which becomes calcified, invaded by host vessels, and replaced by bone (Reddi and Huggins 1972). This highly synchronous sequence of events is analogous to normal endochondral ossification. This principle has been applied in the use of demineralized bone implants in osseous repair, reconstruction, and construction reviewed below.

MATERIALS AND METHODS

Experimental Studies

After 28-day-old rats (male, CD strain) were anesthetized with ether, the pericrania were stripped off the parietal skulls through coronal incisions. A 6 × 9 mm defect was made through each parietal bone with an electric drill and burr. The defects were rinsed with Ringer's solution and were filled with implants or left empty. The skin incisions were closed with interrupted sutures. Isogeneic bone powder was prepared from femoral and humeri of adult rats. Xenogeneic powders were made from bones from humans, chickens, and cows. The cleaned diaphyses were extracted with absolute ethanol (1 h) followed by anhydrous ethyl ether (1 h). The bones were pulverized in a Spex liquid nitrogen impacting mill and sieved to particle sizes 38-75, 75-250, 250-420, and >450 μm (Glowacki, Altobelli, and Mulliken 1981).

Demineralized bone powder (DBP) was prepared by extracting the bone powders with 0.5 M HCl (25 meq/g bone) for 3 h at room temperature followed by washes in distilled water to remove all acid and liberated minerals, and sequential 1 h washes in absolute ethanol and anhydrous ether.

Clinical Studies

Allogeneic bone was obtained from the Interhospital Organ Bank, as part of a multiple organ donor program. Cancellous bone was cut into 6-cm segments or into coarse chips; cortical bone was pulverized and sieved into powder (75-450, >450 μm). These were extracted for 1 h in absolute ethanol and for 1 h in anhydrous ether. The material was demineralized with 0.5 M HCl (25 mmol/g bone); this required 3 h at room temperature for powder and chips and several days at 4°C for the blocks. Acid and dissolved minerals were washed away by copious changes of distilled water. The demineralized bone was sequentially extracted for 1 h in absolute ethanol and 1 h in anhydrous ether. The material was double-wrapped and sterilized by cathode-ray irradiation with 2×10^6 rads or, more recently, by ethylene oxide, and stored at room temperature. Upon rehydration in Ringer's solution, blocks became rubbery and could be carved easily; hydrated powder had the consistency of paste.

Volunteers were entered into the craniofacial, oral, periodontal, hand and orthopedic protocols according to the following criteria: 1) to avoid the harvesting of fresh autografts in infants or patients who had had previous harvestings, 2) to fill a small defect, or 3) to supplement conventional grafting when insufficient autogenous bone was available. The patients' ages ranged from 15 months to 61 years.

Bone healing was documented by clinical and roentgenographic examination, and, when possible, by CT scan and ultrasonographic examination. Biopsy specimens, prepared for undecalcified histologic examination, were obtained in those patients who required further surgery in areas near the demineralized bone implant (Glowacki et al. 1981).

Forty-eight patients (28-61 years) with a variety of periodontal defects volunteered for inclusion in the periodontal study (Sonis, Kaban, and Glowacki, 1983). After standard flap construction and debridement of granulation tissue, allogeneic demineralized bone powder (75-450 μm) was rehydrated and packed into the periodontal osseous defects. The flaps were sutured to approximate primary closure. Pre-operative and monthly postoperative evaluation included radiographic bone height and/or evidence of bony fill, measurement of pocket depth, and tooth mobility.

Twenty-four patients have been entered into orthopedic protocols for treatment of non-union fractures, cysts, congenital pseudarthroses, scoliosis, and staged limb lengthening.

FACTORS INFLUENCING OSTEOINDUCTION

In 1931 Huggins reported that proliferating mucosa of kidney, ureter, or bladder induced bone formation in connective tissue (Huggins 1931). More recently, Ray and Holloway (1957), Urist (1965) and Reddi and Huggins (1972) demonstrated that osteogenesis could also be induced by the devitalized, demineralized matrix of bone or dentin (Figure 13.1). The most important requirement for the matrix is that all acid-soluble components be removed (Glowacki, Altobelli, and Mulliken 1981). Mineral-

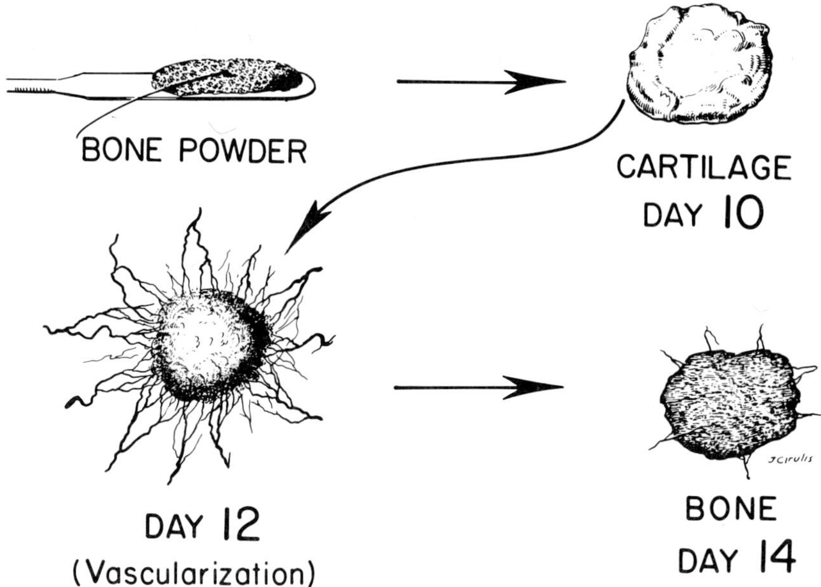

FIGURE 13.1 Following implantation in a subcutaneous pocket, demineralized bone powder induces the proliferation of a cartilagenous button. After vascularization, the cartilage is replaced by bone.

containing powders are not osteoinductive, but rather induce resorption by mono- and multinucleated cells (Glowacki, Altobelli, and Mulliken 1981; Holtrop, Cox, and Glowacki 1982). Following implantation in subcutaneous or intramuscular pockets, demineralized matrix elicits a mild and brief inflammatory phase. Host mesenchymal cells are attracted to the bone powder, attach to its surfaces and by day 7 are phenotypically converted to chondroblasts. These cells produce cartilage matrix for 4 days until vascular invasion, cartilage mineralization, and chondrolysis begin. By the end of the second week, osteoblasts and woven bone with marrow spaces are evident.

The nature of the osteoinductive factor has been extensively investigated by Urist (1980b). Table 13.2 summarizes his evidence for physical, chemical, and enzymatic susceptibility of the osteoinductive factor. Urist's most recent work concerns the characterization of a soluble factor that can initiate osteogenesis, termed bone morphogenetic protein. He characterizes the factor as a hydrophobic glycoprotein (Urist, Mikulski, and Lietze 1979). Reddi has investigated the mitogenic activity of bone matrix

TABLE 13.2

Physical, Chemical and Enzymatic Inactivation of the Osteoinductive Activity in Demineralized Bone Matrix

Physical	Chemical	Enzymatic
Pulverization	Deamination	
Ultrasonication	Dinitrophenylation	Chymotrypsin
>2 mrads irradiation	Cu^{+2}-complex	pronase
100°C	Disulfide cleavage	
	Peptide cleavage at Met	
	Hydrophobic and hydrophilic bond rupture	

Source: Urist, MR, Fundamental and Clinical Bone Physiology, Philadelphia: JB Lippincott, 1980b.

(Rath and Reddi, 1979b) and has extracted a growth factor for fibroblasts but not endothelial cells (Sampath, DeSimone, and Reddi 1982).

Other work points to the importance of surface characteristics of the insoluble demineralized bone matrix for its osteoinductive activity. By treating powders of demineralized bone at low pH with the electronegative polyanion Evans Blue, Reddi and Huggins (1974) found a reduction of osteoinductive activity; this could be restored by treating the inactive material with hexadimethrine. These results were interpreted as evidence for the importance of direct cell-to-bone-matrix contact for osteoinduction. Our observations on the inactivation of demineralized bone implants by presoaking in Povidone-iodine are consistent with this view (Glowacki et al. 1981). Similarly, powders too small (<40 μm) for adequate anchorage for cell spreading have no osteoinductive activity (Reddi 1974). Furthermore, the role of fibronectin, known to be associated with cellular adhesion, has also been demonstrated in matrix-induced osteogenesis (Weiss and Reddi 1980a). We have quantitated osteoinduction in rats by demineralized bone powders of different particles sizes (Table 13.3); the smaller particles, presenting more surface area to the recipient tissue induced more bone per field than did larger particles (Glowacki, Altobelli, and Mulliken 1981). This aspect has importance in designing the most suitable demineralized implant for clinical applications and is discussed later.

The synchrony and homogeneity of osteoinduction, which is endochondral, can be maximized by implanting small particles of narrow size range (75-250 μm). It is therefore possible to predict the amount of cartilage or bone that should be induced at various times following implantation (Glowacki, Altobelli, and Mulliken 1981) and thereby evaluate different materials and the effect of endocrine or drug manipulations. We have shown that demineralized bone powders prepared for human, chicken, rabbit and bovine bones induce bone formation in rats (Mulliken and Glowacki 1980; Glowacki 1982).

Procedures or factors that interrupt the vascularization of cartilage on day 11 appear to freeze induction at the cartilagenous phase (Glowacki 1982). These include 1) transplantation of induced cartilage prior to host vascularization, 2) induction of rickety cartilage in hypocalcemic rats, or 3) administration of medroxy-progesterone during induction. These observations raise the question of the clinical potential for using demineralized bone implants for repair and replacement of cartilage. Acceptable ways of inhibiting vascularization locally would have enormous clinical applications.

The hormonal status of the animal also has expected effects on osteoinduction. The process is dependent on pituitary growth hormone (Reddi and Sullivan 1980; Syftestad and Urist 1980), insulin (Weiss and Reddi 1980b), and normal calcium and vitamin D status (Glowacki 1982). The effects of dexamethasone (Rath and Reddi 1979a) and calcitonin (Weiss et al. 1981; Glowacki and Deftos 1983) have also been studied.

TABLE 13.3

Extent of Osteoinduction at 2 Weeks Following Implantation of Demineralized Bone of Different Particle Size

Particle Size (μm)	Particle Perimeter (mean/mm^2 area)	Induced Bone (% area ± SEM)
38-75	132	42 ± 7
75-250	62	40 ± 6
250-450	33	21 ± 3
>450	4	2

CLINICAL APPLICATIONS OF THE PRINCIPLE OF OSTEOINDUCTION

Following studies documenting the efficacy of demineralized bone implants in animals with experimental cranial (Mulliken and Glowacki 1980) and mandibular (Kaban and Glowacki 1981) defects, a clinical protocol was approved for the use of demineralized cadaver bone in volunteers with craniofacial deformities for whom there were no alternative treatments (Glowacki et al. 1981). After demonstration of the safety of the material, we were able to expand the clinical applications. Table 13.4 summarizes the repair and reconstructive applications of demineralized cadaver bone implants for which follow-up evaluations ranged from 2 to 4 years.

The demineralized bone powder has been used in 3 forms for different clinical situations (Kaban, Mulliken, and Glowacki 1982). Powdered cortical bone provides the largest surface area for osteoinduction and, when rehydrated as a paste, is convenient to use as caulking to fill small irregular defects. Small chips (5 mm) of demineralized cancellous bone provides sufficient surface due to its porous spongy nature and has been used to fill cystic lesions. Segmental defects and contour deficits have been treated with large corticocancellous blocks or strips because they are easy to carve to exact dimensions; the cortical element provides some structural function, and the cancellous portion induces osteogenesis within the porous structure.

Most of the maxillocraniofacial deformities were congenital, such as craniofacial dysostoses, hypertelorism syndromes, oronasal fistulae, nasal and midface hypoplasia, and isolated jaw deformities. In defects that could be stressed or palpated, solid healing was demonstrable by two to three months. Roentgenographic examination showed ossification as early as 10 weeks. Biopsies have been possible in patients who required further surgical procedures in nearby anatomical regions. They showed new bone united to the demineralized implant (Glowacki et al. 1981; Kaban, Mulliken, and Glowacki 1982). We will have to wait 5 years before any comparison can be made between conventional and demineralized bone implants' long-term resorption rates. The results from midface onlay reconstructions are very encouraging, however, because in 11 patients followed up to 18 months, no change in contour was demonstrated. These are sites of rapid resorption of conventional grafts.

The complication rate is less than that in conventional surgery, primarily because of the avoidance of harvesting procedures.

TABLE 13.4

Clinical Applications of Demineralized Bone Implants

Application	Number of Patients
Maxillocraniofacial	
Jaw cysts	3
Maxilla/mandible	39
Clefts, fistulae	14
Craniofacial	16
Orthopedic	
Non-union fractures + pseudarthroses	12
Long bone cysts	7
Scoliosis	5
Limb lengthening	1
Hand	2
Periodontal	48

Urist has the most extensive experience with demineralized bone implants for orthopedic surgery (Urist 1968). We have initiated studies of the efficacy of demineralized bone implants in infants with scoliosis, in documented non-union fractures, in congenital psudarthrosis, in cysts, for phalangeal reconstruction, and for limb lengthening. While the majority of implants have been prepared from cadaver bone, some were of bovine origin.

Demineralized bone implants are safe and easy to use in a variety of surgical procedures. Osteogenesis is rapid, providing stability in maxillofacial regions within weeks. In long-bone fractures or other weight-bearing regions, function may not be restored as rapidly as with conventional mineral-containing bone implants because of the flexibility of demineralized bone. The major advantage of demineralized bone implants is that their use avoids harvesting procedures, which are not always possible in small infants and patients with large defects, nor always justified if only a small amount of bone is needed. The biologic phenomenon of induced osteogenesis does not include an obligatory resorptive phase and may therefore produce bone that undergoes less late resorption. This is a problem especially in contour augmentation in the craniofacial region. Longer follow-ups will be necessary before we can evaluate endurance of induced bone, but our 4-year results indicate maintenance of the corrections.

SUMMARY

The physiological mechanisms of bone grafting vary with different types of implants. New bone can be formed by three basic mechanisms: osteogenesis, osteoconduction, and osteoinduction. In osteogenesis, viable osteoblasts are transplanted from one part of the body (often cancellous marrow of the ilium) to the site where new bone is needed. In osteoconduction, the dead bone or implant acts as a trellis for the ingrowth of vessels, followed by resorption of the implant and deposition of new bone derived from the edges of the defect. Osteoinduction is the conversion of mesenchymal tissue into bone by an appropriate stimulus, such as demineralized bone.

Experimental studies have shown that endochondral bone is induced by demineralized bone. Procedures or factors that interrupt the vascularization of the induced cartilage appear to halt induction at the cartilagenous phase. The hormonal status of the animal also has effects on the timing and extent of osteoinduction. The induced skeletal tissue is under the same physiologic and endocrine regulation as the animal's skeleton.

Demineralized cadaver and bovine bone have been used to spare patients the harvesting procedures required by conventional bone grafting. At Children's Hospital Medical Center, more than 70 patients have received demineralized bone implants for maxillocraniofacial reconstruction, 48 for periodontal defects, and 27 for orthopedic surgery, such as correction of non-union fractures, cysts, and scoliosis. The implants are well tolerated, easy to use, and do not hinder soft tissue healing. Osseous repair and maintenance of the correction have been demonstrated in patients who have been followed for up to 4 years.

REFERENCES

Axhausen, G. Ueber histologischen vorgang vei der transplantation von gelenkenden. Arch. Klin. Chir. 99:1, 1912.

Boyne, PJ. Restoration of osseous defects in maxillofacial casualties. J. Amer. Dental Assoc. 78:767-777, 1969.

Brown, KLB, and Cruess, RL. Bone and cartilage transplantation in orthopedic surgery. J. Bone Joint Surg. 64-A: 270-279, 1982.

Doppelt, SH, Tomford, WW, Lucas, AD, and Mankin, HJ. Operational and financial aspects of a Hospital Bone Bank. J. Bone Joint Surg. 63A:1472-1481, 1981.

Friedlaender, GE. Current concepts review: Bone-banking. J. Bone Joint Surg. 64-A:307-311, 1982.

Glowacki, J. Studies on the regulation of bone synthesis and bone resorption. In Factors and Mechanisms Influencing Bone Growth, Dixon, AD, and Sarnat, BG (eds), pp. 83-91. New York: A. R. Liss, 1982.

Glowacki, J and Deftos, LJ. The effects of calcitonin on bone formation. In The Effects of Calcitonin in Man, Gennari, C, and Segre, G (eds). Milan: Masson Italia Editori, in press, 1983.

Glowacki, J, Kaban, LB, Murray, JE, Folkman, J, and Mulliken, JB. Application of the biological principle of induced osteogenesis for craniofacial defects. Lancet 1:959-963, 1981.

Glowacki, J, Altobelli, D, and Mulliken, JB. Fate of mineralized and demineralized osseous implants in cranial defects. Calcif. Tissue Int. 30:71-76, 1981.

Kaban, LB, Mulliken, JB, and Glowacki, J. Treatment of jaw defects with demineralized bone implants. J. Oral. Maxillo. Surg. 40:623-626, 1982.

Kaban, LB, and Glowacki, J. Induced osteogenesis in the repair of experimental mandibular defects in rats. J. Dent. Res. 60:1356-1364, 1981.

Ham, A, and Gordon, S. The origin of bone that forms in association with cancellous chips transplanted into muscle. Br. J. Plast. Surg. 5:154-160, 1952.

Ham, AW, and Harris, WR. In Biochemistry and Physiology of Bone, Bourne, GH (ed). Vol. III, pp. 338-399. New York: Academic Press, 1971.

Heiple, KB, Chase, SN, and Herndon, CH. A comparative study of the healing process following different types of bone transplantation. J. Bone Joint Surg. 45-A:1593, 1963.

Holtrop, ME, Cox, KA, and Glowacki, J. Cells of the mononuclear phagocytic system resorb implanted bone matrix. Calcif. Tissue Int. 34:488-492, 1982.

Huggins, CB. The formation of bone under the influence of epithelium of the urinary tract. Arch. Surg. 22:377-408, 1931.

Knize, DM. The influence of periosteum and calcitonin on onlay bone graft survival. Plast. Reconstr. Surg. 53:190, 1974.

Mankin, HJ, Fogelson, FS, Thrasher, AZ, and Jaffer, F. Massive resection and allograft transplantation in the treatment of malignant bone tumors. New Eng. J. Med. 294: 1247-1255, 1976.

Mulliken, JB, Glowacki, J, Kaban, LB, Folkman, J, and Murray, JE. Use of demineralized allogeneic bone implants for the correction of maxillocraniofacial deformities. Ann. Surg. 194:366-372, 1981.

Mulliken, JB, and Glowacki, J. Induced osteogenesis for repair and construction in the craniofacial region. Plast. Reconstr. Surg. 65:553-559, 1980.

Murray, JE, Kaban, LB, and Mulliken, JB. Craniofacial abnormalities. In Pediatric Surgery, Ravitch, MM, Welch, KJ, Benson, CD, Aberdeen, E, and Randolph, JG (eds). Vol. 1, pp. 233-248. Chicago: Year Book Medical Publishers, 1979.

Ollier, L. Traite experimental et clinique de la regeneration des os et de la production artificielle du tissu osseux. Paris: Masson, 1867.

Rath, NC, and Reddi, AH. Influence of adrenalectomy and dexamethasone on matrix-induced endochondral bone differentiation. Endocrinology 104:1698-1704, 1979a.

Rath, NC, and Reddi, AH. Collagenous bone matrix is a local mitogen. Nature 278:855-857, 1979b.

Ray, RD, and Holloway, JA. Bone implants: Preliminary results of an experimental study. J. Bone Joint Surg. 39A: 1119-1128, 1957.

Reddi, AH. Bone matrix in the solid state: Geometric influence on differentiation on fibroblasts. Adv. Biol. Med. Phys. 15: 1-18, 1974.

Reddi, AH, and Huggins, CB. Biochemical sequences in the transformation of normal fibroblasts in adolescent rats. Proc. Natl. Acad. Sci. USA 69:1601-1605, 1972.

Reddi, AH, and Huggins, CB. Cyclic inactivation and restoration of competence of bone matrix to transform fibroblasts. Proc. Natl. Acad. Sci. USA 71:1648-1652, 1974.

Reddi, AH, and Sullivan, NE. Matrix-induced endochondral bone formation: Influence of hypophysectomy, growth hormone, and thyroid stimulating hormone. Endocrinology 105:1291-1299, 1980.

Sampath, TK, DeSimone, DP, and Reddi, AH. Extracellular bone-derived growth factor. Exp. Cell Res. 142:460-464, 1982.

Simmons, DJ. Fracture healing. In Fundamental and Clinical Bone Physiology, Urist, MR (ed), pp. 283-330. Philadelphia: J. B. Lippincott, 1980.

Sonis, ST, Kaban, LB, and Glowacki, J. Clinical trial of demineralized bone powder in the treatment of periodontal defects. J. Oral Med. 38:117-121, 1983.

Syftestad, GT, and Urist, MR. Growth hormone dependent matrix-induced heterotopic bone formation. Proc. Soc. Exp. Biol. Med. 163:411-415, 1980.

Taylor, GE, Miller, GDH, and Ham, FJ. The free vascularized bone graft. A clinical extension of microvascular techniques. Plast. Reconstr. Surg. 55:533-544, 1975.

Urist, MR. Bone transplants and implants. In Fundamental and Clinical Bone Physiology, Urist, MR (ed), pp. 331-368. Philadelphia: J. B. Lippincott, 1980a.

Urist, MR. Heterotopic bone formation. In Fundamental and Clinical Bone Physiology, Urist, MR (ed), pp. 369-393. Philadelphia: J. B. Lippincott, 1980b.

Urist, MR. Surface-decalcified allogeneic bone (SDAB) implants. Clin. Orthop. 56:37-50, 1968.

Urist, MR. Bone: Formation by autoinduction. Science 150: 893-899, 1965.

Urist, MR, Mikulski, AJ, and Lietze, A. Solubilized and insolubilized bone morphogenetic protein. Proc. Natl. Acad. Sci. USA 76:1828-1832, 1979.

Weiland, AJ, and Daniel, RK. Microvascular anastomoses for bone grafts in the treatment of massive defects in bone. J. Bone Joint Surg. 61A:98-104, 1979.

Weiss, RE, and Reddi, AH. Synthesis and localization of fibronectin during collagenase matrix-mesenchymal cell interaction and differentiation of cartilage and bone in vivo Proc. Natl. Acad. Sci. USA 77:2074-2078, 1980a.

Weiss, RE, and Reddi, AH. Influence of experimental diabetes and insulin on matrix-induced cartilage and bone differentiation. Am. J. Physiol. 238:200-207, 1980b.

Weiss, RE, Singer, FR, Gorn, AH, Hofer, DP, and Nimni, ME. Calcitonin stimulates bone formation when administered prior to initiation of osteogenesis. J. Clin. Invest. 68:815-818, 1981.

PART IV
Skin Replacement

14
Grafting of Burns with Cultured Epithelium Prepared from Autologous Epidermal Cells II: Intermediate Term Results on Three Pediatric Patients

Nicholas E. O'Connor, Gregory Gallico, Carolyn Compton, Olaniyi Kehinde and Howard Green

INTRODUCTION

The mortality rate in patients sustaining burns of more than 70% of body surface area (BSA) remains high. The major problem is limited availability of donor sites for grafting and the long time needed to cover the burned area completely with the patient's own skin. Many substitutes for autologous skin such as cadaver allografts, pig skin xenografts, amniotic membranes and non-living materials have been used.[1-4] These substitutes have been useful, but the patients require eventual grafting with autologous skin.

Two years ago cultured epithelia prepared from autologous epidermal cells were first used as grafts in two patients.[5] The epidermis regenerated from these grafts was comparable to that resulting from conventional split thickness grafts. In what follows, we describe the use of similar grafts to cover larger areas of burned surface in three younger patients.

MATERIALS AND METHODS

Three patients admitted to the Shriners Burns Institute ranged from two to thirteen years of age, and had burns covering 80% of BSA or greater. All burn wounds were serially

---

These investigations were aided by grants from the National Cancer Institute and a gift from Johnson and Johnson.

The authors wish to express their gratitude to Dr. John Remensnyder for support and advice in the course of these studies.

excised and the excised areas were covered temporarily with frozen cadaver skin allografts. When available, conventional split thickness autologous skin grafts or cultured epithelial grafts were applied to produce permanent coverage.

The methods of cultivation required to produce cultured grafts in sufficient quantity to cover a large surface area have been described earlier.[6,7] Briefly, a full thickness skin sample measuring 2 cm^2 was taken within two days of admission. The tissue samples were placed in culture medium and transferred to the laboratory for cultivation. After removal of as much subcutaneous tissue and dermis as possible, the tissue was minced and trypsinized. Seventy-five cm^2 culture flasks already containing 1.5×10^6 lethally irradiated 3T3 cells were inoculated with over 10^6 epidermal cells each. The cultures were fed with 3:1 mixture of Dulbecco-Vogt modification of Eagle's medium and Ham's F-12 medium.[8] Supplements were as follows: fetal calf serum 10%; hydrocortisone, 0.4 μg/ml; insulin 5 μg/ml; transferrin, 5 μg/ml; triiodothyronine, 2×10^{-9} M; choleragen 10^{-10} M; and adenine 8×10^{-4} M.[9,10] The cultures were incubated at 37°C in an atmosphere containing 10% CO_2. After 3 days, epidermal growth factor (EGF) was added to the medium to 10 ng/ml. The medium was changed twice weekly until the cultures became subconfluent (between 9 and 12 days). Cells from some subconfluent cultures were viably frozen and later subcultured.

To prepare graftable secondary cultures, subconfluent primary cultures were trypsinized and the cells were transferred to flasks of the same size, containing irradiated 3T3 cells. These cultures were maintained in the same way as the primary cultures. One or two days before the cultures were scheduled for grafting, the spent medium was tested for sterility and the cultures were refed with medium from which choleragen was omitted.

When the cultures destined for grafting became confluent, the epithelium was detached intact from the surface of the tissue-culture dish, using the enzyme Dispase II at a concentration of 1.2 u/ml of serum-free medium.[7] The epithelium was then washed with serum-free medium and placed basal side up on a 4.5 × 6.0 cm rectangle of 'Vaseline' gauze in a 100 mm Petri dish. The edges of the epithelium were secured to the gauze with metallic surgical clips. Enough serum-free medium was added to cover the basal surface of the epithelium. The dishes containing the grafts were then placed in an air tight chamber containing ice, and whose gas phase was flushed with 10% CO_2. The sealed jar was transported to the bedside.

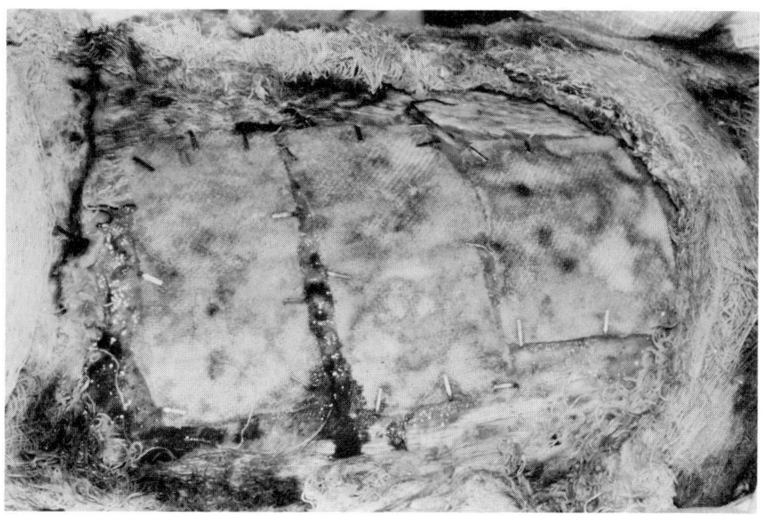

FIGURE 14.1 A close-up photograph of 3 cultured grafts on the left thigh of patient T.H. The vaseline gauze is in place and the epithelium is secured to the gauze with surgical clips.

The recipient sites for the epithelial grafts were prepared by first excising the burn eschar under general anaesthesia, and covering the excised area with cadaver skin allografts. When the epithelial grafts were ready, the cadaver grafts were usually removed at the bedside, and the epithelial grafts with the vaseline gauze covering were placed on the prepared sites with the basal layer directed against the recipient bed (Figure 14.1).

The grafts were not sutured, but were held in place by a single layer of non-impregnated fine mesh gauze overlaid with several layers of coarse mesh gauze; the coarse gauze was changed daily. The fine mesh gauze and the vaseline gauze were usually removed between the 7th and 10th days and the area was redressed with a single layer of vaseline gauze and several layers of coarse gauze. These dressings were changed daily for three to four weeks from the time of the original grafting. Thereafter the grafts were left exposed.

Of the grafts used, 5 were prepared from primary cultures and applied to patient T.H. All other grafts were prepared from secondary cultures.

RESULTS

When formed in culture under these conditions, the epithelium does not possess a stratum corneum, and when applied as a graft is invisible until stratum corneum develops at about 8 days. When the vaseline gauze is removed between 8 and 10 days, the cultured graft is visible as a very thin translucent sheet of epithelium. Over the next 2 to 3 weeks, the graft becomes thicker and begins to resemble a conventional thin split-thickness graft.

In patient T.H., 3 grafts were placed on the left thigh on day 15 following the burn, and on day 40, 7 grafts were placed on the left thigh; 70% of both sets took. These 10 grafts continued to thicken and to merge with each other. On day 78, as there were remaining uncovered areas on both thighs, 4 grafts were placed on the right thigh and 4 on the left thigh. These grafts again had about a 70% take and grew to merge with surrounding conventional and cultured skin grafts (Figure 14.2).

In patient M.D., 4 grafts were placed on the left thigh on day 23. When they were uncovered there was found to be about an 80% take. On day 42, 9 more grafts were placed on the left thigh and again there was take of 80% of the area. Over the next few weeks the grafts began to thicken, to spread outward and merge with each other. For two weeks starting at day 60, the patient developed pulmonary and systemic infection, and during that period of time the grafts began to recede at the edges, leaving open spaces. On day 89, when the infection cleared, 5 more grafts were placed around the periphery of the original 13 grafts. These also showed an 80% take. Over the next several weeks, all the grafts appeared healthy, became thicker and merged with standard meshed autografts on the remainder of the thigh (Figure 14.3).

Patient N.W. received 9 grafts to the right thigh and 5 grafts to the left thigh on day 24. There was about 80% take. The grafts continued to do well, thicken and merge with each other (Table 14.1). At 6 weeks, the resulting epithelial cover was uniformly smooth, moderately thick and pliable.

Patients T.H. and M.D. have had a 6 month follow-up period of observation. In both, the grafts prepared from cultures soon appeared similar to split thickness skin grafts in thickness, durability, texture and appearance. Histological examination of the grafts at 3 months revealed a moderately developed epidermis with a stratum spinosum of approximately 10 cell layers. At this time, the epidermis lacked well-defined

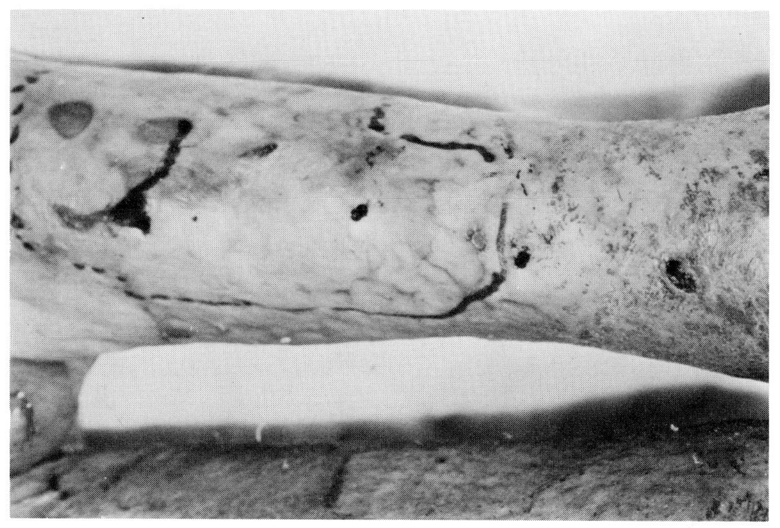

FIGURE 14.2 (above) Left thigh of patient T.H. taken 3 months after grafting. The area covered by cultured grafts is outlined in ink. Standard meshed autografts can be seen on the right thigh.

FIGURE 14.3 (below) Left thigh of patient M.D. 4 months after grafting. The area covered by epithelial grafts is outlined in ink.

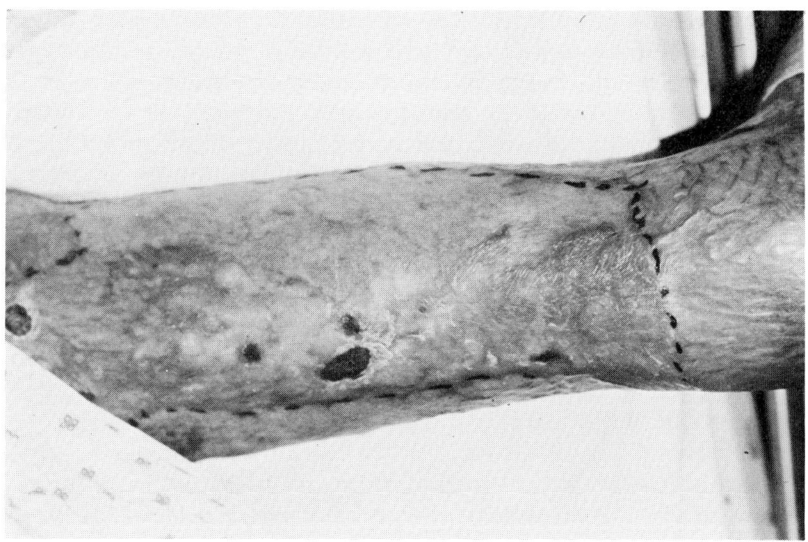

TABLE 14.1

Summary of Results of Grafting with Cultured Epithelia

Patient	Age	Site Covered	No. of Grafts (each 27 cm^2)	Fate of Grafts	% BSA Covered
TH	9	R Ant Thigh	4	70% take	4.0
		L Ant Thigh	14	70% take	
MD	13	L Ant Thigh	18	80% take	3.5
NW	2	R Ant Thigh	9	80% take	5.0
		L Ant Thigh	5	80% take	

rete ridges and had a flat to shallowly undulating contour on transverse section. Basal cells were poorly organized. The basement membrane was well developed and stained with PAS. The subepidermal connective tissue had the appearance of a healing wound with maturing granulation tissue and mild acute and chronic inflammatory infiltrates. Reticulin stain showed the fibers of the subepithelial connective tissue to be composed almost entirely of reticulin (presumptive Type III collagen). No adnexal structures were present.

One region of epidermis regenerated from cultured epithelium on patient M.D. was biopsied at 6 months. Microscopic examination showed an epidermis possessing well differentiated cell layers, but only minimally developed rete ridges. The stratum spinosum contained about 7 cell layers. The dermis showed some distinction between superficial and deep layers, but the superficial layer was more densely collagenized than normal and the vessels were not arborized in a normal fashion. The deep dermis showed increased cellularity and foci of fibrosis (Figure 14.4).

DISCUSSION

The epithelial grafts were derived from cultures which contained foreign proteins (bovine serum, mouse cells and EGF, and choleragen). To remove these proteins as thoroughly as

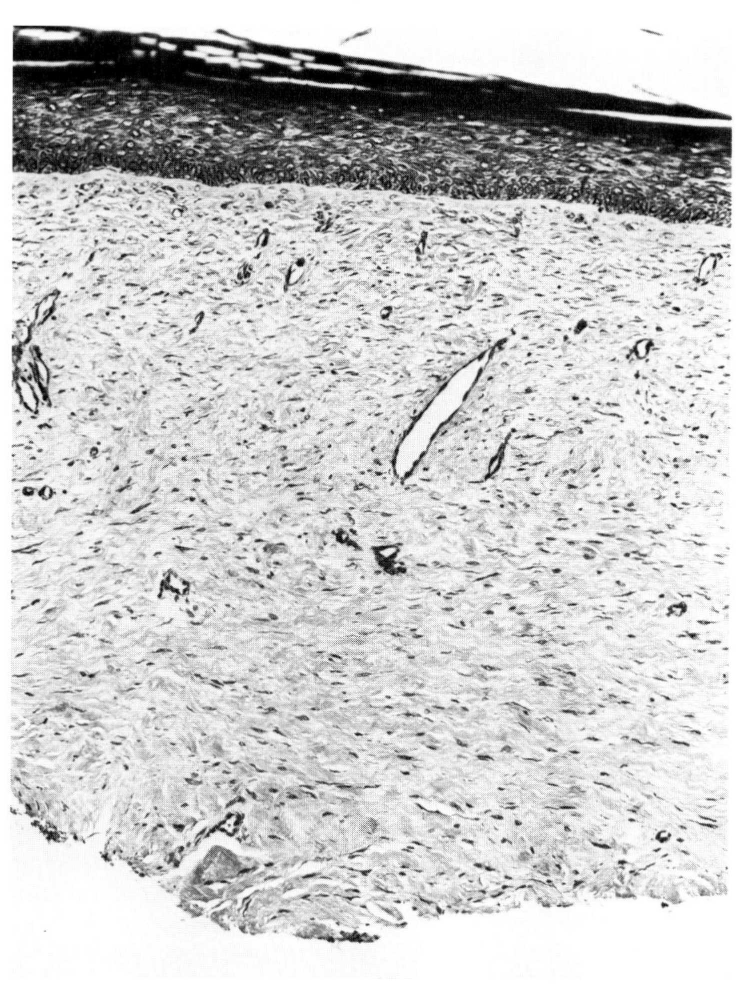

FIGURE 14.4 Histological section through epidermis from cultured epithelium 6 months after grafting to patient M.D. (Trichrome stain).

possible, the grafts were washed several times in serum-free medium both before and after they were removed from the culture vessel. If any of these proteins remained in the grafts, they produced no discernible effects in the three patients in this report, or the two patients reported previously.

In the earlier study,[5] the grafts were made circular and about 2 cm in diameter. In our current technique, we use grafts of rectangular shape measuring 4.5 × 6.0 cm. This size and configuration makes it possible to cover a given surface area completely with fewer grafts. The grafts could be made still larger, but it might become difficult for a much larger graft with its vaseline gauze backing to conform to the irregularities of the burn wound surface. The vaseline gauze is essential because the absence of stratum corneum during the first week after application of the grafts makes them vulnerable to dessication.

In the three patients in this report, the wounds were prepared by excising the burn eschar down to fascia or to bleeding subcutaneous fat, and were temporarily covered with frozen cadaver allografts. These were removed within 24 hours prior to the application of the cultured grafts. The proportion of take was much higher than in our earlier study, in which the grafts were sometimes applied to chronic granulation tissue.[5]

Within the first 3 or 4 weeks after application, the cultured grafts seem to be more vulnerable than standard split thickness skin grafts. For example, when patient M.D. developed systemic sepsis, the epithelial grafts receded, leaving open areas. The conventional grafts also receded but less markedly. As the infection cleared, the performance of the cultured grafts began to improve, and they continued to expand thereafter.

Another possibly important difference between the take of a graft of cultured epithelium and a conventional split-thickness skin graft is that in the former, the plane of union lies between epithelial cells and graft bed rather than between dermal elements and graft bed. Although the nature of this union is poorly understood, the bond between the cultured epithelium and the graft bed seems somewhat slower to develop. By the 10th day after grafting, for example, it is easier to lift the cultured graft from its bed than a conventional graft. By day 20, however, the epithelial graft is firmly adherent.

The samples of skin taken to start cultures were about 2 cm^2. Using mainly secondary subcultures, we have successfully covered 3.5-5% of body surface of these patients. Without modifying the method, a sufficient number of cultures could be prepared to cover wounds of much larger surface area. The total time required to generate graftable secondary cultures is now reduced from about 5 weeks as described earlier[5,7] to about 3 weeks.

F.B. and A.S., the first 2 patients grafted with cultured epithelium,[5] have now been reexamined three and one-half years after the grafting. Both patients had good coverage of the areas to which cultured epithelium had been grafted. In some cases, the circular outline of an epidermal site and its position relative to other sites covered with meshed skin grafts suggested that the epidermis originated from a cultured graft. The quality of the epidermis looked good and no untoward effects could be observed.

It must be assumed that the epidermal coverage produced from the cultured grafts is permanent. There is at present no reason to believe that the long-term quality of the epidermis will be inferior to that produced by conventional split thickness grafts. The intermediate term quality seems to range from satisfactory to excellent.

NOTES

1. Burke, JF, Yannas, IV, Quinby, WC Jr, Bondoc, CC, and Jung, WK. Successful use of a physiologically acceptable artificial skin in the treatment of extensive burn injury. Ann. Surg. 194:413-428, 1981.

2. Robson, MC, Krizek, TJ, Koss, N, and Samburg, JL. Amniotic membranes as a temporary wound dressing. Surg. Gyn. Obstet. 136:904-906, 1973.

3. Bondoc, CC and Burke, JF. Clinical experience with viable human skin and frozen skin bank. Ann. Surg. 174:371-382, 1971.

4. German, JC, Wooley, TE, Achauer, B, Furnas, DW, and Bartlett, RH. Porcine xenograft burn dressings: A critical reappraisal. Arch. Surg. 104:806-808, 1972.

5. O'Connor, NE, Mulliken, JB, Banks-Schlegel, S, Kehinde, O, and Green, H. Grafting of burns with cultured epithelium prepared from autologous epidermal cells. Lancet 1: 75-78, 1981.

6. Green, H, and O'Connor, N. Cultured cells for the regeneration of epidermis by grafting. In Burn Wound Coverings, D. L. Wise (ed). CRC Press, in press, 1983.

7. Green, H, Kehinde, O, and Thomas, J. Growth of cultured human epidermal cells into multiple epithelia suitable for grafting. Proc. Natl. Acad. Sci. USA 76:5665-5668, 1979.

8. Ham, RG. Clonal growth of mammalian cells in a chemically defined synthetic medium. Proc. Natl. Acad. Sci. USA 53:288-293, 1965.

9. Peehl, D, and Ham, R. Clonal growth of human keratinocytes with small amounts of dialyzed serum. In Vitro 16: 526-538, 1980.

10. Wu, Y-J, Parker, LM, Binder, NE, Beckett, MA, Girard, JH, Griffiths, CT, and Rheinwald, JG. The mesothelial keratins: A new family of cytoskeletal proteins identified in cultured mesothelial cells and non-keratinizing epithelia. Cell 31:693-703, 1982.

15
Wound Coverage by Epidermal Cells Grown *In Vitro*

Magdalena Eisinger, Edward R. Kraft and Joseph G. Fortner

INTRODUCTION

The epidermis is an important functional barrier of the body, limiting outward and inward penetration of gasses and liquids as well as providing protection against mechanical and thermal variables in the environment. Because of its crucial functional roles and cosmetic importance, means have been long sought for more suitable ways to replace lost epidermis. Recently acquired abilities to grow epidermal cells in vitro have provided a basis for investigating the feasibility of using tissue culture-derived sheets of epidermal cells to replace large skin losses from burns or other injury. In some individuals a small piece of their own skin could be removed and then enlarged by growth in vitro before use for transplantation.

This chapter will discuss our experiences in using in vitro grown epidermal cells for wound coverage in an experimental model: outbred domestic swine.

COMPOSITION OF THE LATERAL SKIN IN SWINE

Pig skin resembles the skin of man very closely. It varies in thickness and composition depending on its location, age of the animal and breed. Skin on the upper and lower back in outbred domestic swine was used in our studies. Two main

---

This work was partially supported by funds from General Motors and a grant from Johnson and Johnson Products, Inc.

layers of epidermis can be distinguished in this skin: an outer layer of anucleated flattened cells—the stratum corneum, and an inner layer of viable cells—stratum germinativum. The stratum germinativum consists of 4 to 5 layers of nucleated cells covered by laminated cornified cells without nuclei and is 5 to 6 layers thick. The basal layer of epidermis contains irregular ridges (rete ridges) molded against the underlying connective tissue (dermal papillae). Rete ridges on the lateral side of the pig skin are relatively short. The underlying papillary dermis consists of thin collagen bundles and fibers containing many fixed tissue cells, richly vascularized by arterial capillaries and venules. Hair erector muscle and hair follicles and sweat glands are visible. Hair follicles are deeply seated, often reaching to the underlying layer of fatty tissue.

SEPARATION OF THE EPIDERMIS FROM DERMIS

To grow epidermal cells in vitro successfully, it is important to separate the epidermis from underlying dermis in order to obtain a single cell suspension of epidermal cells. The procedure developed by us[1] for separation of human epidermal cells was successfully applied to the separation of pig epidermis. Skin specimens varying in thickness from 0.012 to 0.015 inch were obtained using a Brown dermatome. The graft was meshed using a Collin Ampligraft 2x skin mesher. It was then thoroughly washed in a solution containing antibiotics followed by a brief wash in 0.02% EDTA (SIGMA) solution. The specimen was put in a 0.25% solution of trypsin (DIFCO 1:250) at 4°C for 12 to 15 hours. Manual separation of epidermal sheets from the dermis using watchmaker's forceps was then possible. Following this, the epidermal cells were dissociated using a trypsin-versene solution.

Single cell suspensions obtained by trypsinization were filtered through 3 to 4 layers of gauze and collected in a medium containing fetal bovine serum. The cell suspension was then centrifuged for 10 minutes at 180xg and the cells resuspended in growth medium. This consisted of Eagle's Minimal Essential Medium plus nonessential amino acids, 2 mM L-glutamine, hydrocortisone at 0.4 μg/ml, 10% fetal bovine serum, penicillin, streptomycin and Fungizone, at pH 6.5. The cells were shown to have 90-95% viability by Trypan blue dye exclusion tests.

GROWTH OF PIG EPIDERMAL CELLS *IN VITRO*

The pig epidermal single cell suspension is composed of epidermal cells in different stages of differentiation and a few melanocytes. Viable epidermal cells, 4-5 × 10^6, were used to seed a T25 flask. The seeded cells clumped and became attached to plastic surfaces in 24 to 48 hours. The majority of the cells plated originally became detached during the next 5 to 10 days and were removed when the medium was changed. First growth of isolated colonies of epidermal cells was observed 4 to 5 days after seeding. The growth progressed until a contiguous sheet of cells was obtained. The cells directly attached to the plastic displayed the properties of basal cells. Suprabasal cells were more differentiated keratinocytes. Multilayered sheets ready for transplantation were usually obtained 4 to 5 weeks after initiation of cultures. Since human cells grow better *in vitro*, similar sheets can be obtained in only 2 to 3 weeks after initiation of cultures. In general, pig cells did not plate as well as human cells and also grew more slowly. As shown in Figure 15.1, human cells grew progressively from the sixth day in culture, similar growth with pig cells was not observed until 10 days after the initial seeding. Population doubling time of cultures of human keratinocytes was approximately 48 hours prior to reaching confluency, but 96 hours for pig epidermal cultures. To stimulate the growth of the pig epidermal cells, the medium was supplemented with a soluble extract of the pig dermis. While human epidermal cells could be stimulated, pig cells were only further inhibited in their growth.

REMOVAL OF THE MULTILAYERED EPIDERMAL SHEETS FROM TISSUE CULTURE FLASKS

Thorough washing of epidermal sheets with medium which does not contain fetal bovine serum was done as the first step in removing the cultured cells for use. T25 flasks were then filled with 5 ml of phosphate buffered saline (PBS Ca^{++} Mg^{++} free). The flasks were cut open with a hot scalpel and the edges of the epidermal sheets cut with watchmaker's forceps. The PBS was discarded and a prewetted collagen film was placed on top of the epidermal cell cultures. A collagen sponge soaked in medium without fetal bovine serum was placed on top of this to maintain moisture. The flasks were then placed into the incubator until used for transplantation a short time later.

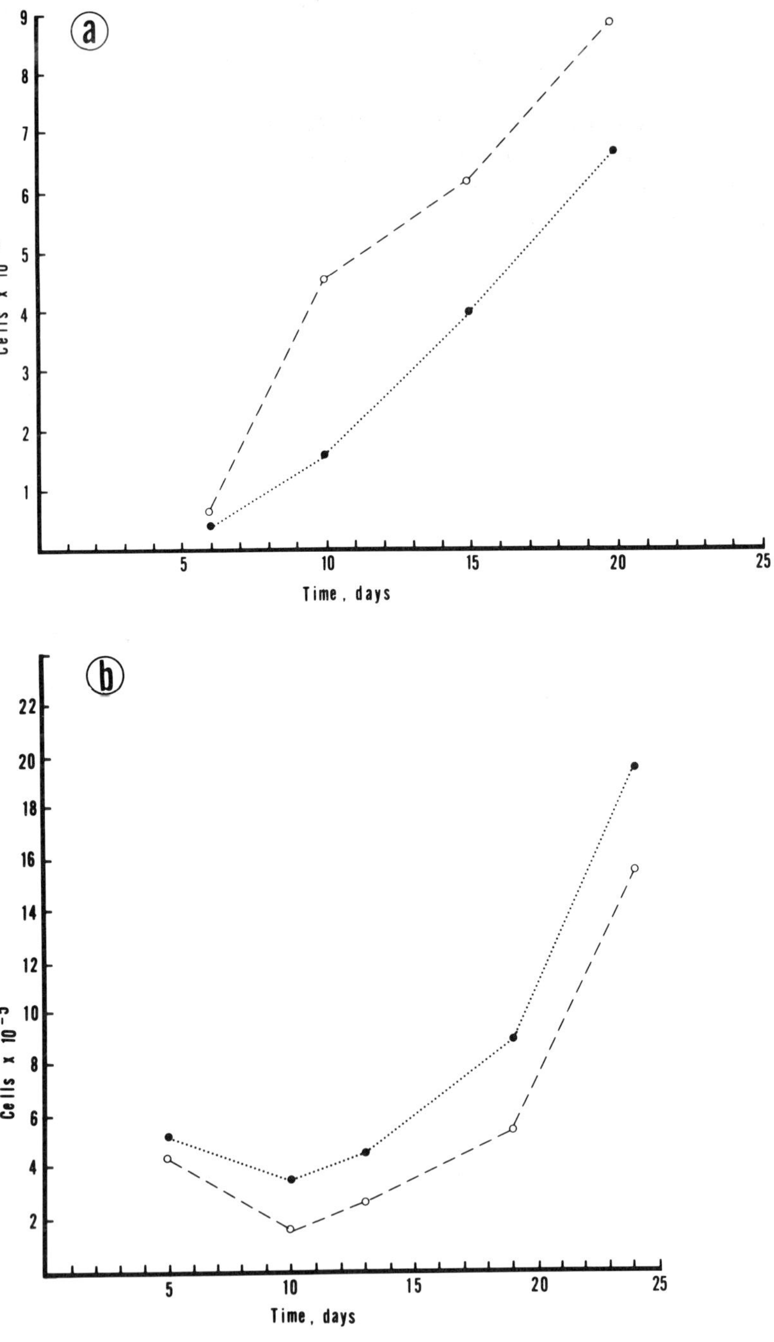

FIGURE 15.1 Growth kinetics of epidermal cells in vitro. a) Human keratinocytes. b) Pig keratinocytes. Both cultures were grown in the medium described in the text and the same medium containing a dermal extract.

PREPARATION OF THE RECIPIENT BED

It was a prerequisite for evaluation of the epidermal graft that the graft bed be prepared so that there was no dermis, hair follicles, sweat glands and sebaceous glands remaining. This defect was achieved by removing the recipient pig's skin at the graft site with a Brown dermatome on the lateral side of the pig. The dermatome setting was 0.075-0.090 inch on the upper lateral side and 0.060-0.075 inch on the lower lateral region. The epidermal grafts were placed on the bed which was just above the fascia.

STERILITY

Adequate information is available to indicate that the wound contaminated with more than 10^5 organisms per specimen will not permit a skin graft to take. This is particularly true of a wound with abundant granulation tissue and in wounds where necrotic tissue remains to support the growth of microorganisms. The recipient bed for the described studies was always a freshly, dermatome-prepared sterile bed. Grafts on granulation tissue were seldom successful.

HEMOSTASIS

Absolute hemostasis in the graft bed was essential for successful take of an epidermal graft. Both hematomas and seromas interfered with success. The recipient bed prepared with dermatome at the thickness described seldom resulted in excessive bleeding or exudation. If minor bleeding occurred, a dry gauze dressing was placed on the wound and pressure applied for 10-15 minutes.

ADDITIONAL TREATMENT OF THE RECIPIENT BED

The surgically-prepared recipient bed was covered with sterile gauze pre-wetted with PBS until the grafts were placed. Silk sutures (3-0 or 2-0) were placed about one and one-half inches apart on both sides of the prepared graft bed to hold a compression stent in place.

PLACING THE EPIDERMAL GRAFT

The epidermal graft was removed from the tissue culture vessel using watchmaker's forceps following removal of the collagen sponge and excess fluid. The epidermis was then peeled off the tissue culture vessel using the collagen as support (Figure 15.2). The peeled epidermis shrank approximately one-tenth of its original size (Figure 15.3). The epidermis was placed on the wound bed (Figure 15.4) with the basal cells facing the wound and the collagen on top. The grafts were covered with petrolatum gauze and "gauze puffs." Silk ligatures were tied so as to provide a compression stent. It was very important to assure that the epidermal graft was not moved and wrinkled during this preparation. It was essential for compression to be tight enough to prevent movement between the graft and the underlying bed. This would dislodge the fibrin clot and prevent the plasmatic stage from being effective.

ATTACHMENT AND GROWTH OF EPIDERMAL CELLS ON THE SURGICALLY PREPARED WOUND BED

The pig epidermal grafts varied in thickness depending on the length of time they were grown in tissue culture. This variation was from 13 to 15 layers after 4 to 5 weeks in vitro to 30 to 40 layers in 3 to 5 months. In general, however, such multilayered sheets had only one or two layers of viable nucleus-containing cells and the other layers were composed of flattened anucleated differentiated cells. Well-developed desmosomal connections between the cells were observed presumably contributing to the elasticity of epidermal sheets. The bottom layer of the cultured epidermal sheets was composed of elongated basal cells which were parallel to the plastic surface of the culture vessel. These cells were larger than basal cells in vivo. When such multilayered epidermal sheets were placed on the wound, the basal cells regained their normal appearance becoming cuboidal or low columnar. Their long axis was perpendicular to the epidermal-dermal interface. In all instances it was found that the graft became attached to the underlying tissue in 48-72 hours. At this point, however, the bonds were weak and the epidermis could be easily damaged. The occasional presence of exudate or fibrin attachment of collagen covering the epidermal cells usually resulted in leaving the collagen on the graft for an additional three days. The epidermis was firmly attached to the underlying tissue six to eight days after transplantation.

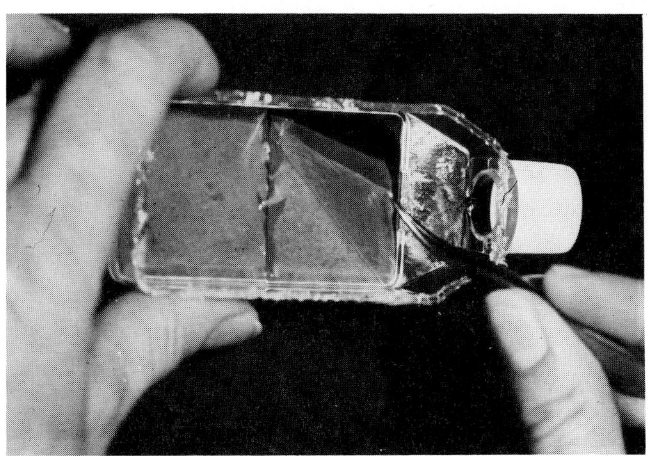

FIGURE 15.2 An epidermal sheet lining the bottom of a tissue culture flask was cut in half and covered by collagen film to allow for the easy removal of the sheet using watchmaker's forceps.

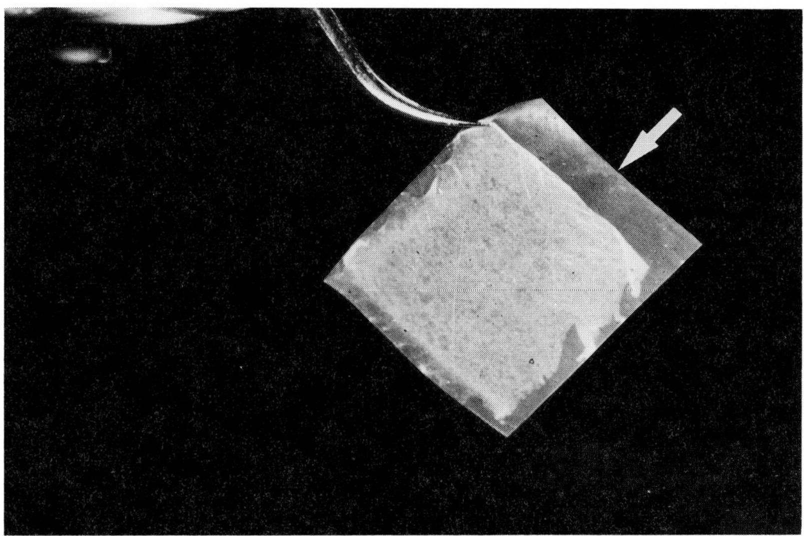

FIGURE 15.3 Epidermal sheet after removal from the tissue culture flask. The peeled epidermis shrank as can be noted by the light border of collagen film (↑).

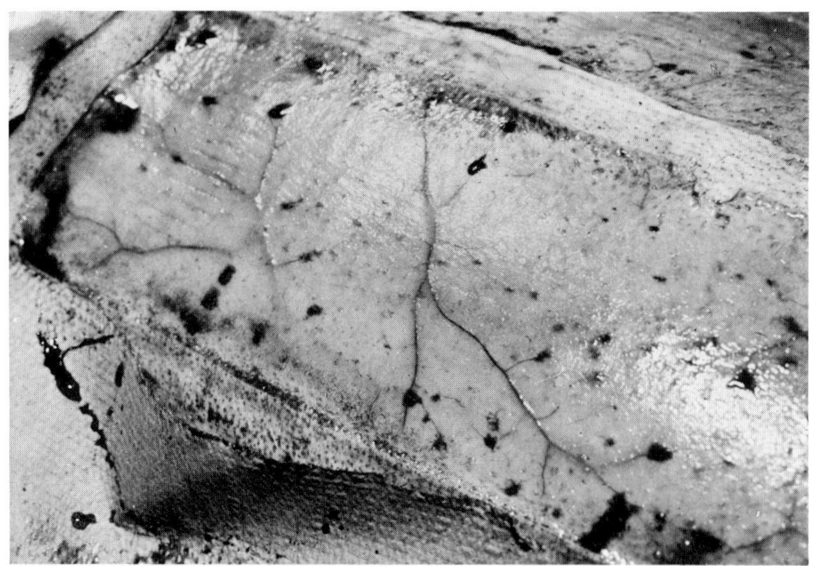

FIGURE 15.4 A typical full-thickness surgically prepared wound bed. Note the vascularity.

When epidermal grafts were placed on the wound bed, leaving areas between them uncovered (Figure 15.5a), the grafts extended considerably (Figure 15.5b) and fused into a confluent epithelial cover. The wound bed usually closed in 15-20 days, reaching the epidermal sheets, and thereafter remained the same size. Epidermal cells proliferated extensively in the first 15 to 20 days with deposition of keratinized cells on the surface. They could be easily peeled off exposing pink viable epidermis. The wounds could be left unbandaged at this time. No bleeding from the wound was observed even though the animals rubbed the wound against the cage.

Epidermal grafts placed on the wound bed to cover the whole area (fitted grafts) fused with the surrounding cells within the first 8 to 15 days, providing uniform coverage (Figure 15.6a). Occasionally a small area was not completely covered as late as 15 days after transplantation (Figure 15.6b). The wounds which were only partially covered by epidermal sheets healed with visible scars in the large areas originally uncovered (Figure 15.5c). On the other hand, no visible scars were formed on the wounds completely covered by epidermal cells grown <u>in vitro</u> (Figure 15.6c).

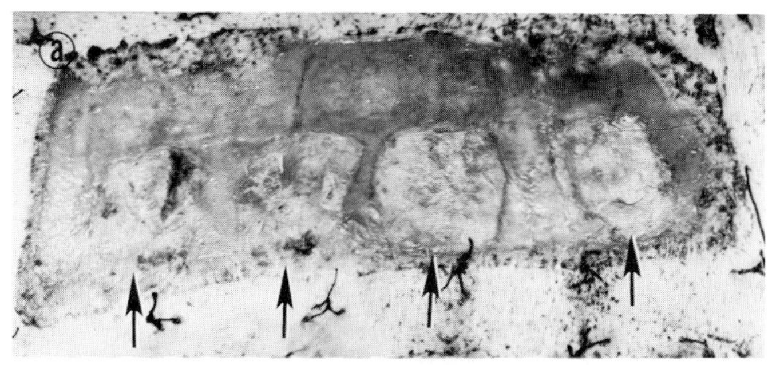

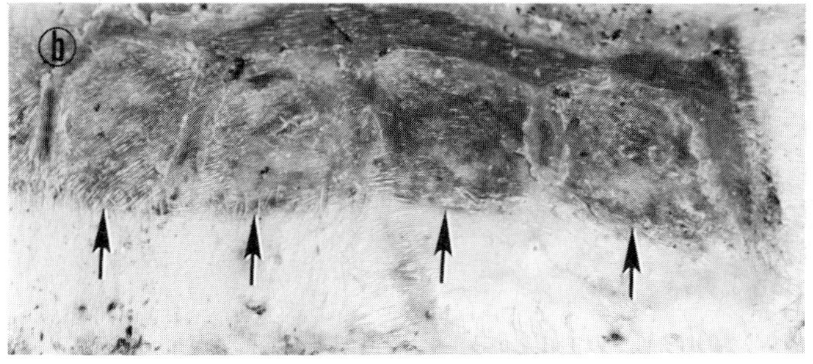

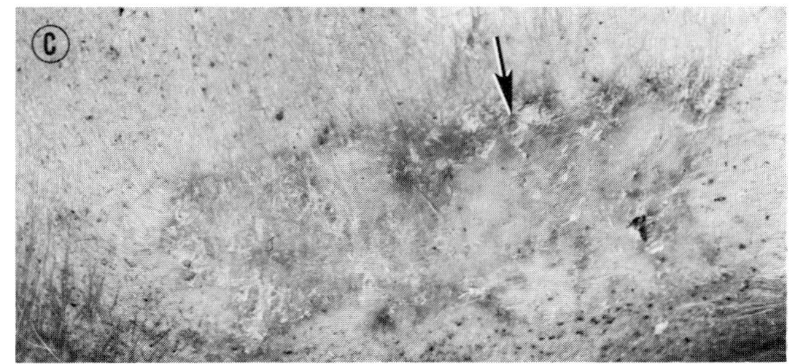

FIGURE 15.5 Appearance of a wound partially covered by epidermal cells grown in vitro. a) Arrows indicate areas covered by epidermal cells, 10 days after transplantation. Four grafts of approximately 15 cm^2 each were originally placed on the full thickness graft bed, leaving spaces between the grafts and large areas of the wound bed uncovered. b) The same wound 5 days later. Note that the epidermal grafts extended and fused into a confluent epithelial cover. The wound bed closed considerably on the distal part, fusing into the surrounding epidermis (↑). c) Healed wound 49 days after transplantation. Note scarring in the areas originally not covered by the epidermal sheets (↑).

FIGURE 15.6 Wound covered by epidermal cells—fitted grafts. a) Full-thickness wound covered by a fitted graft, 10 days after transplantation. b) The same wound 5 days later. Note that the wound is almost completely covered. c) The transplanted area 15 months after transplantation. The skin in the area looks normal, and no scars are noticeable.

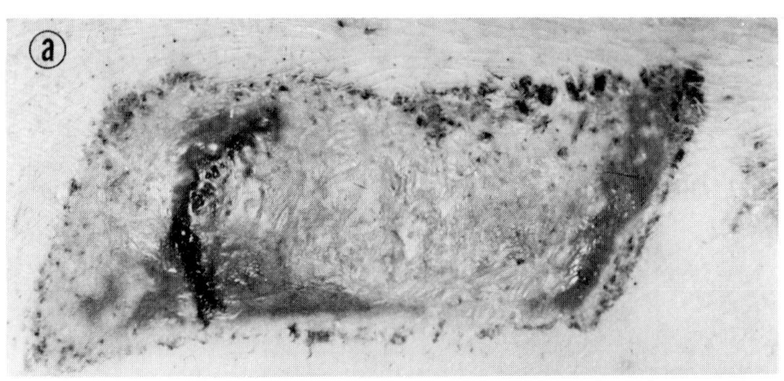

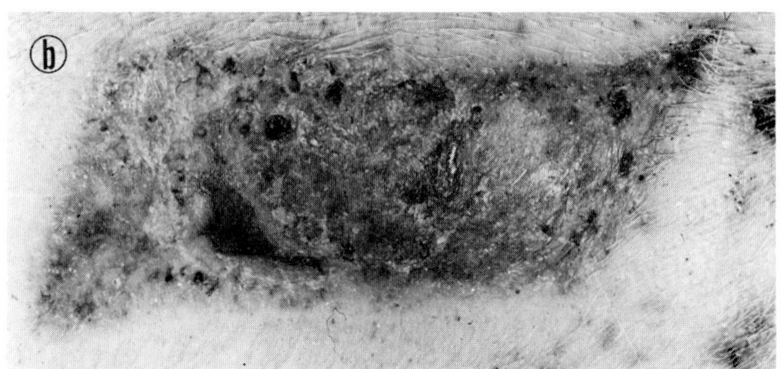

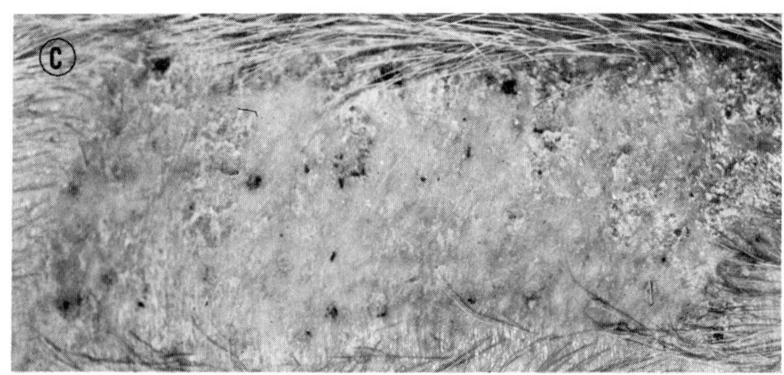

TABLE 15.1

Transplantation of Autologous Epidermal Cells Grown *in Vitro*

Recipient (pig)	Donor (pig)	Time in Culture (days)	Wound Depth (full thickness)	No. of Grafts/ No. of Graft Take
37637	37637	30	+	2/2
55	55	31	+	7/7
28	28	37	+	1/1
37642	37642	38	+	4/3
1032	1032	40	+	2/2
33173	33173	41	+	3/3
1038	1038	45	+	2/2
34250	34250	45	+	2/2
34268	34268	48	+	2/2
34251	34251	51	+	3/3
1046	1046	60	+	2/2
37669	37669	81	+	2/1
1046	1046	86	+	2/2

Successful take of epidermal grafts on surgically prepared, full thickness wound beds was about 94%. As shown in Table 15.1, epidermis of 13 pigs was grown in tissue culture for a period of time varying from 30 to 86 days. In 11 pigs, all applied grafts took and the wounds were properly covered within 10 to 15 days after transplantation. In one pig, one out of four grafts, and on another pig, one of two grafts, did not take. The pigs so transplanted were observed for a minimum of 3 months and a maximum of 18 months post-transplantation.

The healed transplanted areas were covered with soft, pliable skin which could easily be distinguished from the surrounding skin by the lack of hair and pink color (Figures 15.5c, 15.6c). There were no clinical changes noted during the observation period. Histologic examination of samples from long-term epidermal autografts (5-1/2 months and 16 months post-transplantation) have shown that epidermal hyperplasia observed in the first weeks after transplantation ceased; there was still more keratin present than in the normal skin, but its composition was normal. Superficial plexus was restored. The reticular bundles 5-1/2 months after transplantation were a little thicker than normal; 16 months after transplantation the dermis looked normal, but there were no hair follicles and appendages observed.

BEHAVIOR OF ALLOGENEIC EPIDERMAL SHEETS GROWN *IN VITRO*

The initial attachment and growth of allogeneic epidermal cells on the surgically prepared bed resembled that of autologous epidermal cells. As shown in Table 15.2, there was a 100% graft take. Allogeneic epidermal cells within the first week after transplantation underwent a phase of very pronounced hyperplasia. Epidermal cell layers 7 to 9 days after transplantation were 15 to 20 layers thick and a thick cuticle of keratinized cells was formed. As a consequence of this rapid initial growth, wounds with allogeneic grafts were completely covered within 7 to 9 days. Visual inspection of the grafts showed mild swelling starting 7-9 days after transplantation followed by a rapid change in the graft appearance. Its original pink color changed first to a reddish color, then to deep purple. The dry appearance of the graft changed and in most instances empty patches of denuded purple colored swollen granulation tissue were seen followed by a complete disappearance of the grafts ("graft melting"). Histologic examination revealed the presence of inflammatory cells in the immediate graft bed as soon as 9 to 10 days after transplantation. By the 10th to 12th day, there were inflammatory cells also within the epidermis and changes in the appearance of the epidermal cells, such as pronounced vacuolization and beginning necrosis were noticed. The progression of necrosis and accumulation of fluid led to complete separation of epidermis and its lysis. As seen in Table 15.2, complete disappearance of the epidermal graft occurred between days 14 and 16. On the other hand, fresh epidermal grafts (data not shown) were completely rejected in 7 days after transplantation.

DISCUSSION

Tissue culture offers a unique opportunity to induce cells to multiply by providing the necessary nutrients and stimuli. Different cell types, both *in vivo* and *in vitro*, differ in their rate of growth and cumulative numbers of cell generations achieved before senescence, death, or terminal differentiation.

TABLE 15.2

Transplantation of Allogeneic Epidermal Cells Grown *in Vitro*

Recipient (pig)	Donor (pig)	Time in Culture (days)	No. of Grafts/ No. of Graft Take	Graft Rej. (days)
27	59	32	1/1	15
61	27	37	2/2	14
28	29	37	1/1	16
51	55	46	5/5	14
1048	1046	66	2/2	14
65	62	67	1/1	14
37	61	74	2/2	14
55	51	113	2/2	14
65	55	129	3/3	14
37669	34250	175	3/3	13
28	51	184	2/2	14

The best studied cells, fibroblasts (which *in vivo* can be easily stimulated to growth), can be grown *in vitro* for a number of cell generations (over 50) and their growth in tissue culture was accomplished a long time ago. In contrast, epidermal cells, the major constituent of epidermis, are much more fastidious and under suboptimal conditions undergo terminal differentiation. Early attempts to cultivate and multiply epidermal cells *in vitro* met with only partial success. Rheinwald and Green,[2] using an irradiated 3T3 feeder layer and a growth medium containing the epidermal growth factor (EGF), hydrocortisone and fetal bovine serum had the first major success in growing human epidermal cells. Many different approaches to growing human epidermal cells have since been introduced, aiming at successful growth of epidermal cells in the absence of a 3T3 feeder layer.[3,4,5,6] One of them, the method developed by us,[1] enables epithelial cells, under low pH conditions, to plate and replicate (human cells at pH 6-6.2 and pig cells at pH 6.5). Much understanding of the nutrient requirements of epidermal cells has been gained recently by the work of Peehl and Ham,[4,7] thus allowing for better growth of these cells. Availability of these different culturing techniques for epidermal cells provided the opportunity to study their behavior *in vivo* and to evaluate the possibility of their use in skin transplantation. Previous studies[8,9,10] have shown that epidermis grown in vitro, when transplanted into an animal, will acquire morphological and histological characteristics of normal epidermis. New ways have been opened for examining important questions such as the role of epidermis on the deposition of the underlying collagen, and scar formation.

Repair of mammalian skin is brought about mainly by two distinct processes:[11] (1) contraction--closing of the wound by opposition of its original edges; (2) intussusceptive growth--the formation of new tissue upon or within the framework provided by pre-existing tissue. These generalizations apply to the healing wounds in a fully mobile integument. In areas where the skin is more firmly attached to the tissue beneath (as in the greater part of human body, distal ear skin of rabbits or guinea pigs) contraction cannot go to completion so that a fibrous scar covered by epithelium of migratory origin remains.

The skin of pigs, as with human skin, is firmly attached to the tissue beneath. Therefore after initial partial contraction, a fibrous scar is formed. In all our experiments in which fitted grafts of epidermal cells grown in vitro were applied to a full thickness wound bed, only minimal contraction was noted and no visible scars have been formed. Multilayered epidermal sheets prepared in vitro differ from migratory epithelium in that wound contraction is prevented and collagenization of the wound bed is regulated.

In the first clinical trials with human epidermis to cover burn wounds[12] scarring was not evident. It is important to note that the quality of epidermal coverage provided by epidermal cells grown in vitro and applied as large sheets differs from that of migratory epithelium present on spontaneously healing wounds. While migratory epithelium is very fragile and easily wounded, epithelial cells grown in vitro are firmly attached and the wounds are functionally stable 10 to 14 days after transplantation.

These findings lead to several important questions:

1. If large surface areas of the body have to be covered and relatively little skin is available, how soon can this be achieved? Based on our original work[1,9] a 1:20 enlargement of the original surface area could be achieved in the first passage in vitro and 1:60 in the second subculture if the cells are split in a 1:3 ratio. This enlargement required a time period of approximately 20 days. By further splitting of the cultures, enlargement 2000 to 5000 times the original piece of tissue can

be achieved in six to eight weeks.[9,13] As of now, the first and second subcultures of epidermal cells grown in tissue culture proved most applicable for transplantation. Future improvements depend upon determining the specific needs of the rapidly growing and sub-cultured cells, which is now a major subject of investigation.

2. Different types of wounds may require different types of grafts. Our experience with successful healing by cultured epidermal cells was on freshly prepared well-vascularized wound beds, covering a relatively small area of the total body surface. In patients with an extensive body surface damage by third degree burns, it may be necessary to provide dermal components. An artificial dermis has been developed[14] and successfully used in burn patients (see Chapter 16). The question which remains to be answered is whether an artificial framework of collagen is sufficient, or whether the actual presence of dermal cells is required when an _in vitro_ prepared epidermo-dermal graft is applied.

3. An important consideration is the absence of sweat glands and sebaceous glands in the newly formed skin. Early success in the isolation of viable eccrine sweat glands[15] may enable the furtherance of the technology to grow them _in vitro_. Theoretically an artificial matrix seeded with different cell types multiplied _in vitro_ would be a proper skin replacement.

4. A solution to many of the above considerations would be the use of allogeneic skin as the source of tissue for an _in vitro_ expansion. Generally, skin is considered to be one of the most fastidious organs for allogeneic transplantation. Transplantation of split thickness skin among miniature swine homozygous for major histocompatibility complex (MSLA) and matched for all known blood groups showed that MSLA-identical grafts survived only 11.8 days. Skin grafts from animals differing for one or two haplotypes survived 7.0 days.[16] It is therefore of considerable interest that non-cultured allogeneic epidermis was also rejected in 7.0 days, but allogeneic epidermal cells grown _in vitro_ and used for grafting survived 14.1 days.

The findings by Lafferty[17] and Simeonovic[18] that cultivation of thyroid glands and Langerhans islands of pancreas led to allogeneic graft acceptance, could not be applied for pig skin transplantation.

Extensive work on the role of passenger leukocytes and their role in the immunogenicity of skin allograft by Steinmuller[19] and his colleagues suggests that passenger leukocytes and other bone marrow derivatives such as Langerhans cells, probably do not contribute significantly to the immunogenicity of skin allografts. Such cells have proven to be absent in the epidermal cell cultures used in the studies reported here. The tenacious immunogenicity of epidermal cells might be related to the unusually strong organ specific antigens.

We thank A. L. Yu for her excellent assistance with tissue cultures, R. Barters and S. Denecko for assistance with the transplantation experiments.

NOTES

1. Eisinger, M, Lee, JS, Hefton, JM, Darzynkiewicz, Z, Chiao, JW, DeHarven, E. Human epidermal cell cultures: Growth and differentiation in the absence of dermal components or medium supplements. Proc. Natl. Acad. Sci. USA 76:5340-5344, 1979.

2. Rheinwald, JG, Green, H. Epidermal growth factor and the multiplication of cultured human epidermal keratinocytes. Nature 265:421-424, 1977.

3. Price, FM, Camalier, RF, Gantt, R, Taylor, WG, Smith, GH, Sanford, KK. A new culture medium for human skin epithelial cells. In Vitro 16:147-158, 1980.

4. Peehl, DM, Ham, RG. Growth and differentiation of human keratinocytes without a feeder layer or conditioned medium. In Vitro 16:516-525, 1980.

5. Hawley-Nelson, P, Sullivan, JE, Kung, M, Hennings, H, Yuspa, SH. Optimized conditions for the growth of human epidermal cells in cultures. J. Invest. Derm. 75:176-182, 1980.

6. Gilchrest, BA, Calhoun, JK, Maciag, T. Attachment and growth of human keratinocytes in a serum-free environment. J. Cell. Physiol. 112:197-206, 1982.

7. Peehl, DM, Ham, RG. Clonal growth of human keratinocytes with small amounts of dialyzed serum. In Vitro 16:526-538, 1980.

8. Freeman, AE, Igel, HJ, Waldman, NL, Losikoff, AM. A new method for covering large surface area wounds with autografts. I. In vitro multiplication of rabbit-skin epithelial cells. Arch. Surg. 108:721-723, 1974.

9. Eisinger, M, Monden, M, Raaf, JH, Fortner, JG. Wound coverage by a sheet of epidermal cells grown in vitro from dispersed single cell preparations. Surgery 88:287-293, 1980.

10. Banks-Schlegel, S, Green, H. Formation of epidermis by serially cultivated human epidermal cells transplanted as an epithelium to athymic mice. Transplantation 29:308-313, 1980.

11. Billingham, RE, Medawar, PB. Contracture and intussusceptive growth in the healing of extensive wounds in mammalian skin. J. Anat. (London), 89:114-123, 1955.

12. O'Connor, NE, Mulliken, JB, Banks-Schlegel, S, Kehinde, O, Green, H. Grafting of burns with cultured epithelium prepared from autologous epidermal cells. Lancet 1:75-78, 1981.

13. Green, H, Kehinde, O, Thomas, J. Growth of cultured human epidermal cells into multiple epithelia suitable for grafting. Proc. Natl. Acad. Sci. USA 76:5665-5668, 1979.

14. Yannas, IV, Burke, JF. Design of an artificial skin. I. Basic design principles. J. Biomed. Mater. Res. 14:65-81, 1980.

15. Okada, N, Kitano, Y, Morimoto, T. Isolation of a viable eccrine sweat gland by dispase. Arch. Dermatol. Res. 275:130-133, 1983.

16. Leight, GS, Kirkman, R, Rasmusen, BA, Rosenberg, SA, Sachs, DH, Terrill, R, Williams, GM. Transplantation in miniature swine. III. Effects of MSLA and A-O blood group matching on skin allograft survival. Tissue Antigens 12:65-74, 1978.

17. Lafferty, KJ, Cooley, MA, Woolnough, J, Walker, KZ. Thyroid allograft immunogenicity is reduced after a period in organ culture. Science 188:259-261, 1975.

18. Simeonovic, CJ, Bowen, KM, Kotlarski, I, Lafferty, KJ. Modulation of tissue immunogenicity by organ culture. Transplantation 30:174-179, 1980.

19. Steinmuller, D. Passenger leukocytes and the immunogenicity of skin allografts: A critical reevaluation. Transplant. Proc. 13:1094-1098, 1981.

16
Artificial Skin: An Approach to "Regeneration-like" Tissue Repair

John F. Burke

Scar is the material which closes all wounds in animals that have lost the ability to regenerate lost or opened tissue. From the standpoint of survival it is effective, for it preserves life. However, from the standpoint of function (both mechanical and cosmetic) it is wanting more often than not. Nowhere are the deficiencies of scar more evident than in the spontaneous healing of a large thermal burn particularly those involving the hand or face. The deficiencies of scar, however, though less noticeable, are apparent through the entire province of repair.

Scar is always associated with loss of function, whether it be the healing of an injured common bile duct, the repair of a simple laceration of the skin, the result of spontaneous healing, or the most sophisticated of surgical intervention. The scar seems a small price to pay for survival until biologic science could provide an alternative.

It is surely possible to close a wound with exact preservation of normal function; regeneration of the lost or injured tissue is the key. One might wonder at the size of the effort made to induce, speed, or otherwise manipulate the natural process of wound healing (since it always leads to scar), compared to that expended on inducing and controlling regeneration (which would avoid the problems of scar). There are at least two connected explanations: first, wound healing provides a process where the cell biologist can study cellular behavior and control (a very important research activity); these processes are studied in well developed wound healing models; and second, there appears to be insufficient information on cellular behavior and control necessary to mount a broad-based investigation of regeneration. Understanding of healing may well be a prerequisite for an understanding of regeneration. Today wound healing and regeneration are studied by different groups of biologists, many of whom do not see scar and are not pressed to develop methods of healing which would avoid it. The pressure to bring these two areas of study together is not as strong as it could be.

Although there is general agreement that regeneration is the mode that would effectively retain normal function, it is not achievable at present. Attempts to substitute auto- and allo-transplantation or nonbiologic, mechanical replacement parts (such as hip prostheses), have met with considerable success, but they are complex. So specific solutions to problems which are rigidly-defined are of limited usefulness.

To provide a general solution for skin replacement and in an attempt to obtain tissue repair without scar formation in the treatment of burn patients, we have attempted to develop an artificial skin. It would replace normal physiologic and cosmetic function by utilizing a combination of mechanical and quasi regenerative processes. It would be mechanical in the sense of providing a template which would: 1) induce mesenchymal ingrowth without inflammation or immunologic rejection, and 2) direct the incoming connective tissue matrix into a pattern resembling normal dermis, and not scar, with controlled biodegradation of the manufactured artificial dermis resulting in a neodermis which would then function more as dermis than scar. Our experiments were carried out in close collaboration with Prof. Ionas Yannas of the Department of Mechanical Engineering at Massachusetts Institute of Technology with the biomaterials studies carried out in Prof. Yannas' laboratories.

In this work, we formulated several hypotheses which could be tested by experiment. These hypotheses are: 1) a material consisting of a collagen glycosaminoglycan composite made into an open fibrillar lattice would induce the migration of mesenchymal cells and the synthesis of new connective tissue resembling dermal connective tissue fibers, without inducing an inflammatory reaction or immunologic rejection. 2) If the artificially constructed fibrillar lattice were constructed in a manner similar to the third-dimensional distribution of connective tissue fibers in normal dermis, the incoming mesenchymal cells and microvasculature would use the artificial template as a scaffolding and lay down newly synthesized connective tissue matrix in a pattern resembling normal dermal structure, rather than the structure of scar. 3) If a neodermis could be created whose structure resembled more normal dermal architecture than scar, it would function both physically and cosmetically more like dermis in the clinical setting than like scar. 4) That the newly formed neodermis, if covered with the patient's epidermal cells, would function as normal skin with conventional antibacterial and reparative properties, remaining intact through the same type of remodeling processes as normal dermis for the remainder of the individual's life.

Our plan incorporated two phases. First, a mechanical phase represented by the Silastic epidermis and artificial dermis, and a second biologic phase where the patient's mesenchymal cells migrated into the artificial matrix, biodegraded it and replaced it with a neodermis and the ingrowth of epidermis through the seeding of the neodermis with the patient's epidermal cells. In short, this type of two-phase wound repair would provide a permanent skin replacement without scar through the initial use of a biodegradable synthetic template which organized the incoming cellular and connective tissue components into a dermal-like structure which could be covered by auto-epithelium and function as normal skin.

Our studies have led to the development of a physiologically acceptable bilayer artificial skin composed of a temporary Silastic® epidermis, to be replaced at a time of election by the patient's own epidermal cells, and a porous collagen chondroitin-6 sulfate fibrillar dermis whose third dimensional structure resembles the normal dermal collagen fiber pattern.[1,2,3,4] Application of this material to an open wound induces the migration of cells, the synthesis of new connective tissue, and the subsequent invasion of microvasculature, all of which are processes of great importance. All migration occurs shortly after the artificial matrix is placed in contact with the open wound and takes place without histologic signs of inflammation—that is, without white cell infiltration or detectable increases in vascular permeability. Whether the initial cells entering the matrix are macrophages or fibroblasts, or both, is an unsettled question. It is our view that both cell lines are present. Here again, the question concerning the initial events in tissue repair are raised.

On the basis of the fragmentary evidence at hand, it is our view that the initial phases of classic inflammation are only required as the first step in wound healing if there is debris or foreign material present which must be removed before new connective tissue formation can take place. This "clean up" process leaves a volume of tissue without appropriate structure and when fibroblasts move in to create a new connective tissue matrix, there is no model to copy and the matrix pattern of scar is produced. Where there is no debris or foreign material to be removed, the migration of connective tissue cells and the synthesis of new connective tissue are both preceded by macrophage migration but without inflammation. This set of responses may well be important to the replacement of tissue without scar formation.

This artificial skin has been tested clinically over the past two-and-one-half years in more than 40 patients with extensive burn injuries treated at the Massachusetts General Hospital and the Shriners Burns Institute in Boston.[4] It has been used to successfully close burn wounds up to 60% of the body surface, following prompt excision of the burn and immediately grafting with the artificial skin. Following grafting, the dermal portion is populated with mesenchymal cells and vessels migrating from the wound bed, as described above. The third-dimensional structure of the artificial dermis fibrillar matrix resembles fibrillar matrix in normal dermis and has been seen to serve as a template for the synthesis of new connective tissue and the formation of a "neodermis." The artificial template is slowly biodegraded over a period of approximately 60 days, as it is replaced by newly formed connective tissue. Following vascularization, the temporary Silastic® epidermis is removed at a time of clinical election and immediately replaced with an epidermal graft harvested from the patient himself. This procedure is performed at seven to 46 days following artificial skin grafting. Clinical and histologic experience indicates that the newly formed neodermis retains many of the anatomic characteristics and mechanical behavior of normal dermis, thus promising improvement in the functional and cosmetic results following repair of burn injuries.

The artificial skin is prepared in a sterile state and may be stored for long periods of time. It is capable of being produced in a large scale. It would be immediately available for use as a skin substitute for what we believe can be an effective method of wound closure. How successful this method will be in avoiding scar formation, and providing mechanical and cosmetic function, is not yet established.

NOTES

1. Burke, JF, Yannas, IV, Quinby, WC, Bondoc, CC, Jung, WK. Successful use of a physiologically acceptable artificial skin in the treatment of extensive burn injury. Ann. of Surg. 1981: 194: 413-28.

2. Dagalakis, N, Flink, J, Stasikelis, P, Burke, JF, and Yannas, IV. Design of an artificial skin. III. Control of pore structure. J. Biomed. Mat. Res. 1980: 14:511-528.

3. Yannas, IV, Burke, JF. Design of an artificial skin. I. Basin design principles. J. Biomed. Mater. Res. 1980: 14: 65-81.

4. Yannas, IV, Burke, JF, Gordon, PL, et al. Design of an artificial skin. II. Control of chemical composition. J. Biomed. Mater. Res. 1980: 14:107-32.

17
Dressings and Wound Healing

William H. Eaglestein
and Patricia M. Mertz

INTRODUCTION

In his 1955 monograph, The Mechanisms of Healing in Human Wounds, Shattuck W. Hartwell,[1] M.D., Ph.D. says that while in training he "came to feel that many surgical dressing procedures demanded by different surgeons were more ritualistic than necessary. The dressing was always outside the wound. . . ." Since then, a large body of information has been developed showing that dressings which prevent a dry crust from forming on a wound have many effects on wound healing. These dressings are known collectively as "occlusive or semiocclusive dressings" and healing beneath them is called "moist wound healing." At this time occlusive dressings are probably best defined by the biologic effect they produce, that is, as dressing materials which maintain tissue hydration or avoid tissue dehydration. Table 17.1 presents a number of currently available occlusive dressings and a description of their properties. Although some of the dressings vary considerably in their chemical composition and their physical properties, they all keep the healing tissues moist. This chapter is devoted to a discussion of the effects of occlusive dressings on the epidermis and the dermis during healing, and the effects on the microflora of healing wounds. Throughout, the word "open" will refer to air-exposed, non-dressed wounds and "covered, closed or occluded" will refer to wounds covered with an occlusive dressing.

THE EFFECT OF OCCLUSIVE DRESSINGS ON EPIDERMAL HEALING

Winters[2] (1962), studying wounds in pigs, and Hinmann and Maibach[3] (1963), studying human wounds, were among the

TABLE 17.1

Properties of Occlusive Dressings

	Bioclusive®	Duoderm®	Op-Site®	Tegaderm®	Vigilon®
Transmits oxygen	+	-	+	+	?+
Transmits moisture vapor	+	-	+	+	?-
Excludes bacteria	+	+	+	+	?-
Absorbs fluids	-	±	-	-	+
Transparent	+	-	+	+	±
Adhesive to normal tissue	+	+	+	+	-

Note: Bioclusive®, Op-Site® and Tegaderm® are polyurethane films with adhesives. Vigilon® is a polyethylene oxide hydrogel (95%) water sandwiched between two polyethylene films. Duoderm® is composed of hydrocolloid particles surrounded by a hydrophobic polymer.

first to demonstrate the increased rate of epidermal resurfacing produced by occlusive dressings. Winters found that shallow wounds covered with polythene film were protected from dehydration and had an altered pattern and speed of epithelization. Beneath the film, epidermal cells began to migrate sooner and completed their resurfacing sooner. The migrating cells were elongated and moved in or through a moist exudate rather than through a wound bed of dessicated tissue. The "sheet" of migrating epidermal cells was thinner than in an open wound.

Epidermal resurfacing is primarily a function of epidermal cell movement, although cell division is important in providing cells for remodeling and extensive resurfacing. In studies of human forearm wounds, Rovee et al.[4] (1972) found that occlusive dressings reduced the magnitude and duration of the mitotic response occuring in the wounded tissue. This may be because more cells are lost in open wounds than in wounds covered with an occlusive dressing. Occlusive dressings reduced the resurfacing time but did not shorten the time interval between wounding and the onset of mitosis, clearly indicating that resurfacing is dependent primarily upon epidermal cell migration rather than mitosis.

The effect on re-epithelialization of some of the newest occlusive dressings (Table 17.1) has been studied. May[5] (1981) compared healing of human donor sites beneath Op-Site®, porcine xenografts and Scarlet Red impregnated gauze. In the twenty-two patients he studied, the healing time in days was 6.7 ± 2.7, 11 ± 1 and 10 ± 0.8 respectively. In May's studies, re-epithelialization was evaluated by clinical inspection of the healing donor sites. When Barnett et al.[6] (1983) compared resurfacing in human donor sites beneath Op-Site®, Tegaderm® and fine mesh gauze, the days to healing were 6.9, 6.7, and 10.5 respectively.

In studies of partial thickness wounds in domestic swine, evaluated by serial histologic sections, Winters[7] found a greater percent of wound re-epithelialization at the second and third days in Tegaderm®-dressed compared to Op-Site®-dressed wounds: 85% ± 21.7 compared to 58.7% ± 15.7. These two dressings are very similar. They are both made of polyurethane and transmit gases and moisture vapor. It might be helpful to know why these slight differences in the re-epithelialization rate occur beneath them. Ultimately, at seven days, Winters[7] found 100% re-epithelialization beneath both Op-Site® and Tegaderm®. Geronimus[8] studied Vigilon®, a polyethylene oxide hydrogel dressing in swine partial thickness wounds. Epidermal healing was evaluated after separating the epidermis from the dermis. Four days after wounding, 100% of the Vigilon®-dressed wounds were healed compared to 32% of the air-exposed wounds. Vigilon® is a gel covered on both sides by a polyethylene film. Geronimus removed the film from the side placed on the wound. The polyethylene film was left attached to the gel on the exposed side of the gel and the film's edges were taped to the nonwounded skin. Vigilon® transmits oxygen but in contrast to the polyurethane films it absorbs fluids.

We compared re-epithelialization in partial thickness swine wounds beneath Duoderm®, Op-Site® and wet to dry gauze dressings and open air treatment.[9] We expressed our results as the number of days needed for half the wounds to heal (HT_{50}). In our studies the HT_{50}s were: Duoderm® 2.5, Op-Site® 3.1, gauze wet-to-dry 4.1 and open 3.9 days. Using these data, the relative rates of healing [(Air Exposed HT_{50} - Treatment HT_{50})/(Air Exposed HT_{50}) × 100] are Duoderm® + 36%, Op-Site® + 21% and gauze wet-to-dry -5%. Duoderm® is a hydrocolloid gel which does not transmit oxygen or water vapor. Its effects on re-epithelialization were surprising because a correlation between the wound surface oxygen tension and re-epithelialization has been reported. Silver[10] (1972) measured different oxygen tensions beneath different occlusive and nonocclusive dressings and suggested the rate of re-epithelialization might be a function of a dressing's ability to increase wound surface oxygen tension. Rovee[11] has been unable to relate a dressing's oxygen permeability to re-epithelialization rate. Duoderm® absorbs wound fluids, becoming a semi-solid "paste" at the wound surface. This soft material allows the dressing to be removed with little trauma to the newly resurfaced wound. In contrast, in our studies Op-Site® tended to adhere to the newly re-epithelialized areas so that when the dressing was removed the new epidermis was sometimes torn away from the wound with the dressing. We suspected some of the difference seen in the re-epithelialization rates in our studies could be related to this re-injury. To study this possibility we studied the effect of changing the Op-Site® dressing every day. When Op-Site® was changed daily, the percent of healed wounds decreased from 92% on day three to 75% on day four, probably because of re-wounding.

THE EFFECT OF OCCLUSIVE DRESSINGS ON DERMAL HEALING

Based on his histologic studies of shallow wounds in swine, Winters concluded that connective tissue regeneration begins about 3 days earlier in occluded wounds.[2] In addition, he noted an earlier appearance in the dermis of mononuclear cells, fibroblasts and collagenous material. Rather than accumulate in the dermis, the polymorphonuclear leukocytes migrated out of the dermis into the moist serous material beneath the occlusive film. In histologic studies of incisional wounds in guinea pigs, Linsky et al.[12] (1981) also found that occlusive dressings produced a markedly altered pattern of dermal repair. In open wounds there was a wide area of dermal repair containing lymphocytes and many tightly packed fibroblasts. In contrast, wounds covered for seven days had a much narrower zone of repair and did not contain many lymphocytes or fibroblasts. Pulse labeling with L-[5-^{3}H]-Proline followed by autoradiography produced high grain counts in the dermis of open wounds. The dermal grain count of covered wounds was no higher than in adjacent non-wounded dermis. Histologically (and clinically) the inflammatory response was reduced in the covered wounds. When the force needed to break strips of 7-day old incisional wounds was evaluated, they found that less force was needed to break the open wounds than the covered. Placing and removing dressings at different times, they found the dressing's effect on breaking strength was related to its being on the wound during the second or third day after wounding. It is generally concluded that some component of the inflammatory response to wounding is essential in stimulating regeneration. To test the idea that the observed reduced rate of gain of wound breaking strength beneath occlusive dressing was related to a reduction in inflammation, they irritated healing guinea pig wounds. Seven days after wounding, the breaking strength of irritated wounds was greater than that of non-irritated wounds.

In our studies of partial thickness swine wounds,[9] the dermis beneath occlusive dressings had a greater biosynthetic capacity than the dermis of open wounds. After separating the dermis from the epidermis of the excised wounds, the 7 × 10 mm dermal wound area was minced and incubated with ^{14}C Proline in HEPES buffered Krebs Ringer medium supplemented by ascorbate. Using a modification of the methods described by Petekofsky and Diegelmann,[9] we determined the collagen biosynthetic capacity of the wounded tissues. The dermis from occlusively dressed wounds synthesized significantly more collagen than the dermis of wounds left open. The increased collagen biosynthetic capacity was found in tissues dressed with Duoderm® and in tissues dressed with Op-Site®. Fibroblasts incubated with Duoderm® "granules" did not synthesize more collagen. It is possible Duoderm® stimulated the biosynthetic capacity in a special way which overcame the adverse effect of its not transmitting oxygen. However, we believe the best current interpretation of our results is that in our model atmospheric oxygen transmission is not important to obtain increased dermal collagen biosynthetic capacity. An increased collagen biosynthesis is not incompatible with the decreased breaking strength and the decreased number of cells in occluded wounds at 7 days. Breaking strength is related to collagen maturity (intermolecular cross linking) rather than to the amount of collagen synthesized. It is important to realize that wound breaking strength in occluded, compared to open wounds, at various times after 7 days has not been studied. It is probable that the ultimate breaking strength of healed open and closed wounds will be similar and, as is well known, lower than that of nonwounded skin.

THE MICROBIOLOGIC EFFECT OF OCCLUSIVE DRESSINGS

In large measure, occlusive dressings have not been utilized because of the fear that they will produce wound infections. Clinically, the appearance of many white blood cells in the serous wound fluid (pus) sustains this concern. On normal skin, microorganisms flourish beneath occlusive films.[13,14] Buchan et al.[15,16] (1981) reported a series of experiments evaluating the antibacterial activity of the cells and fluids which accumulate in wounds covered by Op-Site®. They studied partial thickness wounds in humans and in swine. At various times the cell population, neutrophil antibacterial activity, protein content and type and the lysozyme content of the wound exudate were determined. Swab cultures of the wounds were taken throughout the studies. The cell type and numbers of cells in the exudate were typical of a normal inflammatory response and the protein content of the exudate was indistinguishable from the plasma. The neutrophils in the exudate four and twenty-four hours post operatively killed S. aureus at a rate greater than that of blood neutrophils from the same patient or animal. By 48 hours the exudate neutrophils had a decreased bactericidal effect. The lysozyme concentration was elevated at 24, 48 and 72 hours. Only 7% of the swab cultures taken 24 and 48 hours after wounding grew bacteria.

In partial thickness swine wounds we cultured more microflora from Op-Site® occluded wounds than from exposed wounds.[17] (1983) Our cultures were taken with the scrub technique which is more sensitive than the swab technique.[18] (1981) As seen in Fig. 17.1, the number of organisms in covered and open wounds was similar at 24 hours. At 48 hours there were 5 logs more organisms in the Op-Site® wounds. The increased number of organisms seen at 48 hours but not at 24 hours might be related to the bactericidal effect of the neutrophils during the first 24 hours. In addition to the increased number of organisms, we found a shift toward gram-negative organisms in the occluded compared to open wounds. These effects are similar to those produced by occlusive dressings on non-wounded skin: an increase in the number of organisms and a shift toward gram-negatives. Microflora recovery is increased with the scrub technique compared to the swab technique, and this difference

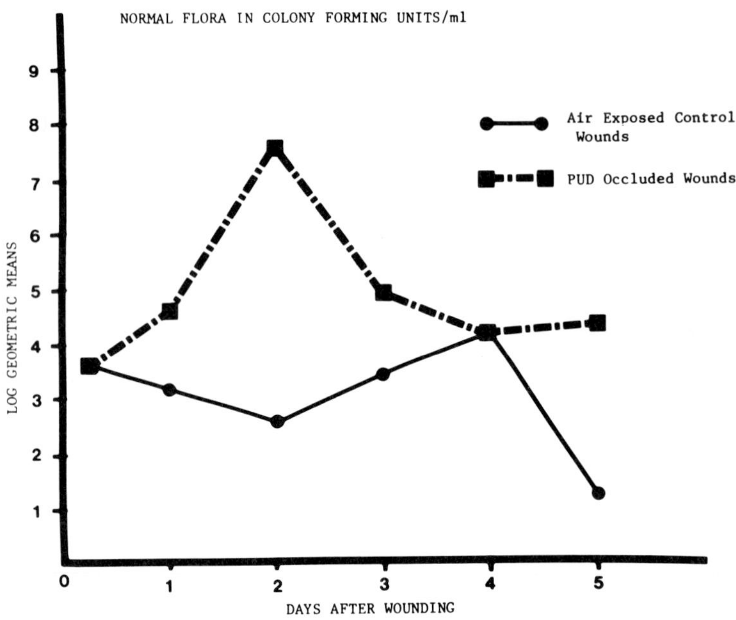

FIGURE 17.1

in culturing technique probably accounts for the large number of microflora we found compared to Buchan's[16] results. Finding large numbers of bacteria in these wounds which resurface rapidly is consistent with our conclusion that large numbers of normal skin flora do not interfere with re-epithelialization. The possibility that they contribute to the increased healing rate is unstudied.

Several of the occlusive dressings exclude bacteria. In order to evaluate the adhesive edge and surface barrier properties of Duoderm®, we applied Duoderm® to partial thickness swine wounds.[9] We subsequently bathed the surface of the dressing and all the adjacent skin with a 10^8 CFU per ml suspension of Staphylococcus aureus. The marker S. aureus was not recovered from wounds protected with the Duoderm®; however, large numbers of S. aureus were recovered from the surface of the dressing and adjacent non-dressed, non-wounded skin.

In standardized in vitro studies evaluating only the barrier surface properties, occlusive film dressings are placed over an opening between two fluid filled chambers. One chamber contains sterile fluid while the other chamber contains fluid and bacteria. The sterile fluid is monitored at varying time intervals for the presence of bacteria. Both Tegaderm® and Op-Site® are barriers to bacterial penetration in this system. However, this in vitro method does not address the penetration of bacteria at the edge of the dressing.

GENERAL EFFECTS OF OCCLUSIVE DRESSINGS ON WOUNDS

Almost all documented clinical experiences with these dressings note that occlusively dressed wounds are less painful, less tender, less erythematous and less swollen. Both Linsky[12] and Eaton[20] (1980) evaluated the cosmetic results of human incisional wounds covered with occlusive dressing. Eaton's patients and nurses preferred the appearance of the Op-Site® treated wounds. Linsky found the covered half better than the open half.

CONCLUSION

In the past five years, an assortment of occlusive dressings has been made available. They are promoted for use as post-operative dressing, donor site dressings, ulcer treatments, covers for minor skin abrasions, backings for skin donor tissues, covers for cutdown sites and IV sites and for prevention of pressure sores. Their different properties, for example, transparency, opacity, ability to exclude bacteria, adhesiveness and flexibility, make different dressings more useful in one set of circumstances than another. Their ultimate acceptance and role will depend upon the results of empiric and controlled use and the promotional abilities of the producers. One of their most important contributions has been to stimulate the study of wound healing.

NOTES

1. Hartwell, SW. 1955. The Mechanisms of Healing in Human Wounds. Springfield: Charles C. Thomas, pp. 4-5.

2. Winters, GD. 1962. Formation of scab and the rate of epithelialization of superficial wounds in the skin of the young domestic pig. Nature 193:293-294.

3. Hinman, CD, Maibach, H, and Winters, GD. 1963. Effect of air exposure and occlusion on experimental human skin wounds. Nature 200:377-378.

4. Rovee, DT et al. 1972. Effect of local wound environment on epidermal healing. In Epidermal Wound Healing. Edited by H. I. Maibach and D. T. Rovee. Chicago: Year Book Medical Publishers, pp. 159-81.

5. May, SR. Physiology, immunology and clinical efficacy of an adherent polyurethane wound dressing: Op-Site™. In Burn Wounds Covering, Vol. II, CRC Press, Boca Raton, Fl. In press (July 1984).

6. Barnett, A, Bekowitz, RL, Mills, R, Vistnes, LM. 1983. Comparison of synthetic adhesive moisture vapor permeable and fine mesh gauze dressings for split-thickness skin graft donor sites. American J of Surg 145:379-381.

7. Winters, GD. Transparent adhesive dressing for superficial wounds. In Clinical Investigator's Brochure. Medical Products Division, 3M.

8. Geronimus, RG and Robins, P. 1982. The effect of two new dressings on epidermal wound healing. J Dermatol Surg Oncol 8:850-852.

9. Alvarez, OM, Mertz, PM, and Eaglstein, WH. 1983. The effect of occlusive dressings on collagen synthesis and re-epithelialization in superficial wounds. J Surg (in press).

10. Silver, IA. 1972. Oxygen tension and epithelialization. In Epidermal Wound Healing. Edited by H. I. Maibach and D. T. Rovee. Chicago: Year Book Medical Publishers, pp. 291-305.

11. Rovee, DT. Unpublished personal communication.

12. Linsky, CB, Rovee, DT, and Dow, T. 1981. Effect of dressing on wound inflammation and scar tissue. In The Surgical Wound. Edited by P. Dineen and G. Hildick-Smith. Philadelphia: Lea and Febiger, pp. 191-205.

13. Leydon, JL, Steward, R, and Kligman, AM. 1979. Updated in vivo methods for evaluating topical antimicrobial agent on human skin. J Invest Dermatol 72:165-170.

14. Aly, R. 1982. Effect of occlusion on microbial population and physical skin conditions. Seminars in Dermatology 1 (2):137-142.

15. Buchan, IA, Andrews, JK, and Lang, SM. 1981. Clinical and laboratory investigation of the composition and properties of human skin wound exudate under semi-permeable dressing. Burns 7:326-334.

16. Buchan, IA, Andrews, JK, and Lang, SM. 1981. Laboratory investigation of the composition and properties of pig skin wound exudate under Op-Site®. Burns 8:39-46.

17. Mertz, PM and Eaglstein, WH. 1983. The effect of a semi-occlusive dressing on the microbial population in superficial wounds. Arch of Surg (Submitted).

18. Noble, WC and Somerville, D. 1981. Methods for examining the skin flora. In Microbiology of Human Skin. Edited by Noble. London: Lloyd-Luke, Ltd., ch. 18, pp. 401-408.

19. E.R. Squibb & Sons, Inc. 1982. Duoderm® Hydroactive Dressings Technical Booklet.

20. Eaton, AC. 1980. A controlled trial to evaluate and compare a sutureless skin closure technique (Op-Site® Skin Closure) with conventional skin suturing and clipping in abdominal surgery. Br J Surg 67:857-860.

PART V
Inflammation and Wound Healing

18
Mesenchymal Cell Proliferation in Wound Repair: The Role of Macrophages

Samuel Joseph Leibovich

INTRODUCTION

When an organism is injured, a complex series of events is initiated, which results ultimately in the reconstitution of the injured tissue. In animals other than mammals, this often occurs by a process of regeneration, with the reformation of tissues or limbs which are identical or near identical to the original. (See Chapter 29.) In mammals, however, the capacity to regenerate has been largely lost, and the restoration of tissue integrity is by a process of repair, with the formation of a connective tissue scar. This scar tissue is generally similar, whatever the site of injury, and many of the characteristics which differentiate a particular tissue or organ from another are absent from this scar tissue. For example, hair follicles, sweat glands, taste buds, and other specialized epithelial structures are not usually regenerated following injury.

The events following injury have been subdivided into several stages (Arey 1936; Schilling 1968; Ross and Benditt 1961). These have been termed (a) the inflammatory phase of repair, (b) the proliferative or fibroblastic phase, and finally, (c) the remodelling phase of repair.

The inflammatory phase commences immediately following injury, and is characterized by the events of a typical acute inflammatory response. These events will be discussed in some detail below.

This work was supported in part by a grant from the United States Public Health Service, number RO1-GM 29135.

The proliferative or fibroblastic phase is characterized by the controlled migration and proliferation of fibroblastic cells into and within the wounded area, and the controlled directional migration and proliferation of endothelial cells from local capillaries and small blood vessels adjacent to the wound into the wound area. Combined, this fibroblastic proliferation and neovascularization results in the formation of granulation tissue. These processes result in the amplification of the connective tissue forming factory, the connective tissue fibroblastic cells, which synthesize the collagen, proteoglycans, glycoproteins and other connective tissue constituents, which together reconstitute the integrity and continuity of the injured tissue, with the formation of a connective tissue scar.

The remodelling phase of repair, in contrast to the inflammatory and proliferative phases, is an extended process. During the remodelling phase to form the mature scar, the highly cellular granulation tissue gradually changes into an avascular, relatively acellular connective tissue, with the disappearance of the majority of the capillaries, blood vessels and fibroblasts. With maturation of the scar tissue, controlled degradation and resynthesis of connective tissue matrix takes place, with the acquisition of increasing structural order, and increasing tensile strength of collagen fibers. While these various phases of the wound repair process have been considered separately, it has become clear that these events are not at all separable in ways other than descriptive, and each is intimately involved in controlling that which follows it. Nature has evolved, in response to injury, a remarkable cascade of interacting processes, each dependent on others preceding it, which stem bleeding, protect the injured tissue, combat infection by foreign organisms, and restore the integrity of the injured tissue.

In this brief review, I will consider the events of the acute inflammatory response that are involved in stimulating and controlling the events of the subsequent proliferative, fibroblastic phase of repair. In particular, I will consider the role played by the monocyte/macrophage cells in stimulating the migration and proliferation of fibroblasts and capillaries, and the mechanisms by which these functions are carried out by these cells.

ACUTE INFLAMMATORY PHASE OF REPAIR

The acute inflammatory response following wounding is typical of acute inflammatory responses seen in many other situations. The cellular and humoral reactions which follow wounding serve several functions. Initial vasoconstriction, mediated by vasoactive humoral factors such as histamine, generated locally at the wound site, aids in preventing blood and fluid loss due to rupture of blood vessels. Platelet adhesion, with formation of retractile platelet plugs (microthrombi) at the damaged, or cut ends of microvessels serves to seal the damaged ends of these vessels, stemming blood loss. Platelets play an important role in the blood coagulation process. Interaction with exposed matrix sites on damaged vessels, induces platelet degranulation aggregation and thrombus formation, and results in the production of a variety of substances which are involved either in the process of coagulation, mediation of vascular permeability or the control of cell proliferation. Production of growth factors by platelets which stimulate fibroblast and smooth cell growth will be considered in more detail below (Ross et al. 1974; Ross, Raines and Bowen-Pope 1982). Formation of fibrin filaments, by activation of the clotting cascade serves to provide a fibrillar matrix which binds together the edges of the wound, resulting in temporary restoration of tissue continuity and the provision of an initial wound dressing in the form of a clot. Platelets play an important role in clot retraction, excluding plasma and fluid from the clot. The fibrin matrix—which appears always to be a copolymer of fibrin and fibronectin (Kurkinen et al. 1980), also acts as a substrate for the migration of fibroblasts, epithelial cells, and possibly also of endothelial cells into the wound area. (See Chapter 2.) Complement cleavage product serve to protect the wound against infection and invasion by foreign organisms. In particular, C_3b, generated either by the classical or alternative complement activation pathways, serves to opsonize foreign particles and organisms by binding to them, and promoting their recognition and phagocytosis by polymorphonuclear neutrophilic leukocytes (PMNs) and monocytes/macrophages. The anaphylotoxins, C_3a and C_5a, also generated as products of complement activation, act as chemoattractants for PMNs and monocytes, as well as having profound effects on microvascular tone and permeability.

Following the initial coagulation and microvascular permeability changes, which result in clot formation and plasma exudation into the wound area, migration of leukocytes into the extravascular wound area from the local microvasculature commences. The cells which migrate most rapidly are the PMNs which, in a linear skin wound, for example, reach an optimal level, and constitute the predominant cell type by 8 to 18 hours following injury. These cells perform an important role in protecting the wound site against infection by foreign organisms. Many bacteria activate and bind the C_3 component of complement directly on their cell surfaces. Both PMNs and monocytes have receptors for bound C_3a, and C_3b. Coated organisms can thus be recognized, bound and phagocytized by these cells. The uptake of opsonized organisms activates the oxidative respiratory burst, a transient hyperenergetic state of the PMNs, in which toxic oxygen radicals are rapidly generated within phagolysosomes. The generation of these toxic radicals plays an important role in the cytocidal mechanisms of PMNs (Klebanoff 1975; Clark 1983). In patients with chronic granulomatous disease, for example, PMNs do not exhibit the normal oxidative respiratory burst, and toxic oxygen radicals are not generated. Phagocytosis of bacteria appears to proceed normally in these patients, but once within phagolysosomes, the organisms are not killed and continue to grow, often resulting in chronic infections and granuloma formation. In addition to their cytocidal capacity, PMNs are equipped with a potent array of lysosomal enzymes, enabling them to digest foreign organisms and tissue debris. In wounds, degranulation of PMNs is often observed, with release of granular constituents into the extracellular milieu. PMNs clearly play an important role as a first line of defense against host invasion by foreign organisms. In the absence of overt infection, however, PMNs do not appear to be vital to the wound repair process. In experimental animals, depleted of neutrophils by treatment with anti-neutrophil sera, immigration of monocytes, fibroblasts and capillaries, and other events of the proliferative phase of repair occurred in the same way and on the same schedule as in control wounds (Simpson and Ross 1972). These results, as well as those of others, suggest that PMNs are not involved *in vivo* in the production of substances which stimulate migration and/or proliferation of fibroblasts or endothelial cells. In contrast, the other prominent cell type of the acute inflammatory response, the monocyte/macrophage, appears to play a much more significant role in this regard. Depletion of macrophages from healing wounds in guinea pigs resulted in a marked inhibition of fibroplasia, granulation tissue formation and wound repair (Leibovich and Ross 1975), and macrophages have been shown to produce a substance(s) termed "Macrophage-Derived-Growth-Factor" (MDGF), which stimulates the proliferation of a variety of mesenchymal cells *in vitro* (Leibovich and Ross 1976; Martin et al. 1981). In addition, we have recently demonstrated that macrophages actively synthesize a potent angiogenic activity which specifically induces the growth of new blood vessels *in vivo* and stimulates the growth of vascular endothelial cells *in vitro* (Polverini and Leibovich

1983). Evidence for the role of macrophages in controlling events of the proliferative phase of repair will be discussed in detail below.

FIBROBLASTIC, PROLIFERATIVE PHASE OF REPAIR

The proliferative phase of repair is characterized by the migration of fibroblasts from the uninjured tissues adjacent to the wound into the wound area and their subsequent proliferation, and the directional migration and growth of capillary blood vessels from uninjured vessels adjacent to the wound into the wound area. Migration and proliferation of fibroblasts and capillaries can be seen in experimental skin wounds as early as one to three days following injury, but this proliferative response does not become significant until the acute inflammation begins to resolve after 3-7 days. Wound fibroblasts originate from quescent perivascular connective tissue cell adjacent to the wound. Wound capillaries originate largely from pre-existing capillaries and small venules in the periwound area. Induction of fibroplasia in wound repair is a complex process. Activation of resting cells, induction of migration through normal extracellular matrix towards the wound, migration on a fibrin/ fibronectin meshwork and stimulation of mitosis within the wound are all required for a fibroproliferative response. Once present within the wound, synthesis of extracellular matrix components including collagen, glycosaminoglycans, proteoglycans, and structural glycoproteins must also be controlled. Induction of neovascularization is also an extremely complex process. Endothelial cells must be disturbed from their normal physiological location in the intact wall of capillaries and small venules. Intercellular junctions must be disrupted; basement membrane, which bounds these small vessels, must be degraded, and directional migration of the cells must be induced. The migrating cells must be stimulated to proliferate, to generate the new cells required for vessel formation, and resealing of cell junctions with generation of endothelial tubes must take place. Anastomosis of newly formed capillary sprouts to pre-existing blood vessels must also occur, to generate capillary loops which are capable of acting as conduits for blood (or lymph) flow. These various processes must all be induced in a highly controlled and coordinated fashion to result in successful repair. While the detailed mechanisms involved in control of the fibroproliferative response are far from being well understood, a few pertinent observations which relate to these mechanisms will be described here. In particular, the role of the monocyte/macrophage in controlling fibroblast and endothelial cell migration and proliferation will be discussed.

Macrophages and the Fibroproliferative Response

Macrophages present within wounds, as in other inflammatory lesions, are derived from blood-borne monocytes, which, in turn, are derived from precursor cells in the bone marrow (Van Furth 1970). Monocytes migrate into the wound area, presumably in response to chemotactic stimuli, by a process of diapedesis. This involves margination of leukocytes within the microcirculation, adhesion to endothelial cell surfaces, active migration between the junctions of adjacent endothelial cells, and degradation of the subendothelial basement membrane. During diapedesis, and within the wound area, maturation of monocytes to macrophages takes place, with the acquisition of particular morphologic features and of specific cell surface antigenic markers characteristic of mature and activated macrophages. Leibovich and Ross (1975) studied the role of macrophages in the wound repair process using linear full thickness skin wounds in guinea pigs as an experimental model. By using a combination of systemic hydrocortisone to induce a circulating monocytopenia, thus removing the main source of macrophage precursor cells, and of local injection of specific antimacrophage serum to destroy residual macrophages from the wounds, almost complete elimination of macrophages from these experimental wounds was achieved. Under these conditions, very marked inhibition of fibroblast proliferation, capillary regeneration, and collagen and connective tissue synthesis was observed. In addition, wound debridement was severely inhibited, with accumulation of large amounts of fibrin. These studies suggested two important functions for macrophages in the repair process. Firstly, macrophages seemed to be the principal phagocytic cell in wound repair, responsible for the clearance of tissue debris, including dead and damaged cells, fibrin, serum proteins, effete red blood cells and dead and dying PMNs. Secondly, macrophages seemed to be required to stimulate, either directly or indirectly, the subsequent proliferative phase of repair. These <u>in vivo</u> experiments led to studies <u>in vitro</u> (Leibovich and Ross 1976), which demonstrated the production by macrophages of an activity which stimulated the proliferation of fibroblasts in culture. This activity was originally termed "Macrophage-dependent Fibroblast-Stimulating-

Activity" (M-FSA), but in the light of more recent experiments, which clearly demonstrate this growth promoting activity to be a direct, biosynthetic product of macrophages, this activity has been renamed "Macrophage-Derived Growth-Factor" (MDGF) (Martin et al. 1981). MDGF will be discussed in detail below.

The Macrophage-Derived Growth Factor

In 1976, Leibovich and Ross demonstrated that macrophages cultured in vitro produce into the supernatant medium an activity that stimulates the proliferation of fibroblasts in vitro. Initial experiments utilized guinea pig macrophages derived from either unstimulated peritoneal cavities, or macrophages elicited by the prior intraperitoneal injection of sterile mineral oil. Fibroblast target cells were primary cell cultures derived from guinea pig skin wound granulation tissue. Production of this growth promoting activity was shown to be specific for macrophages. Neither PMNs nor lymphocytes derived from mesenteric or popliteal lymph nodes produced any activity under similar conditions. The system utilized the fact that plasma-derived serum (that is, serum prepared from plasma free of any cells, in particular, platelets) does not stimulate the growth of fibroblasts in culture, but maintains them in a state of physiological quiescence. It has been demonstrated that most, if not all, of the growth-promoting activity of normal serum is produced as a result of the release of growth factors from platelets during the clotting process (Ross et al. 1974). Some properties of the platelet-derived-growth-factor (PDGF) will be discussed below. Because of its ability to maintain cells in a state of physiological quiescence without stimulating cell division, plasma-derived serum (PDS) was used as a base for studying the production of growth factors by macrophages. Production of MDGF was shown to require the culture for several hours of viable macrophages. Some storage of MDGF was found within cells, as freeze-thawing produced a small amount of activity. Production of MDGF was increased although not markedly, by phagocytosis in vitro of either latex, zymosan or opsonized sheep red blood cells. Further studies by Leibovich (1978) demonstrated that MDGF was produced by macrophages for at least five days in culture, with regular medium changes, but that optimal activity was produced into a particular batch of medium within 6-8 hours. In addition, macrophages also produced in culture low molecular weight factors, which inhibit the incorporation of [^{3}H]-thymidine into the DNA of dividing cells. Production of these low molecular weight factors was highly dependent on macrophage concentration. One of these factors is certainly thymidine, produced as a result of macrophage biosynthetic activity. This aspect has been studied in detail by Calderon, Williams and Unanue (1974) and by Stadecker et al. (1977). In addition to thymidine, other low molecular weight inhibitors of [^{3}H]-thymidine incorporation into DNA are also produced by cultured macrophages. These low molecular weight factors do not necessarily inhibit DNA synthesis and cell division. Thymidine merely interferes with the [^{3}H]-thymidine assay commonly used for measuring DNA synthesis, by competing with the radio-labelled material for incorporation into newly synthesized DNA. If present in sufficiently high concentration, it will also inhibit cell division.

Since the initial demonstration of MDGF production by Leibovich and Ross (1976), production of MDGF has been demonstrated by monocytes and macrophages from a variety of sources. These include: mouse and rat peritoneal macrophages, human peritoneal macrophages, human lung and rabbit wound macrophages, human monocytes, rabbit vitreal macrophages and a number of macrophage-like cell lines (Polverini et al. 1977; Greenburg and Hunt 1978; Grumm and Armstrong 1979; Wall et al. 1978; Wahl, Wahl and McCarthy 1980; Martin et al. 1981; Burke 1980; Wharton et al. 1982; Wharton 1983; Jalkanen 1981; Schmidt et al. 1982; DeLustro, Sherer and LeRoy 1981; DeLustro and LeRoy 1982; Rutherford, Steffin and Sexton 1982; Glenn and Ross 1981; Hunt and Van Winkle 1977; Martin et al. 1983; Bitterman et al. 1982). While MDGF has not yet been purified to homogeneity, a number of features concerning its mode of production, mechanism of action and biochemical properties have been described. These will be discussed in detail below.

Biochemical Characteristics of MDGF

The biochemical characteristics of MDGF are summarized in Table 18.1. This table is a combination of data obtained in my own laboratory, as well as that of others. MDGF appears to be a polypeptide, as it is trypsin-sensitive, but resistant to ribonuclease, DNA-ase and phospholipase A_2. Using gel filtration chromotography on Sephacryl S-200, we find two peaks of activity. The major peak (>80%) has an apparent molecular weight of around 80,000, under both isotonic and hypertonic (2M.NaCl) conditions. The minor peak (<20%) has a molecular weight of 15-20,000. These results are essentially in agreement with those of Martin et al. (1981). Our assay for routine detec-

TABLE 18.1

1. Trypsin sensitive, Ribonuclease, DNA-ase, Phospholipase A_2 resistant.
2. Destroyed by boiling for 3 mins., or heating at 80°C for 15 mins.
3. Resistant to heating at 56°C for 30 mins.
4. Resistant to freeze-thawing.
5. Sensitive to reducing agents.
   (20mM mercaptoethanol, 5 mins.
   20mM dithiothreitol, 30 mins.)
6. Not inhibited by protease inhibitors (PMSF, N-ethyl maleimide, benzamidine, E-amino-caproic acid, pepstatin, leupeptin, aprotinin).
7. Binds to DEAE-Biogel (or DEAE-Sephadex) at neutral pH. Elutes between 0.25 and 1.1 M NaCl.
8. Does not bind to DM-Sephadex.
9. Iso-electric point (pI) of 4.8 (4.6-5.3) by isoelectric focusing.
10. Molecular weight, by gel permeation chromatography on Sephacryl S-200: 80,000 (>80%)
    15-20,000 (<20%)
11. Produced by macrophages and stimulated monocytes. Production increased by macrophage activators (LPS, latex, PMA, Con-A).
12. Produced by macrophage-like cell lines NCTC-3749, J-774-2, WEHI-2, and U937-1, but not by either differentiated or undifferentiated HL-60 cells.
13. Stimulates proliferation of fibroblasts, smooth muscle cells, 3T3 cells and endothelial cells.
14. Acts as a "competence factor."
15. Induces neovascularization *in vivo* in the rat cornea.

tion of MDGF utilizes a ^{3}H-thymidine incorporation assay using 96 well culture plates, in which target cells (routinely Balb-c 3T3 cells) are induced to quiesce in 5% PDS. It is important in this assay of MDGF to test several serial dilutions of MDGF. This is because at high concentrations, saturation of the growth-stimulating effects are observed. Above saturation, increasing concentrations of MDGF do not yield further increases in cell growth or ^{3}H-thymidine incorporation. By testing serial dilutions of MDGF, the dilution at which 50% maximal ^{3}H-thymidine incorporation by target cells is induced can be determined, and comparisons of the amounts of MDGF present within various test media and column fractions can be made. Without the use of serial dilution assays, it is easy to assume that two fractions from a column have similar amounts of activity, whereas, because maximal stimulation of target cells is induced by both fractions, one fraction could have many times the content of MDGF of the other. Similar problems in quantitation of Interleukin I production have been described (Mizel and Mizel 1981). The interrelationship of the two peaks of activity, of high and low molecular weight, is not yet clear. The high molecular weight peak could be either a unique entity, an aggregate of smaller subunits, or an association of a smaller molecule with a carrier protein. This aspect remains to be clarified. On the basis of isoelectric focusing, MDGF (high molecular weight peak) has a pI of 4.9 (4.6-5.3). It has at least one disulfide group required for activity, as its growth stimulating properties are destroyed by 20mM mercaptoethanol or dithiothreitol. MDGF binds to phenyl sepharose, but to date, we have not been able to elute successfully significant amounts of activity, using polyethyleneglycol concentrations of up to 20% as eluant. MDGF binds to DEAE Biogel or DEAE-Sephadex at low ionic strength (0.01M sodium phosphate, pH 7.4) and can be eluted with increasing concentrations of sodium chloride. DEAE ion exchange chromatography provides a useful concentration step for analyzing MDGF from macrophage supernatant culture media. MDGF does not bind to DM-cellulose. Using a combination of ammonium sulfate precipitate, DEAE-Biogel ion exchange chromatography, Sephacryl S-200 gel permeation chromatography and iso-electric focusing, we have achieved to date an 8-9000 fold purification of MDGF from crude supernatant media of mineral-oil induced, latex-stimulated rat peritoneal macrophages with a recovery of 31% of initial activity. MDGF does not appear to be a proteolytic enzyme, as it is not inhibited by a variety of protease inhibitors (Table 18.1). Although this seems unlikely to us, the possibility that MDGF might have metallo-proteinase properties has not been ruled out. The effects of chelating agents such as EDTA on MDGF activity cannot be rigorously tested, because metal ions must be added back to MDGF for assay in cell culture. MDGF retains activity following repeated freezing and thawing and heating at 50°C for 20 minutes. It is rapidly destroyed by heating at temperatures above 80°C.

Relationship of MDGF to Other Growth Factors

Platelet-Derived-Growth-Factor (PDGF)

Following the initial description of PDGF production (Ross et al. 1974), PDGF has been purified to homogeneity in several laboratories. Its properties are rapidly becoming understood in some depth. PDGF differs markedly from MDGF in several respects. PDGF is a protein with a molecular weight in the unreduced form of approximately 32,000, consisting of two polypeptide chains of approximately 17,000 and 14,000. These chains are joined by disulfide bonds, which are essential for its activity. PDGF is a basic protein (pI 9-8), and binds strongly to CM-Sephadex. In contrast, MDGF is acidic, with a pI of 4.8. MDGF is reported not to compete with PDGF for PDGF receptor sites on fibroblasts (Ross, Raines and Bowen-Pope 1982) and does not crossreact with antibodies to PDGF. Also, PDGF is not mitogenic for endothelial cells in culture, these cells apparently lacking receptors for PDGF (Wall et al. 1978; Haudenschild et al. 1976; Thorgeirsson and Robertson 1978). In contrast, MDGF is a potent mitogen for these cells. It thus appears that MDGF and PDGF are distinct biochemical entities, with clear structural and functional differences. The ability of MDGF to stimulate endothelial cell growth *in vitro*, as well as to stimulate neovascularization *in vivo* will be considered in detail below.

Interleukin I (IL-1)

Interleukin I (IL-1) was until recently referred to as "Lymphocyte-activating factor" (LAF). At the 2nd International Lymphokine Workshop held at Ermatingen, Switzerland, in 1979, new nomenclature was introduced, in an attempt to introduce standard nomenclature into a field in which extensive literature proliferation had occured, with little firm biochemical data, namely that of lymphokine and monokine research. IL-1 was defined as a macrophage-derived factor with a molecular weight of 12-16,000, which enhanced lymphocyte proliferation (Mizel and Farrar 1979). IL-1 is a genetically unrestricted, antigen non-specific and species-unrestricted peptide that stimulates a variety of T-lymphocyte dependent processes, such as thymocyte proliferation (Farrar et al. 1978; Chen and DiSabato 1976; Gillis and Mizel 1981), *in vitro* antibody responses (Wood and Gaul 1974; Farrar and Hilfiker 1982) and allo-antigen specific T-cell mediated cytotoxicity (Farrar, Mizel and Farrar 1979). IL-2 was defined as a polypeptide of molecular weight 30,000D, which could support the continuous proliferation of cytotoxic

T-lymphocytes (Watson et al. 1982; Larsson, Iscove and Coutinho 1980). While the original definition dealt with single molecular entities, and, indeed Mizel and Mizel have recently reported the apparent purification to homogeneity of a unique molecular species designated IL-1 from a "superinduced" P-388DI macrophage-like cell line (Mizel and Mizel 1981), the term IL-1 is being used in circumstances where it refers, not to a distinct molecular species, but to macrophage-derived activities (Rosenwasser, Dinarella and Rosenthal 1979). It is not clear whether many of the activities assigned to IL-1 [such as endogenous pyrogen activity (Rosenwasser, Dinarello and Rosenthal 1979; Sipe et al. 1979) which increases murine serum amyloid A concentrations (Kampschmidt, Pulliam and Upchurch 1980), fibrinogen and C-reactive protein, and "mononuclear cell factor" (MCF), which stimulates collagenase and prostaglandin production by rheumotoid synovial cells in culture (Dayer et al. 1979; Mizel et al. 1981)], are attributable to a single molecular species, or to closely related polypeptides. Schmidt et al. (1982) have suggested that MDGF is also related to IL-1, and demonstrated that MDGF and IL-1 copurify through a series of purification steps, including ammonium-sulfate precipitation, Sephacryl S-200 gel filtration, and flat bed isoelectric focusing. While data of this type suggest marked similarities between IL-1 and MDGF, it is clear that many polypeptides could copurify through these purification steps. Our own data, as well as that of others, clearly indicates that MDGF (as assayed by fibroblast stimulation) and IL-1 (as assayed by thymocyte stimulation) can be readily separated by ion exchange chromatography on DEAE-cellulose or DEAE-Biogel. Thus, while clear similarities do exist between IL-1 and MDGF, it seems likely that they are not the same polypeptide (Martin et al. 1981; Bitterman et al. 1982; Wharton et al. 1982). This problem will be resolved ultimately by the isolation of sufficient quantities of MDGF to enable full structural studies to be carried out.

Cells Stimulated by MDGF

MDGF is a potent mitogen for a variety of mesenchymal cells *in vitro*. These include fibroblasts from a variety of sources (fetal and adult), smooth muscle cells, and vascular endothelial cells. In addition to stimulating cell growth *in vitro*, MDGF also acts as a potent angiogenic agent *in vivo* (Polverini and Leibovich 1983). The angiogenic potential of macrophages was first demonstrated by Polverini et al. (1977), using the rat corneal implantation assay for angiogenesis. This procedure assesses the growth of new blood vessels into the normally avascular cornea induced by materials implanted in the corneal pocket. New blood vessels develop from the pre-existing vasculature at the limbus of the cornea, and neovascularization can be monitored regularly by viewing with a slit lamp and dissecting microscope. Permanent records of the microvascular network can be made by intravascular perfusion with colloidal carbon prior to sacrifice. Using this technique, we have demonstrated that partially purified MDGF is a potent angiogenic agent in vivo, in addition to stimulating bovine aortic endothelial cell proliferation in vitro (Polverini and Leibovich 1983). While we do not yet know for certain that the angiogenic activity, and the in vitro growth stimulating activities reside in the same molecule, these activities clearly copurify through several fractionation procedures. Ultimate resolution of this question will depend on the purification to homogeneity and characterization of the various stimulatory activities.

Production of MDGF by Monocytes, Macrophages and Macrophage-Like Cell Lines

Since the initial demonstration of MDGF production by Leibovich and Ross (1976) production of growth-promoting activity by macrophages from a variety of sources has been demonstrated. These include: guinea pig resident and induced peritoneal macrophages, murine resident and activated peritoneal macrophages, rat peritoneal macrophages, macrophages from human peritoneal dialysis washings, rabbit and human wound fluids, murine bone marrow macrophages and rabbit and human alveolar macrophages. In addition, monocytes from human peripheral blood have been shown to produce MDGF when activated in vitro with either lipopolysaccharide (endotoxin) or Concanavalin-A. In general, activation of macrophages either in vivo (mineral-oil, thioglycollate, protease-peptone, LPS, BCG) or in vitro (LPS, latex Con-A, phorbol-myrystate acetate, PMA and fibronectin), stimulates the production of MDGF in culture.

Production of MDGF by Macrophage-Like Cell Lines

We have utilized mineral oil-induced, latex-stimulated rat peritoneal macrophages as a source of culture media for purification of MDGF. Peritoneal macrophages, as is the case for most normal macrophages, do not grow in culture, but can be maintained as a static, biosynthetically active population. It is thus not possible to propagate large quantities of normal macrophages in vitro for the preparation of large quantities of culture media. This has been a severe handicap in our attempts to purify MDGF. Recently, we have obtained several macrophage-like cell lines, and have studied their ability to produce MDGF activity. Many macrophage-like cell lines are currently available. We have tested the following: NCTC-3749—an adherent subline of P-388DI, derived from a murine lymphoid neoplasm; J-774-2—a murine line derived from a spontaneous tumor; HL-60—a human promyeloid leukemic cell line that can be induced to differentiate to either granulocytic or monocytic macrophagic cells in vitro, and U-937—a human monocytic cell line. In accord with the recent experiments of Wharton et al. (1982) we confirm that the NCTC-3749, J-774-2, WEHI-2 and U-937 cell lines are all producers of a growth promoting activity for fibroblasts which resembles MDGF. In addition, we have demonstrated, using the purification procedures outlined above, that the growth promoting activity produced by NCTC-3749 and by U-937 cells behaves similarly to the MDGF produced by rat peritoneal macrophages through several purification steps. These results suggest that these cell lines should prove extremely valuable for the production of large scale cultures for the preparation of large batches of conditioned medium for detailed purification and characterization of MDGF. In contrast to U-937 cells, the human promyeloid HL-60 cells did not produce detectable MDGF activity, even when stimulated with PMA. Under these conditions, the HL-60 cells rapidly attach to the plastic substratum, spread, cease proliferation, and develop morphologic, functional and surface receptor characteristics of mature macrophages. These include the ability to phagocytize latex, opsonized RBC and C_3b coated RBC. It thus appears that production of MDGF is separable from other biological characteristics of macrophage differentiation and activation. In addition to stimulating fibroblast growth in vitro, we have demonstrated that medium from NCTC-3749 and U-937 cells stimulates growth of vascular endothelial cells in vitro. These cells, and their conditioned media also potently induce neovascularization in vivo in the rat corneal angiogenesis assay. The activities which stimulate fibroblast proliferation, endothelial cell growth and corneal angiogenesis appear to be closely related biochemically, copurifying through several purification procedures, as discussed earlier.

Role of Macrophage in Angiogenesis

Neovascularization, the growth and formation of capillary blood vessels, is a process that occurs in several normal and pathological situations, including growth, wound repair, inflammation, fibrosis, and tumor development. Angiogenesis, the directed outgrowth of new capillaries toward a specific stimulus, is an intrinsic part of these processes, and the characterization of angiogenesis-inducing factors is of great importance to our understanding of them. Macrophages have been implicated in the induction of microvascular proliferation in several pathophysiologic processes, including inflammation, wound repair, and immune responses. This angiogenic potential of macrophages appears to be closely related to the production of MDGF by these cells. We have recently demonstrated that, in addition to mediating neovascularization in wound repair and inflammation, macrophages also contribute significantly to the neovascularization induced by tumors (Polverini and Leibovich 1983). Using a methylcholanthrene-induced fibrosarcoma of rats, we were able to fractionate macrophages directly from the tumors, and to examine directly their angiogenic potential in the rat cornea, as well as their ability to promote endothelial cell proliferation in culture. Tumor associated macrophages (>98% pure) were potent inducers of angiogenesis, in a manner similar to that of normal activated peritoneal macrophages (Polverini et al. 1977). Tumor cells depleted of macrophages were considerably less potent inducers of angiogenesis than whole tumor cell suspensions, which normally consist of a mixed population of tumor cells and macrophages. Reconstitution of macrophage-depleted tumor cells with the purified tumor associated macrophages resulted in the restoration of the angiogenic activity of the original whole tumor cell preparations. These experiments indicate clearly that much of the tumor-induced angiogenesis is in fact a function of the tumor associated macrophages. The angiogenic activity produced by the tumor-associated macrophages has properties in common with MDGF. There is increasing evidence that macrophages may contribute to tumor growth (Gabizon, Leibovich and Goldman 1980; Evans 1979). Our observations support this view, and document a mechanism by which macrophages may mediate this effect. Recent work by Montovani (1981) suggests that tumor associated macrophages may also stimulate tumor cell proliferation directly.

As discussed earlier, neovascularization is an extremely complex process involving many distinct processes. Recently,

Banda et al. (1982) have isolated an angiogenic factor from rabbit wound fluid, which they believe also to be of macrophage derivation. This factor has a molecular weight between two and 14,000 on the basis of dialysis through membranes of different molecular weight cut-off. Interestingly, this factor does not possess mitogenic activity for endothelial cells _in vitro_, but will induce directed migration of endothelial cells through gelatin coated 10 μm-pore-diameter polycarbonate filters in Boyden blind well chambers. The factor is also angiogenic _in vivo_ in the corneal assay in rabbits. The relationship of this low molecular weight, nonmitogenic angiogenesis factor to the high molecular weight MDGF which we are studying is not yet clear. Production of this low molecular weight factor from wound fluid requires dialysis against 0.1M acetic acid. This acid dialysis has also been utilized in preparation of angiogenesis activity from tumors (Fenselau, Watt and Mello 1981). It could be that the acid dialysis liberates low molecular weight material from a higher molecular weight carrier protein, or, it could be that lysosomal proteases present in wound fluid are activated by the reduced pH, and cleave a larger molecule, into fragments yielding the small nonmitogenic factor. This interrelationship of MDGF and other angiogenic factors should prove to be an interesting line of investigation.

Our demonstration that macrophages play an important role in tumor-induced angiogenesis suggests that angiogenesis in this process is analogous to that in other pathophysiological processes, such as wound repair and fibrosis, where macrophages also appear to play a key role in inducing new blood vessel growth. Our results suggest that macrophage products, either alone, or in conjunction with other mediators, play a central role in stimulating neovascularization in a variety of conditions where fibrovascular proliferation is a distinct component.

SUMMARY

In this chapter, I have emphasized the role played by macrophages in the wound repair process, in particular, in terms of the production by macrophages of a growth factor for mesenchymal cells, termed the Macrophage-Derived-Growth-Factor (MDGF). Clearly, the interactions between events of the acute inflammatory response of the wound repair process and those of the subsequent fibroblastic, proliferative phase of repair have a broader significance than that of wound repair alone. Macrophages and MDGF are believed to serve important functions in those situations where macrophage infiltration is accompanied by a fibroproliferative response and granulation tissue formation. These include wound repair, chronic inflammations, such as rheumatoid arthritis and pulmonary fibrosis, atherosclerosis, tumor neovascularization, granulomatous diseases, graft versus host disease, systemic sclerosis, glomerular nephritis, and many others. The importance of macrophages and macrophage derived products in induction of fibroblast proliferation and neovascularization has been demonstrated, and in our hands, partially purified MDGF is active in stimulating fibroblast, smooth muscle and endothelial cell growth *in vitro*, and angiogenesis *in vivo*. Ultimate demonstration that the endothelial cell stimulating activity is biochemically identical with the fibroblast stimulating activity must await complete purification of MDGF as must the ultimate demonstration of the importance of MDGF *in vivo*.

ACKNOWLEDGMENTS

We express grateful appreciation to Dr. Peter Polverini for helpful discussions, and Ms. Kristi Novak for expert technical assistance. I also wish to thank Ms. Alice Stepney for preparing the manuscript.

REFERENCES

Arey, LB. Wound healing. Physiol. Rev. 16 (1936):327-406.

Banda, MJ, Knighton, DR, Hunt, TK, and Werb, Z. Isolation of a nonmitogenic angiogenesis factor from wound fluid. Proc. Nat. Acad. Sci. USA 79 (1982):7773-7777.

Bitterman, PB, Rennard, SI, Hunninghake, GW, and Crystal, RG. Human alveolar macrophage growth factor for fibroblasts. J. Clin. Invest. 70 (1982):806-822.

Burke, JM. Phagocytes that invade the vitreous after injury stimulate DNA synthesis in neural retina in vitro. Ophthalmologie 24 (1980):223-227.

Calderon, J, Williams, RT, and Unanue, ER. An inhibitor of cell proliferation released by cultures of macrophages. J. Immunol. 119 (1974):4273-4277.

Chen, DM, and DiSabato, G. Further studies on the thymocyte stimulating factor. Cell Immunol. 22 (1976):211-224.

Clark, RA. Extracellular effects of the myeloperoxidase-hydrogen peroxide-halide system. In Advances in Inflammation Research, Ed. Weissman, G. (1983). V.5, pp. 107-146. New York: Raven Press.

Dayer, JM, Breard, J, Chess, L, and Drane, SM. Participation of monocytes-macrophages and lymphocytes in the production of a factor that stimulates collagenase and prostaglandin release by rheumatoid synovial cells. J. Clin. Invest. 64 (1979):1386-1392.

DeLustro, F, Sherer, GK, and LeRoy, EC. Human monocyte stimulation of fibroblast growth by a soluble mediator(s). J. Reticuloendothel. Soc. 28 (1980):519-532.

DeLustro, F, and LeRoy, EC. Characterization of the release of human monocyte regulators of fibroblast proliferation. J. Reticuloendothel. Soc. 31 (1982):295-305.

Evans, R. Host cells in transplanted murine tumors and their possible relevance to tumor growth. J. Reticuloendothel. Soc. 26 (1979):427-437.

Farrar, JJ, Simon, PL, Koopman, WJ, and Fullur-Bonar, J. Biochemical relationship of thymocyte mitogenic factor and factors enhancing humoral and cell-mediated immune responses. J. Immunol. 121 (1978):1353-1360.

Farrar, WL, Mizel, SB, and Farrar, JJ. Initiation of alloantigen specific cytotoxic T-lymphocyte responses by lymphocyte-activating (LAF). Fed. Proc. 38 (1979):1006.

Farrar, JJ, and Hilfiker, ML. Antigen-non-specific helper factors in the antibody response. Fed. Proc. 41 (1982): 263-268.

Fenselau, A, Watt, S, and Mello, RJ. Tumor-angiogenic-factor. Purification from the Walker 256 rat tumor. J. Biol. Chem. 256 (1981):9605-9611.

Gabizon, A, Leibovich, SJ, and Goldman, R. Contrasting effects of activated and nonactivated macrophages and macrophages from tumor-bearing mice on tumor growth in vivo. J. Nat. Canc. Inst. 65 (1980):913-920.

Gillis, S, and Mizel, SB. T-cell lymphoma model for the analysis of Interleukin 1-mediated T-cell activation. Proc. Nat. Acad. Sci. USA 78 (1981):1133-1137.

Glenn, KC, and Ross, R. Human monocyte-derived growth factor(s) for mesenchymal cells: activation of secretion by endotoxin and concanavalin-A. Cell 25 (1981):603-615.

Greenburg, GB, and Hunt, TK. The proliferative response in vitro of vascular endothelial and smooth muscle cells exposed to wound fluids and macrophages. J. Cell. Physiol. 97 (1978):353-360.

Grumm, FG, and Armstrong, PB. Proteases are mitogenic to mesenchyme in vivo. A study using the chick chorioallantoic membrane. Exp. Cell. Res. 110 (1979):317-326.

Haudenschild, CC, Zahniser, D, Folkman, J, and Klagsburn, M. Human vascular endothelial cells in culture. Lack of response to serum factors. Exp. Cell. Res. 98 (1976):175-183.

Hunt, TK, and Van Winkle, W Jr. In Fundamentals of Wound Management in Surgery (1977) Chirurgecom Inc., New Jersey, pp. 1-8.

Jalkanen, M. Connective tissue activating macromolecules in macrophage culture medium. Connect. Tiss. Res. 9 (1981): 19-24.

Kampschmidt, RF, Pulliam, LA, and Upchurch, HF. The activity of partially leukocytic endogenous mediator in endotoxin-resistant C_3H/HeJ mice. J. Lab. Clin. Med. 95 (1980):616-623.

Klebanoff, SJ. Antimicrobial mechanisms in neutrophilic polymorphonuclear leukocytes. Semin. Hematol. 12 (1975):117-142.

Kurkinen, M, Vaheri, A, Roberts, PJ, and Stenman, S. Sequential appearance of fibronectin and collagen in experimental granulation tissue. Lab. Invest. 43 (1980):47-51.

Larsson, E-L, Iscove, NN, and Coutinho, A. Two distinct factors are required for induction of T-cell growth. Nature 283 (1980):664-666.

Leibovich, SJ, and Ross, R. The role of macrophages in wound repair. A study with hydrocortisone and antimacrophage serum. Am. J. Pathol. 78 (1975):71-100.

Leibovich, SJ, and Ross, R. A macrophage-dependent factor that stimulates the proliferation of fibroblasts in vitro. Am. J. Pathol. 84 (1976):501-513.

Leibovich, SJ. Production of macrophage-dependent fibroblast stimulating activity (M-FSA) by murine macrophages. Exp. Cell. Res. 113 (1978):47-56.

Mantovani, A. In vitro effects on tumor cells of macrophages isolated from an early-passage chemically-induced murine sarcoma and from metastases. Int. J. Cancer 27 (1981): 221-228.

Martin, BM, Gimbrone, MA Jr, Unanue, ER, and Cotran, RS. Stimulation of non-lymphoid mesenchymal cell proliferation by a macrophage-derived growth factor. J. Immunol. 126 (1981):1510-1515.

Martin, BM, Gimbrone, MA, Majeau, GR, Unanue, ER, and Cotran, RS. Stimulation of human monocyte/macrophage-derived growth factor (MDGF) production by plasma fibronectin. Am. J. Pathol. 111 (1983):367-373.

Mizel, SB, and Farrar, JJ. Revised nomenclature for antigen non-specific T-cell proliferation and helper factors. Cell Immunol. 48 (1979):433-436.

Mizel, SB, Dayer, JM, Krane, S, and Mergerhagen, S. Stimulation of rheumatoid synovial cell collagenase and prostaglandin production by partially purified lymphocyte-activating-factor (Interleukin I). Proc. Nat. Acad. Sci. USA 78 (1981): 2474-2477.

Mizel, SB, and Mizel, D. Purification to apparent homogeneity of murine Interleukin 1. J. Immunol. 126 (1981):834-838.

Polverini, PJ, Cotran, RS, Gimbrone, MA Jr, and Unanue, ER. Activated macrophages induce vascular proliferation. Nature 269 (1977):804-806.

Polverini, PJ, and Leibovich, SJ. Macrophage cell-lines induce neovascularization and endothelial cell proliferation. Submitted for publication.

Polverini, PJ, and Leibovich, SJ. Neovascularization and endothelial cell proliferation: Induction by tumor-associated macrophages. Submitted for publication.

Rosenwasser, LJ, Dinarello, CA, and Rosenthal, AS. Adherent cell function in murine T-lymphocyte antigen recognition. IV. Enhancement of murine T-cell antigen recognition by human leukocytic pyrogen. J. Exp. Med. 150 (1979):709-714.

Ross, R, and Benditt, ER. Wound healing and collagen formation I. Sequential changes in components of guinea pig skin wounds observed in the electron microscope. J. Biophys. Biochem. Cytol. 11 (1961):677-700.

Ross, R, Glomset, B, Kariya, B, and Harker, L. A platelet-dependent serum factor that stimulates the proliferation of arterial smooth muscle cells in vitro. Proc. Nat. Acad. Sci. USA 71 (1974):1207-1210.

Ross, R, Raines, E, and Bowen-Pope, D. Growth factors from platelets, monocytes and endothelium: Their role in cell proliferation. Annals N.Y. Acad. Sci. 397 (1982):18-24.

Rutherford, B, Steffin, K, and Sexton, J. Activated human mononuclear phagocytes release a substance (s) that induces replication of quiescent human fibroblasts. J. Reticuloendothel. Soc. 31 (1982):281-293.

Schilling, JA. Wound healing. Physiol. Rev. 48 (1968):374-423.

Schmidt, JA, Mizel, SB, Cohen, D, and Green, I. Interleukin 1, a potential regulator of fibroblast proliferation. J. Immunol. 128 (1982):2177-2182.

Silver, IA. The physiology of wound healing. In Wound Healing and Wound Infection. Theory and Surgical Practice. Ed. Hunt, TK, pp. 11-28. New York: Appleton-Century-Crofts, 1980.

Simpson, D, and Ross, R. The neutrophilic leukocyte in wound repair: A study with anti-neutrophil serum. J. Clin. Invest. 51 (1972):2009-2023.

Sipe, JD, Vogel, SW, Ryan, JL, McAdam, JKPW, and Rosenstreich, DL. Detection of a mediator derived from endotoxin-stimulated macrophages that induces the acute phase serum amyloid A response in mice. J. Exp. Med. 150 (1979):597-606.

Stadecker, MJ, Calderon, J, Karnofsky, ML, and Unanue, ML. Synthesis and release of thymidine by macrophages. J. Immunol. 119 (1977):1738-1743.

Thorgeirsson, G, and Robertson, AL. Platelet factors and the human vascular wall, part 2. Such factors are not required for endothelial cell proliferation and migration. Atherosclerosis 31 (1978):231-238.

Van Furth, R. Origin and kinetics of monocytes and macrophages. Sem. Haematol. 7 (1970):125-141.

Wahl, LM, Wahl, SM, and McCarthy, JB. Adjuvant activation of macrophage functions. In Regulatory Role of the Macrophage in Immunity. Eds. Rosenthal, A, and Unanue, E, pp. 491-504. New York: Academic Press, 1980.

Wall, RT, Harker, LA, Quadracci, LJ, and Striker, GE. Factors influencing endothelial cell proliferation in vitro. J. Cell. Physiol. 96 (1978):203-214.

Watson, J, Barton Frank, M, Mochizuki, D, and Gillis, S. The biochemistry and biology of Interleukin-2. In *Lymphokines* Ed. Mizel, SB. V. 6, pp. 95-116. New York: Academic Press, 1982.

Wharton, W, Gillespie, GY, Russell, SW, and Pledger, WJ. Mitogenic activity elaborated by macrophage-like cell lines acts as competence factor(s) for BALB/c 3T3 cells. *J. Cell. Physiol*. 110 (1982):93-100.

Wharton, W. Human macrophage-like cell line U937-1 elaborates mitogenic activity for fibroblasts. *J. Reticuloendothel. Soc*. 33 (1983):151-156.

Wood, DD, and Gaul, SL. Enhancement of the humoral response of T-cell-depleted murine spleens by a factor derived from human monocytes *in vitro*. *J. Immunol*. 113 (1974):925-933.

19
Macrophage Factors Affecting Wound Healing

Charles E. Olsen

INTRODUCTION

Wound healing requires a complex series of events involving many different cell types. Not all the cells seen in the normal course of wound healing are absolutely necessary for successful healing. Simpson and Ross (1972) showed that the neutrophil is not required for normal wound healing, even though this cell predominates in the early stages of repair. On the other hand, the macrophage is required for healing. When animals were depleted of macrophages by hydrocortisone and antimacrophage serum, wound healing was delayed (Leibovich and Ross 1975). The macrophage has been found to have so many functions that it is not difficult to imagine that it plays an important role in many stages of wound repair. This cell is a phagocytic cell capable of producing many enzymes such as collagenase (Wahl et al. 1974), elastase (Werb and Gordon 1975), and proteoglycan degrading enzymes (Laub et al. 1982) which would be useful in debridement of the wound. Macrophages also produce fibronectin which is chemotactic to fibroblasts (Tsukamoto et al. 1981). Once the fibroblasts are attracted to the wound, macrophage factors could stimulate collagen synthesis in these cells (Wahl et al. 1979; Leibovich 1978). In addition, macrophages are capable of stimulating neovascularization (Polverini et al. 1977). Because the macrophage has the potential to degrade connective tissue as well as stimulate its formation, it may be the key cell in controlling wound healing. It might be possible to influence the course of wound healing by altering the function of the macrophage. For example, Leibovich and Danon (1980) attracted macrophages to a wound site using glucan and found this simulated wound healing.

We have compared macrophages obtained from wound cylinders (Schilling et al. 1959; Hunt et al. 1967) with peritoneal exudate macrophages in the production of PGE_2 and collagenase, and found them to respond the same. In addition, we have investigated the effect of retinoids on macrophage function and found that PGE_2 and collagenase production can be inhibited.

METHODS AND MATERIALS

Preparation of Cells

Peritoneal exudate cells were obtained by injecting guinea pigs with sterile mineral oil, then harvesting by lavage with phosphate buffered saline (PBS) 4 days later. Cells were collected by centrifugation, resuspended in ammonium chloride lysing buffer to lyse the red blood cells, diluted with Dulbecco's Modified Eagle's media (DME), recentrifuged, then suspended in DME. Wound macrophages were harvested from fluid collected in stainless steel wire mesh cylinders implanted subcutaneously in guinea pigs (Hunt et al. 1967). Fluid was collected by aspirating with a needle through the skin. The cells were prepared in the same manner as the peritoneal macrophages.

Culture of Cells

Cells were added to tissue culture flasks and allowed to adhere for 4 hours. At this time, the flasks were washed twice to remove non-adherent cells and fed with DME. Any additions to the cultures were made at this time. After 24 hours at 37°C, media was poured off, centrifuged to remove any cells, and saved for assay. The cells were refed with DME without additions, unless otherwise indicated, and cultured for 24 hours. The media were again saved for assay.

PGE Assay

Media from the first 24 hour culture were assayed for PGE_2 by radioimmunoassay using rabbit anti-PGE_2 serum, goat anti-rabbit 7S-globulin, and ^{3}H-PGE. PGE_2 was used as the standard.

Collagenase Assay

Media from the second 24 hours of culture were dialyzed against distilled water, lyophilized, then dissolved in 0.3 ml of 0.2M NaCl, 50mM Tris, 5mM $CaCl_2$, pH 7.5. This material was assayed for collagenase activity by release of radioactivity from ^{14}C-acetylated collagen (Gisslow and McBride 1975) or from collagen labelled in vivo with ^{14}C-glycine. Results are expressed as cpm released with background levels subtracted. Trypsin at 100 μg/ml was used to indicate the proportion of substrate susceptible to non-specific proteases.

Materials

Endotoxin (E. coli 055:B5) was obtained from Difco Laboratories, Detroit, MI. Retinoic Acid was obtained from Roche Laboratories, Nutley, NJ. N-4-Hydroxyphenylretinamide was prepared by Dr. R. J. Gander at Johnson & Johnson Products, Inc.

RESULTS

Macrophages were isolated from the wound fluid of cylinders, and oil-induced peritoneal macrophages were cultured in vitro. The media from the first 24 hours of these cultures were assayed for PGE_2 and the media from the second 24 hours of culture were assayed for collagenase activity. The results are shown in Table 19.1. The wound macrophages behave the same as peritoneal exudate cells. Both synthesized low levels of PGE_2 and collagenase in control cultures and many-fold higher levels in endotoxin stimulated cultures.

Retinoids affect wound healing, especially in hosts compromised by steroids (Ehrlich and Hunt 1968). Since steroids exert some of their effects on macrophages, the effects of retinoic acid on macrophage PGE_2 synthesis and collagenase production were determined. Figure 19.1 shows a dose response curve. Retinoic acid inhibits both collagenase and PGE_2 synthesis, and in this case collagenase was more inhibited than PGE_2. This is not always the case. Although inhibitors of prostaglandin synthesis inhibit collagenase production (Wahl et al. 1977) this is not the mode of action of retinoic acid since PGE_2 added to the cultures does not reverse the effect of retinoic acid (Table 19.2). Hydroxyphenylretinamide, a less toxic retinoid, was also found

TABLE 19.1

Prostaglandin and Collagenase Production by Macrophages[1]

Source	Endotoxin (30 μg/ml)	PGE_2 (pg/10^6 cells)	Collagenase Activity[2] (cpm/10^6 cells)
Peritoneal exudate	-	35	1
	+	1,350	181
Wound cylinders	-	34	28
	+	959	250

[1] Peritoneal exudate macrophages (60×10^6) and wound cylinder macrophages (35×10^6) were cultured in 10 milliliters of DME as described in Materials and Methods.

[2] A total of 20,000 cpm of ^{14}C-acetylated collagen was used in the assay. The most active sample digested 64% of the collagen before the reaction was stopped.

TABLE 19.2

PGE_2 Does Not Reverse Inhibition of Collagenase Synthesis by Retinoic Acid[1]

Additions	Collagenase Activity[2] (cpm)
None	70
Endotoxin (30 μg/ml)	611
Endotoxin + Retinoic Acid (10^{-7}M)	129
Endotoxin + Retinoic Acid + PGE_2 (10^{-6}M)	144
Endotoxin + Indomethacin (10^{-6}M)	151
Endotoxin + Indomethacin + PGE_2 (10^{-6}M)	1,767

[1] 60×10^6 peritoneal exudate macrophages were cultured in 10 milliliters of DME as described in Materials and Methods.

[2] Collagenase activity was assayed using <u>in vivo</u> labelled collagen. Total radioactivity in the assay was 3,750 cpm.

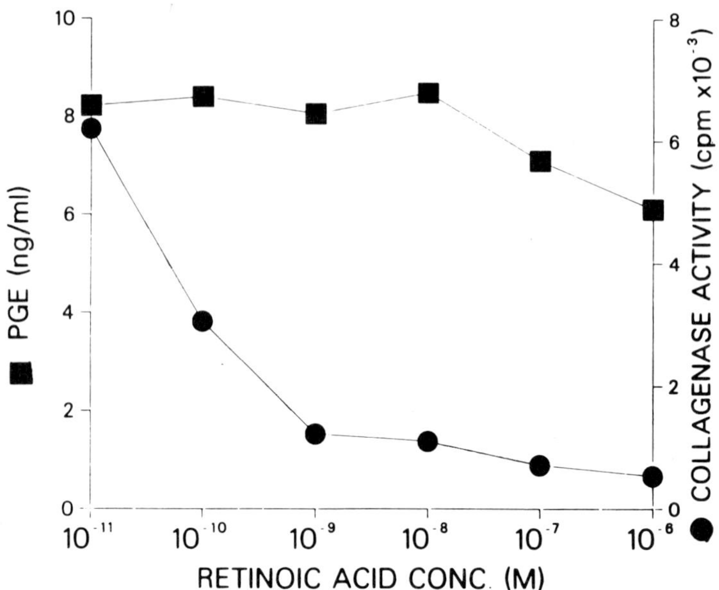

FIGURE 19.1 Retinoic acid inhibition of peritoneal exudate macrophage PGE_2 and collagenase synthesis. 50×10^6 macrophages were cultured in 10 milliliters of DME in the presence of 30 μg/ml endotoxin and various concentrations of retinoic acid. Media was changed at 24 hours and retinoic acid was also added at this time. A total of 21,000 cpm of ^{14}C-acetylated collagen was used for the collagenase assay with an incubation time of 25 hours.

to have similar effects, although it is not as potent as retinoic acid (Figure 19.2).

DISCUSSION

Macrophages differ in their activities depending on their local environment. For example, oil-induced peritoneal exudate cells are more active than resident peritoneal cells (Polverini et al. 1977). However, peritoneal exudate cells are still not fully active since they can be stimulated by a number of substances to secrete proteases such as collagenase (Wahl et al. 1974). In this respect, the wound macrophage behaves like peritoneal exudate cells. They produce little prostaglandin or collagenase unless stimulated by endotoxin. Therefore, it is

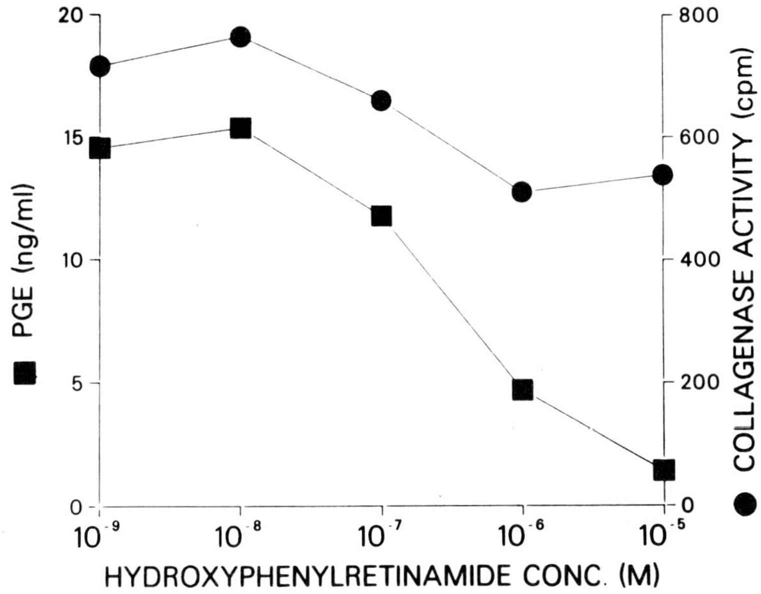

FIGURE 19.2 Hydroxyphenylretinamide inhibition of peritoneal exudate macrophage PGE_2 and collagenase synthesis. 50×10^6 macrophages were cultured in 10 milliliters of DME in the presence of 30 μg/ml endotoxin and various concentrations of hydroxyphenylretinamide. Media were changed at 24 hours and hydroxyphenylretinamide was also added at this time. A total of 23,000 cpm of ^{14}C-acetylated collagen was used for the collagenase assay with an incubation time of 24 hours.

likely that in the wound, the macrophage is not synthesizing large amounts of collagenase. Yet it can respond to stimuli such as lymphokines or endotoxin.

Retinoic acid inhibits macrophage function, namely PGE_2 and collagenase synthesis. Indomethacin blocks the production of macrophage collagenase by inhibiting prostaglandin synthesis. When PGE_2 is added to these indomethacin treated cultures, collagenase synthesis is restored (Wahl et al. 1977). The action of retinoic acid is not by that mechanism since the addition of PGE_2 does not restore collagenase synthesis. The mechanism of action is not known at this time. Hydroxyphenylretinamide also inhibits both collagenase and PGE_2 synthesis by peritoneal exudate macrophages, but it is not as potent. It is a better inhibitor of PGE_2 synthesis (Levine 1980) than retinoic acid but not as strong an inhibitor of collagenase synthesis. Brinckerhoff et al. (1982) found similar results on the synthesis of PGE_2 and collagenase by synovial fibroblasts using these two compounds. Retinoic acid enhances wound healing in both cortisone-treated (Ehrlich and Hunt 1968) and normal animals (Klein and Schmidt-Vogel 1972). It is difficult to explain how retinoic acid inhibits the macrophage, yet stimulates wound healing. However, retinoic acid stimulates other cell types such as epidermal cells (Christophers 1974) and these stimulating effects may compensate for any inhibition of the macrophage. On the other hand, it is conceivable that the collagenase secreted by macrophages may delay wound healing and that by inhibiting collagenase production retinoic acid stimulates wound healing.

REFERENCES

Brinckerhoff, CE, Nagase, H, Nagel, JE, and Harris, ED Jr. 1982. Effects of all-trans-retinoic acid (retinoic acid) and 4-hydroxyphenylretinamide on synovial cells and articular cartilage. J. Am. Acad. Dermatol. 6:591-602.

Christophers, E. 1974. Growth stimulation of cultured post-embryonic epidermal cells by vitamin A acid. J. Invest. Dermatol. 63:450-455.

Ehrlich, HP, and Hunt, TK. 1968. Effects of cortisone and vitamin A on wound healing. Ann. Surg. 167:324-328.

Gisslow, MT, and McBride, BC. 1975. A rapid sensitive collagenase assay. Anal. Biochem. 68:70-78.

Hunt, TK, Jawetz, E, Hutchinson, JGP, and Dunphy, JE. 1967. A new model for the study of wound infection. J. Trauma 7:298-306.

Klein, P, and Schmidt-Vogel, W. 1972. Experimental investigation of the relationship between wound healing and local applications of vitamin A acid. Zeit. Exp. Chir. 5/6:417-425.

Laub, R, Huybrechts-Godin, G, Peeters-Joris, C, and Vaes, G. 1982. Degradation of collagen and proteoglycan by macrophages and fibroblasts. Biochem. Biophys. Acta 721:425-433.

Leibovich, SJ. 1978. Production of macrophage-dependent fibroblast-stimulating activity (M-FSA) by murine macrophages. Exp. Cell Res. 113:47-56.

Leibovich, SJ, and Danon, D. 1980. Promotion of wound repair in mice by application of glucan. J. Reticuloendothiel. Soc. 27:1-11.

Leibovich, SJ, and Ross, R. 1975. The role of the macrophage in wound repair. A study with hydrocortisone and anti-macrophage serum. Am. J. Pathol. 78:71-98.

Levine, L. 1980. N-(4-hydroxyphenyl)retinamide: A synthetic analog of vitamin A that is a potent inhibitor of prostaglandin biosynthesis. Prostaglandins Med. 4:285-296.

Polverini, PJ, Cotran, RS, Gimbrone, MA Jr, and Unanue, ER. 1977. Activated macrophages induce vascular proliferation. Nature 269:804-806.

Schilling, JA, Joel, W, and Shurley, HM. 1959. Wound healing: A comparative study of the histochemical changes in granulation tissue contained in stainless steel wire mesh and polyvinyl sponge cylinders. Surg. 46:702-719.

Simpson, DM, and Ross, R. 1972. The neutrophilic leukocyte in wound repair. A study with antineutrophilic serum. J. Clin. Invest. 51:2009-2023.

Tsukamoto, Y, Helsel, WE, and Wahl, SM. 1981. Macrophage production of fibronectin, a chemoattractant for fibroblasts. J. Immunol. 127:673-678.

Wahl, SM, Olsen, CE, Sandberg, AL, and Mergenhagen, SE. 1977. Prostaglandin regulation of macrophage collagenase production. Proc. Natl. Acad. Sci. 74:4955-4958.

Wahl, LM, Wahl, SM, Mergenhagen, SE, and Martin, GR. 1974. Collagenase production by endotoxin-activated macrophages. Proc. Natl. Acad. Sci. 71:3598-3601.

Wahl, SM, Wahl, LM, McCarthy, JB, Chedid, L, and Mergenhagen, SE. 1979. Macrophage activation by mycobacterial water soluble compounds and synthetic muramyl dipeptide. J. Immunol. 122:2226-2231.

Werb, Z, and Gordon, S. 1975. Elastase secretion by mouse macrophages. Characterization and regulation. J. Exp. Med. 142:361-377.

20
Effects of Inflammation on Wound Healing: *In Vitro* Studies and *In Vivo* Studies

M.F. Graham, R.F. Diegelmann, W.J. Lindblad, R. Gay, S. Gay and I. Kelman Cohen

INTRODUCTION

During the past decade, the Plastic Surgery Research Laboratory at the Medical College of Virginia has been involved in a variety of studies focused on the regulation of collagen metabolism during normal[1-6] and abnormal tissue repair.[7-10] This chapter describes two studies designed to gain a better understanding of the interaction of the inflammatory process and the process of fibroplasia.

The first series of studies define an in vitro model designed to analyze fibroplasia. The basic model consists of chicken tendon biopsies cultured in an "inflammatory" environment provided by a fibrin clot. This in vitro system can be used to simultaneously analyze the influence of various factors on fibroblast proliferation, migration and collagen synthesis.

The second section of this chapter describes preliminary observations of early collagen deposition in the rat open wound model. These initial findings suggest that cells in the residual skin appendages at the margin of the wound, such as hair follicles and sebaceous glands, produce Type IV collagen as early as 12 hours post-wounding. In addition, Types IV and V collagens were observed around the cells in the clot region by 24 hours post-wounding. The possible physiological significance of these findings are discussed in this second section.

These studies were supported by NIH Grants GM-20298, DE-02570, and HL-11310.

In Vitro Studies

The phenomenon of fibroplasia consists of three major events: the proliferation and migration of fibroplastic cells and collagen synthesis by these cells. The study of fibroplasia requires the quantitation of each of these three processes. Our current understanding of the factors thought to influence these events and the interrelationships between them has been somewhat limited by the lack of suitable models. *In vivo* studies, although providing the most realistic environment, do not allow for control of the myriad factors and interactions at play. Cell culture techniques provide a controllable system for study, but place the cell in a foreign environment out of the natural tissue biomatrix in which it is programmed to perform. We have thus attempted to develop a model that would, on the one hand, permit the study of these fibroplastic cells while they remain in their native tissue matrix and at the same time have the versatility of an *in vitro* system.

Because fibroblast proliferation, migration, and collagen synthesis are proceeding synchronously, and because there is a possibility of interrelationships between these events, the model was designed to allow all three fibroplastic parameters to be quantitated synchronously. This capability would then permit the determination of the interrelationship between the three events in response to a single modulator.

This section of the chapter describes how such a model was developed and how this *in vitro* system was used in some initial studies to examine the influence of humoral and cellular inflammatory mediators on fibroplasia.

The basic design of the model was to place a tissue explant in a controllable inflammatory environment, observe and measure the migratory response of the fibroplastic cells into this *in vitro* "wound," and at the same time measure rates of proliferation and collagen synthesis. Manipulation of the inflammatory environment would then allow one to determine the factors which affect each of these events. The tissue chosen for the model was tendon. This is because it contains an exclusively homogenous population of cells (tenoblast)[11] and it was observed that given a favorable inflammatory milieu, such as a plasma clot, the migratory response of these cells was prompt and could be seen and measured within three days of culture.[5,6]

The design of the model was as follows: two mm punch biopsies of isolated chicken tendons were placed in the chambers of multi-well culture plates and embedded in 50 μl of fibrinogen which was allowed to clot (Fig. 20.1). The preparations were then incubated at 37°C in 1 ml of Dulbecco's Modified Eagle Medium (DMEM) containing fresh ascorbate (0.1 mM) and 10% fetal calf serum.

Fibroblasts were observed migrating out of the plug into the plasma clot after 48 hours of culture (Fig. 20.2). After five days incubation, the tendon fibroblasts had migrated several millimeters from the edge of the tendon biopsy (Fig. 20.3). Fibroblast migration was quantitated by projecting the radiating fan of fibroblasts onto a screen and measuring this area of migration with an automatic planimeter (Fig. 20.4).

Tendon fibroblast proliferation was quantitated by the incorporation of [^{125}]iododeoxyuridine (^{125}IUDR, 2,000 Ci/mmol), into DNA. Cultures were incubated for various times with 1 μCi/ml of ^{125}IUDR.[12] Control specimens were pre-incubated with 25 mM hydroxyurea, a specific inhibitor of DNA synthesis.[13] There was a linear rate of ^{125}IUDR incorporation from 10 to 17 hours of isotope incubation and therefore in all subsequent experiments, the preparations were incubated with isotope for 12 hours. Control specimens incubated in the presence of hydroxyurea showed less than 10% of the level of radioactivity incorporated into the test specimens. Determination of fibroblast proliferation was then measured on days three, five, and seven of culture and shown to be maximal by the fifth day.[6] Therefore, in all subsequent experiments, comparisons were made on the fifth day of exposure to various modulators.

Collagen synthesis by these tendon fibroblasts was quantitated by determining the susceptibility of newly synthesized protein to purified bacterial collagenase.[14] On days five and seven of incubation, tendon explants embedded in plasma or fibrin clots were incubated with serum-free DMEM containing fresh ascorbate (0.1 mM) and 10 μCi of ^{3}H-proline (43 Ci/mmol). After four hours, the incubation was stopped by rapid freezing, the explants and medium were removed, the tissue was homogenized, and the radioactive protein was precipitated in the cold with trichloroacetic acid (TCA) (5%) prior to digestion with a highly specific bacterial collagenase as previously described.[1,14] After digestion of the collagen, the noncollagenous protein was re-precipitated with 5% TCA-0.25% tannic acid. Supernatants containing collagen-derived peptides and pellets containing the noncollagenous protein were then counted separately for radioactivity. Radioactivity released by collagenase is represented by the value in the numerator and the percent collagen synthesized as a function of total protein synthesized is calculated according to the following formula:

IN VITRO FIBROPLASIA MODEL

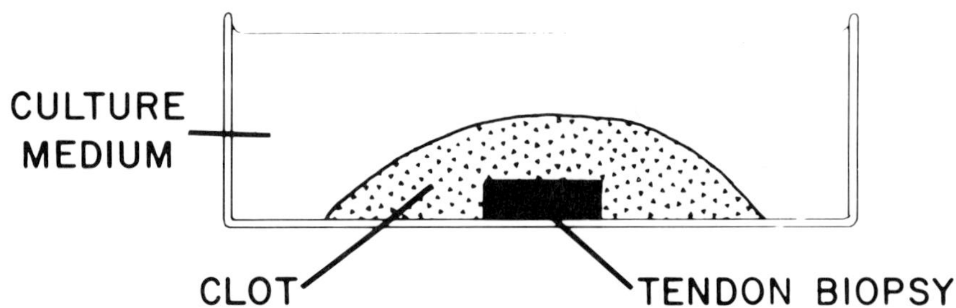

FIGURE 20.1 (above) Tendon explants were prepared from the chicken flexor digitorum profundus tendon using a 2 mm dermal trephine and placed in multiwell culture plates (Costar No. 3524, Cambridge, MA). The tendon biopsies were covered with 50 μl of fibrinogen which was allowed to clot before 1 ml of tissue culture medium was added.

FIGURE 20.2 (below) Phase contrast photomicrograph of tendon fibroblasts migrating out of the tendon biopsy at 48 hours (200X).

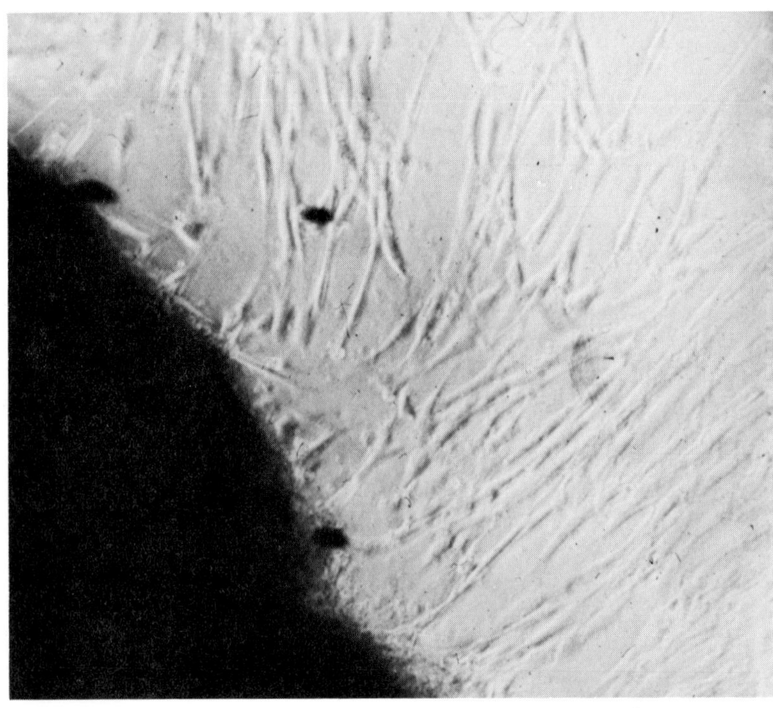

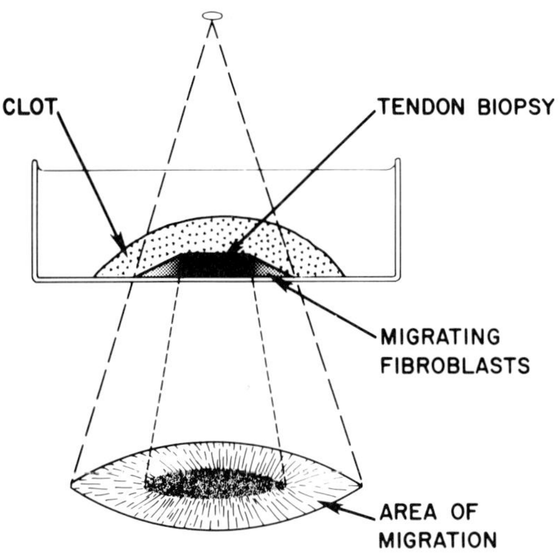

FIGURE 20.4 (above) Diagram of the technique used to quantitate tendon fibroblast migration. The profile of the tendon explant and rim of migrating tendon fibroblasts are projected onto a piece of paper. The area of migration is quantitated using an area subtraction technique on a Zeiss MOPP III automatic planimeter. Reprinted with permission, J. Orthoped. Res.[6]

FIGURE 20.3 (below) Photomicrograph made in the sagittal plane at the junction of the edge of the tendon explant (lower right) and fibrin clot after 5 days in culture (64X). Reprinted with permission, J. Orthoped. Res.[6]

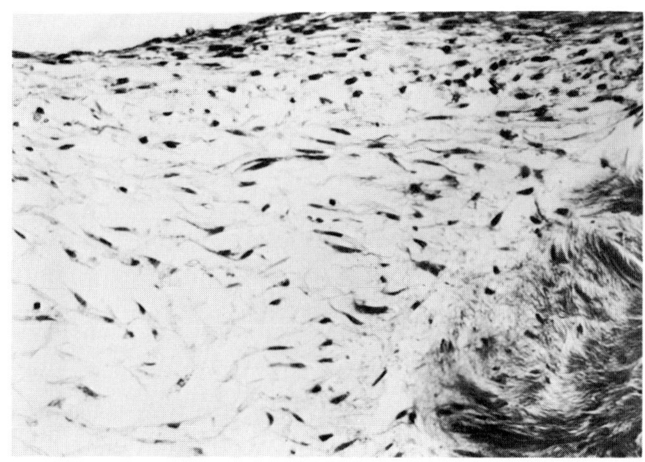

$$\% \text{ Collagen} = \frac{\text{cpm in collagen}}{[\text{cpm in non-collagen protein} \times 5.4] + \text{cpm in collagen}} \times 100$$

The factor of 5.4 represents the enriched content of proline and hydroxyproline in collagen versus proline in noncollagen protein.[15] Analysis of the radioactive proteins synthesized by the tendon explants in culture indicated that approximately 6.5% of the total protein produced was represented by collagen (Table 20.1).

Once it had been demonstrated that this model could indeed quantitate in reproducible fashion, tenoblast migration, proliferation, and collagen synthesis studies were then performed to determine which inflammatory factors could modulate these processes and if these processes were interrelated or independ-

TABLE 20.1

Collagen Synthesis by Tendon Explants in the In Vitro Fibroplasia Model

	cpm in Assay		
Experiment	Collagen	Non-Collagen Protein	Relative Collagen Synthesis (%)[a]
1	1977	5237	6.5
2	1252	3171	6.9
	1185	4507	4.7
3 (n=6)	1117 ± 307	3050 ± 889	6.7 ± 0.8
Mean of 9 observations			6.5 ± 0.5

Analysis of collagen synthesis was made after two weeks in culture in experiment 1,[5] and after five days in experiments 2 and 3. The tendon explant cultures were embedded in a plasma clot in experiments 1 and 3 and in a fibrin clot in experiment 2. All were incubated with DMEM containing 10% fetal calf serum. Where indicated, values represent ± S.E.M.

[a] The value for relative collagen synthesis is derived from a calculation to correct for the enriched imino acid content found in collagen compared to noncollagen protein.[15]

ent. The first experiment was designed to examine the influence of the plasma clot and its cellular elements.[6] With a control clot consisting of agarose gel alone, there was no tendon fibroblast migration and only a modest rate of proliferation was observed (63% of maximum). Addition of cells from the plasma to the agarose did not induce migration or stimulate proliferation (58% of maximum). When the agarose gel was substituted by a plasma clot, migration was observed (3.5 mm^2) and proliferation was maximal (125×10^3 cpm per explant).

Reconstitution of the plasma clot with its cellular elements further stimulated migration (6.8 mm^2), but had no additional effect on proliferation (103×10^3 cpm per explant). These findings demonstrated that the plasma clot was absolutely necessary for migration and stimulated proliferation.[6] It was interesting to note that the cellular elements could stimulate migration without a concomitant effect on proliferation, thus suggesting the independence of these two events.

The next study was performed to determine which humoral constituents of the plasma clot were responsible for these observations. In this study components of clot were added back individually to an agarose base.[6] The addition of serum or thrombin did not induce migration and had no significant effect on proliferation (84% and 68%, respectively of maximum). If fibrinogen was added, however, migration proceeded (3.7 mm^2), but without a significant effect on proliferation (97% of maximal). The addition of whole plasma to the agarose base, likewise, induced migration (2.1 mm^2) without an effect on proliferation (80% of maximum). Plasma clot alone showed the greatest effect on migration (5.1 mm^2) and tendon fibroblast proliferation (140×10^3 cpm per explant).

Having established that fibrin was the only constituent of the clot that was absolutely necessary for tendon fibroblast migration out of the tissue explant and into the simulated "wound" environment, all subsequent experiments were performed using a reconstituted fibrin clot. To achieve this, fibrinogen (KABI, Grade L) was prepared in DMEM to give a final concentration of 3 mg/ml.

Having optimized the conditions to observe and measure the potentiation of the system, the next experiments were then designed to examine the interrelationships of the three fibroplastic events in response to various modulators. When the tendon explants were incubated in the presence of various concentrations of fetal calf serum, it became apparent that the three parameters of fibroplasia responded independently (Table 20.2). Low concentrations of fetal calf serum (0.1 to 0.5%)

TABLE 20.2

Independent Effects of Fetal Calf Serum on Tendon Fibroblast Migration, Proliferation and Collagen Synthesis

Fetal Calf Serum (%)	Proliferation, ^{125}IUDR (cpm × 10^3/explant)	Migration (mm^2)	Relative Collagen Synthesis (%)
0.1	6.1	0.7	20.0
0.5	4.7	0.9	19.0
2.0	9.9	4.0	6.5
10.0	60.6	9.9	5.8

(n=6)

favored production of collagen relative to total protein synthesis but were suboptimal for tendon fibroblast proliferation and migration. In contrast, 10% fetal calf serum was highly stimulatory for proliferation and migration at the expense of differential collagen synthesis (Table 20.2).

In other experiments, it was observed that if the fetal calf serum was heat-treated (56°C for 15 minutes) and dialyzed, it could still stimulate fibroblast proliferation in a dose-response fashion, but no fibroblast migration was observed.

Platelet-poor plasma (PPP) and platelet extract were prepared from human blood by a procedure described by Pledger et al.[16] Incubation of the tendon explants in 2% PPP provided a quiescent but stimulatable system.[6] Under these static conditions, platelet lysate was then titrated into the culture medium and the effect on migration and proliferation was analyzed. A linear dose response curve for fibroblast proliferation was observed from 1 to 5 μg/ml of platelet lysate. There was no further significant increase in proliferation up to a concentration of 100 μg/ml. In contrast, in a background, quiescent environment of 2% PPP, platelet lysate was without effect on fibroblast migration at concentrations between 5 and 50 μg/ml. Only at a concentration of 100 μg/ml did the platelet lysate stimulate migration (45% of maximal obtained with 10% fetal calf serum). Studies of the effect of these mediators on collagen synthesis have not yet been performed.

We present here a model for the study of fibroplasia that will enable investigators to gain a better understanding of the many factors responsible for the fibrotic response to inflammation. The model is dynamic, reproducible, and responsive. With the use of this model we have shown that: 1) proliferation and migration are two discrete events with independent responses to modulating factors; 2) these events may occur at the expense of the specialized production of collagen; 3) fibrin appears to be essential for the migration of fibroplastic cells out of the tendon biomatrix and into the area of "inflammation"; 4) whole fetal calf serum contains a heat-sensitive or possibly dialyzable factor required for fibroblast migration; and 5) platelet lysate appears to have disparate and concentration-dependent effects on fibroblast proliferation and migration.

Based upon these observations, we have developed a working model for the interrelationship between inflammatory factors and the response of fibroblastic cells (Fig. 20.5). The mode (proliferation versus migration versus collagen synthesis) and the degree of response are both dependent upon the nature and concentration of the factor, and a reciprocal relationship between the three cellular events. This *in vitro* model now provides a means of more clearly defining the various regulatory influences involved in wound healing.

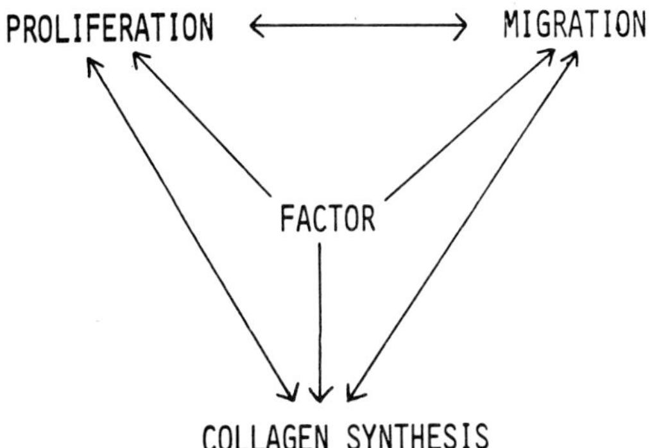

FIGURE 20.5 Interrelationship of inflammatory factors and the response of fibroblastic cells.

In Vivo Studies

Prior studies have demonstrated enhanced levels of collagen biosynthesis in dermal wound healing, as early as 24 hours post-injury.[3] These studies using an open wound model in the rat indicated that this early synthetic activity was localized to the granulating wound center, particularly in the panniculus carnosis.[3] These experiments were performed employing an in vitro labeling period which requires placing the tissue into an environment dissimilar from the in vivo state.[1] This makes it difficult to relate this synthetic rate to the in vivo situation. In addition to this problem, this approach could only localize the site of collagen biosynthesis in a gross manner and could not identify the cells contributing to the elevated rates of collagen synthesis.

The study presented here was designed to localize the early biosynthetic activity to specific locations within the wound area and to identify the cell type(s) involved with this synthesis. An immunohistochemical approach was taken in an attempt to obviate the necessity for in vitro labeling and therefore obtain information on in vivo deposition.

The open wound model was again used in which a 3 mm punch wound was inflicted on the dorsal side of male Wistar rats (∿200 g). At various times post-wounding, the wound area was excised using an 8 mm trephine (Fig. 20.6). The tissue was immediately divided in half, embedded in Ames™ O.C.T. compound and 8 micron sections were prepared from the blocks and placed on ovalbumin-coated slides. The sections were processed for light microscopy with hematoxylin-eosin (H&E) and for immunochemical staining using antibodies specifically directed against collagen Types I, III, IV, and V.[17-19] An immunofluorescent procedure was employed using monospecific rabbit anti-collagen primary antibodies followed by goat anti-rabbit IgG conjugated with fluorescein. Several tissue samples were prepared by paraffin embedding followed by standard sectioning and staining with H&E. This method produces much clearer definition of cell morphology.

The orientation of the tissue sections is demonstrated in Figure 20.7. This H&E section shows tissue removed at 24 hours post-injury and demonstrates the clot containing degenerated erythrocytes and inflammatory cells (Fig. 20.7). These inflammatory cells are principally polymorphonuclear cells, although some monocytic cells are apparent. The cell population at this time represents cells trapped in the clot at the time of

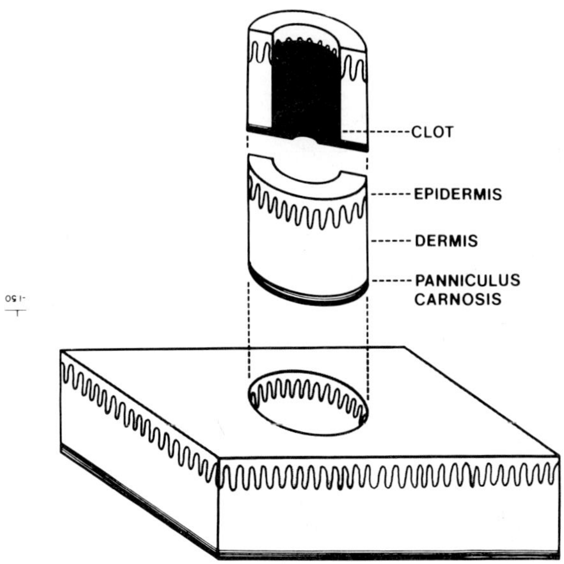

FIGURE 20.6 Schematic representation of the removal of wound tissue for immunohistochemical analysis. The inner cylinder represents a 3 mm core which provides the standard injury.

hemostasis and it does not appear to contain fibroblasts or epithelial cells.

Staining for collagen Type IV deposition at 12 hours post-wounding revealed extensive staining of various structures in the wound margin (Fig. 20.8). At this time, the clot was devoid of fluorescence; however, the cells of the skin appendages (hair follicles and sebaceous glands) within a few millimeters of the wound margin were associated with intense staining of proliferating epithelial cells and possibly endothelial cells. By 18-24 hours post-injury, fluorescent staining was observed for collagen Type IV in the base of the clot (Fig. 20.9). The staining was found intracellularly in certain mononuclear cells and was also localized to the immediate vicinity of the cells. Somewhat fainter, but with true positive staining, was the staining of the clot for collagen Type V at 24 hours following injury (Fig. 20.10). The deposition of collagen Type III was discerned at 24 hours post-wounding in the wound margin immediately adjacent to the clot (Fig. 20.11). This staining

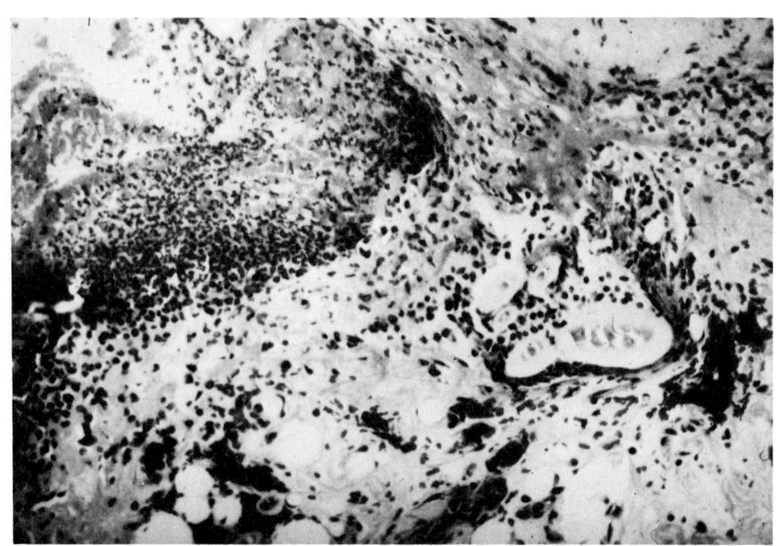

FIGURE 20.7 H&E stained section of a paraffin embedded tissue removed 24 hours post-wounding (40X). A residual hair follicle can be seen on the right and the base of the clot is on the upper left.

FIGURE 20.8 Anti-Type IV collagen staining of dermis adjacent to the wound at 12 hours post-wounding. There was extensive staining of epidermal cells in the skin appendages (160X).

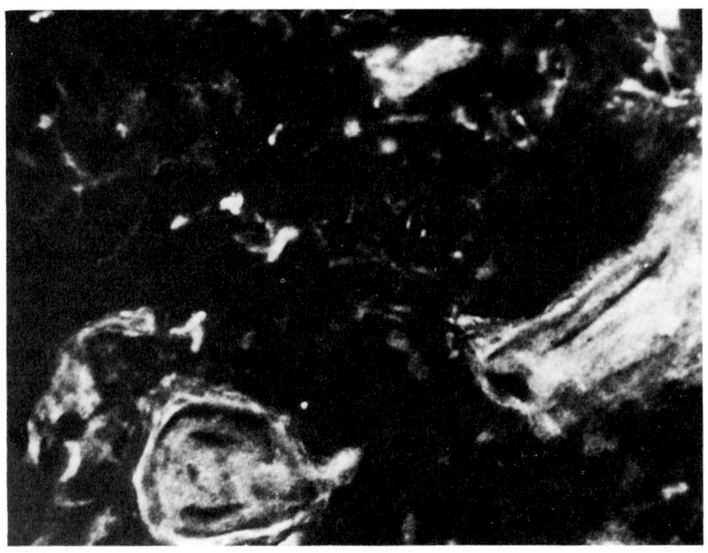

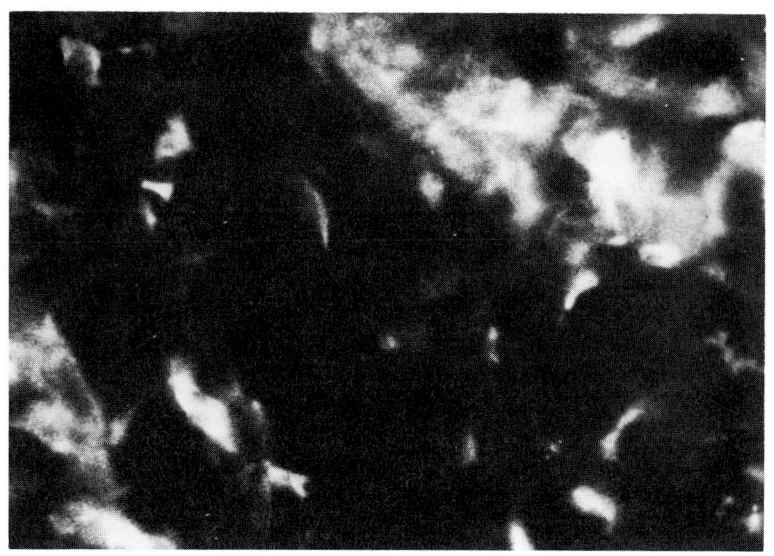

FIGURE 20.9 Anti-Type IV collagen staining of the clot at 24 hours postwounding. The outline of cell nuclei can be discerned of cells which are staining positive (160X).

FIGURE 20.10 Anti-Type V collagen staining in the clot at 24 hours post-injury. This staining was quite faint compared to the response for Type IV collagen (160X).

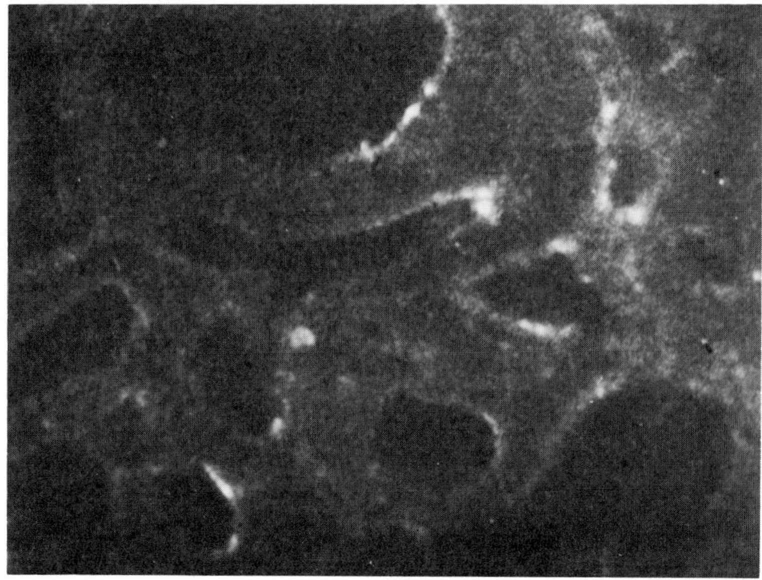

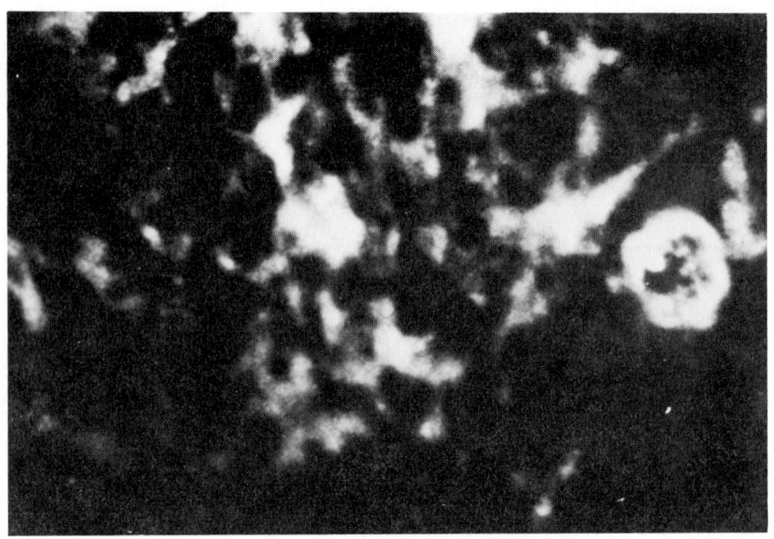

FIGURE 20.11 Anti-Type III collagen staining of the clot/dermis junction at 24 hours post-injury. The intensity of the staining of the dermis (bottom of photo) appeared to diminish in a gradient manner (160X).

FIGURE 20.12 Anti-Type IV collagen staining within the clot at 60 hours post-wounding was quite extensive. At this time, the intensity of positive staining in the dermis was declining (160X).

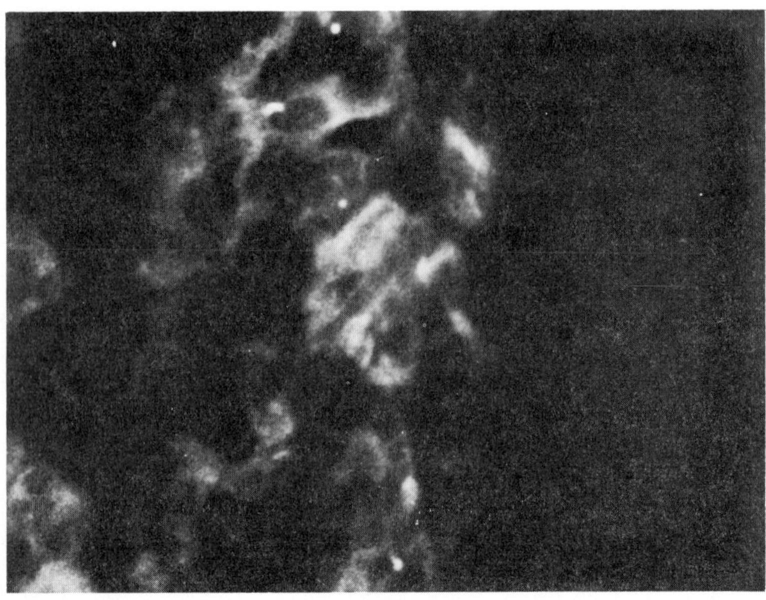

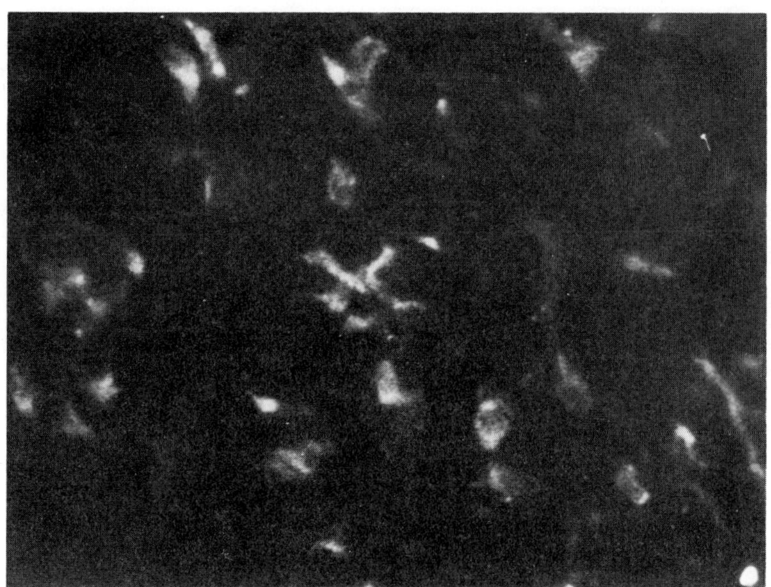

FIGURE 20.13 Anti-Type V collagen staining in the clot following 60 hours can clearly discern cells which are positive in addition to the pericellular matrix (160X).

FIGURE 20.14 Anti-Type III collagen staining at 60 hours post-injury was very extensive throughout the clot. At this time Type I collagen was also localized throughout the clot (64X).

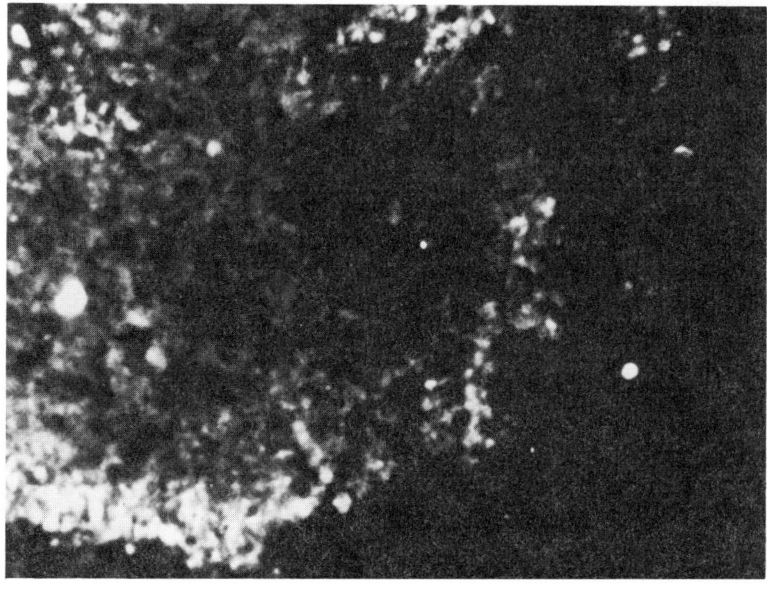

TABLE 20.3

Identification of Collagen Types in Dermal Granulation Tissue by Immunohistochemical Staining

Time Post-Wounding (hr)	Intensity of Staining for Collagen Type			
	I	III	IV	V
0	-	-	-	-
12	-	-	(3+)/-[a]	-
18	-	-	1+	1+
24	(+)	1+	2+	1+
36	1+	1+	1+	
48	2+	3+	1+	
60	2+ - 3+	1+	1+	1+
72	2+ - 3+	1+	1+	

[a] At 12 hours 3+ staining for collagen Type IV was observed only around cells in residual skin appendages. The clot and other wound areas were negative for Type IV at 12 hours. (+), weak; 1+, moderate; 2+, marked; and 3+, very marked staining intensity.

diminished in intensity in sections taken further into the dermis. At this time no collagen Type III was detectable within the clot.

Following 60 hours of tissue repair, the clot was extensively infiltrated with Type IV collagen (Fig. 20.12). This collagen was distributed throughout the clot and initial organization of this collagen was observed. By this time, Type V collagen was readily detected within the clot (Fig. 20.13). Cell nuclei were clearly discernible and a network of collagen Type III was localized throughout the clot in a very intense staining profile (Fig. 20.14). The deposition of Type I collagen, which was initially found at 36 hours was also uniformly distributed in the clot at this time.

Examination of serial sections of these immunofluorescent sections with H&E staining revealed a cell population at 60 hours post-injury consisting mainly of inflammatory cells. Examination of the wound area for epithelial cells showed a marked proliferation of cells in the skin appendages at this time, but there was no visible migration of these cells into the clot environment.

Therefore, the cells within the clot were most likely inflammatory cells trapped at the time of hemostasis.

The total series of time points examined is summarized for all the collagen Types in Table 20.3. The principal collagen Type found early in wound healing was Type IV which was initially localized to skin appendages, specifically to sites of proliferating epithelium. At this time the dermal stroma and clot were negative. Subsequent to 18 hours, deposition of Type IV and Type V collagen in the clot was detected. By 48 hours post-injury, the Type IV collagen staining intensity in the dermis at the wound margin was starting to lose intensity, although the clot was still highly fluorescent.

Type IV collagen staining was initially found in the dermal-wound margin at 24 hours post-wounding, with subsequent infiltration of the clot with this collagen Type. Type I collagen was the final collagen detected with the initial appearance in the dermis at 24-36 hours post-injury. This was followed by a significant deposition of Type I collagen as previously demonstrated by biochemical analysis.[4]

A working hypothesis has been formulated to facilitate further studies in this model system. It is reasonable to postulate that the initial association of Type IV and Type V collagens around certain mononuclear cells in the blood clot provides a primative organization matrix which allows for latter cell attachment and migration into the clot. In addition, degradation of the collagen may then produce chemotactic fragments which would draw other connective tissue cells into the wound leading to subsequent wound healing events.

ACKNOWLEDGMENTS

The authors wish to thank Mrs. Rae Spivey for excellent secretarial assistance in preparing this chapter.

NOTES

1. Diegelmann, RF, Rothkopf, LC, and Cohen, IK. Measurement of collagen synthesis during wound healing. J. Surg. Res. 19:239-243, 1975.

2. Cohen, IK, Diegelmann, RF, and Johnson, ML. Effect of corticosteroids on collagen synthesis. Surgery 82:15-20, 1977.

3. Cohen, IK, Moore, CD, and Diegelmann, RF. Onset and localization of collagen synthesis during wound healing in open rat skin wounds. Proc. Soc. Exp. Biol. Med. 160:458-462, 1979.

4. Clore, JN, Cohen, IK, and Diegelmann, RF. Quantitation of collagen Types I and III during wound healing in rat skin. Proc. Soc. Exp. Biol. Med. 161:337-340, 1979.

5. Becker, H, Graham, M, Cohen, IK, and Diegelmann, RF. Intrinsic tendon cell proliferation in tissue culture. J. Hand Surg. 6:616-619, 1981.

6. Graham, MF, Becker, H, Cohen, IK, Merritt, W, and Diegelmann, RF. Intrinsic tendon fibroplasia: Documentation by in vitro studies. J. Orthoped. Res., 1984. (In press)

7. Diegelmann, RF, Bryant, CP, and Cohen, IK. Tissue alpha globulins in keloid formation. Plast. Reconstr. Surg. 59:418-423, 1977.

8. Diegelmann, RF, McCoy, BJ, and Cohen, IK. Growth kinetics and collagen synthesis by keloid fibroblasts in vitro. J. Cell. Physiol. 98:341-346, 1979.

9. Clore, JN, Cohen, IK, and Diegelmann, RF. Distribution of Type III collagen in keloid biopsies and fibroblasts in culture. Biochem. Biophys. Acta 586:384-390, 1979.

10. Diegelmann, RF, Cohen, IK, and Kaplan, AM. Effect of macrophages on fibroblast DNA synthesis, proliferation and collagen synthesis. Proc. Soc. Biol. Med. 169:445-451, 1982.

11. Lindsay, WK, and Thomson, HG. Digital flexor tendons: Experimental study. (Part 1). Br. J. Plast. Surg. 12:289-316, 1960.

12. Cohen, AM, Burdick, JE, and Ketcham, AS. Cell-mediated cytotoxicity: An assay using ^{125}I-iododeoxyuridine-labeled target cells. J. Immunol. 107:895-898, 1971.

13. Pfeiffer, SE, and Tolmach, LJ. Inhibition of DNA synthesis in HeLa cells by hydroxyurea. Cancer Res. 27:124-129, 1967.

14. Peterkofsky, B, and Diegelmann, RF. The use of a mixture of proteinase-free collagenase for the specific assay of radioactive collagen in the presence of other proteins. Biochemistry 10:988-994, 1971.

15. Diegelmann, RF, and Peterkofsky, B. Collagen biosynthesis during connective tissue development in chick embryo. Dev. Biol. 28:443-453, 1972.

16. Pledger, WJ, Stiles, CD, Antoniades, HN, and Scher, CD. Induction of DNA synthesis in BALB/c 3T3 cells by serum components: Re-evaluation of the commitment process. Proc. Natl. Acad. Sci. USA 74:4481-4485, 1977.

17. Gay, S, Kresina, TF, Gay, R, Miller, EJ, and Montes, F. Immunohistochemical demonstration of basement membrane collagen in normal human skin and in psoriasis. J. Cutaneous Pathol. 6:91-95, 1979.

18. Timpl, R, Wick, G, and Gay, S. Antibodies to distinct types of collagens and procollagens and their application in immunohistology. J. Immunol. Methods 18:165-182, 1977.

19. Gay, R, Buckingham, RB, Prince, RK, Gay, S, Rodman, GP, and Miller, EJ. Collagen types synthesized in dermal fibroblast cultures from patients with early progressive systemic sclerosis. Arth. Rheumatol. 23:190-196, 1980.

21
The Role of Platelets in Wound Healing: Demonstration of Angiogenic Activity

Dov Michaeli, Thomas K. Hunt and David R. Knighton

INTRODUCTION

The process of wound repair comprises a sequence of interrelated biochemical and cellular events. The first phase involves the formation of a hemostatic plug, followed within hours by the migration of neutrophils into the traumatic space. These inflammatory cells are replaced within three to four days by macrophages, which remain in the central dead space until repair is complete. Concomitant with the process of debridement by the inflammatory cells, the process of fibroplasia is initiated. Resting fibroblasts at the wound edge begin to proliferate and migrate into the periphery of the wound space. These cells secrete collagen and proteoglycans to make the new connective tissue that eventually organizes into a scar. To sustain this increased proliferative and synthetic activity, capillary and venular endothelial cells at the wound edge migrate, proliferate and form new capillary loops.[1]

This highly ordered, interrelated sequence of events suggests a high degree of regulation. Indeed, several powerful regulatory macromolecules that are important in initiation of the repair process have been identified.

Injured cells release "tissue factor" (thromboplastin, factor III), a phospholipoprotein. This factor forms a complex with factor VII, resulting in acceleration of the coagulation cascade.[2]

This work was supported in part by a grant from Collagen Corp.

In addition, fibers at the wound surface cause activation of Hageman factor (factor XII), which in turn initiates the intrinsic coagulation system and the formation of a fibrin clot.

Fibrin and fibrin-split products have been shown to be chemotactic for leukocytes in vitro and to cause platelet-release reaction and aggregation.[3] Platelets have also been shown to participate in clot retraction,[4] thereby approximating the sides of a wound.

One of the most powerful regulatory macromolecules in wound healing is platelet-derived growth factor (PDGF). This protein has been shown to be chemotactic and mitogenic for fibroblasts and smooth muscle cells in vitro.[5] In addition, there is evidence for PDGF chemotactic activity for monocytes and neutrophils.[6]

Knighton et al.[7], have shown that thrombin-activated platelets have angiogenic activity, as demonstrated by corneal neovascularization following their injection into rabbit corneas. This paper reports some preliminary investigations on platelet angiogenic activity and its possible role in the repair process.

MATERIALS AND METHODS

Fractionation of Platelet-Rich Plasma

The procedure for preparation of defibrinogenated, platelet-poor plasma (plasma serum) is largely based on the one described by Raines and Ross.[8] Outdated units of platelet-rich plasma were treated either with thrombin (1 U/ml), or were freeze-thawed three times, pooled, heat-defibrinogenated at 55°C for 10 min, and allowed to stand overnight at 4°C. Following centrifugation at 30,000 × g for 30 min at 4°C, the pellet was washed, first with 0.01 M Tris and 0.39 M NaCl, pH 7.4, and then with 0.01 M Tris and 1.09 M NaCl, pH 7.4. All the supernatants (plasma serum and the pellet washings) were pooled, and the pH was adjusted to 7.4 with 1.0 M Tris base.

CM-Sephadex™ Chromatography

Chromatography on CM-Sephadex™ was a modification of the procedure described by Raines and Ross.[8] Elution with 0.01 M Tris and 0.09 M NaCl, pH 7.4, yielded fraction I, a large and broad peak. Elution with 0.01 M Tris and 0.19 M NaCl, ph 7.4, yielded fraction II. Fractions III and IV were obtained by elution with a gradient of 0.01 M Tris and 0.14-1.0 M NaCl, pH 7.4 (see Figure 21.1).

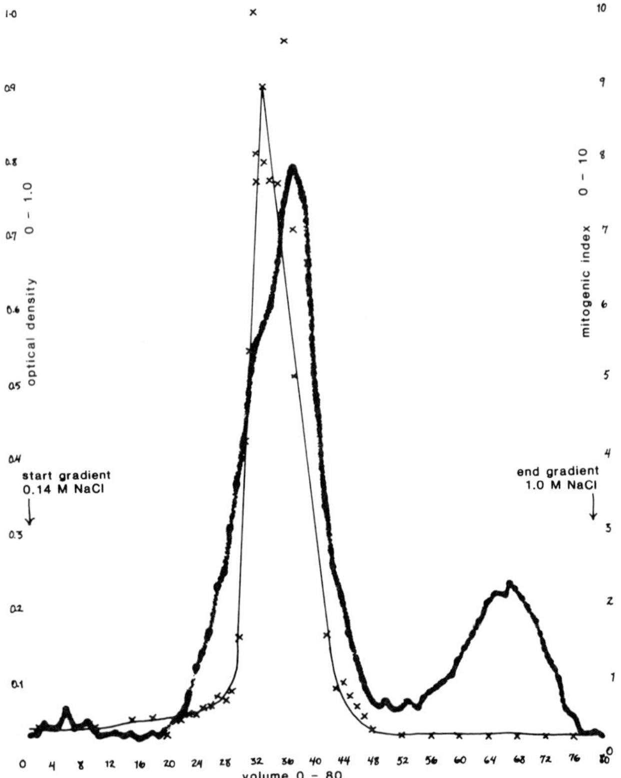

FIGURE 21.1 CM-Sephadex chromatography of plasma serum. Fractions III and IV were eluted with a salt gradient of 0.14-1.0 M NaCl. Peaks I and II were eluted with 0.09 M NaCl and 0.19 M NaCl, respectively (not shown).

Dialysis

Production of plasma serum was done as described above, except that the pellet was not washed further after centrifugation. Plasma serum, 100 ml, was placed in a standard M_r 14,000-limit dialysis bag and dialyzed against three changes (24 hr each) of 1000 ml deionized water at 4°C. The three-liter dialysate and 100-ml retentate fractions were lyophilized.

Corneal Implant Assay

This was carried out as described by Gimbrone et al.[9] Equal volumes of the fraction to be assayed and of Hydron were mixed and 20-μl aliquots of the mixture placed on a polypropylene sheet for drying and polymerization under reduced pressure.[10] The pellet was then implanted in rabbit corneas, 2 mm proximal to the superior limbus. Eyes were evaluated on the third through fourteenth days after implantation. Angiogenic response was scored blindly on a scale of 0-4+. A negative or normal eye was rated zero and a maximum response was 4+. Eyes that were positive for angiogenesis were removed, fixed and processed for histologic examination.

Ivalon™ Sponge Implantation

Ivalon (polyvinylchloride) sponge discs were prepared from a stock sheet 5-mm thick using a cork punch 7 mm in internal diameter. The discs were washed extensively in deionized water to remove residual formaldehyde used in their manufacture and were then sterilized by autoclaving in deionized water. Before implantation the sponges were squeezed dry and injected with 100 μl of the test materials.

Test materials were prepared by mixing 1.0 ml of pepsin-treated, bovine skin collagen (Zyderm®, Collagen Corp.) 8.5 mg/ml in phosphate-buffered saline, pH 7.2, with the platelet fraction. Group A had collagen, plus 10^9 outdated, A-positive, human platelets. Group B had plasma serum (A_{280} = 1.040). Group C was plasma-serum dialysate (A_{280} = 1.540). Group D was plasma-serum retentate (A_{280} = 1.150). The sponges were implanted subcutaneously in 200-gm Sprague-Dawley rats. Each rat received 12 sponge implants, arranged as in Figure 21.2.

Each of the above materials was tested with four sponges per animal, in three locations on the long axis (cephalad, middle and caudad), and each location was repeated on three animals. Thus, each material was tested in a total of 36 sponges. Sponges were collected at five days after implantation. One sponge of each test material and its surrounding capsule was used for histologic examination with H&E staining. The other sponges were stripped of surrounding tissue, cut in half, and dispersed for chemical assays. Each assay was conducted on one-half of a sponge.

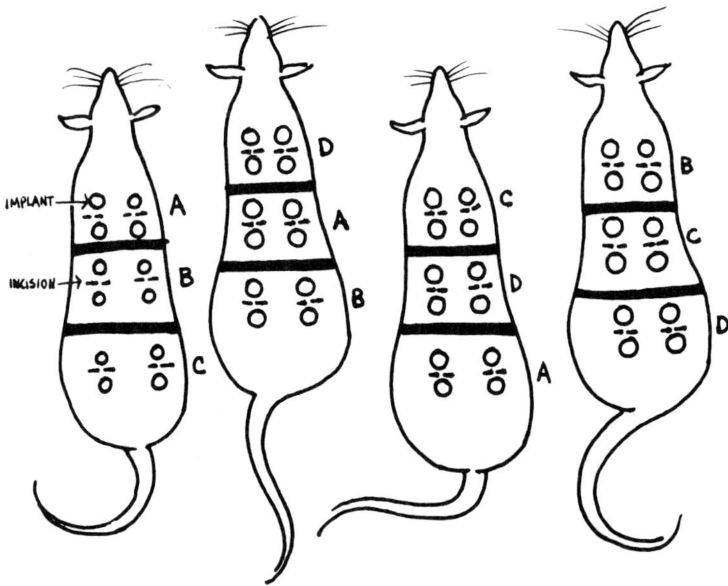

FIGURE 21.2 Design of Ivalon™ sponge implant experiment. Each rat received a total of 12 implants, four-sponge sets of three of the four test materials per rat. The sponges were implanted subcutaneously bilaterally on the dorsolateral aspects of the back. Each experiment consisted of three groups of four rats each. Thus, each test substance was tested in four sponges per animal, at three locations on the long axis of the body, and each repeated three times, for a total of 36 sponges for each test material.

^{3}H-Thymidine Uptake

This was done as described by Gospodarowicz,[11] using confluent, serum-starved, rabbit skin fibroblasts. Cells (10^5 per well) were grown for five days in 24-well plates (Costar®), in 1 ml Dulbecco's modified Eagle's medium (DMEM), supplemented with 2% heat-inactivated, bovine calf serum. On day 6 the medium was replaced with 50-100 µl of test material diluted to 1 ml in the same medium. On day 7, 0.5 µCi of ^{3}H-thymidine (specific activity 11 Ci/mM) was added to each well. After an additional 24 hr the cells were washed twice with saline, lysed, and the radioactivity determined by liquid scintillation counting. Data are expressed as a mitogenic index obtained by ^{3}H-thymidine uptake in the experimental material divided by that of the control.

Chemotaxis Assay

This was done as previously described.[12,13] Solutions to be tested were diluted from 1:10 to 1:10,000, to a final volume of 300 μl, in DMEM medium, and placed in the bottom of Boyden blind-well chambers. Gelatin-coated, 5 μm-pore diameter, polycarbonate filters (Nucleopore®) were placed over the test solution, and 2.5×10^5, low-passage (<10), fetal rabbit skin explant fibroblasts, suspended in DMEM, were added to the top compartment. Chambers were incubated for 4.5 hr at 37°C. At the end of the incubation, the tops of the filters were wiped clean. The filters were fixed, stained and evaluated by counting the number of cells that had migrated to the bottom side of the filter.

RESULTS

CM-Sephadex Chromatography

Plasma serum was chromatographed on CM-Sephadex and eluted with 0.01 M Tris and 0.09 M NaCl (fraction I), 0.01 M Tris and 0.14 M NaCl (fraction II), and 0.01 M Tris and a gradient of 0.14-1.0 M NaCl (fractions III and IV). Fractions I, II and IV were devoid of significant angiogenic activity. Fraction III displayed a strong mitogenic activity, as well as angiogenic activity (see Table 21.1). It should be noted that although the starting material (plasma serum) induced angiogenesis in the rabbit cornea, this reaction was accompanied by intense inflammatory cell infiltration. This causes an uncertainty whether the angiogenic effect was direct or whether it was indirect, via the inflammatory cells.

Figure 21.3 shows the histology of rabbit corneas implanted with Hydron containing CM-Sephadex fraction III. Figure 21.3a shows the growth of the vessels from the limbus toward the Hydron implantation site. Figure 21.3b demonstrates the lack of any significant inflammatory infiltration around the neovascular growth, suggesting a direct effect of the implanted material on the angiogenic process.

Dialysis

In a separate experiment, plasma serum, as well as its retentate and dialysate fractions, was assayed for mitogenic,

TABLE 21.1

Mitogenic and Angiogenic Activity of CM-Sephadex Fractions

Fraction	Mitogenesis μg Protein Added	Mitogenesis Index[1]	Angiogenesis[2]
Plasma serum	257.8	4.5	2[3]
CM-Sephadex I	169.9	3.1	—
CM-Sephadex II	69.0	1.5	—
CM-Sephadex III	20.5	10.0	2
CM-Sephadex IV	52.4	1.9	—

1 ^{3}H-thymidine uptake (experimental ÷ control).
2 Scale 0-4.
3 Accompanied by intense inflammatory response.

TABLE 21.2

Mitogenic, Chemotactic and Angiogenic Activity of Dialysis Fractions of Plasma Serum

Fraction	Mitogenic Index[1]	Chemotaxis[2]	Angiogenesis[3]
Plasma serum	4.5	15	2[4]
Retentate	1.0	34	2-3
Dialysate	2.9	3	2-3

1 ^{3}H-thymidine incorporation (experimental ÷ control).
2 Net number fibroblasts/field (experimental - control).
3 Scale 0-4.
4 Accompanied by intense inflammatory response.

chemotactic (for fibroblasts) and angiogenic activity. Table 21.2 summarizes the results of these experiments. Plasma serum had a mitogenic index (experimental/control) of 4.5 and significant chemotactic activity. The retentate, containing proteins of $M_r > 14{,}000$, had a mitogenic index of 1.0 and strong chemotactic activity. The dialysate showed a mitogenic index of 2.9, but no significant chemotactic activity over the control. However, both retentate and dialysate showed angiogenic activity, as assessed by the cornea assay.

Histology

The cellular response at day 5 to implanted Ivalon™ sponges impregnated with collagen and plasma-serum retentate was a prominent capsule forming around the sponge. The cells in the capsule were primarily fibroblast-like, with scattered inflammatory cells also present. A moderate degree of angiogenesis was evident. In contrast, the predominant cell type in the capsule around the sponge impregnated with collagen and plasma-serum dialysate was inflammatory. There was a striking abundance of blood vessels in the capsule (see Figures 21.4a and 21.4b). Moreover, unlike the sponge impregnated with collagen and plasma-serum retentate (Figure 21.3), a remarkable degree of cellular infiltration and neovascularization occurred inside this sponge at day 5 (see Figures 21.4c and 21.4d). Grossly, we observed that sponges impregnated with collagen-plus-plasma serum dialysate were encapsulated by connective tissue containing a rich network of blood vessels.

Table 21.3 summarizes the histologic findings of the various preparations in the sponge and the surrounding capsule. In general, most of the histologic changes occur in the capsule at five days. Of note is the remarkable degree of neovascularization in the capsule surrounding the plasma-serum dialysate/collagen-impregnated sponge, and the cellular (inflammatory cells and fibroblasts), vascular, and connective tissue infiltration into this sponge.

DNA and Collagen Synthesis

The synthetic activity of cells in the sponge was measured by ^{3}H-thymidine incorporation and ^{14}C-proline incorporation (see Table 21.4). DNA synthesis was elevated in the capsules impregnated with collagen-plus-plasma serum and with collagen-

FIGURE 21.3 Histologic section of rabbit cornea implanted with Hydron containing CM-Sephadex fraction III. L (limbus), I (implantation site), V (blood vessel), Ep (epithelial surface of cornea), En (endothelial surface of cornea).

a. Low magnification (25x), showing the site if implantation, the limbus, and the limbal vessels penetrating the cornea.

b. Higher magnification (100x), demonstrating the penetrating vessels and the lack of any surrounding inflammation.

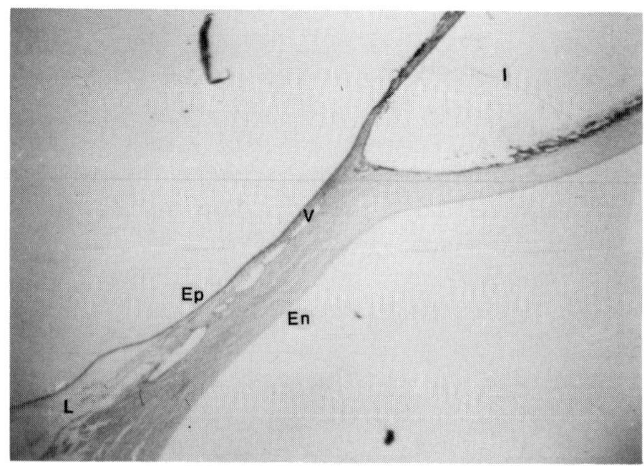

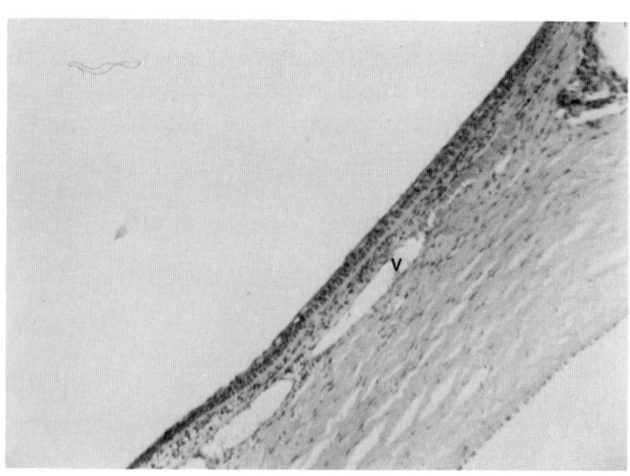

FIGURE 21.4 Histologic sections of a five-day Ivalon™ sponge implant impregnated with collagen-plus-plasma serum dialysate. S (sponge), C (capsule), V (capillaries).

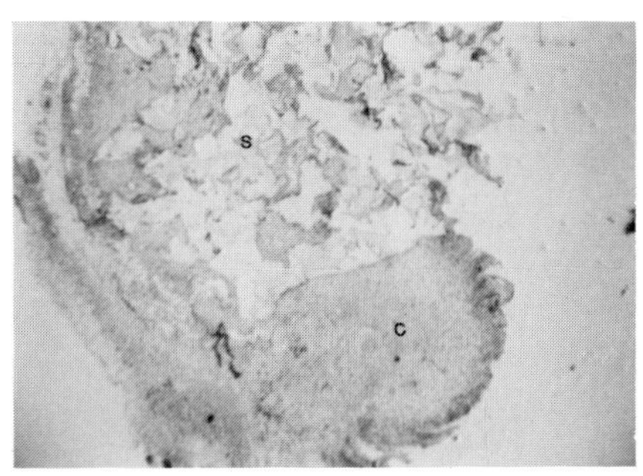

a. Low magnification (25x). Note the extensive capsule and the rich cellular infiltration into the capsule and sponge.

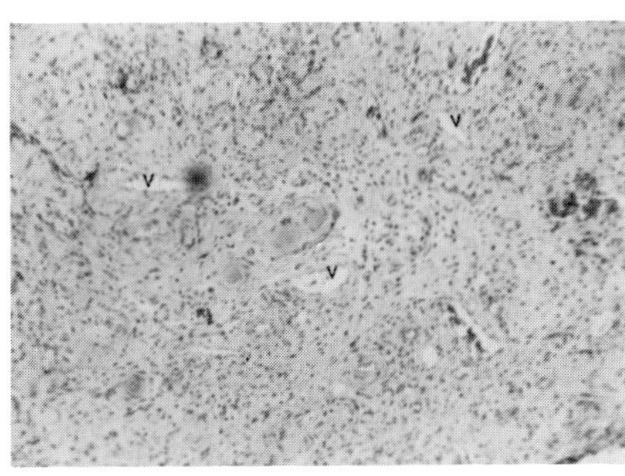

b. Higher magnification (100x) of the capsule. Extensive inflammatory cell infiltration and many capillaries are evident.

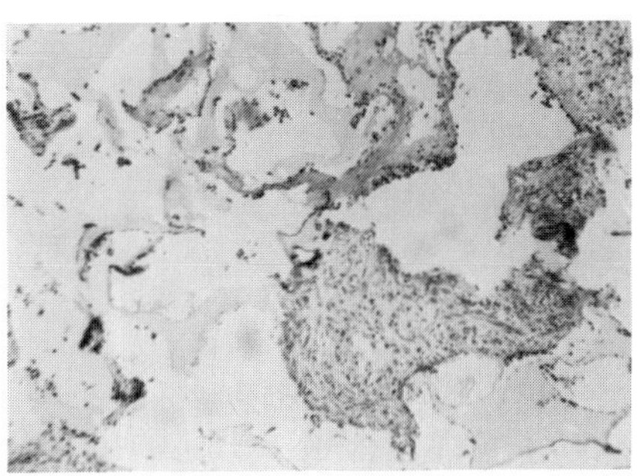

c. Cellular infiltration inside the sponge (magnification 100x).

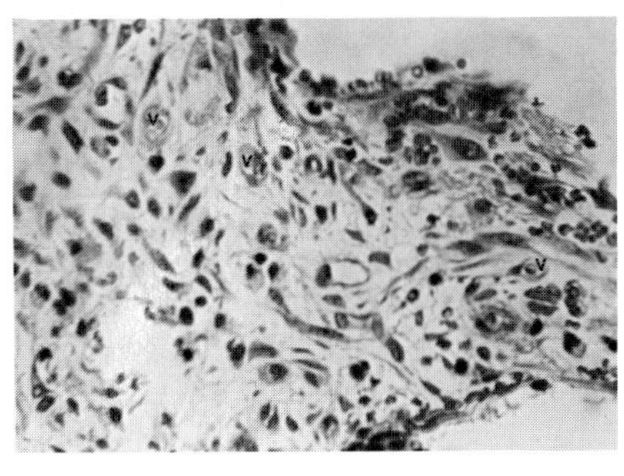

d. Higher magnification (400x) of the cellular infiltrate inside the sponge. Note the inflammatory cells and the numerous capillaries.

TABLE 21.3

Histologic Assessment[1] of Dialysis Fractions of Plasma Serum

Preparation	Capsule Vascularity	Capsule Cellularity	Connective Tissue	Sponge Cellularity	Sponge PMN/macrophages
Collagen	2	2[2]	2	2-3	8/2
10^9 platelets/collagen	2	4[3]	2	4	9/1
Plasma serum/collagen	3	4[2]	2	4	5/5
Retentate/collagen	2	1-2[2]	3	2	7/3
Dialysate/collagen	4	3[2]	3	3	8/2

[1] Scale 0-4 (graded blindly by two observers).
[2] Primarily fibroblasts; few inflammatory cells.
[3] Prominent inflammatory infiltration.

TABLE 21.4

Effect of Plasma Serum Dialysis Fractions on DNA and Protein Synthesis in Ivalon™ Sponges

Preparation	Mitogenic Index[1]	^{14}C-proline Incorporation[2] Total	^{14}C-proline Incorporation[2] Collagenase-Sensitive
Collagen	1.00	8,901	1,822
10^9 platelets/collagen	1.15	7,675	1,395
Plasma serum/ collagen	1.54	11,277	1,662
Retentate/collagen	1.15	7,972	1,468
Dialysate/collagen	1.59	8,114	1,654

[1] Collagen + addition ÷ collagen only.
[2] Counts per minute/sponge.

plus-plasma serum dialysate, which is in accord with the histologic picture (Figure 21.4). On the other hand, retentate plus collagen did not elicit cellular proliferative activity to a significantly higher degree than collagen alone or collagen-plus-whole platelets. Collagen synthesis was essentially the same at day 5 in all the treatment groups.

DISCUSSION

Two methods of plasma serum fractionation were employed. The first, chromatography of CM-Sephadex, is also the first step in the isolation procedure of PDGF.[8] It was, therefore, not surprising to find that CM-Sephadex fraction III, which contains PDGF, had the highest mitogenic index when tested with fetal rabbit fibroblasts (Table 21.1). However, the finding that the same fraction showed significant angiogenic activity when assayed by the corneal test (Table 21.1, Figure 21.3) was unexpected. Platelet-derived growth factor has been shown to have specific receptors on cells like fibroblasts, smooth muscle cells and glial cells,[14,15] but not on endothelial cells. The most likely explanation, therefore, is that another component which cochromatographed with PDGF on CM-Sephadex contained the angiogenic activity.

An important issue to address is whether the angiogenic activity of platelets affects capillary endothelial cells directly, or whether it acts indirectly via other cell types, such as the macrophage. A definitive answer will have to await purification of the platelet-derived angiogenic factor. However, Figure 21.2 offers preliminary evidence that the effect may be direct. Plasma serum-Hydron implantation in the cornea elicited both a 2+ angiogenic response and a strong inflammatory infiltrate. CM-Sephadex fraction III-Hydron implantation, on the other hand, elicited a strong angiogenic response without significant inflammation.

In a separate series of experiments, plasma serum was dialyzed and the resultant fractions, dialysate and retentate, were assessed for their effect on wound healing. After a five-day implantation period, sponges impregnated with the dialysate showed a 2.9 mitogenic index, whereas the retentate showed no increase of mitogenesis over the control. Chemotactic activity was present in the retentate only, and angiogenic activity was present in both fractions (Table 21.2). These data are puzzling, since PDGF, with molecular weights of 27,000 to 31,000, would be expected to show mitogenic activity in the retentate fraction.

It should be borne in mind, however, that unlike the in vitro assay for PDGF this assay was carried out in vivo, where many other factors, some of them, probably countervailing, are in operation. Moreover, unlike the close contact between PDGF and the target cell in the in vitro assays for mitogenicity, the close cells in this assay are at a relatively great distance from the PDGF, which was placed in a totally acellular environment. Last, the in vitro effect of PDGF is measured within hours, while in the Ivalon™ sponge assay measurements were made at five days after implantation.

More informative, albeit less amenable to quantitation, is the histologic assessment of the sponges and their surrounding capsules. Since the experiment was terminated at day 5, most of the histologic events were localized in the capsule. A marked difference between the retentate and dialysate fractions is evident. The retentate sponge was surrounded by a thick capsule, rich in fibroblasts and collagen, with only moderate vascularity and infrequent inflammatory cells. The capsule of the dialysate sponge, on the other hand, was heavily infiltrated with inflammatory cells and had a rich network of new blood vessels evident both grossly and microscopically. Moreover, even within the short space of five days, the sponge was already infiltrated with connective tissue, inflammatory cells and many capillaries (Figure 21.4d). Clearly, a qualitative difference in cell type, degree of angiogenesis, and rate of repair exists between the retentate and dialysate fractions. This conclusion is further bolstered by the data summarized in Table 21.4. DNA synthesis, which reflects cellular proliferation, was markedly elevated in the dialysate sponge, but not in the retentate sponge.

The fact that platelets have a chemotactic/mitogenic factor (PDGF) and angiogenic activity makes these cells extremely important in the regulation of the repair process. Through these factors, as well as through their hemostatic functions, platelets can control the processes of fibrin deposition, neutrophil and macrophage chemotaxis, fibroplasia, and angiogenesis. Since these are probably also the first cells at the site of injury, especially if the injury is accompanied by vascular disruption, it seems increasingly likely that platelets regulate the initiation and progression of repair.

ACKNOWLEDGMENTS

Acknowledgments to Heinz Scheuenstuhl and Ted Lowenkopf for excellent technical assistance, and to Cherry Elliott for typing the manuscript and for the illustration for Figure 21.2.

NOTES

1. Hunt TK (ed). Fundamentals of wound management in surgery. Wound Healing: Disorders of Repair. Chirurgicom, South Plainfield, N.J., 1976.

2. Nemerson Y, Pitlick FA. Extrinsic clotting pathways. In Spaet TH (ed), Progress in Hemostasis and Thrombosis, Vol. 1, pp. 1-37. New York: Grune & Stratton, 1972.

3. Orloff KG, Michaeli D. Fibrin-induced release of platelet serotonin. Am J Physiol 231:344-350, 1976.

4. Diminno G, Bertele V, Cerletti C, Gaetano G, Silver MY. Arachidonic acid induces human platelet-fibrin retraction: The role of platelet cyclic endoperoxides. Thromb Res 25:299-306, 1982.

5. Grotendorst GR, Seppa HEJ, Kleinman HK, Martin GR. Attachment of smooth muscle cells to collagen and their migration toward platelet-derived growth factor. Proc Natl Acad Sci USA 78:3669-3672, 1981.

6. Deuel TF, Senior RM, Huang JS, Griffin G. Chemotaxis of monocytes and neutrophils to platelet-derived growth factor. J Clin Invest 69:1046-1049, 1982.

7. Knighton DR, Hunt TK, Thakral KK, Goodson WH III. Role of platelets and fibrin in the healing sequence. Ann Surg 196:379-388, 1982.

8. Raines EW, Ross R. Platelet-derived growth factor. I. High yield purification and evidence for multiple forms. J Biol Chem 257:5154-5160, 1982.

9. Gimbrone MA, Cotran RS, Leapmann SB, Folkman J. Tumor growth and neovascularization: An experimental method using the rabbit cornea. J Natl Cancer Inst 52:413-427, 1974.

10. Langer R, Folkman J. Polymers for the sustained release of proteins and other macromolecules. Nature (London) 263:797-800, 1976.

11. Gospodarowicz D. Purification of a fibroblast growth factor from bovine pituitary. J Biol Chem 250:2515-2520, 1975.

12. Seppa H, Grotendorst G, Seppa S, Schiffmann E, Martin GR. Platelet-derived growth factor is chemotactic for fibroblasts. J Cell Biol 92:584-588, 1982.

13. Postlethwaite AE, Snyderman R, Kang AH. The chemotactic attraction of human fibroblasts to a lymphocyte-derived factor. J Exp Med 144:1188-1203, 1976.

14. Heldin GH, Wasteson A, Westermark B. Interaction of platelet-derived growth factor with its fibroblast receptor. J Biol Chem 257:4216-4221, 1982.

15. Bowen-Pope DF, Ross R. Platelet-derived factor. II. Specific binding to cultured cells. J Biol Chem 257:5161-5171, 1982.

PART VI
Orthopaedic Implants

22
The Effects of Chemotherapy and Radiation Therapy on Physiologic Bone Turnover and Fracture Repair

Gary E. Friedlaender, Roland Baron, Richard R. Pelker and Andrew C. Doganis

INTRODUCTION

Aggressive primary neoplastic diseases and metastatic lesions of the skeleton or surrounding soft tissues are often treated, in part, with systemic chemotherapy or local irradiation. In addition to their anti-tumor activity, both modalities would be expected to exert direct effects on bone, and this secondary influence may be reflected in physiologic turnover of intact bone, fracture repair or bone graft incorporation. The concern for intact bone homeostasis and healing of pathologic fractures is clear, and the increasing enthusiasm for use of osteochondral allografts in limb-sparing tumor resections adds clinical significance to evaluation of this therapeutic modality as well. This chapter summarizes our experience with the influence of two chemotherapeutic agents, adriamycin and methotrexate, and palliative doses of radiation therapy on histologic and histomorphometric aspects of intact bone biology, as well as histologic and biomechanical aspects of fracture repair in an animal model.

Supported, in part, by N.I.H. grant #CA-30169 and Naval Medical Research and Development Command contract #N00014-77-C-0442. The opinions or assertions contained herein are the private ones of the authors and not to be construed as official or reflecting the views of the U.S. Naval Department or the Naval Service at large.

BACKGROUND

Methotrexate is a folic acid antagonist, and consequently interferes with production of nucleic acids required for DNA and RNA synthesis (Bertino et al. 1964). Adriamycin exerts its anti-metabolic effect through intercalation between adjacent nucleotide base pairs, resulting in interference with DNA replication (Di Marco 2975). Both drugs inhibit protein synthesis, not only of neoplastic cells, but of all metabolically active cell types. Irradiation also disrupts the normal reproductive integrity of cells, presumably through a direct effect on the DNA molecule (Hellman 1982).

Most past reports of chemotherapeutic drug-induced effects on bone have been limited to macroscopic levels of inquiry, usually clinical observations, and often anecdotal (Aarskog and Hexeberg 1968; Au and Raisz 1972; Karnofsky and Lacon 1964; Nesbit et al. 1976; O'Regan et al. 1973; Prosnitz et al. 1981; Ragab et al. 1970; Robins and Jowsey 1973; Singh and Sanyal 1974; Stanisavljevic and Babcock 1977; Vahlsing 1965). For example, chronic methotrexate chemotherapy in the treatment of childhood leukemias has been associated with bone pain, osteoporosis and spontaneous fractures (O'Regan 1973; Ragab 1970; Stanisavljevic 1977). There has also been a clinical impression that chemotherapy and irradiation slow down facture repair (Hellman 1982). Relatively little experience exists with the use of massive osteochondral allografts in patients also receiving high dose chemotherapy or irradiation to the operative site. Most of the available information describes a high complication rate in these situations and, in general, has discouraged this approach (Grant et al. 1982; Mankin et al. 1982). Systemic chemotherapy has been associated with a high rate of failure of bony union at the anastomotic site, delayed or inadequate incorporation resulting in graft fragmentation and collapse and an increased incidence in deep-wound infection. This latter point has also been confirmed in experimental studies of soft tissue healing (Cohen et al. 1975a; Cohen et al. 1975b) and susceptibility to infection (Ariyan et al. 1980) in animals receiving chemotherapy. More recently, Mankin (1983) has been using frozen massive bone allografts in patients receiving multi-drug chemotherapy following limb-sparing tumor resections, and the early results have been encouraging. One explanation for this apparent difference may be related to the use of freeze-dried allografts in the earlier experience as well as reflect the surgical expertise gained from over 175 osteochondral transplants performed by Dr. Mankin and his colleagues.

INTACT BONE STUDIES

The influence of a drug or other treatment modality on bone can be evaluated at various levels of structure from cell biology to mechanical properties of large segments. Further perspective may relate to studies of routine physiologic homeostasis (turnover or remodeling), fracture repair or graft incorporation. All of these points of view are important and clinically significant. In the studies to be discussed, we have concentrated on intact bone turnover and fracture repair, and anticipate expanding this methodology to evaluate autograft and allograft incorporation in the future.

Histomorphometry

Central to defining the effect of any extrinsic influence on bone is an objective method for quantitating the induced change. For intact bone, the net result may be reflected in measurement of bone volume or mass, but effects on the dynamic interaction between bone formation and resorption activities (physiologic turnover) cannot be fully appreciated without assessing these independent but coupled aspects of the bone-remodeling cycle. Thus, measurement of bone volume alone may be misleading in identifying the presence and magnitude of changes in resorption and formation activity. For example, bone volume or mass will remain unchanged despite increased or decreased formation, provided resorption is coupled in both direction and magnitude.

Physiologic turnover of bone has been described by Frost (1980) as a sequence of activities by different cell populations collectively referred to as "the basic multi-cellular unit (BMU)" of bone remodeling. The events, which occur at each remodeling site, can be summarized as follows (Baron 1977; Baron et al. 1980; Frost 1980):

1. Activation—a resting area of the trabeculum, for reasons yet unknown, becomes an active site of remodeling.
2. Resorption—active osteoclasts appear, resorption of a finite quantity of bone occurs, and then these cells disappear from resorptive cavities (Howship's lacunae).
3. Reversal—empty lacunae fill with mononuclear cells which are not yet functionally recognizable as osteoblasts, but more likely represent mononuclear phagocytes. It is speculated the cement line is generated during this phase (Tran Van et al. 1982a; Tran Van et al. 1982b).

4. Formation—a population of osteoblasts appears in the lacunae and they deposit osteoid which subsequently is mineralized to complete the bone formation phase of the cycle prior to returning to a resting state.

Frost has further described a system for evaluating bone turnover in which characteristics are either directly measured or calculated from direct measurements, reflecting both formation and resorption activity in addition to net bone volume (mass) (Frost 1977). Using an optical planimeter with a digitizing tablet and eyepiece micrometer, the parameters listed in Table 22.1 can be directly assessed and the additional characteristics

TABLE 22.1

Directly Measured Histomorphometric Parameters of Trabecular Bone

1. Total Sampling Area (WTBT): area occupied by the trabecular bone tissue, that is, trabeculae plus marrow area.
2. Trabecular Area: area of WTBT occupied by trabeculae.
3. Osteoid Area: area of WTBT occupied by osteoid.
4. Trabecular Perimeter (TP): total surface length of all trabeculae.
5. Osteoid Perimeter: that portion of TP covered by osteoid.
6. Osteoblast Perimeter: that portion of TP covered by active osteoblasts.
7. Osteoclast Perimeter: that portion of TP covered by osteoclasts in Howships' lacunae.
8. Empty Lacunae Perimeter: extent of Howships' lacunae without osteoclasts or osteoid, but lined with mononuclear cells (reversal phase).
9. Number of Osteoclasts: number of osteoclasts in tissue sampled.
10. Single Labeled Perimeter: that portion of TP covered by one fluorescent label.
11. Double Labeled Perimeter: that portion of TP covered by two fluorescent labels.
12. Interval Between Labels: distance between the two labels in double labeled areas.
13. Thickness of Complete Remodeling Foci: distance between the reversal cement line and the bone surface in non-resorbing and non-osteoid areas.

TABLE 22.2

Calculated Histomorphometric Parameters of Trabecular Bone

1. Percent trabecular bone volume (%TBV)
2. Trabecular surface (TS)* - millimeters^2
3. Bone formation rate (BFR) - 10^{-2} millimeters^3/millimeters^2
4. Percent TS covered by osteoid (%OS)
5. Absolute osteoid volume (%AOV)
6. Osteoid thickness (OT) - microns
7. Percent TS covered by active osteoblasts (%OBS)
8. Mineralization rate (MR) - microns/day
9. Percent TS covered by double fluorescent labels (%DL)
10. Percent TS covered by osteoclasts (%OCS)
11. Osteoclasts per millimeter TS (OC/mm) - number/millimeter
12. Percent TS covered by reversal surfaces, total lacunae (%RevS)

* Trabecular surface (TS) is the measured trabecular perimeter (TP) expressed as an area, such that TS and TP are interchangeable terms.
Units indicated when other than percent.

defined in Table 22.2 can be calculated. Rates of bone formation and mineralization can also be determined by in vivo pulse-labeling with a fluorescent compound prior to retrieval of the bone specimen.

Animal Model

We have evaluated the effects of adriamycin and methotrexate on physiologic turnover of bone in rat tail vertebrae. The acute effects reflect daily intraperitoneal administration of either 1 mg/kg of Adriamycin or 0.75 mg/kg of methotrexate for 5 days in 250 ±25 gram Wistar-Lewis rats. These animals were pulse-labeled with calcein (30 mg/kg) 7 and 13 days following initiation of chemotherapy and sacrificed on the 14th day. Constant segments of proximal tail vertebrae were recovered and compared with similar specimens obtained from animals not receiving treatment.

Chronic effects of these same chemotherapeutic agents were determined following 16 weeks of treatment with adriamycin at a dose of 1.0 mg/kg once a week intravenously until sacrifice or with methotrexate 0.1 mg/kg intraparitoneally 5 of every 7 days for 16 weeks. These doses were at, or near, the maximal tolerated amount for these animals, since treated animals failed to gain weight normally and slight increases caused mortality. Lewis rats (250-300 grams) were used for the long-term studies and compared to age and weight matched controls.

Irradiation effects were determined by deliveryying 10 daily fractions of 250 rads each to the tail and both hindlimbs of Lewis rats. The remainder of their body was lead-shielded. Animals were pulse-labeled with calcein (30 mg/kg) 8 and 1 day prior to sacrifice at several intervals between 4 and 16 weeks after initiation of the radiation therapy.

Bone specimens were fixed immediately after sacrifice in 40% ethanol at 4°C, dehydrated in graded solutions of alcohol and embedded undecalcified in methylmethacrylate (Baron et al. 1983). Longitudinal sections, 4 microns thick, were prepared using a Jung-K microtome and stained with toluidine blue. The parameters listed in Table 22.1 were measured using a Zeiss MOP 3 Optical Planimeter. A minimum of 20 fields were evaluated in each specimen, avoiding the region of the growth plate and a 1 mm band including the primary spongiosa in the metaphysis and also excluding cortical periosteal and endosteal surfaces. This was done to minimize the effect of rapid growth, although there is nothing intrinsically misleading about the qualitative evaluation of these regions other than the quantitative amplification of the turnover response.

Decalcified sections were used to measure the mean wall thickness (the distance from the cement line to trabecular surface), and additional nondecalcified sections, 10 microns thick, were used to measure the distribution of fluorescent labels and the distance between pulses.

Histomorphometric Results

Our results are shown in Table 22.3. Short-term treatment caused significant changes in physiologic turnover of intact tail vertebrae in this rat model (Friedlaender et al. [in press]; Tross et al. 1979; 1980). Methotrexate resulted in a 27% reduction in cancellous bone volume and adriamycin lead to a 12% decline. As previously discussed, observation of bone volume alone provides only the net result of formation and resorption activities.

TABLE 22.3

Acute and Chronic Effects of Adriamycin and Methotrexate on Bone Remodeling in Rat Tail Vertebrae

	Adriamycin		Methotrexate	
	1 week	16 weeks	1 week	16 weeks
Whole Tissue				
bone volume	-12%	ns	-27%	-26%
Osteoblast Dependent				
% osteoid surfaces	ns	-85%	ns	-23%
% absolute osteoid volume	-29%	ns	-36%	-42%
osteoid thickness	-21%	+20%	-24%	-24%
bone formation rate	-59%	-42%	-58%	-42%
Osteoclast Dependent				
% osteoclast surfaces	ns	ns	ns	ns
total lacunae	ns	ns	ns	ns

Note: ns indicates not statistically different from control values.

Both drugs caused significant decreases in the volume and thickness of osteoid; adriamycin-treated animals demonstrated a 29% and 21% decrease in these respective parameters, while methotrexate reduced absolute osteoid volume 36% and osteoid thickness 24%. Neither drug, however, caused a decrease in the percent trabecular surface covered by osteoid or osteoblasts, although the amount of synthetic activity per cell was diminished with respect to osteoid production. This was confirmed by significant decreases in the bone formation rate, 59% with adriamycin and 58% with methotrexate, and decreases of similar magnitude in the percent trabecular surfaces covered by doubled-labeled new bone. Once the osteoid matrix was synthesized, it was mineralized at a rate not statistically different from control animals. There was a suggestion of increased resorption activity in methotrexate-treated animals, but the osteoclastic-dependent parameters measured by this approach do not allow quantitation of rates of resorption.

On the other hand, two of the three elements of the bone remodeling equation (net mass = formation + resorption) were determined: net bone mass and formation, so resorption activity can be derived. In the acute treatment protocol for methotrexate, the decreased osteoblastic activity must have been accompanied by a relatively smaller decrease (or no change from control levels) in the rate of resorption to produce a substantial decrease in net bone volume. Adriamycin, on the other hand, must have significantly decreased resorption (to a greater degree than methotrexate) since the profound decrease in the measured rate of bone formation was not as strikingly manifest in reduced mass.

Measurement of drug effects on an acute basis allows little time for compensatory mechanisms to exert an influence, but evaluation of animals following 16 weeks of chemotherapy reflects both the influence of the drugs as well as whatever physiologic compensation is possible.

Chronic administration of adriamycin was not associated with a diminished bone volume; however, the bone formation rate remained depressed by approximately 42% and the mineralization rate was also reduced (approximately 31% of control values) (Friedlaender et al. 1983a). In this case, measurement of the bone volume alone would suggest there was no effect of the drug or that it has been adequately compensated for by otherwise uneffected physiologic responses. Indeed, the persistent decrease in bone forming activity was coupled to a decrease in resorption activity of similar magnitude, the net result being no change in mass. Whether the effect on resorption is a direct effect of the drug or a compensatory effort (or both) could not be answered by these data, although speculation would favor a direct toxic effect on osteoclastic activity.

The decreased bone volume induced acutely by methotrexate persisted throughout the 16 weeks of treatment, remaining approximately 26% below control levels (Friedlaender et al. 1982). The bone formation rate remained depressed by approximately 42%. Methotrexate, therefore, appears to diminish bone formation more than it depresses resorption activity (resulting in a net decrease in mass), but with time, a new equilibrium is established such that the initial loss is held constant. Again, it cannot be determined, at this point, how much of the influence on resorption at 16 weeks is direct toxicity or a physiologic response.

Histomorphometric analysis of tail vertebrae from rats receiving palliative doses of irradiation is not yet complete. Preliminary observations pertain only to bone volume 2, 4, 8 and 10 weeks following initiation of treatment (Friedlaender et al. 1981), and to a subjective glance at the fluorescent labeling pattern in the 4 week group. With these shortcomings in mind, it was noted that bone volume was slightly, but insignificantly decreased compared to control levels at 2 weeks, reduced by nearly 50% at 8 weeks and restored to normal by 10 weeks. Virtually no double labeled osteoblastic surfaces could be identified in the animals sacrificed at 4 weeks and there was a suggestion that single labels were wider and more intense than usually observed. This suggests the bone formation rate was profoundly reduced, causing the interval between the 2 pulses to be too small to distinguish and measure (consequently both pulses appeared superimposed). If bone formation was reduced and the mass (volume) did not change from control levels, then resorption was also diminished to a commensurate degree. The loss of bone volume in the 8 week group and return of this parameter to normal at later intervals may indicate that osteoclasts recover or repopulate the vertebra faster than osteoblastic cells. Radiation therapy is known to interfere with cell replication (Hellman 1982), even at low doses, so the postulated sensitivity of both osteoblasts and osteoclasts is tenable. It must be kept in mind, however, our data are preliminary and offered in that context.

FRACTURE REPAIR STUDIES

The influence of chemotherapy on fracture repair has not been objectively studied in humans, although there is a subjective impression that anti-neoplastic agents delay union in patients with pathologic fractures who are also receiving chemotherapy. There are often, of course, multiple contributing factors in these individuals including general cachexia, persisting influence of the tumor at the fracture site and the use of local irradiation. Spontaneous fractures have been reported in children receiving chronic methotrexate for treatment of leukemia (Ragab et al. 1970). A small number of animal studies have been accomplished. Hajj et al. (1981) evaluated healing of rat femoral fractures by failure in bending and comparison to intact contralateral limbs. This group demonstrated that animals receiving methotrexate regained only 50% of their biomechanical strength at the fracture site over the period of observation, compared to untreated controls. Langendorff et al. (1981) did not detect any change in mechanical properties of intact rabbit bone but did note a significant decrease in load-bearing capacity of surgical fractured femurs and mineral content after 4 weeks of treatment with cyclophophamide.

There are few studies available demonstrating the effect of irradiation on bone, all accomplished in animals and all limited by lack of sensitive objective methods of evaluating induced effects. These studies suggest that fracture healing occurs after small or moderate amounts of radiation therapy, but delays in repair can be anticipated as doses increase (Bonarigo and Rubin 1967; Hayashi and Suit 1971).

We have evaluated the repair of fractures in rats receiving systemic adriamycin or methotrexate or local irradiation with the effects judged histologically and biomechanically (Friedlaender et al. 1983b; Pelker et al. 1983).

Histology

Open surgical fractures were created in the mid shaft femur of 300 gram Lewis rats and then internally fixed with an intramedullary K-wire. Chemotherapy was administered as described earlier in this report (adriamycin, 1.0 mg/kg once each week; and methotrexate, 0.1 mg/kg 5 of every 7 days). Irradiation was delivered in 10 daily doses of 250 rads (2500 rads total) beginning 3 days after surgery (see Table 22.4). Groups of of approximately 5 animals each were sacrificed and evaluated 1, 2, 4, 8 and 12 weeks after fracture (Friedlaender et al. 1983b). Longitudinal paraffin-embedded sections were stained with hematoxylin and eosin, and then an arbitrary scale was

TABLE 22.4

Histology of Fracture Repair in Rats Receiving Adriamycin, Methotrexate or Irradiation*

	Weeks**				
	1	2	4	8	12
Control	2.2	4.6	5.3	5.8	8.7
Methotrexate	2.6	4.8	5.0	6.2	5.8
Adriamycin	2.0	—	3.9	—	5.8
Irradiation	2.0	2.2	2.6	3.4	4.0

*See text for explanation of arbitrary grading criteria.
**Weeks following initiation of treatment.

used to quantitate fracture repair in treated animals compared to untreated controls. Three phases of repair were designated with a maximum of three points ascribed to each phase, depending upon the degree of progress observed. The most immature phase of repair was characterized by a fibrovascular response at the fracture site with minimal subperiosteal reactive new-bone formation adjacent to the fracture. Intermediate repair included a cartilagenous response at the fracture site with increased reactive bone at the periphery of the callus. Advanced repair included abundant new-bone formation at the fracture site and early cortical remodeling. Thus, in this model, one point indicated the least mature and 9 points the most advanced healing.

Both adriamycin and methotrexate interfered with the normal progression of fracture repair as observed in the control group. The initial callus response was indistinguishable from normal; but after 12 weeks, chemotherapy-treated animals were clearly impaired in terms of histologic characteristics of healing. Conversion of this semi-quantitative scale into verbal terms would indicate that the average fracture in the chemotherapy-treated groups plateaued at the end of the cartilagenous phase of repair.

An even greater influence was seen following irradiation. Repair in these animals plateaued at a late fibroblastic or early cartilagenous stage. However, it is not known if these observations represented an end point of healing or delay in an eventually satisfactory response. That question could be resolved with longer periods of observation.

Biomechanical Evaluation

Biomechanical testing by machining bone specimens to a uniform size emphasize the bone's material properties. Whereas, the structural, anatomical spatial distribution, properties of bone are emphasized by testing intact bone. In reality, both forms of testing address structural and material properties, but to different degrees. The nature in which bone is stressed, and consequently mechanical properties recorded, can occur in a variety of modes including torsion, bending, shear or combinations of each of these. Furthermore, results obtained are dependent upon the rate and magnitude of loading, as well as the end point chosen for the test.

Our studies in torsion were carried out over frequent intervals between 4 and 24 weeks after surgical fracture (Pelker et al. 1983). The rat model (internally fixed femoral fractures) and therapeutic programs already described were also used for these experimental approaches. Specimens were tested to failure in torsion at a rate of 13.2 radians per second (following removal of the intramedullary fixation), and the torque, stiffness, energy absorption and angle to failure were calculated from the resultant load-deformation curve. The value for each parameter was normalized to that obtained from the intact contralateral limb, and a "least squares fit" was calculated using the formula $Y = A + B \exp^{CX}$ where (Y = torque and X = healing time in weeks).

Fractures in untreated animals regained normal biomechanical strength in this testing mode by 10 to 12 weeks, perhaps slightly delayed compared to other investigations that used closed methods for producing fractures. Chemotherapy-treated animals failed to heal mechanically through 16 weeks of observation and irradiated fractures plateaued far short of normal despite 24 weeks of time (Figure 22.1).

BONE GRAFT STUDIES

Burchardt et al. (1983) have evaluated the effects of adriamycin and methotrexate on bone graft incorporation using histomorphometric and biomechanical analysis in a canine model. In their experimental approach, a 4 cm segment of fibular served as the graft; no internal fixation being required in this non-weightbearing bone (although there are undoubtedly forces exerted by muscular attachments).

Burchardt has described his methodology and results in detail elsewhere, including extensive evaluation of fresh and freeze-dried autografts and allografts (Burchardt et al. 1978a; Burchardt et al. 1978b; Enneking et al. 1975). A summary of his findings will follow.

In previous descriptions by these investigators of the normal sequence of events associated with cortical autograft repair, osteoclastic activity predominated in the early phase and resulted in increasing porosity of the peripheral cortex and internal graft architecture. This loss of mass was associated with at least a transient decrease in mechanical strength until the second, or osteoblast-dependent, phase of repair was established. In control and methotrexate-treated dogs (20 mg/M^2 - twice per week), internal porosity was increased in a similar (and by definition, normal) fashion as seen in control animals, but adriamycin-treated animals (30-50 mg/M^2 - every 3 weeks) failed to demonstrate this degree of resorption activity. This suggests that adriamycin (versus methotrexate) inhibited osteoclastic activity.

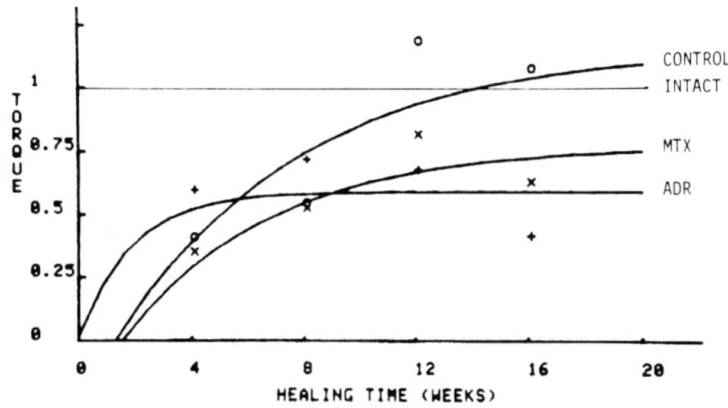

FIGURE 22.1A Chemotherapy/FX healing.

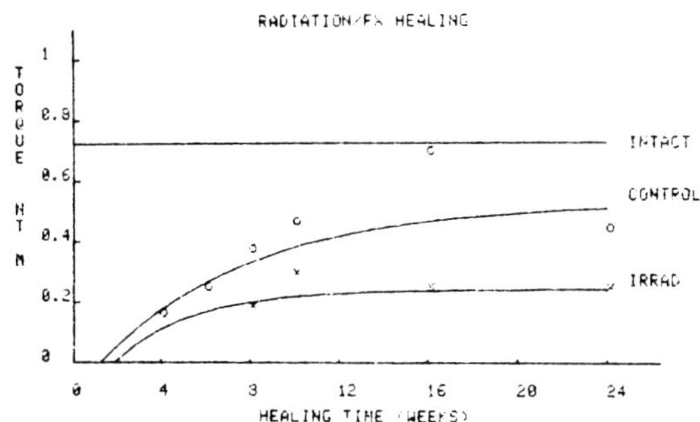

FIGURE 22.1B Radiation/FX healing.

Both methotrexate and adriamycin caused a decrease in new-bone formation, presumably a direct toxic effect on osteoblastic cells or their precursors. This pattern of effect on bone formation and resorption was similar to that observed by us in intact bone turnover (Friedlaender et al., unpublished; Friedlaender et al. 1983a; Friedlaender et al. 1982).

Radiographic union of grafts occurred quantitatively and temporally identical to controls in animals receiving methotrexate or lower doses of adriamycin (30 mg/M^2), but higher doses of adriamycin (40-50 mg/M^2) delayed, or perhaps prevented, union in this model.

Mechanical strength, measured in torsion to failure, was affected in both adriamycin and methotrexate-treated dogs. Normally, autografts in untreated animals demonstrated increased strength compared to sham operated (intact) bone. The magnitude of this increase was not statistically significant in the treated animals, perhaps a reflection of diminished new-bone activity and decreased resorption.

There has been little attention to the effects of irradiation on the biologic properties of bone allograft incorporation. A recent pilot study by Pellet et al. (1983) suggests that sterilizing doses of irradiation (2.5 megarads and greater) adversely influence repair judged by x-rays and cursory routine histology. Doses between 10 kilorads and 1 megarad appeared to improve the rate of incorporation of frozen segmental allografts in a rat model compared to nonirradiated frozen allogeneic controls, but this observation requires confirmation using more objective and thorough methodology.

SUMMARY

Available studies in animal models, and limited clinical observations, indicate that systemic chemotherapeutic agents and local irradiation have toxic effects on bone. This adverse influence may become manifest in biologic and biomechanical parameters of intact bone, repair of fractures and graft incorporation. Specifically, adriamycin and methotrexate substantially decrease new-bone formation in both acute and chronic treatment protocols and adriamycin, more than methotrexate, also has a profound inhibitory effect on the resorptive activity within intact bone. The net result over time is a significant but static decrease in bone mass during methotrexate administration and a normal bone volume associated with adriamycin treatment.

The influence of irradiation has not been as well defined but significant suppression of bone formation and resorption appears to occur rapidly, with a faster recovery seen by osteoclastic cells causing a transient loss of bone mass.

There is ample evidence that these same treatment modalities adversely effect fracture repair and reasonable speculation (although scant data) would lead to the conclusion that graft incorporation is also substantially retarded.

The approaches now being applied to evaluate the effects of drugs and physical factors on the skeleton are reasonably objective and appear sound in their ability to quantitate the observed effects. Knowledge of the nature and magnitude of these induced changes on bone healing and repair is of practical concern and should lead to improved methods for administering therapy and minimizing adverse effects. This may be accomplished by altered treatment protocols, early detection of potential but recognized toxic effects, compensatory therapeutic approaches and alterations in postoperative rehabilitation programs. The scope of agents evaluated must expand in terms of specific drugs and additional classes of therapeutic agents (including immunosuppressants), and recovery times from toxic insults and the efficacy of compensatory or protective therapeutic approaches must also be defined. This is a laborious but rewarding direction, and we look forward to increased activity by others.

ACKNOWLEDGMENTS

The technical assistance of N. Troiano, J. McKay, Jr. and M. Kaplan is gratefully acknowledged.

REFERENCES

Aarskog, D and Hexeberg, A. 1968. Actinomycin D and transverse lines of growing bones. Acta Paediat. Scand. 57:463-467.

Ariyan, S, Kraft, RL, and Goldberg, NH. 1980. An experimental model to determine the effects of adjuvant therapy on the incidence of postoperative wound infection: II. Evaluating preoperative chemotherapy. Plast. Reconstr. Surg. 65:338-345.

Au, WYW and Raisz, LG. 1972. Drugs toxic to bone. Seminar in Drug Treat. 2:137-146.

Baron, R. 1977. Importance of the intermediate phase between resorption and formation in the measurement and understanding of bone remodelling sequence. In Bone Histomorphometry, PJ Meunier (editor), pp. 179-183. Lab. Paris: Armour Montagu.

Baron, R, Vignery, A, Neff, L, Silverglate, A, and Santa Maria, A. 1983. Processing of undecalcified bone specimens for bone histomorphometry. In Bone Histomorphometry: Techniques and Interpretation, RR Recker (editor), Florida: CRC Press.

Baron, R, Vignery, A, and Tran Van, P. 1980. The significance of lacunar erosion without osteoclasts: Studies on the reversal phase of the remodeling sequence. Metab. Bone Dis. Rel. Res. 2S:35-40.

Bertino, JR, Boothe, BA, Cashmore, A, Bieber, AL, and Sarorelli, AC. 1964. Studies of the inhibition of dihydrofolate reductase by the folate antagonist. J. Biol. Chem. 239:479-485.

Bonarigo, BC and Rubin, P. 1967. Nonunion of pathologic fractures after radiation therapy. Radiology 88:889-898.

Burchardt, H and Enneking, WF. 1978a. Transplantation of bone. Surg. Clin. North America 58:403-427.

Burchardt, H, Glowczewskie, FP, and Enneking, WF. 1983. The effects of adriamycin and methotrexate on the repair of segmental cortical autografts in dogs. J. Bone Joint Surg. 65A:103-108.

Burchardt, H, Jones, H, Glowczewskie, F, Rudner, C, and Enneking, WF. 1978b. Freeze-dried allogeneic segmental cortical-bone grafts in dogs. J. Bone Joint Surg. 60A: 1082-1090.

Cohen, SC, Gabelnick, HL, Johnson, RK, and Goldin, A. 1975a. Effects of cyclophosphamide and adriamycin on the healing of surgical wounds in mice. Cancer 36:1277-1281.

Cohen, SC, Gabelnick, HL, Johnson, RK, and Goldin, A. 1975b. Effects of antineoplastic agents on wound healing in mice. Surgery 78:238-244.

DiMarco, A. 1975. Adriamycin (NSC-123127): Mode and mechanism of action. Cancer Chemother. Rep. 6:91-106.

Enneking, WF, Burchardt, H, Puhl, JJ, and Pietrowski, G. 1975. Physical and biological aspects of repair in dog cortical-bone transplants. J. Bone and Joint Surg. 57-A: 237-252.

Friedlaender, GE, Baron, R, Doganis, AC, Hausman, M, and Kirkwood, J. 1983a. Chronic effects of adriamycin on bone volume in rats. Transact. Orthop. Res. Soc. 8:297.

Friedlaender, GE, Doganis, AC, Baron, R, Kapp, D. 1981. Histomorphometric changes in cancellous bone following palliative doses of radiation. Transact. Orthop. Res. Soc. 6:310.

Friedlaender, GE, Doganis, AC, Baron, R, and Kirkwood, J. 1982. Histomorphometric changes in the rat bone following chronic methotrexate chemotherapy. Transact. Orthop. Res. Soc. 5:98.

Friedlaender, GE, Goodman, A, Hausman, M, and Troiano, N. 1983b. The effects of methotrexate and radiation therapy on histologic aspects of fracture healing. Transact. Orthop. Res. Soc. 8:244.

Friedlaender, GE, Tross, RB, Doganis, AC, Kirkwood, JM, and Baron, R. Effects of chemotherapeutic agents and bone.

I. Short-term methotrexate and doxorubicin (adriamycin) treatment in a rat model. (Submitted for publication.)

Frost, HM. 1980. Skeletal physiology and bone remodeling. In Fundamental and Clinical Bone Physiology, MR Urist (editor), pp. 208-241, Philadelphia: J. B. Lippincott.

Frost, HM. 1977. A method of analysis of trabecular bone dynamics. In Bone Histomorphometry, PJ Meunier (editor), pp. 445-476. Paris: Lab Armour Montagu.

Grant, TT, Eilber, FR, Johnson, EE, and Mirra, JM. 1982. Limb salvaging in osteosarcoma. Presented at the 49th Annual Meeting of the American Academy of Orthopaedic Surgeons, Las Vegas.

Hajj, A, Mnaymneh, W, Ghandur-Mnaymneh, L, and Latta, LL. 1981. The effects of methotrexate on the healing of rat femora. Transact. Orthop. Res. Soc. 6:79.

Hayashi, S and Suit, HO. 1971. Effects of fractionation of radiation doses on callus formation at site of fracture. Radiology 101:181-186.

Hellman, S. 1982. Principles of radiation therapy. In Cancer: Principles and Practice of Oncology. DeVita, VT, Jr, Hellman, S, and Rosenberg, SA (editors), pp. 103-131. Philadelphia: J. B. Lippincott.

Karnofsky, DA and Lacon, CR. 1964. Effects of drugs on skeletal development of the chick embryo. Clin. Orthop. 33:59-79.

Langendorff, HU, Sauer, HD, Schottle, H, Ringe, JD, and Jungbluth, KH. 1981. The influence of cyclophosphamide upon the healing of fractures in the rabbit. Unfallchirurgie 7:231-235.

Mankin, HJ. Personal communication, 1983.

Mankin, HJ, Doppelt, SH, Sullivan, TR, and Tomford, WW. 1982. Osteoarticular and intercalary allograft transplantation in the management of malignant bone tumors. Cancer 50: 613-630.

Nesbit, M, Krivit, W, Heyn, R, and Sharp, H. 1976. Acute and chronic effects of methotrexate on hepatic, pulmonary and skeletal systems. Cancer 37:1048-1057.

O'Regan, S, Melhorn, B, and Neuman, A. 1973. Methotrexate-induced bone pain in childhood leukemia. Am. J. Dis. Child. 126:489-490.

Pelker, RR, Friedlaender, GE, Markham, T, Hausman, M, Doganis, AC, and Panjabi, M. 1983. Effects of adriamycin and methotrexate on fracture healing biomechanics. Transact. Orthop. Soc. 8:186.

Pellet, S, Strong, DM, Temesi, A, and Matthews, JG. 1983. II: Effects of irradiation on frozen corticocancellous bone allograft incorporation and immunogenicity. In Osteochondral Allografts: Biology, Banking and Clinical Applications. Friedlaender, GE, Mankin, HJ and Sell, KW (editors), pp. 353-361. Boston: Little, Brown and Co.

Prosnitz, LR, Lawson, JP, Friedlaender, GE, Farber, LR, and Pezzimenti, JF. 1981. Avascular necrosis of bone in Hodgkin's disease patients treated with combined modality therapy. Cancer 47:2793-2796.

Ragab, A, Frech, R, and Vietti, T. 1970. Osteoporotic fractures secondary to methotrexate therapy of acute leukemia in remission. Cancer 25:580-585.

Robins, PR and Jowsey, J. 1973. Effect of mithramycin on normal and abnormal bone turnover. J. Lab. Clin. Med. 82:576-586.

Singh, S, and Sanyal, AK. 1974. Abnormal patterns of ossification in the hands of foetuses produced by cyclophosphamide administration to pregnant rats. Acta Anat. 89:121-133.

Stanisavljevic, S, and Babcock, AL. 1977. Fractures in children treated with methotrexate for leukemia. Clin. Orthop. 125: 139-144.

Tran Van, P, Vignery, A, and Baron, R. 1982a. An electron microscopic study of the bone-remodeling sequence in the rat. Cell. Tiss. Res. 22S:283-292.

Tran Van, P, Vignery, A, and Baron, R. 1982b. Cellular kinetics of the bone remodeling sequence in the rat. Anat. Rec. 202:445-451.

Tross, RB, Friedlaender, GE, Baron, R, and Panjabi, MM. 1980. The effects of adriamycin and methotrexate on bone remodeling. Transact. Orthop. Res. Soc. 5:223.

Tross, RB, Friedlaender, GE, Baron, R, and Panjabi, MM. 1979. The effects of chemotherapy on bone volume and strength. Transact. Orthop. Res. Soc. 4:262.

Vahlsing, HL, Feringa, ER, Britten, AG, and Kinning, WK. 1965. Dental abnormalities in rats after a single large dose of cyclophosphamide. Cancer Res. 35:2199-2202.

Vietti, T, and Ragab, A. 1975. Complications and total care of the child with acute leukemia. Cancer 35:1007-1014.

Wie, H, Engesaeter, LB, and Beck, EJ. 1979. Effects of cyclophosphamide on mechanical properties of bone and skin in rats. Acta Orthop. Scand. 50:629-634.

23 Soft Tissue Repair and Replacement with Carbon Fiber-Absorbable Polymer Composites

John R. Parsons, Harold Alexander and Andrew B. Weiss

INTRODUCTION

Carbon has been used successfully as an implant material in a number of applications (Benson 1971; von Fraunhofer et al. 1971; Mooney et al. 1974). Jenkins et al. (1977, 1978), Wolter et al. (1977), Neugebauer et al. (1979A, 1979B, 1980), and Claes et al. (1978) have shown that tendons and ligaments can be replaced by filamentous carbon implants which act as scaffolds for the development of new fibrous tissue. Carbon succeeds as a scaffolding material for a number of reasons. It provides mechanical strength on implantation, allowing early return of function. The material is extremely compatible, permitting the ingrowth of new, aligned fibrous tissue. Finally, the carbon fiber may degrade mechanically as the new tissue matures, allowing for the gradual transfer of load to the regrown tissue structure.

Forster et al. (1978) and Jenkins et al. (1977, 1978) used spun carbon fiber tows as replacement anterior cruciate ligaments and medial collateral ligaments in sheep. They have since proceeded to use this raw, uncoated carbon in humans for various ligament reconstruction (Jenkins et al. 1980). Similarly, Wolter et al. (1977), Claes et al. (1978), and Kinzl et al. (1979) used thick woven tows of carbon to replace medial collateral ligaments in sheep and extra-articular knee and ankle ligaments in humans. In the work of these groups, as well as in animal studies conducted by the authors, raw carbon fiber was found to partially fragment during and immediately after the operative procedure. This permitted carbon to migrate from the implant site before the new fibrous tissue could encapsulate it. Carbon fragments were found in the lymph nodes of the animals and it is most likely in the humans into whom the uncoated carbon was implanted.

Although not shown to be detrimental in any way, spread of carbon fiber fragments to nearby lymph nodes is clearly undesirable.

This chapter reports a program of research in which the authors addressed the problem of the mechanical degradation of the brittle filamentous carbon during its implantation and during the early phases of tissue growth. This premature mechanical degradation, and the resulting migration of carbon fragments from the implant site, was largely eliminated by utilizing a composite of carbon fiber and polylactic acid polymer (PLA) or a copolymer of PLA and Poly ε-caprolactone (copolymer). The composite has greatly improved handling characteristics when compared with raw carbon fiber. The composite, in a ribbon-like configuration, was used in a variety of animal models, several of which are reported herein. In these studies, the implant material was successful as a scaffold for the development of new soft tissue. The implants allowed early resumption of activity and eventual growth of new structures histologically and mechanically similar to the natural structures.

The high initial strength, rapid ingrowth, and benign tissue reaction of the composite suggested that this new material might be useful in the treatment of tendon and ligament injuries in humans. Consequently, human clinical trials were initiated. As part of a Food and Drug Administration (FDA) sanctioned multi-center trial, over 250 patients have had implant surgery for the repair of extensor mechanisms, knee ligaments, Achilles tendons, shoulder rotator cuffs, and other soft tissue problems. At this writing, 18 months of follow-up is available on some patients. Early results are encouraging and expanded multi-center trials continue.

MATERIALS AND METHODS

Ligament and Tendon Replacement Materials

Absorbable polymer-filamentous carbon tissue scaffolding ribbons are produced by coating uniaxial filamentous carbon with either PLA or co-polymer. The individual carbon fiber tows typically contain 10,000 fibers, 6 to 10 microns in diameter. The fibers are pyrolized from a polymer fiber precursor. The resulting material is almost pure elemental carbon with mechanical strength and rigidity greater than steel. It has a modulus of over 200 GPa and an ultimate tensile strength of approximately 2.5 GPa.

The polylactic acid polymer is produced from L(-) lactide. This cyclic diester, the lactide of lactic acid, polymerizes by an ionic ring-opening addition mechanism to a high polymer which can be cast into films, spun into fibers, or extruded into rods similar to the industrial polyesters, such as Dacron. It is a thermoplastic and can also be dissolved readily in a number of solvents. Poly ε-caprolactone alone is similar in character. However, the co-polymer of PLA and Poly ε-caprolactone is, interestingly, elastomeric in nature. As such, it is tough and flexible.

Fabrication of coated fiber tows is accomplished by first preparing PLA or co-polymer solution. The fibers are coated with the polymer by solution dipping or spraying. For attachment to soft tissues, suture needles are attached to the ends of the fiber tows. The device is then sterilized in ethylene oxide gas, through a dry heating cycle, or with appropriate gamma irradiation techniques.

The biocompatibility of carbon fiber and polylactic acid and polycaprolactone have previously been demonstrated. Finely divided carbon particles have been shown to be well tolerated; they do not cause formation of foreign body giant cells in the synovial lining of joints, nor do they produce cytotoxic effects (Haubold 1977). Studies of tissue tolerance of carbon materials by Christel et al. (1980) have also indicated that carbon materials are well accepted by connective tissues. Filamentous carbon has been used as a component of implants currently in human use, and studies in rabbits and mice indicated good short and long-term biocompatibility of this material. The question of foreign body or physically-induced carcinogenicity was addressed in studies using carbon fiber connective tissue implants conducted by Jenkins (1982) and Claes (1982). To date, investigators found no abnormal tumor formation in their studies.

The short and long-term response to polylactic acid has been studied by Cutright et al. (1971), Brady et al. (1973), and Kulkarni et al. (1966). Polylactic acid has been found to be a biocompatible material that elicits little immunological response, probably due to the absence of peptide linkages. It biodegrades by undergoing hydrolytic de-esterification to lactic acid, a normal metabolic intermediate. The compatibility of poly ε-caprolactone has been studied by a number of researchers (Rice et al. 1978; Pitt et al. 1981). The polymer and its degradation product, hydroxycaporic acid, are compatible. Biological response to and degradation of PLA/polycaprolactone co-polymers have been investigated by Schimdler et al. (1977).

Canine Patellar Tendon Study

To investigate the response of this tissue scaffold replacement material in a full load-bearing situation, a canine patellar tendon study was conducted in which patellar tendons were removed from 14 adult beagle dogs (Alexander et al. 1981). In one series of 6 dogs, two received patellar tendon prostheses of PLA-coated filamentous carbon tows in one leg and the other leg was unoperated, 2 received prostheses of uncoated carbon in one leg and the other leg was unoperated, and 2 received PLA-carbon prostheses in one leg and nylon suture prostheses in the other. These 6 dogs were sacrificed at 2 months post-implantation. An identical series of six dogs were sacrificed at four months post-implantation. Two dogs with PLA-carbon prostheses in one leg and one leg unoperated were sacrificed at one year post-implantation for a total of 14. All of the implants were passed through drill holes in the tibia and through the quadriceps tendon above the patella to form a continuous figure-of-eight repair (Figure 23.1). The implant was tensioned manually such that the distance between the original tendon insertions was maintained. The ends of implants were tied to each other. Post-operatively, the animals were unprotected and allowed to move freely in their cages. Upon sacrifice, half of the specimens were subjected to mechanical testing in a tensile mode, while the other half were histologically evaluated.

Rabbit Achilles Tendon Study

Another factor in the evaluation of the utility of the composite is its ability to encourage rapid development of secure soft tissue anastomosis. A study was conducted in 54 adult male rabbits (Parsons et al. 1983a). In 48 rabbits, the proximal third of the Achilles tendon was removed and replaced by either a PLA-carbon composite, a carbon co-polymer composite, or a control PLA-Dacron fiber composite. The anastomoses were achieved by use of a new anastomosis technique, the locking weave, which allows the replacement tendon to act as its own suture. This yields a strong juncture between the small diameter composite tendon and the larger diameter muscle or tendon remnant (Figure 23.2). Six rabbits underwent sham procedures in which the proximal third of the Achilles tendon was removed and no replacement was provided. In all animals, the contralateral limb served as a control. No immobilization was applied to the operated limbs, and the animals were free to move about their cages. The animals were sacrificed according to the

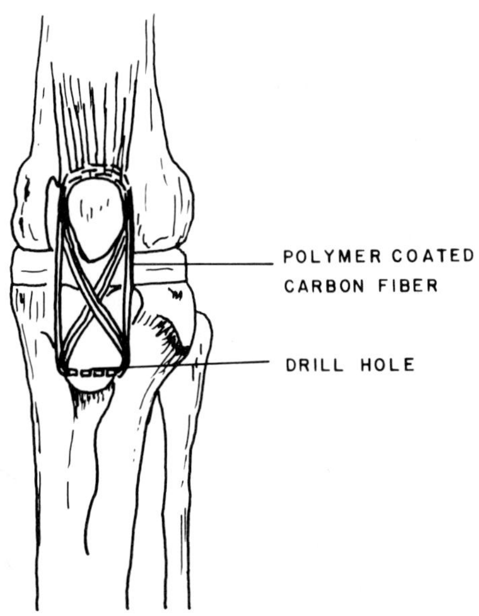

FIGURE 23.1 Patellar tendon replacement with PLA-coated filamentous carbon tows.

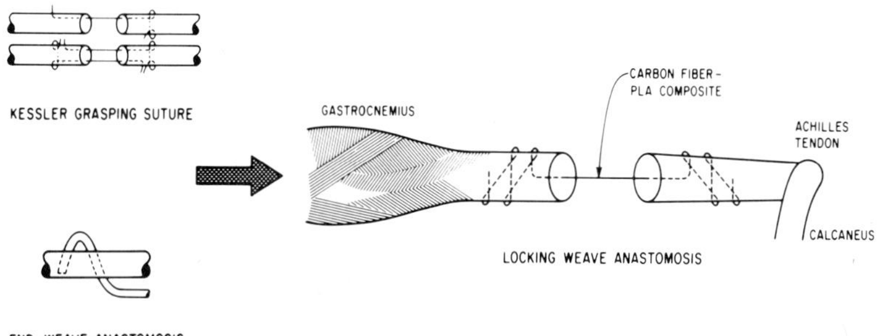

FIGURE 23.2 The techniques of the Kessler grasping suture and the end-weave anastomosis are combined to form the locking-weave anastomosis.

TABLE 23.1

Sacrifice Schedule, Rabbit Achilles Tendon Study

	Acute	1 Wk.	2 Wks.	4 Wks.	8 Wks.	16 Wks.
Carbon -PLA	1	3	3	3	3	3
Carbon-copolymer	1	3	3	3	3	3
Dacron-PLA	1	3	3	3	3	3
Sham	1	1	1	1	1	1

Legend: Sacrifice schedule for rabbits used in the Achilles tendon repair model. One rabbit from every group of three was sacrificed for histology; the other two were used for mechanical tests. All "acute" and "sham" rabbits were mechanically tested.

schedule shown in Table 23.1. In each group, at each time period (except post-op), one animal was sacrificed strictly for histology and 2 were mechanically tested. All "shams" and all "post-ops" were mechanically tested. The mechanical test was a uniaxial test to failure.

Canine Medial Collateral Ligament Study

In this study (Parsons et al. 1981), the medial collateral ligament of adult male beagle dogs was chosen for replacement with the composite material. Under appropriate anesthesia and using sterile technique, the medial aspect of the knee was exposed. The medial collateral was excised from its origins on the femur and tibia. In addition, the medial side of the joint capsule was excised to produce a gross valgus instability. The implant was placed across the joint in an anatomic position and secured using soft tissue attachment techniques developed in other experiments (see Rabbit Achilles Tendon). The contralateral knee served as a control. A second group of animals served as "shams." These dogs were subjected to identical surgery, only no implant was installed. The surgical wounds were closed in layers in a standard fashion and a bulky "Jones-type" dressing was applied. This dressing provided some immobilization and remained in place for 2 weeks.

After periods of 4 weeks, 8 weeks, 12 weeks, and 26 weeks, the dogs were sacrificed and the regrown medial collateral structures were tested mechanically. All mechanical tests were conducted on a custom MTS servo-hydraulic test machine. The mechanical test procedure included a low force cantilever bending test and a uniaxial tension test to failure. The low force cantilever bending was designed to simulate a clinical valgus stress test for stability. The measure of stability was the opening of the joint at a calculated ligament force of 25 N (Figure 23.3). The joint was then mounted so a uniaxial tension test could be performed to determine ultimate strengths of the regrown tissue. For this test, all ligamentous and capsular structures were cut, except those in the medial collateral position. The ligaments were tested to failure and the ultimate strengths and slope of the load-elongation curves recorded.

Canine Anterior Cruciate Ligament Study

To evaluate the growth of tissue into the implant within a synovial joint, a canine anterior cruciate replacement study was initiated (Alexander et al. 1982). This study involved 8 different experiments utilizing 73 dogs. Various combinations

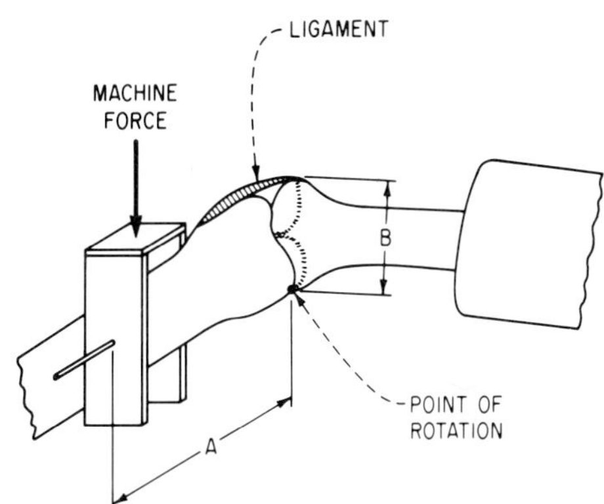

FIGURE 23.3 Cantilever Bending Test—This low force, non-destructive mechanical test simulates a clinical valgus stress test. Laxity is measured as the opening of the joint in millimeters at a calculated ligament force of 25 N.

of carbon fiber, polylactic acid polymer, autogenous tissue structures, and fixation methods were investigated. The experiments involved: 1) polymer-coated carbon fibers alone, 2) fascia lata detached proximally, reinforced with PLA-coated carbon fiber, 3) fascia lata alone, 4) PLA-coated carbon fiber that was implanted subcutaneously for 2 weeks and then transplanted to the joint, 5) uncoated carbon fibers alone, 6) free tendon graft, flexor halluxes longus reinforced with polymer-coated carbon fiber, 7) primary repair of a severed anterior cruciate ligament with PLA-coated carbon fiber, and 8) medial third patellar tendon graft reinforced with PLA-coated carbon fiber.

The animals were immobilized in a cast for 2 weeks. They were then periodically evaluated for clinical laxity. After periods of 4, 8, 12, and 26 weeks, the dogs were sacrificed and the ligament structures were examined grossly and tested mechanically. The mechanical test involved a machine controlled in vitro anterior drawer test to establish joint laxity, ligament stiffness, and ultimate strength.

Synovial Joint Debris Study

The question of carbon fragmentation and the consequences of such debris residing in the body for long periods remains troublesome. This is particularly true when carbon debris may be released within a synovial joint as with the repair or replacement of a cruciate ligament. In this environment, carbon fiber debris may cause direct abrasion of the articular cartilage. Alternately, the carbon fragments may be picked up by the synovial lining of the joint. Particulate matter residing in the synovium can produce a synovitis. Often a consequence of synovitis is degradation of the articular cartilage through release of enzymes by the inflamed synovium.

In this study (Parsons et al. 1983b), the consequence of carbon fiber debris residing within the rabbit knee joint was examined. As a positive control, a well-defined magnesium tetrasilicate (talc) particle-induced synovitis model was used (Gershuni et al. 1980).

A canine knee joint with a failed carbon fiber anterior cruciate ligament was available for histologic study. From examination of the synovium, a carbon fragment size distribution was obtained (range = 10ν - 80ν, mean = 50ν).

Carbon fragments having a similar size distribution were produced. Talc particles having a similar distribution were obtained commercially.

In the right knee of white New Zealand rabbits, 1.0×10^{-4} kg of sterile carbon particles suspended in 1.0×10^{-3} M^3 of saline was injected. In groups of 5, these animals were sacrificed at 4 days, 2 weeks, 4 weeks, 8 weeks, and 16 weeks post-injection.

The medial articular surfaces of the knees of these rabbits were tested mechanically using an indentation technique. The lateral articular surfaces and synovium were examined histologically.

Additional groups of rabbits were treated in a similar fashion. These groups of rabbits, however, received an injection of 1.0×10^{-4} kg of talc particles in 1.0×10^{-3} M^3 of saline in the right knee. These groups were sacrificed at 4 days, 2 weeks, and 4 weeks.

Early Clinical Trials

After extensive pre-clinical testing, this implant system was placed in Phase I clinical trials with one of the authors (ABW) as sole investigator for a one-year period. It has recently been approved for Phase II multi-center clinical trials. Those trials are now ongoing at 15 centers around the United States and Europe. The implant in clinical use is a double-armed uniaxial tow of 10,000 fibers coated with PLA. More recently, a co-polymer coating has been adopted to further improve surgical handling characteristics. The system has been used initially with soft tissue attachment only, using the locking-weave anastomosis shown in the animal studies. More recently, bone attachment has been accomplished through the use of a newly designed composite material attachment device (expandable rivet).

At our institution, substantial data has been amassed on 89 patients. Of these 89 patients, 72 have had repairs about the knee, 8 have had Achilles tendon repairs, and 9 have had other repairs. The majority of the injuries treated were old, chronic injuries (87%). The age of injury ranged from acute to 22 years, with an average of 4.8 years. The mechanism of injury was sports activity in 31% of the patients, vehicular accident in 26%, job related in 20%, and miscellaneous in 21%. The patients had 0 to 13 previous operations, with the average number of previous operations being 2. The operations performed were lateral knee stabilization, medial knee stabilization, Achilles tendon repair, extensor mechanism repair, and collateral plus cruciate ligament repair.

For the lateral knee repairs, the material was sutured through the soft tissues on the lateral side of the knee, replacing the function of the lateral collateral ligament. The locking-weave anastomosis, as demonstrated in the animal studies, was used. Medial knee stabilization was accomplished in a similar way.

Achilles tendon repairs have been performed by weaving the material through the distal and proximal remnants of the damaged Achilles tendon exactly as was done in the rabbit study.

Extensor mechanisms were repaired in a similar fashion as that done in the dog study. The material was woven through the quadriceps tendon above the patella, using the patella as a rip stop. Then it was woven through the tissues to the tibial tuberosity. If necessary, it was passed through a drill hole in the tibial tuberosity.

Cruciate ligament repair has been done using the carbon composite as a stent in conjunction with either the iliotibial band or the medial third of the patella tendon as a soft tissue cover for the carbon fiber. Utilizing the iliotibial band, the composite is passed through the iliotibial band tissue which is then tubed around the implant, completely enveloping it. The composite and tubed tissue are then placed in a plastic tendon passer which is threaded "over the top" into the joint and through a tibial drill hole (Figure 23.4). After the implant is in place, the plastic tube is pulled back, leaving only natural tissue exposed within the joint. This avoids carbon fiber ever being presented to the joint tissue. The implant tows may then be passed around an expandable rivet and tightened. The rivet central pin is driven home, locking the fibers in place and maintaining the ligament tension. As an extra precaution, the fibers are then passed through the soft tissues using the soft tissue anastomosis technique. In essence, the composite is used to augment a standard repair procedure.

The patients have been evaluated through an orthopaedic evaluation scheme rating stability, pain, function, strength, range of motion, and deformity for a total score from 0 to 100. They have also been evaluated on a Cybex isokinetic testing machine with percent deficits noted for both high and low speed measurements. Each patient has been evaluated pre-operatively, at 3 months, 6 months, 9 months, and 1 year. Evaluation every 6 months is planned thereafter to a total of 5 years.

RESULTS

Canine Patellar Tendon Replacement

All of the knees initially regained good function. However, with time, 2 of the raw carbon fiber prostheses became infected

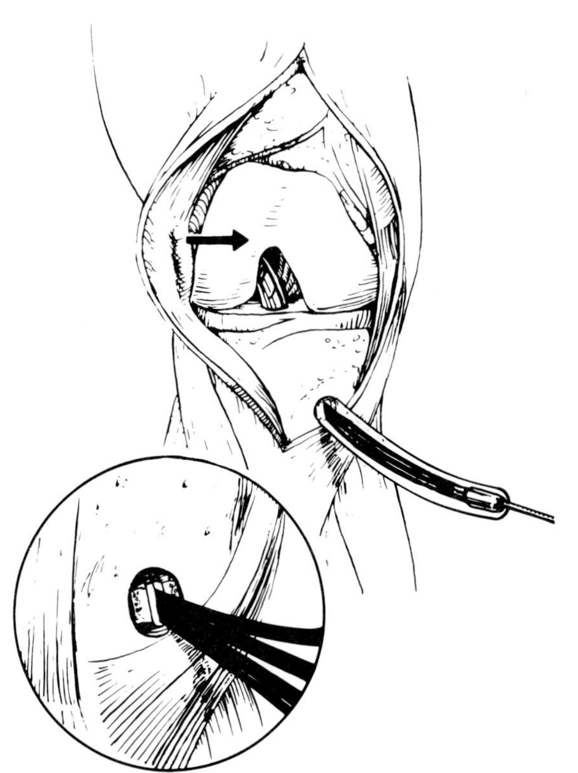

FIGURE 23.4
Anterior cruciate ligament replacement using polymer coated carbon reinforced iliotibial band. Implant is shown still inside plastic tendon passer after having been passed through the joint.

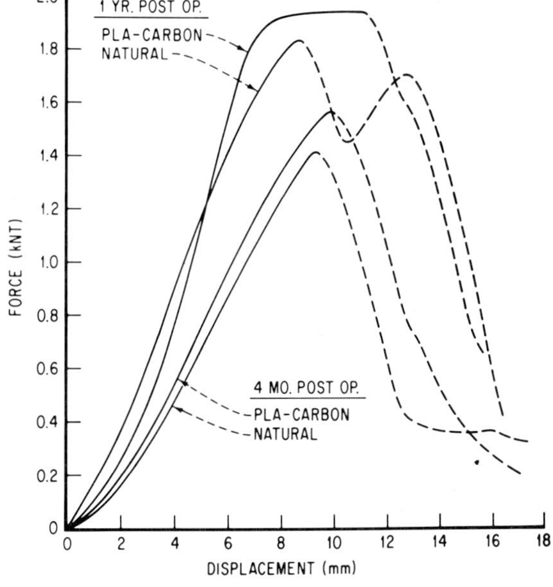

FIGURE 23.5
Load-extension response comparison for regrown and contralateral natural patellar tendons at 4 and 12 months.

due to migration of the carbon. This unprotected, brittle carbon was found to migrate from its implantation area and in some cases formed sinus tracks through the skin.

The dogs with nylon prostheses ultimately developed limps and passive range of motion was restricted in flexion.

The PLA-carbon prostheses appeared to provide a more consistent return of function than did the other 2 types. Passive range of motion was normal. In particular, the dogs retained for 12 months both walked with no discernable limp.

The results of mechanical tests are presented in Table 23.2. The mechanical tests appeared to be valid in that no slippage was detected and the specimens all failed within the central tendon region, away from the grips or tibial attachment.

The PLA-carbon regrown tendons were found to have mechanical properties similar to the contralateral unoperated patella tendons. For both the 4 month and 12 month data, shown in Figure 23.5, the slopes of the force-extension curves of the regrown and the natural patella tendons are quite similar. The regrown tendons both have slightly higher ultimate strengths due presumably to some still intact carbon fibers. It appears that the soft tissue remodeling process has resulted in a regrown structure almost mechanically identical to the original patella tendon.

Absolute values of strength and stiffness for the raw carbon fiber replacements were somewhat lower than for the composite replacements. However, on a paired basis they appeared to be similar to their contralateral normal controls.

The nylon suture prosthesis was successful in that scar tissue growth in combination with the intact suture resulted in acceptable levels of strength. However, mechanical testing suggested most of the load was being carried by the nylon suture. Failure was always preceeded by a loud "snap." The broken suture, which was not biologically attached to the tissue, would slide out of the tissue as the much weaker tissue gradually failed.

Upon sacrifice, gross histological evaluation indicated that the PLA-carbon fiber tendon replacements were freely moveable with no adhesions to adjacent tissue. The carbon was well contained within the regrown tissue. The tissue appeared grossly normal. By contrast, 2 of the 4 unprotected carbon prostheses were clearly infected and showed a serous discharge. Carbon fiber had spread to the adjacent subcutaneous tissue. The multi-stranded nylon suture prosthesis elicited an intense fibrous tissue reaction with the development of bulky, space-filling granulation tissue. This tissue reaction most probably led to the unsatisfactory functional results of these replacements.

TABLE 23.2

Test Results of Study Specimens

Dog	Sacrifice (mo)	Leg	Prosthesis	Stiffness (N/mm)	Ultimate Strength (N)
1	2	L	None	157	1350
		R	PLA-Carbon	Error in Mech, Test Specimen Destroyed	
2	4	L	None	272	1545
		R	PLA-Carbon	267	1420
5	2	L	None	160	1290
		R	Unprotected Carbon	150	960
6	4	L	None	154	780
		R	Unprotected Carbon	150	780
9	2	L	Nylon Suture	211	1800
		R	PLA-Carbon	167	1380
10	4	L	Nylon Suture	200	1210
		R	PLA-Carbon	208	1560
13	12	L	None	267	1825
		R	PLA-Carbon	367	1940

Legend: Mechanical test results from the study of canine patellar tendon replacement.

Microhistology of the carbon-PLA replacements at 2 months and 4 months revealed that developing fibrous tissue has well-infiltrated the implant, aligning along the axis of the fibers. This infiltration of tissue has spread the fibers and greatly increased the cross-sectional area of the original carbon fiber tow. The implant was well tolerated. No inflammatory or giant cell reaction was evident. At 12 months (Figure 23.6), the new tissue was similar in appearance to natural aligned patellar tendon collagen with the exception of the embedded carbon fibers. The fibers appear somewhat fragmented, but completely contained. It is unclear whether the fibers had fractures *in vivo* or if the fractured appearance is a sectioning artifact. The microhistology of the raw carbon replacements which did not become infected was similar to that of the composite replacements. In contrast, microhistology of the nylon implants demonstrated at both 2 months and 4 months a disorganized, space-filling granulation tissue.

Scanning electron micrographs of the central tendon region of the patellar tendons regrown about the carbon-PLA scaffold demonstrated extensive ingrowth. A collagen fiber network similar to that of the corresponding region of a normal patellar tendon was found (Figure 23.7). The developing collagenous network appeared to grow about the carbon fibers as it would about a naturally occurring collagen fiber bundle. The normal collagen fiber bundles of the patellar tendon of the dog were similar in size to the individual fibers.

Bone attachment is a serious concern in all ligament and tendon replacement attempts. At 2 months, the drill holes in all the tibias were found to have enlarged. However, at 4 months and 12 months, no additional enlargement was found. At 12 months, microhistological evaluation of tissue showed bone growing in and around the carbon fibers in both the uncoated and polymer-coated replacements. This finding is similar to that reported by Minns and Flynn (1978).

By contrast, the tissue regrown in the bony cavity around the multi-stranded nylon suture material was unorganized granulation tissue. There was no bony growth about the nylon suture and a complete lack of attachment was apparent.

Rabbit Achilles Tendon

Prior to testing it was noted that no composite tendons pulled out of their anastomoses and none had ruptured. There were no infections. The rabbits actively used their limbs by the

FIGURE 23.6 Longitudinal view of connective tissue growth about the PLA-carbon prosthesis after 12 months. (1000x)

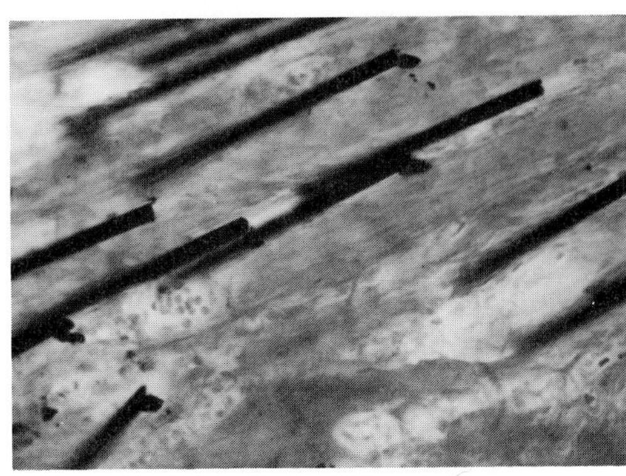

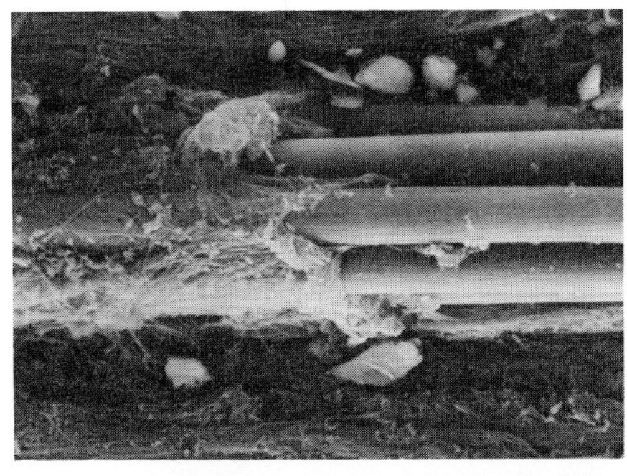

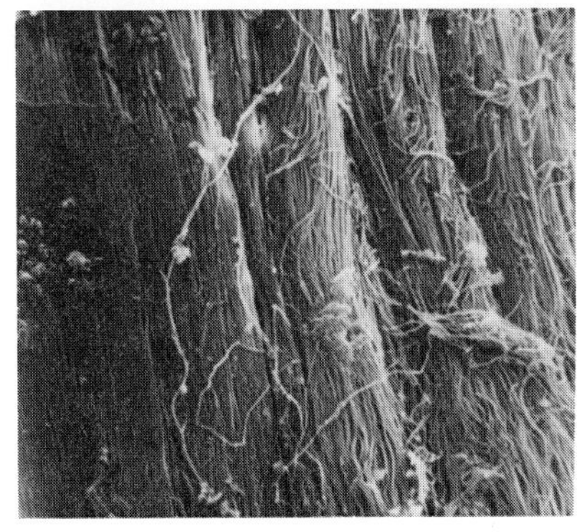

FIGURE 23.7 SEM comparison of natural and regrown tendons 7 months post-implantation. a) A regrown tendon. Tissue has been stripped away to expose carbon fibers. b) Natural.

fourth post-operative day. Sham procedures resulted in a slower, less predictable return of function with considerable muscle atrophy.

The unoperated gastrocnemius mechanisms of the control limbs failed in tension by rupture through the belly of the gastrocnemius muscle. The average force of failure was 399 N.

At all time periods, the mechanical response of PLA-carbon implants and co-polymer-carbon implants was equivalent (Table 23.3). Consequently, the mechanical data from carbon fiber composites has been lumped together. During the early post-operative period up to 2 weeks, the gastrocnemius mechanisms with carbon composite implants failed by pullout of the carbon composite from the proximal soft tissue anastomosis. At 4 weeks, 8 weeks, and 12 weeks, the carbon composites failed via a mechanism similar to that of the contralateral normal. That is, failure of the gastrocnemius well proximal to the repair site. The Dacron composites at all time periods were weaker than the repairs receiving carbon fiber implants. Further, the Dacron composites continued to fail through the area of resection at all times.

The shams always failed by rupture of the paratendinous soft tissue in the region of resected tendon. The mechanical behavior of carbon composites, Dacron composites, and shams are illustrated in Figure 23.8.

Examined grossly, the carbon fiber composites and the Dacron composites were rapidly incorporated into the proximal and distal soft tissue anastomoses. At one week post-operatively

TABLE 23.3

Achilles Tendon/Muscle Unit, Strength (Newtons) vs. Time

Time, Weeks	1	2	4	8	12
Carbon/PLA	119	185	329*	230	310*
Carbon/Co-polymer	124	186	294*	290*	315*

* Average value within 95% C.I. for normal Achilles tendon/muscle unit strength (339 + 50N).

Legend: Rabbit Achilles tendon/muscle unit strength (Newtons) vs. time. The repair strengths of carbon fiber-PLA and carbon fiber co-polymer are equivalent.

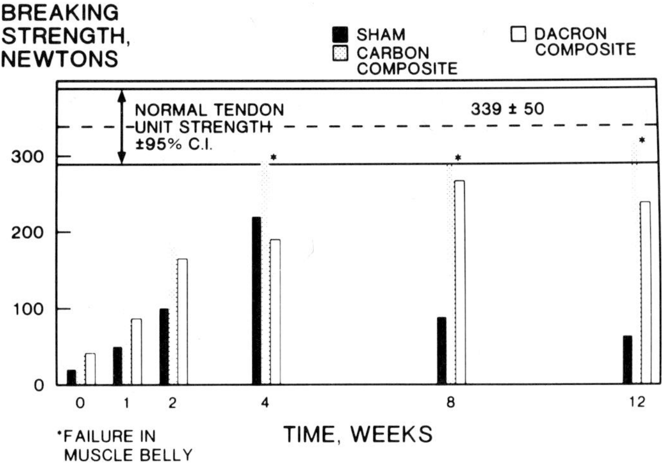

FIGURE 23.8 Ultimate strength vs. time for rabbit Achilles tendon repairs using carbon fiber absorbable polymer composites and Dacron fiber absorbable polymer composites. The strength of sham procedures (scar) is shown for comparison.

in the area of the resected tendon, a large volume of space-filling soft tissue had formed about the implants. In the regions of anastomosis, the implants had likewise been covered with tissue. At one week, the appearance of the sham procedure specimen was similar to that of the carbon and Dacron implant specimens.

All implant specimens at two weeks post-operatively had increased volumes of enveloping soft tissue. This tissue appeared to be slightly more organized. The sham specimen appearance was similar.

For the implant groups and the sham group, surrounding soft tissue appeared to reach a maximum volume at four weeks post-operatively.

Eight weeks post-operatively, remodeling of the soft tissues about all the implants had begun to occur. The volume of soft tissue in the area of resected tendon had been reduced. This was true of both the carbon and Dacron implant specimens and the sham specimens. The tissue about the implants was firm and organized; whereas, the tissue of the sham specimen was thin and attenuated. In all animals, some muscle atrophy was evident but this was not quantitated.

Soft tissue remodeling progressed rapidly. At 12 weeks post-operatively, the gastrocnemius systems with implants (carbon or Dacron) closely resembled their unoperated contralateral controls (Figure 23.9). The tissue in the region of anastomosis appeared normal. Sham specimens had only a filmy, attenuated tissue in the region of resected tendon.

At one week post-operatively, microscopic studies revealed a disorganized space-filling tissue forming about the area of all implants. Implant specimens demonstrated little ingrowth into the composite materials at this time.

At 2 weeks, the surrounding tissue appeared more organized. Some tissue ingrowth was noted about the periphery of both the carbon composite and the Dacron composite. Minimal foreign body response was apparent with the carbon implant, whereas the Dacron elicited a stronger response.

After four weeks, infiltration of tissue in the implants was significant in the anastomosis region as well as in the area of resected tendon. This tissue ingrowth caused separation of the carbon fibers or Dacron fibers and hence a volumetric expansion of the composite implants.

Tissue remodeling after eight weeks was extensive. All the implants were fully infiltrated with oriented collagenous tissue. The volume of scar tissue in the region of resected tendon was reduced. Fibroblasts about the implants appeared mature and well aligned.

Tissue remodeling after 12 weeks of implantation was even more pronounced. With both carbon and Dacron, the volume of collagenous tissue making up the regrown tendon section appeared normal. The carbon fiber composite was completely infiltrated (Figure 23.10).

Canine Medial Collateral Ligament

All knees with implants healed uneventfully with no infections. All joints appeared to have a full range of motion and no lameness was detected. Gross inspection of the implants after 4 weeks <u>in vivo</u> revealed an implant infiltrated with, and covered by, collagenous tissue. There was no obvious spread of carbon fiber beyond the initial site of implantation. The implants examined after 8 weeks, 12 weeks, and 26 weeks were similar in appearance. There were, however, increasing amounts of collagenous tissue about the implants with increasing time <u>in vivo</u>. No adverse reactions were noted. Similarly, animals having had sham procedures healed uneventfully. Gross inspection of the site of ligament and capsule resection revealed healing with a space-filling scar tissue.

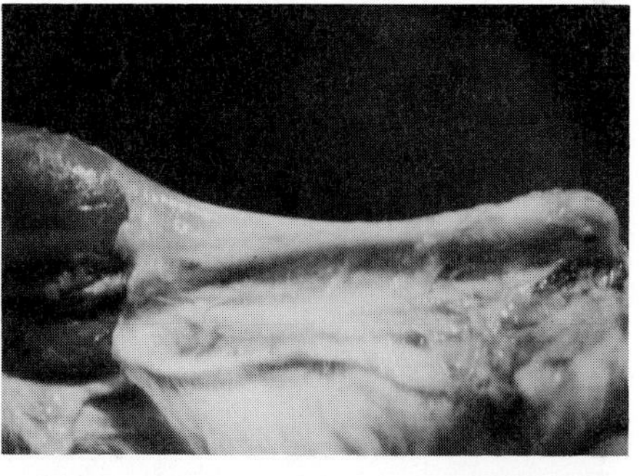

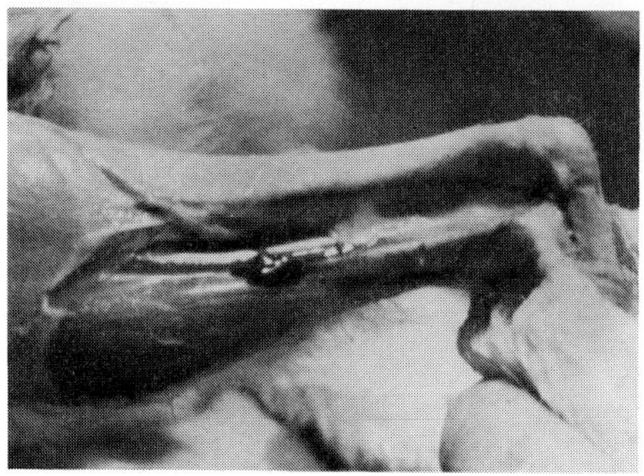

FIGURE 23.9 Gastrocnemius systems in situ. a) A normal rabbit gastrocnemius system. b) A rabbit gastrocnemius system twelve weeks following implantation of the carbon-PLA composite.

After 26 weeks *in vivo*, infiltration of tissue into the implant was significant. This tissue ingrowth caused separation of the carbon fibers and, hence, a volumetric expansion of the composite. Histologic appearance was similar to that of the rabbit Achilles tendon at 12 weeks. Viewing under polarized light revealed no trace of residual polymer. The tissue reaction to the implant was remarkably benign in terms of foreign body inflammatory response.

For each time period the sham and implant groups contained 4 animals. It is difficult to determine with certainty the statistical significance of alterations in mechanical behavior based on samples this small. For this reason, the mechanical data are presented strictly as mean values. The contralateral control joints of these animals, on the other hand, represent a large group (N = 32). Thus, for comparison, mean values and 95% confidence intervals are presented for this group.

The stability of all joints was evaluated quantitatively in a low force cantilever bending test that simulates a clinical valgus

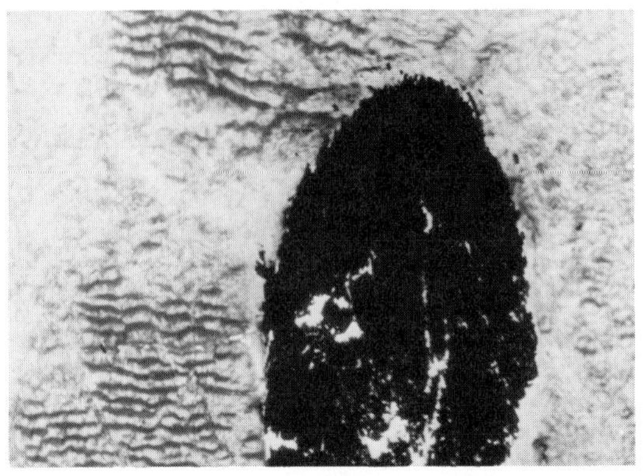

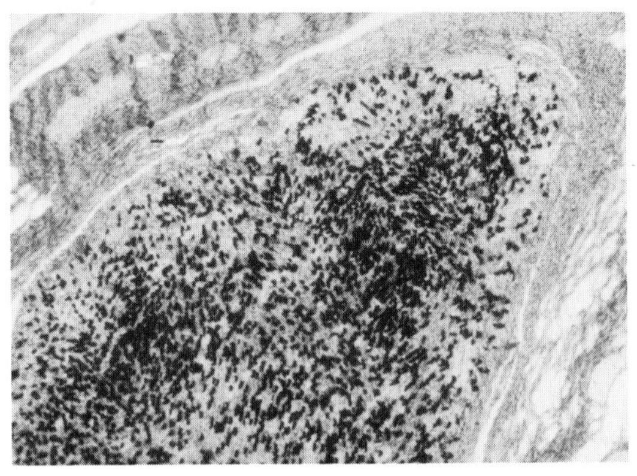

FIGURE 23.10 Microhistology of the carbon-PLA Achilles tendon implants. a) Cross-section of the implant at the level of the myotendinous anastomosis at one week. There is little tissue ingrowth. The carbon remains in intimate contact with the surrounding soft tissue. There is minimal inflammatory response (200x). b) Cross-section of the implant at the level of the myotendinous anastomosis at 12 weeks. There is significant tissue ingrowth spreading the individual carbon fibers of the implant. The ingrown tissue is highly cellular. There is minimal foreign body or inflammatory response present. This tissue ingrowth provides a secure physiologic bond between the carbon-fiber scaffold and surrounding soft tissue.

stress test. The measure of stability was the laxity, or "opening," of the joint in millimeters at a calculated ligament force of 25 N. The results of this non-destructive mechanical test are shown in Figure 23.11. At all time periods, the knees with implants were more stable than were the sham knees.* In fact, the mean laxity of the joints with implants fell very near or within the 95% confidence interval of the mean for all contralateral normal joints.

Following the non-destructive cantilever bending tests, the joints were positioned so that a uniaxial tension test could be performed. All ligamentous and capsular structures were cut, except for a 1 cm band regrown in the medial collateral position. In this configuration the regrown structures were tested to failure and the ultimate strengths and slope of the load-elongation curves recorded. Figure 23.12 compares the ultimate strengths of medial collateral ligaments regrown about the composite implants and scar regrown in the sham procedure. At all times, the mean ultimate strengths of implant groups were higher than those of the sham group. The mean strengths of the implant groups rose monotonically over the entire period of implantation. A strength three-quarters that of normal was present at 26 weeks. This strength is well beyond the "working" range of the normal canine MCL. The tissue regrown following the sham procedure remained weaker, never achieving strengths equivalent to the implants.

Stiffness of the implant system also increased with time (Figure 23.13). After 26 weeks <u>in vivo</u> the implant group had a mean stiffness 90% that of normal. The sham groups for all time periods displayed mean stiffness values less than those of the corresponding implant groups.

Canine Anterior Cruciate Ligament

The complete results of this study were recently presented (Alexander et al. 1982). In clinical evaluation, almost all of the dogs had minimal anterior drawer when compared to their

---

*The behavior of the implant group in terms of joint stability was so different from that of the sham ($p < 0.01$, Student's t-test) that assignment of statistical significance seems justified despite the small number ($N = 4$) of experimental animals per group.

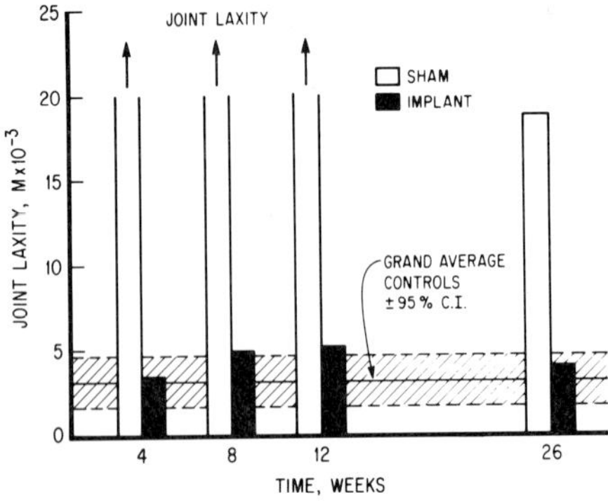

FIGURE 23.11 Medial Collateral Joint Laxity—These measurements were made using a low force, non-destructive cantilever bending test which simulates a clinical valgus stress test. Laxity was defined as the opening of the joint in millimeters at a calculated ligament force of 25 N.

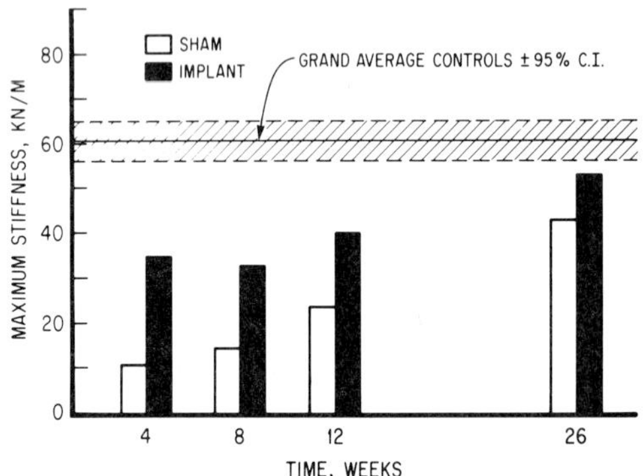

FIGURE 23.12 Medial Collateral Ultimate Strength—Ultimate strength of the regrown structures was determined in a uniaxial tensile test. All ligament and capsular structures were cut except a 1 cm band in the medial collateral position.

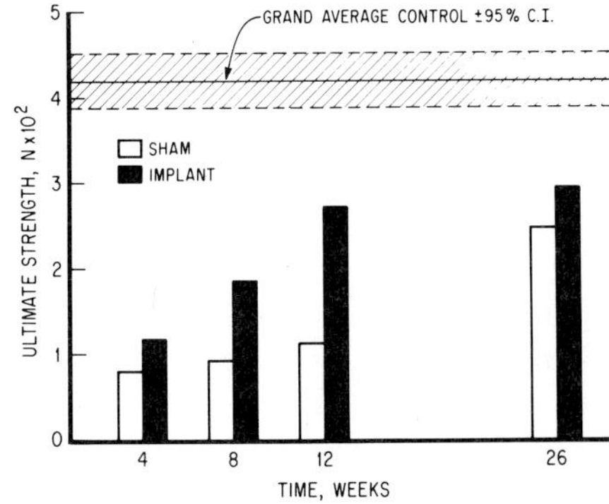

FIGURE 23.13 Medial Collateral Maximum Stiffness—The maximum stiffness of the regrown structures is the maximum slope of the force-elongation curve generated in the uniaxial tensile test.

contralateral normal legs. However, upon sacrifice it was found that, in many instances, this was due to hypertrophy of the medial capsule. This hypertrophy appears to be a natural reaction to anterior cruciate insufficiency in the canine. Gross histological examination provided extremely variable results. For the early time periods in all experiments (less than 8 weeks) and for the later time periods in the fiber reinforced autogenous graft experiments, a structurally sound regrown anterior cruciate ligament was noted. However, for later time periods in the non-autogenous graft experiments, a thin, whispy tissue structure was found.

Mechanical testing indicated high laxity, low stiffness, and low ultimate strength for the non-autogenous graft experiments. The reinforced autogenous graft experiments produced better results. This was particularly true for the primary repairs, for the repairs using the central one-third of the patellar tendon, and the flexor halluxes longus repairs. However, long term these too were only marginally successful with some joint laxity developing and ultimate strengths of 400-500 Newtons (compared with 1300-1400 Newtons for the contralateral normals). We (the authors) have abandoned the canine cruciate as a viable cruciate model.

Synovial Joint Debris

No carbon or talc particles were seen to be embedded in the cartilage layer. Instead, most particulate matter appeared to reside in the synovium, particularly in the supra-patellar region and posterior aspects of the knee.

Histologically, all positive controls revealed talc particles in the synovium. These birefringent particles are easily identified under polarized light. Throughout the study, these particles elicited a strong inflammatory response in the synovial tissue directly adjacent to the particles. The cartilage from these knees demonstrated some loss of metachromasia at 2 weeks and 4 weeks. This loss of metachromasia (and presumably proteoglycan) was most prevalent near the surface of the cartilage, but varied greatly from animal to animal.

Carbon fiber particles also elicited an inflammatory response from the synovium throughout the study period. The response was relatively mild in comparison to that produced by talc. The cartilage from these joints appeared to be normal.

At 2 weeks, the talc induced synovitis had maximally altered the measured mechanical parameters. At 4 weeks, the talc synovitis appeared to be resolving and mechanical parameters began to approach normal.

Throughout the 16-week study, the cartilage from knees with carbon fiber debris appeared to be mechanically normal. Of the parameters measured, none was significantly different ($p < 0.05$) from contralateral controls.

Early Clinical Trials

Since the study is more than 2 years old, some results are now available. Microhistologically one sees collagen grown around the carbon fibers very similar to that experienced in the animal testing. A scanning electron micrograph of tissue grown in the patellar tendon of one patient (Figure 23.14) shows this very vividly. Grossly and through arthroscopy, regrown tissue structures have been identified. This ACL replaced by PLA-carbon reinforced central third of the patellar tendon demonstrates this point six months post-operatively (Figure 23.15).

To illustrate the progress of the patients (most of whom are knee patients), the orthopaedic evaluation of all 72 patients having received implants about the knee are summarized in Table 23.4.

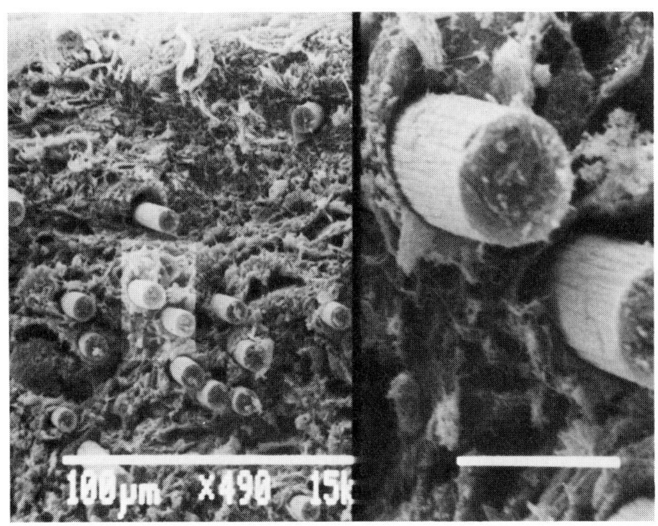

FIGURE 23.14 Scanning electron micrograph of tissue from a human patellar tendon replacement, six months post-operatively.

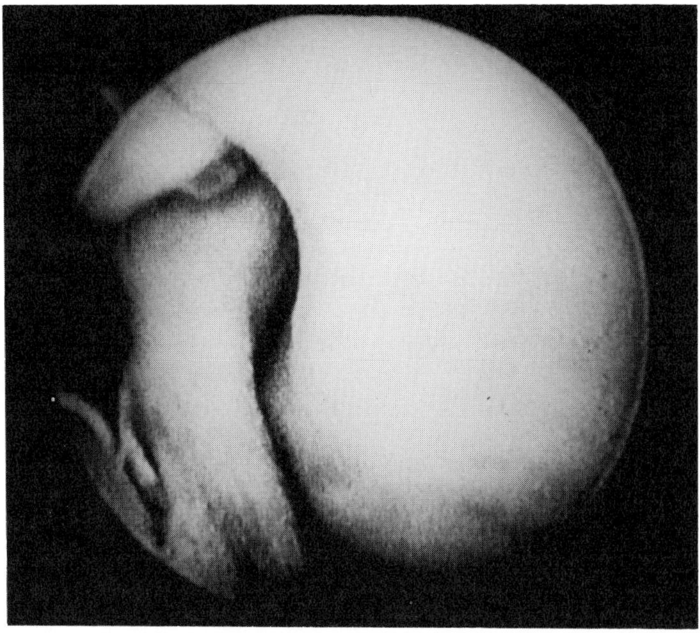

FIGURE 23.15 Arthroscopic view of a patellar tendon graft reinforced with polymer coated carbon fiber used as an anterior cruciate ligament replacement. Six months post-operatively.

TABLE 23.4

Orthopaedic Evaluation, Knees

Category	Evaluation Time					
	Pre-Op	3 Mos.	6 Mos.	9 Mos.	12 Mos.	18 Mos.
Stability	8	14*	15*	12*	14*	15*
20 pts.	N=72	N=28	N=27	N=10	N=10	N=9
Function	10	13	16*	19*	20*	19
25 pts.	N=72	N=25	N=27	N=10	N=11	N=9
Pain	7	11*	10*	11*	12*	11
15 pts.	N=71	N=28	N=27	N=10	N=11	N=9
Range of motion	8	7	8	9	8	8
10 pts.	N=72	N=28	N=27	N=10	N=11	N=9
Deformity	13	12	13	13	13	14
15 pts.	N=72	N=28	N=27	N=10	N=11	N=9
Strength	10	10	11	10	11	10
15 pts.	N=72	N=28	N=27	N=10	N=11	N=9
Total	56	67	74*	74*	78*	78*
100 pts.	N=72	N=28	N=27	N=10	N=11	N=9

*Significantly different from pre-op values, paired t-test ($p < 0.05$).

Legend: Orthopaedic evaluation scores for patients having knee ligament repairs using the carbon fiber composite.

TABLE 23.5

Cybex Evaluation, Knees

	Pre-Op	6 Mos.	9 Mos.	12 Mos.	18 Mos.
		% Deficit,* Low Speed			
Extension	53	43	8	-4	8
	N=71	N=18	N=7	N=6	N=4
Flexion	49	17	-11	-15	7
	N=71	N=18	N=7	N=6	N=4
		% Deficit,* High Speed			
Extension	54	27	9	0	12
	N=61	N=16	N=7	N=6	N=4
Flexion	54	19	-4	-25	-11
	N=61	N=16	N=7	N=6	N=4

* % deficit is the difference (%) in the maximum torque values generated by the affected leg at the time periods indicated and the maximum torque generated by the contralateral normal leg pre-operatively.

Legend: Quantitative Cybex evaluation for patients having knee ligament repairs using the carbon fiber composite.

Cybex evaluation of knees demonstrated a dramatic decrease in percent deficit in as little time as 6 months in both high and low speed testing. This is illustrated in Table 23.5.

DISCUSSION

Canine Patellar Tendon

Replacement of the canine patellar tendon proved to be a complex experimental system with many variables. However, the success of the carbon fiber-PLA composite in such an elementary design serves to demonstrate the usefulness of this new material.

The carbon fiber PLA scaffold replacements monotonically increased in stiffness and ultimate strength over the 12 month post-operative period. Stiffness increased from 1.57×10^5 N/M at two months to 3.67×10^5 N/M at one year. Ultimate strength increased from 1.38 KN at 2 months to 1.94 KN at one year. We believe this increase in strength and stiffness with time is indicative of the regrowth and organization of collagenous tissue on the scaffold replacement. A permanent prosthetic replacement will only become weaker with time. The scaffold approach to replacement permits strengthening with time to some optimal level and maintenance thereafter. On a paired or absolute basis, the mechanical properties of these regrown patellar tendons appear to be indistinguishable from normal.

The ultimate strengths of these replacements are lower than the projected immediate post-operative strength. We must assume some fiber fracture has occurred. It is this gradual mechanical failure of the carbon fiber which transfers load to the developing tissue. We believe this gradual transference of load is critical in the proper development of a well-organized, remodeled structure. The rate of mechanical degradation and transference of load is not known in either the unprotected or polymer-protected replacements. As there were no catastrophic failures of the implants, it seems that the degradation rate is sufficiently slow as to allow adequate regrowth.

Scanning electron micrographs of regrown and natural patellar tendons indicate that the carbon fibers are approximately the same diameter as the naturally occurring collagen fiber bundles. The developing collagen fibers seem to grow around the carbon fibers as they would about a naturally occurring fiber bundle. The result is a structure mechanically and histologically very similar to the natural structure.

Certainly, protection of the carbon fiber with a resorbable polymer is desirable to improve handling characteristics and to prevent the spread of carbon fiber into adjacent tissue. This PLA-carbon fiber structure provides mechanical strength upon implantation, allows ingrowth of new tissue, and is thought to mechanically degrade as the new tissue matures. It has been demonstrated, even in this "elemental design" form, to be an acceptable patellar tendon replacement in dogs. The dogs retained for 12 months regained and maintained normal function as a result of this surgery.

Rabbit Achilles Tendon

In the initial 2 week post-operative period, the mode of failure in tension of the systems with implants was pullout of the composite from its proximal soft tissue anastomosis. Since no implant separated from its anastomosis prior to testing, it would appear that the "locking-weave" technique of anastomosis provided adequate initial strength (approximately 60N) to maintain the anastomosis while tissue ingrowth progressed. The progressive increase in strength with time would seem to correspond with early tissue ingrowth as determined histologically. In addition, there is the formation of a loose, disorganized scar in the region of resected tendon which contributes significantly to these early strengths.

During this same period, the sham procedures failed by separation through the area of resected tendon. This sham procedure produced a regrown structure significantly weaker than systems with implanted composites. As with the implant group, a loose, disorganized scar formed about the area of resected tendon. This volume of scar accounts for the early strength of the shams.

During the 4 to 12 week post-operative period, an important change occurred in mode of failure of the carbon composites. These implants no longer failed by pull-out of the composite from the soft tissue anastomosis. Failure now occurred by rupture through the belly of the gastrocnemius system. This rupture occurred proximal to the anastomosis site. This mode of failure was identical to the failure mode of the unoperated limbs. That is, the ultimate strength of the gastrocnemius muscle is the limiting factor in the gastrocnemius system. The anastomosis between implant and soft tissue was no longer the region of failure. Tensile tests at 4 and 12 weeks indicate that the strength of the systems with implants were equivalent to the strengths of the unoperated systems. The Dacron composite repairs continued to fail through the area of resection and at lower forces than the carbon composites.

During this 4 week to 12 week post-op period, the sham procedure continued to fail through the area of resected tendon, as in Weeks 1 and 2. No tensile strength value of a sham or a Dacron composite repair fell within the 95% confidence interval of the normal group. Scar tissue surrounding the sham resulted in a maximum strength at 4 weeks. During the eight week to 12 week period, this scar resorbed resulting in a weak attenuated and disorganized tissue corresponding to the area of resected tendon. Repairs made with the Dacron composite remained relatively strong.

Comparison of force-extension curves for implant and unoperated systems at 12 weeks showed a mechanically similar response. This mechanical behavior of the implant systems (both carbon and Dacron) suggests that due to biological fixation and tissue remodeling along the composite scaffold, a structure similar mechanically to the contralateral normal has been regenerated.

The canine patellar tendon replacement proved successful in a highly loaded situation. However, this replacement was a continuous loop of composite material initially anchored in bone. Therefore, this experiment yielded little information regarding the rapidity and security of soft tissue attachment to the composite. A secure soft tissue attachment may be required for many ligament and tendon repairs. The successful replacement of a major portion of the rabbit Achilles tendon utilizing only soft tissue attachment demonstrates this is possible.

Canine Medial Collateral Ligament

Based on the success of earlier soft tissue repairs in animals, human clinical trials of carbon fiber-PLA composites seemed feasible. A human replacement procedure would likely involve the extra-articular ligaments of the knee. Damage to any of the ligaments of the knee is a serious clinical problem. Instability in this joint is debilitating and often leads to chronic progressive osteoarthritis if left unchecked.

Before a replacement procedure could be considered in the human, it was necessary to demonstrate the usefulness of a similar procedure in an animal model. In this study, the medial collateral ligaments and medial capsular structures of canines were resected and replaced with a carbon fiber-polylactic acid polymer tissue scaffold or allowed simply to "scar in." After 4 weeks, 8 weeks, 12 weeks, and 26 weeks in vivo, the stability of the knees was quantitatively evaluated and the mechanical properties of the regrown structures determined. Histologic sections of the regrown structures were examined after 26 weeks in vivo.

At all time periods, operative knees receiving implants were quantitatively judged to be considerably more stable than sham knees. Further, the structures regrown about the carbon fiber-PLA scaffolds were consistently stronger and stiffer than tissue resulting from the sham procedure. We believe this increase in strength and stiffness with time is indicative of the regrowth and organization of collagenous tissue on and within the scaffold replacement. This concept is supported by the microhistologic appearance of the implant after 26 weeks in vivo. The soft tissue attachment technique utilized appears to form a strong, rapid bond as ingrowth proceeds. No adverse tissue reactions were noted and the function of the joints receiving implants was excellent.

In short, the test results presented suggest that carbon fiber-PLA composite ligament replacements may aid significantly in the stabilization of an acutely damaged joint. The improved mechanical performance of implant groups over sham groups suggests repair with a carbon fiber tissue scaffold is superior to simply allowing the ligament deficit to "scar in."

Canine Anterior Cruciate Ligament

Within the synovial joint, protection of the carbon fiber with autogenous tissue appears to be necessary. This not only seems to prevent abrasion and premature failure of the carbon fiber, but also seems to promote a more rapid regrowth of tissue. Mechanically, the results from use of carbon augmented autogenous tissue were superior to that of the composite alone. It appears that a bed of autogenous tissue (vascular if possible) is absolutely necessary to counteract the slower soft tissue growth rates in the synovial environment. Finally, it is our impression that the anatomy of the canine knee represents an overly severe model for ACL replacement and we have abandoned it. However, these experiments were valuable in demonstrating the efficacy of using autogenous tissue with the composite in these repairs.

Synovial Joint Debris

When a carbon implant is used in the repair or replacement of an anterior cruciate ligament, there is naturally concern that some carbon debris may ultimately find its way into the joint. In this environment, such debris was found to be rapidly picked up by the synovium. The residence of this debris within the synovium produced a mild synovitis. No changes in mechanical properties or histology of the cartilage was noted. In our opinion, loss of a ligament and the resulting instability will produce more joint damage than carbon debris as used in this experiment.

Early Clinical Trials

Early clinical trials have been very encouraging. This is particularly true of the patients having undergone repair of knee ligaments. This group, which represents most of the patients treated (81%), showed continuous improvement in total orthopaedic evaluation scores, going from a pre-op value of 56 points to 78 points 18 months post-operatively. Improvements in score were statistically significant ($p < 0.05$) when compared to pre-op values (paired t-test) at 6 months, 9 months, 12 months, and 18 months. This continuous improvement is due to better stability and function and less pain. Range of motion, deformity, and strength appeared to remain constant.

Cybex testing revealed a quantitative improvement in joint function. That is, the percent deficit of the affected leg fell to within normal limits by 9 months and essentially maintained that level at 12 months and 18 months.

CONCLUSIONS

This series of animal experiments and early clinical trials suggests that carbon fiber-absorbable polymer composites may be useful in soft tissue repair. Fibrous tissue ingrowth appears to be consistent in extra-articular locations with some organization of the tissue evident as early as four weeks. Complete envelopment of the implant by aligned collagen fibers has been noted at eight weeks. Bone ingrowth around the carbon fibers in the drill holes in beagle tibias (Patellar Tendon Study) was also evident. However, this process is clearly much slower than soft tissue ingrowth, requiring upward of one year. Within the synovial joint, protection of the carbon fiber with autogenous tissue appears to be necessary to counteract the slower growth rates in this environment.

Carbon fiber composite clinical implants have, to date, demonstrated ingrowth potential similar to that seen in the animal studies. Two year evaluation results have likewise been encouraging. Most patients have shown significant improvement with many demonstrating good to excellent stability and function.

The carbon composite has high strength and reasonable flexibility. It is highly biocompatible and encourages rapid tissue ingrowth. It can be fashioned into a variety of shapes for different applications. Potential forms and applications include mesh sheets for hernia repair or other soft tissue defects. In addition to ligament and tendon replacement, the combination of absorbable polymer and carbon fiber may find other applications in orthopaedic implants. These components, in a different composition, are being explored as a possible bone plate or intra-medullary device for fracture fixation. In this application, the composite would function as a temporary prosthesis, rather than as a scaffold. It would be rigid upon implantation, but then gradually degrade. This would prevent the stress protection atrophy which results from the use of currently available metallic devices. Additional advantages include radiolucency, no need for surgical removal, and the excellent biocompatibility of the material.

SUMMARY

Two avenues of research have dominated ligament replacement. The first is that of an adequately designed permanent prosthetic replacement. Such a replacement must be constructed of a biocompatible material. It must have sufficient mechanical strength, with some promise of surviving the millions of fatigue cycles associated with normal ligament use. It is the view of the authors that no material currently available can adequately fulfill these requirements.

The second concept utilizes a scaffold replacement approach that allows the ingrowth of new collagenous tissue. This latter technique provides only temporary mechanical integrity until the new tissue can assume the mechanical function. Working along these lines, the authors have found composites of filamentous carbon fiber and absorbable polymer to be a new and useful class of orthopaedic biomaterials. Ribbon-like composite structures have been utilized in the repair and replacement of both tendons (Achilles and patellar) and ligaments. When used in this way, the composite acts as a scaffold upon which new collagenous tissue can grow.

These materials have proven successful in a variety of animal models and human clinical trials have been initiated.

REFERENCES

Alexander, H, Parsons, JR, Smith, G, Fong, R, Mylod, A, and Weiss, AB. 1982. Anterior cruciate ligament replacement with filamentous carbon. Trans. Orthop. Res. Soc. 7:45.

Alexander, H, Parsons, JR, Strauchler, ID, Corcoran, SF, Gona, O, and Mayott, CW. 1981. Canine patellar tendon replacement with a polylactic acid polymer-filamentous carbon tissue scaffold. Orthop. Review 10:41-51.

Aragona, J, Parsons, JR, Alexander, H, and Weiss, AB. 1981. Soft tissue attachment of a filamentous carbon-absorbable polymer tendon and ligament replacement. Clin. Orthop. Rel. Res. 160:268-278.

Benson, J. 1971. Elemental carbon as a biomaterial. J. Biomed. Mater. Res. 5:41-47.

Brady, JM, Cutright, DE, Miller, RA, Battistone, GC, and Hunsuck, EE. 1973. Resorption rate route elimination and ultrastructure of the implant site of polylactic acid in the abdominal wall of the rat. J. Biomed. Mat. Res. 7:155-166.

Christel, P, Buttazzoni, B, Leray, JL, and Morin, C. 1980. Tissue tolerance of carbon materials. Trans. World Biomat. Congress 1:4, 7, 9.

Claes, L. 1982. Private communication.

Claes, L, Wolter, D, Gistinger, G, Rose, P, Huttner, W, and Fitzer, E. 1978. Physical and biological aspects of carbon fibres in the ligament prosthesis. 3rd Conf. on Mech. Prop. of Biomat., Keele Univ. (personal communication).

Cutright, DE, and Hunsuck, EE. 1971. Tissue reactions to the biodegradable polylactic acid suture. Oral Surg. 31:134-139.

Forster, IW, Ralis, ZA, McKibbin, B, and Jenkins, DHR. 1978. Biological reaction to carbon fibre implants. Clin. Orthop. Rel. Res. 131:299-307.

Gershuni, DH, Kuei, SC, Woo, SL-Y, Thibodeaux, JI, and Akesom, WH. 1980. Articular cartilage deformation following experimental synovitis in the rabbit hip. Trans. Orthop. Res. Soc. 5:63.

Haubold, A. 1977. Carbon in prosthetics. Ann. New York Acad. Sci. 283:383-395.

Jenkins, DHR. 1978. The repair of cruciate ligaments with flexible carbon fibre. J. Bone Jt. Surg. 60B:520-522.

Jenkins, DHR. 1982. Private communication.

Jenkins, DHR, Forester, IW, McKibbins, B, and Ralis, ZA. 1977. Induction of tendon and ligament formation by carbon implants. J. Bone Jt. Surg. 59B:53-57.

Jenkins, DHR, and McKibbin, B. 1980. The role of flexible carbon-fibre implants as tendon and ligament substitutes in clinical practice—A preliminary report. J. Bone Jt. Surg. 62B:497-499.

Kinzl, L, Wolter, D, and Claes, L. 1979. Aspects of coated carbon fibres in the ligament prostheses. Trans. Soc. for Biomat. 3:71.

Kulkarni, RK, Moore, EG, Hegyeli, AF, and Leonard, F. 1966. Polylactic acid for surgical implants. Arch. Surg. 93:839-843.

Minns, RJ, and Flynn, M. 1978. Intra-articular implant of filamentous carbon fibre in the experimental animal. J. Bioengineering 2:279-286.

Mooney, V, Hartman, DB, McNeal, D, and Benson, J. 1974. The use of pure carbon for percutaneous electrical connector systems. Arch. Surg. 108:148-153.

Neugebauer, R, Burri, C, Claes, L, Helbing, G, and Wolter, D. 1979A. The replacement of the abdominal wall by a carbon-cloth in rabbits. Trans. Soc. for Biomat. 3:135.

Neugebauer, R, Burri, C, Claes, L, Helbing, G, and Wolter, D. 1979B. The anchorage of carbon fibre strands into bone; A biomechanical and biological evaluation on knee joints. Trans. European Soc. of Biomat., Vol. 2, p. 64.

Neugebauer, R, Burri, C, Claes, L, and Helbing, G. 1980. The trap door; A possibility of fixation of carbon fibre strands into cancellous bone. Trans. World Biomat. Congress 1:4, 7, 5.

Parsons, JR, Alexander, H, Ende, LS, and Weiss, AB. 1983. Fiber reinforced absorbable polymer tissue scaffolds: A comparison of carbon fiber and dacron fiber systems. Trans. Orthop. Res. Soc. 8:86.

Parsons, JR, Aragona, J, Alexander, H, and Weiss, AB. 1981. Medial collateral ligament replacement with a partially absorbable tissue scaffold. Proc. 9th Northeast Bioengineering Conf. Pergamon Press, pp. 29-32.

Parsons, JR, Byhani, S, Alexander, H, and Weiss, AB. 1983b. Carbon fiber debris within the synovial joint: Time-dependent mechanical and histological studies. Trans. Orthop. Res. Soc. 8:9.

Pitt, CG, Gratzl, MM, Kimmel, GL, Surles, J, and Schindler, A. 1981. The degradation of poly[DL-lactide] poly[E-caprapectone] and their copolymers M-V in-vivo. Biomaterials 2:215.

Rice, RM, Hegyeli, AF, Gourlay, SK, Wade, CW, Dillon, JG, Jaffe, H, and Kulkarni, RK. 1978. Biocompatability testing of polymers: in-vitro studies with in-vitro correlation. J. Biomed. Mater. Res. 12:43-54.

Schindler, A, Jeffcoat, R, Kimmel, GL, Pitt, GG, Wall, ME, and Zweidinger, R. 1977. Biodegradable polymers for sustained drug delivery. In Contemporary Topics in Polymer Science, E. Pearce and J. Schaefgen (eds.), Vol. II, pp. 251-289. New York: Plenum Press.

von Fraunhofer, JA, L'Estrange, PR, and Mask, AO. 1971. Materials science in dental implantation and a promising new material—vitreous carbon. Biomed. Eng. 6:114-118.

Wolter, D, Fitzer, E, Helbing, G, and Goldaway, J. 1977. Ligament replacement in the knee joint with carbon fibers coated with pyrolitic carbon. Trans. Soc. for Biomat. 1:126.

PART VII
Infection

24

Impairment of Microbicidal Function in Wounds: Correction with Oxygenation

Thomas K. Hunt, Betty Halliday, David R. Knighton, Finn Gottrup, David C. Price, Stephen J. Mathes, Ning Chang and David C. Hohn

INTRODUCTION

No surgeon of good judgment would consider removing a benign skin lesion from the foot of a patient with severe peripheral arteriosclerosis. On the other hand, few surgeons would hesitate to remove the same lesion from the earlobe of the same patient. In the absence of obvious evidence to the contrary, no one would doubt the immune competence of this patient, but clearly one would expect a wound in his foot to become infected.

Though the immune system is enormously complex, one acceptable generalization about it is that the polymorphonuclear leukocyte, its phagocytic action and its intracellular killing, are the mainstay of resistance to infection in injured tissue. Clearly, a polymorphonuclear leukocyte can seek out and kill organisms in the ear of this patient, but cannot seek out and kill organisms in his foot. Is it simply that blood flow is inadequate in the foot? If so, what component is inadequate? Do white cells reach that area? If they do, why don't they kill bacteria there?

Recent years have seen great advances in the appreciation of immune-suppression in surgical patients, especially traumatized, malnourished, diabetic or cancer patients. We have recognized that every operation or trauma produces transient immune suppression. Many studies have shown lymphocytic dysfunction or inadequate antibody production, but the clinical significance of most of these findings is as yet unclear. Comparatively little attention has been paid to granulocyte phagocytic function, although Meakins and others have used the medium of delayed hypersensitivity to demonstrate that one unifying factor in immune suppression in these patients is impaired leukocyte migration.[1] None of the current tests, however, measures the ability of phagocytes in the environment of injured tissue to kill contaminating bacteria.

Phagocytic killing is usually conceived of as having two major pathways. The first is degranulation, in which ingested bacteria are exposed to various antimicrobial compounds carried in leukocyte granules and poured onto the bacteria by fusion of granules with the phagosome. The enzyme "packages" are carried by the leukocyte from its point of origin to the scene of phagocytosis, and the efficacy of this system seems to be unrelated to the environment of the wound in which the leukocyte engulfs the bacteria. The second mechanism is called "oxidative killing" and depends upon the ability of the leukocyte to capture molecular oxygen from its environment and convert it to high-energy oxygen radicals such as superoxide, hydroxyl radical, peroxide, aldehydes, hypochlorite, hypoiodite, and others which are toxic to bacteria. These two pathways represent a considerable dichotomy of function, since motility of polymorphs and the act of phagocytosis both rely exclusively on anaerobic metabolism and occur uninhibited in the absence of oxygen, while the oxidative microbicidal pathway absolutely requires relatively-abundant oxygen to work at maximum speed and efficacy.[2]

Our previous finding of the hypoxic nature of wounds led us to establish their susceptibility to anaerobic organisms. As controls, we tested resistance to aerobic organisms. That, too, was impaired, and subsequently we found that rabbits which were breathing high concentrations of oxygen cleared their wounds of bacteria much more rapidly than animals with the same, standard wounds breathing an hypoxic atmosphere[3,4,5,6,7] (Figure 24.1). During these studies, Halliday noted that infected wounds in hypoxic animals contained twice as many leukocytes as infected wounds in hyperoxic animals.[8]

More recently, literally dozens of investigators have begun to dissect the basic elements of the oxidative microbicidal pathway. The mechanism was first suggested by the discovery of the "respiratory burst" more than fifty years ago. When white cells ingest bacteria their consumption of oxygen rises as much as twenty times that of basal rates, consequent upon the activation of a primary oxygenase located in the white cell membrane and activated by phagocytosis. The energy requirements for the step are furnished largely by the hexosemonophosphate shunt.

Genetic absence of the primary enzyme is responsible for the disease called "chronic granulomatous disease of childhood (CGD), which is characterized by frequent bacterial infections.

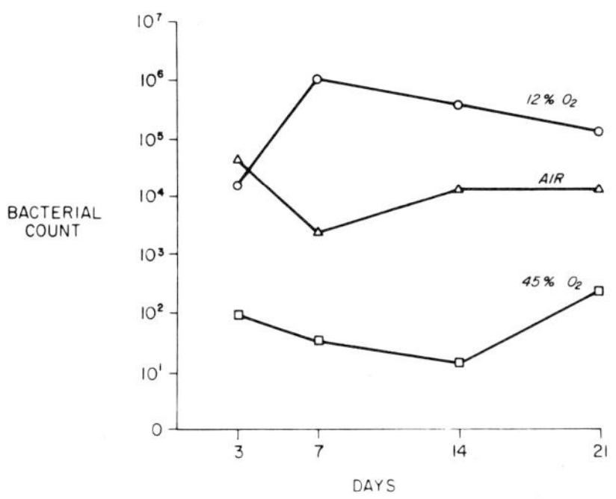

FIGURE 24.1 (above)
Average bacteria count with given breathing gas vs. day (10^6 bacteria).

FIGURE 24.2 (right)

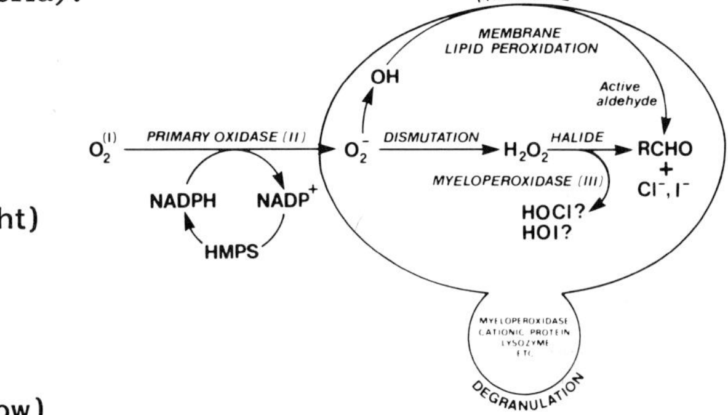

FIGURE 24.3 (below)

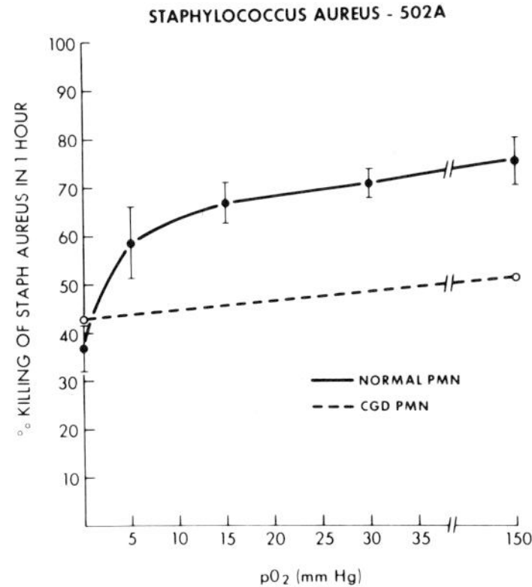

Before antibiotics, CGD always led to an early death. The appreciation that leukocytes from CGD patients failed to mount a respiratory burst led to the discovery that the respiratory burst following phagocytosis coincides with a period of intense bacterial killing. The sequence can be replicated in vitro by incubating susceptible bacteria in cell culture fluid in the presence of chloride, hydrogen peroxide, and myeloperoxidase, all of which are portions of the oxidative killing mechanism. In this case, hypochlorite, which is lethal to many test organisms, is generated. A schema of the present concept is given in Figure 24.2. The bacteria which are killed more by the oxidative than the nonoxidative pathway include Staphylococcus aureus, many Klebsiellae, many E. coli, Serratia marcescens, and Salmonella, most of the well-known wound pathogens.[9]

The absence of an enzyme is equivalent to the absence of the substrate on which that enzyme acts. The absence of the primary oxidase (as in CGD) which reduces oxygen to superoxide (the first of the toxic oxygen radicals) should be mimicked by anoxia. Therefore, hypoxia should induce in a granulocyte the equivalent of chronic granulomatous disease. A simple confirmation was made of this prediction by my colleague, David Hohn, by comparing CGD cells with normal cells, measuring bacterial killing rates at various oxygen tensions from zero to 150 mm Hg. For the test organism, Staphylococcus 502A at 150 mm Hg pO_2, CGD cells have approximately half the killing capacity of normal white cells. As shown in Figure 24.3, normal white cells lose their killing capacity as pO_2 falls. Below about 20 mmg Hg rapid loss of killing function occurs, to the point that normal cells and CGD cells have equivalent microbicidal activity at zero oxygen tension, exactly as the laws of chemistry predict. Therefore, white cells which fall into a zone of hypoxic tissue "acquire" CGD to a degree dictated by the extent of hypoxia.[10]

As noted above, hypoxic rabbits clear common wound-infecting organisms from wire-mesh cylinder wounds much less rapidly than normoxic or hyperoxic animals. We predicted that hyperoxia would enhance bacterial killing in other models. We employed the model of Burke and Miles[11] for confirmation because that model had correctly predicted the rules for prophylactic antibiotic use in man and, even more to the point, predicted approximately the degree or clinical efficacy of antibiotics as prophylactic agents in man.

THE EFFECTS OF SYSTEMIC HYPOXIA AND HYPEROXIA

Methods

Escherichia coli, wild strain, were placed on tryptose blood agar base plates and incubated aerobically at 37°C for 24 hr. Ten separate colonies were selected and put into 10 cc tryptose phosphate broth for 18 hr at 37°C. Part of the 1:2 diluted bacterial suspension was autoclaved in order to determine influence of bacterial proteins on lesion size.

Young-adult, female, Hartley guinea pigs weighing 285-310 gm were prepared for injection by removing the hair on the back and sides with a commercial depilatory. This agent was carefully washed away, and care was taken to ensure uniform exposure of all animals (overexposure results in chemical irritation, making later reading variable and difficult). Before injection all animals were kept in room air and then randomly assigned to test atmospheres.

Escherichia coli were injected into the dermis of the guinea pig back using an air-injection gun designed for human mass immunization. Eleven sites on the back of each animal were injected, ten with bacterial samples of about 10^8 organisms from the same culture. The eleventh site was randomly chosen as a control, where heat-killed bacteria in the same concentration were injected.

Injected guinea pigs were then placed in cages with different oxygen tensions for varying lengths of time. Plexiglass cages were constructed to house four guinea pigs each. One cage was ventilated with an oxygen-air mixture (providing a constant high-flow, 45% oxygen environment) and the second cage with a nitrogen-air mixture (to provide a constant high-flow 12% oxygen environment). The high flow of gases assured CO_2 levels below 0.5% and normal levels of water vapor. The third oxygen environment was obtained by piping the same volume of air through the same chambers. In later experiments, the air-exposed animals were kept in the vivarium, since we could detect no changes in results between animals living in normal cages and the controlled environment cages ventilated with air. Animals received their usual food and water.

In the first set of experiments, injected guinea pigs were divided into six groups. Group I was exposed to 12% oxygen for 48 hr. Group II was exposed to 45% oxygen for 1.5 hr, followed by 12% oxygen for 46.5 hr. Group III was exposed to 12% for 24 hr, followed by 45% oxygen for 48 hr, and group IV was exposed to 12% oxygen for three hours, followed by 45% oxygen for 45 hr. Group V was exposed to room air for 48 hr, and group VI was exposed to 45% oxygen for 48 hr.

The guinea pigs were removed from the controlled environments at 24 and 48 hr and the dimensions of infectious necrosis measured. The indurated area was larger, but this area, which has been the major item of measurement by others using the technique, was ignored in favor of the more precisely measurable area of necrosis. Necrosis was identified as the visibly infarcted and discolored skin centering on the injection site. The lesion diameter was recorded as the square root of Dd, where D and d are the lengths of the major and minor axes. Measurements were made to the nearest millimeter. Statistical analysis was performed using the Wilcoxen rank sum for lesion diameter and by chi-square analysis for presence or absence of necrosis.

In a further series of experiments, using _E. coli_, half the animals were injected with ampicillin (6 mg intraperitoneally) at the same time as they were injected with bacteria. They were then placed in the same test oxygen environments. In these experiments, _E. coli_ 25922 (ATCC) were used, the 18-hour broth culture was diluted 1:2 in tryptose phosphate broth, and the readings of both induration and necrosis were made with a peak scale loupe (7x magnification) to the nearest 0.1 mm.

Results

Results for injection of _E. coli_ are summarized in Figure 24.4. Obviously, the degree of necrosis and the number of lesions showing any necrosis at all were inversely proportionate to the percentage of oxygen in the mixture breathed. Exposure to 45% oxygen for one and a half hours, before exposure to 12% for the rest of the observation period, resulted in a 36% reduction in mean lesion diameter and a 48% reduction in the number of necrotic lesions. Exposure to 12% oxygen for three hours, and then 45% for 45 hr, gave similar results as the initial exposure to 45% oxygen for one and a half hours, followed by 12% oxygen for 46.5 hr. Longer exposure to 12% oxygen (for 24 hr), followed by 45% oxygen for 48 hr, resulted in a 24% reduction in lesion size, but only a 6% reduction in the number of necrotic lesions. When compared to 48-hr exposure to 12% oxygen, 48-hr exposure to 21% oxygen gave a 50% reduction in lesion size and a 30% reduction in their number. Exposure to 45% oxygen for 48 hr, compared with 12% oxygen for 48 hr, gave a 63% reduction in lesion diameter and a reduction of 57% in the number

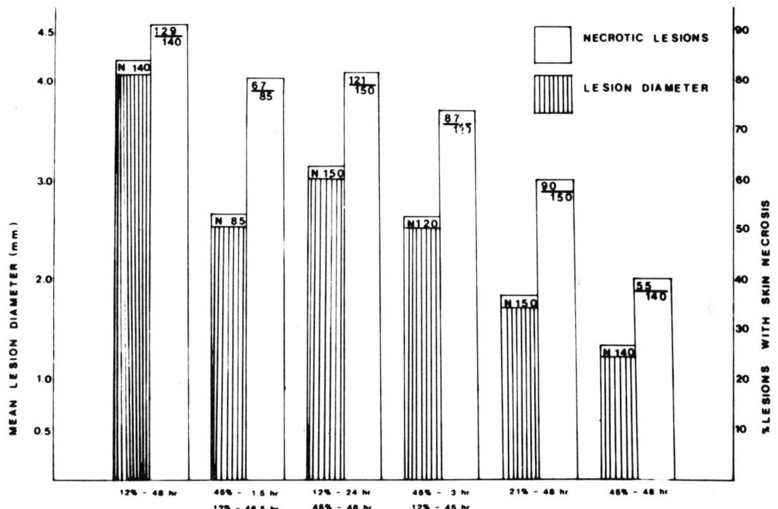

FIGURE 24.4

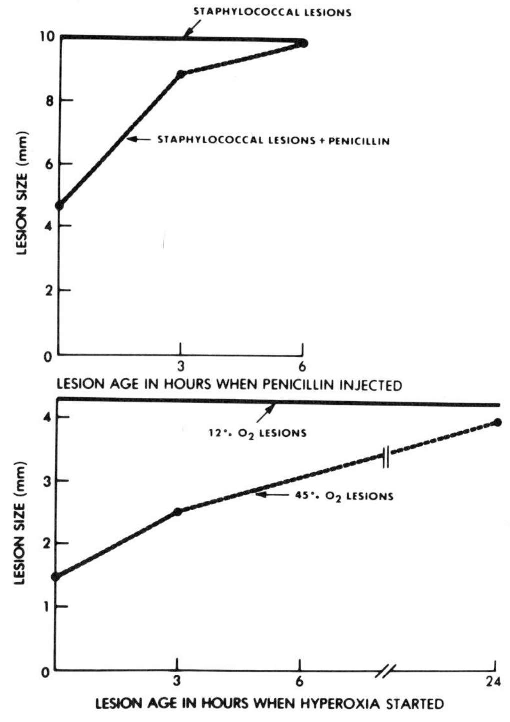

FIGURE 24.5

of necrotic lesions. Statistical analysis shows that all groups are significantly different from the 12%-for-48-hr group in lesion size at $p < 0.010$ or smaller. The number of necrotic lesions was significantly less for groups exposed for 48 hr, compared to 12% oxygen exposure for 48 hr ($p < 0.001$).

Injections of Staphylococcus aureus yielded similar data, except that hyperoxia improved little on normoxia. Nevertheless, both hyperoxic and normoxic groups were significantly improved beyond the 12% oxygen group.

In the second series of experiments, in which a change in oxygen from 12% to 21% was compared to a timely, properly sized dose of specifically effective antibiotic, both the antibiotic group and the 21%-oxygen group were significantly better than a group of animals breathing 12% oxygen. Significantly, the effect of raising the oxygen tension was marginally superior to that of giving antibiotics. Hypoxia and antibiotics proved additive, so that only rarely was any evidence of infection seen in animals treated with both, whereas 100% infections occurred in hypoxic animals getting no antibiotics!

Discussion

The results clearly show that resistance to two clinically important wound pathogens is proportionate to the oxygenation of the tissues surrounding the area of inoculation. As opposed to antibiotics whose effective period ends within four hours of inoculation, the effect of oxygenation appeared to last at least 24 hr with, however, the greater effect exhibited in the first three hours. Furthermore, the effect of correcting tissue oxygenation from that produced by 12% oxygen-breathing to that corresponding to normal air was equivalent to the effect of an adequately-sized, appropriately timed dose of specifically effective antibiotic (Figure 24.5).

Silver has demonstrated that the injection of bacteria into tissue is followed by vasodilation and then vasospasm, with major corresponding changes in oxygen supply. The effects of changes in arterial pO_2 are passed on in terms of quantity of available oxygen at the site of infection.[12] Thus, the cycle seems to be complete.

THE EFFECTS OF LOCAL HYPOXIA

The above experiments do not distinguish between strictly local and potentially systemic effects of hypoxia and hyperoxia.

Experiments in which the whole animal is exposed to an artificial atmosphere are subject to some reservations about other potential effects of hypoxia or hyperoxia on endocrine function, hemodynamics, catecholamines, and so on. For the purpose of eliminating these effects we devised a dog model, in which a standard, random pattern (RP) flap (in which tissue hypoxia is measurable) was compared to a symmetrical, identically-sized, simultaneously-made musculocutaneous (MC) flap,[13] whose circulation and oxygenation were demonstrable equal to nearby control tissues. A diagram of the experiment is in Figure 24.6.

Methods and Results

The flaps were raised and replaced immediately. The RP flap was dissected from the deeper tissue in a plane deep to the subcutaneous muscle, while the MC flap was designed to include the rectus abdominus muscle, leaving intact its major vessels, the superficial epigastric artery and vein.

Oxygen tensions were measured by the implanted Silastic® sheath method of Chang[14] and Niinikoski et al.[15] in the distal and proximal thirds of both flaps, as well as in corresponding positions in the normal, unwounded tissue on each side.[14,15] Oxygen tension in the normal tissue and both levels of the MC flap was approximately 50 mm Hg. Oxygen tension in the distal aspect of the RP flap was approximately 20 mm Hg, while the pO_2 in its proximal portion was approximately 40 mm Hg.

Inoculations of 10^9 Staphylococcus aureus were made by a tuberculin syringe with a 26g needle, three in each level of each flap, with corresponding controls laterally. Lesion size was measured in the next 24 and 48 hours.[14] Results are charted in Figure 24.7. Infection of the distal (hypoxic) area of the RP flap resulted in such large areas of necrosis that confluent gangrene was the rule. Histologic examination of the gangrene showed many white cells, some bacteria, no abscess formation, and considerable intravascular thrombosis. Lesion in the MC flap and control tissues were smaller than in the RP flap and were essentially similar to each other. Histological examination revealed abscess formation without gangrene and without intravascular thrombosis. Control flaps, without injections, survived in toto without exception.

Injections were made in the distal part of flaps raised in a set of three animals. At the same time, 30 cc blood was withdrawn. The ACD blood was sedimented with hydroxyethyl starch for one hour, when the supernatant was centrifuged

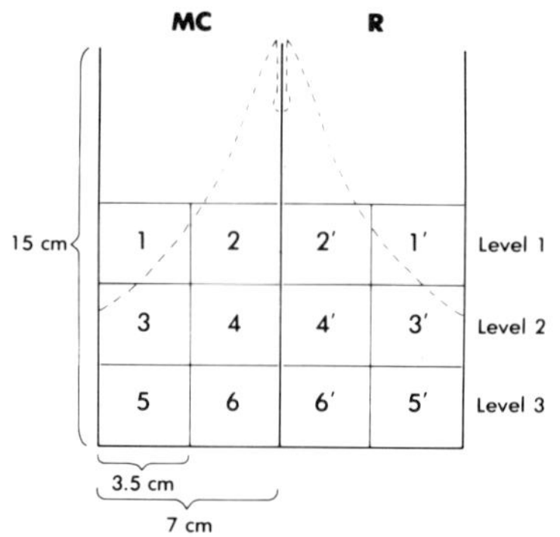

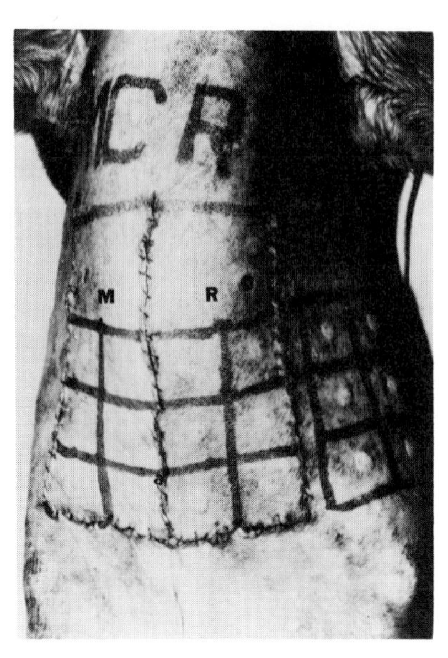

FIGURE 24.6 Intradermal bacteria injection. (Left) Each flap contains six 3.5 × 3 cm rectangles for bacteria injection. Corresponding numbers and levels form the basis for the paired sample analysis. (Right) Skin wheals produced with intradermal injection of bacteria in the musculocutaneous flap (M), random pattern flap (R), and normal skin (C).

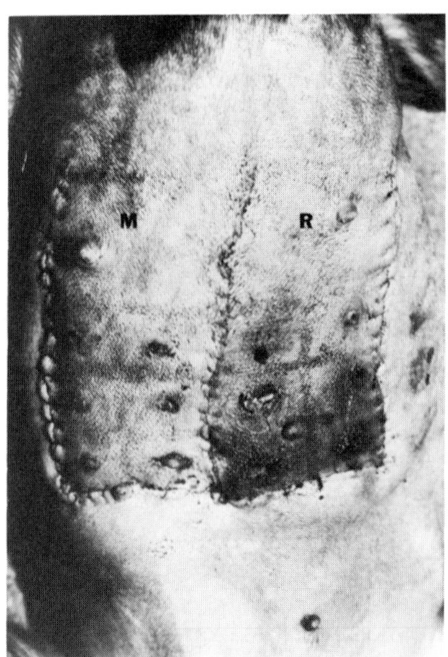

FIGURE 24.7

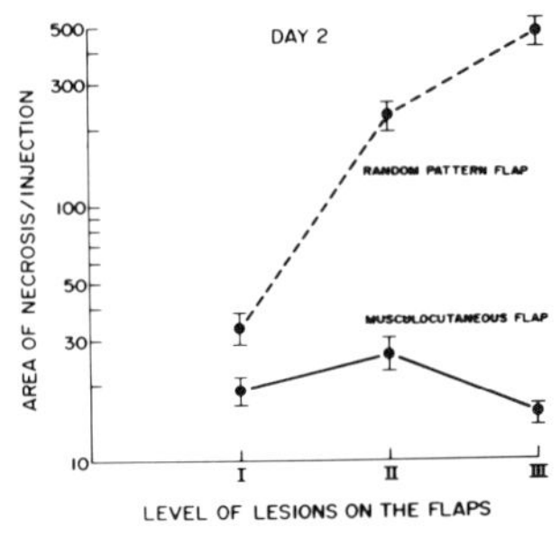

slowly to separate granulocytes, but not platelets. Granulocytes were resuspended in normal saline and 0.3 mCi ^{111}indium-oxine sulfate was added. After 15 min incubation, the cells were sedimented by low-speed centrifugation and resuspended in plasma, washed once, and injected in 10 cc plasma into a peripheral vein in the anesthetized donor animal. Forty-eight hours after the flaps were raised, the dogs were killed and the excised flap imaged and calibrated against a known standard in a standard field scintillation camera interfaced to a DEC computer.[16] Isotope uptakes were expressed as percent of the total dose of ^{111}indium given. The flaps were excised and rescanned. The amounts of radioactivity found in control injections, RP flap injections and MC flap injections were essentially the same, although, for unknown reasons, the MC flap received more than did the normal tissue.

Percent Injected Dose

Normal tissue	RP flap	MC flap
0.272 ± 0.296	0.368 ± 0.320	0.695 ± 0.779

Discussion

These last experiments are not yet finished, but certain conclusions are already obvious. First, ischemic, hypoxic tissue is far more susceptible to infection than normal tissue. Infection in this tissue spreads rapidly and seems unlimited by the abscess formation which hinders spread of infection in the immediately adjacent normal tissue and in the MC flap. Infection in the ischemic tissue causes intravascular thrombosis and infectious gangrene, which appear indistinguishable from what we had thought was simple ischemic gangrene due to inadequate flap design.

The more surprising finding, however was that leukocytes enter the ischemic tissue, as easily as they enter the well-perfused tissue. One must conclude, therefore, that the white cells which do arrive become inefficient in the hypoxic tissue. The oxygen tension of the tissue in which these white cells find themselves engulfing bacteria is well below the critical levels shown in Figure 24.4, and, as a first approximation, we submit that these white cells are probably inefficient because they lack oxygen for killing purposes. This conclusion will not be fully warranted until we make changes in the tissue oxygen tension in the locally hypoxic tissue model and produce concordant changes in infectability. (These experiments are essentially complete and confirm this statement. They are not yet published.[17]) However, the guinea pig experiments leave us with a strong hypothesis that hypoxic white cells, though able to migrate and engulf bacteria, are unable to kill them. *In vitro* studies show that decreasing or increasing pO_2 has relatively less effect on leukocyte function.[10]

The answer to the question which these experiments were originally designed to answer is that local hypoxia is at least as effective in enhancing infection as systemic hypoxia. The immediate conclusion is that leukocytes in wounds need oxygen to kill clinically important wound-infecting organisms, such as *Staphylococcus aureus* and *E. coli*, and the absence of oxygen clearly interferes with this ability.

In Chapter 30 William H. Goodson will report systematic measurement of oxygen tension in human wounds by an easily applicable technique. Oxygen tensions near and below the critical levels are common in our clinical experience and equally commonly undetected by other techniques. We might note that results in Figure 24.3 were obtained with human leukocytes and that they clearly predict that the results obtained in guinea pigs and dogs reflect accurately the physiology of man. Despite a prejudice to the contrary, Chapter 30 will document the fact that tissue oxygen increases proportionately to arterial pO_2 even above the full-saturation point of hemoglobin.

Surgical wound infections represent a failure to mount an adequate defense against the infecting agent. The problem, excluding systemic changes in host resistance, reduces to a simple equation: if the number or type of infecting agent overwhelms the host's ability to contain and destroy it, a clinically significant infection results. Again, in the absence of systemic disorders of immunity the solution seems equally simple: either the number of infecting organisms presented to the host must be decreased or the host defences must be made more efficient. As a first approximation, it appears that the simple provision of more oxygen to a contaminated surgical wound can fulfill the latter condition. We do not mean to condense all immunity to infection into failures of the oxidative microbicidal mechanism of granulocytes. However, in wounds this mechanism must be one of the most common breaks in the human armor, and certainly it is one of the most easily correctable.

NOTES

1. Meakins JL. Host defense mechanisms, wound healing, and infection. In Hunt TK, Dunphy JE (eds) Fundamentals of Wound Management in Surgery. New York: Appleton-Century-Crofts, 1979, pp. 242-285.

2. Klebanoff S. Oxygen metabolism and the toxic properties of phagocytes. Ann Int Med 93:480-489, 1980.

3. Connolly WB, Hunt TK, Sonne M, Dunphy JE. Influence of distant trauma on local wound infection. Surg Gynec Obstet 128:713-718, 1969.

4. Hunt TK, Linsey M, Grislis G, Sonne M, Jawetz E. The effect of differing ambient oxygen tensions on wound infection. Ann Surg 181:35-39, 1975.

5. Hohn DC, MacKay RK, Halliday B, Hunt TK. The effect of O_2 tension on the microbicidal function of leukocytes in wounds and in vitro. Surg Forum 27:18-20, 1976.

6. Hohn DC, Ponce B, Burton RW, Hunt TK. Antimicrobial systems of the surgical wound. I. A comparison of oxidative metabolism and microbicidal capacity of phagocytes from wounds and from peripheral blood. Am J Surg 133:597, 1977.

7. Hunt TK. Disorders of repair and their management. In Hunt TK, Dunphy JE (eds), Fundamentals of Wound Management in Surgery. New York: Appleton-Century-Crofts, 1979, pp. 68-169.

8. Halliday B, unpublished data, 1983.

9. Mandell G. Bactericidal activity of aerobic and anaerobic polymorphonuclear neutrophils. Infect Immun 9:337-341, 1974.

10. Hohn DC. Host resistance of infection: Established and emerging concepts. In Hunt TK (ed), Wound Healing and Wound Infection: Theory and Surgical Practice. New York: Appleton-Century-Crofts, 1980, pp. 264-280.

11. Burke J, Miles A. The sequence of vascular events in early infective inflammation. J Pathol Bact 76:1-19, 1958.

12. Silver I. Tissue pO_2 changes in acute inflammation. Adv Exp Med Biol 94:769-774, 1978.

13. Gottrup F, Firmin R, Hunt TK, Mathes SJ. Dynamics of tissue oxygen in healing flaps. Surgery (in press), 1983.

14. Chang N, Mathes SJ. Comparison of the effect of bacterial inoculation in musculocutaneous and random-pattern flaps. Plast Reconstr Surg 70:1-10, 1982.

15. Niinikoski J, Heughan C, Hunt TK. Oxygen tensions in human wounds. J Surg Res 12:77, 1972.

16. Price DC, Hartmeyer JA, Prager RJ, Lipton MJ. Evaluation of *in vivo* thrombus formation in dogs using Indium-111-oxine labeled autologous platelets. In Thakur ML, Gottschalk A (eds). *Indium-111 Labeled Neutrophophils, Platelets and Lymphocytes*. New York: Trivirum Pub. Co., 1980, pp 183-186.

17. Jonsson K, verbal communication, 1983.

25
Combination of Hyperbaric Oxygenation, Surgery, and Antibiotics in the Treatment of Anaerobic Gas-Producing Wound Infections

Juha Niinikoski

INTRODUCTION

Anaerobic gas-producing wound infection of both clostridial and nonclostridial origin are serious infections, often life-threatening, and frequently associated with increased morbidity, cost, disability, and cosmetic disfigurement. These infections are spectacular lesions with an acute onset and rapid progression leading to considerable destruction of involved tissues.

CLOSTRIDIAL WOUND INFECTIONS

Gas gangrene or clostridial myonecrosis is among most dreaded complications of traumatic and surgical wounds. The rapid, fulminating course, profound toxemia, tissue destruction, and high mortality have continued to stimulate investigation of new methods of therapy. In the past, advances in the treatment of clostridial myonecrosis were limited to variations of antibiotics or to the method and extent of surgical debridement. If the disease progressed rapidly upward in the extremity, an emergency high amputation or even high exarticulation was the only alternative. Recovery was unusual in patients with primary involvement of or extension to the trunk. The advent of hyperbaric oxygen therapy and its use in the management of clostridial gas gangrene, pioneered by Brummelkamp, Hogendijk and Boerema (1961), has provided a therapeutic medium for the control and cure of this devastatingly rapid-spreading infection.

Hyperbaric oxygen therapy, antibiotics and surgery are regarded as complementary modes of treatment. Necrotic tissue requires excision but the use of hyperbaric oxygen therapy, by halting the spread of infection and reducing toxemia, diminishes the amount of tissue requiring excision and provides time for a balanced assessment of this requirement (Slack, Hanson and Chew 1969; Roding, Groeneveld and Boerema 1972).

Large patient series, in which hyperbaric oxygen therapy has been included in the treatment program of clostridial gas gangrene, show an overall mortality rate of 22 to 27% and a case fatality rate from the primary clostridial infection of 13 to 15% (Davis et al. 1973; Holland et al. 1975; Heimbach et al. 1977).

In cases with diffuse spreading myonecrosis or toxic spreading cellulitis, a survival of 78% has been observed for patients receiving hyperbaric oxygen therapy, surgical excision, and antibiotics, in contrast to a survival of 55% for patients receiving surgical excision and antibiotics alone (Hitchcock, Demello and Haglin 1975).

Evaluation of surgery, antibiotics and hyperbaric oxygen used singly and in different combinations as therapy for experimental gas gangrene in dogs demonstrated that hyperbaric oxygen therapy was an effective ancillary form of treatment that complemented the effects of surgery and antibiotics (Demello, Haglin and Hitchcock 1973).

As with any new therapeutic approach, some observers have been skeptical regarding the reported benefits of hyperbaric oxygen therapy for this disease (Altemeier and Fullen 1971).

Bacteriology and Pathogenesis

Clostridia are gram-positive, obligately anaerobic, spore-forming bacilli. They are found in the soil, clothing and intestinal flora of the majority of humans.

Clostridium perfringens is the most common etiologic agent. Clostridia must germinate before the organisms begin to multiply and produce toxins. Germination of clostridial spores requires an abnormally low tissue oxidation-reduction potential. This can be generated by tissue hypoxia and acidosis, which are frequently encountered in traumatic wounds and fractures with devitalized muscle and retained foreign bodies, tissues with severely impaired blood supply, and aerobic infections where the organisms consume the available oxygen.

The clostridia become effective pathogens through production of numerous exotoxins. The most important toxin produced by C. perfringens is the α toxin, which is chemically a lecithinase C.

The clostridial exotoxins destroy and liquefy surrounding tissues producing a rapid spread of the infection. Intense edema develops quickly, interfering with the circulation of tissues encased in fascial compartments. This may result in completely anoxic tissue environment, which further enhances growth of the organisms. A malignant phase may follow, with successive stages of rapid muscle disintegration and bacterial invasion, progressing to involve groups of muscles, an entire extremity, or the trunk in a matter of few hours. Gas bubbles may be seen coming from the wound, and crepitus may be palpable in affected areas. The defense mechanisms of the host can be completely overwhelmed within a period of 12 to 24 hours, and the patient succumbs from the disease.

Posttraumatic gas gangrene may also occur as a complication of minor wounds that have been closed primarily after incomplete debridement. The diseased gallbladder and colon can harbor a large population of clostridia; postsurgical gas gangrene of the abdominal wall is encountered most commonly after biliary and colorectal operations. Gas gangrene may also occur in anorectal and perineal areas as a complication of local wounds or abscesses (Bubrick and Hitchcock 1979). Factors that predispose to the development of clostridial crepitant infections include diabetes mellitus, vascular insufficiency, and malignant neoplasms (Hitchcock, Demello and Haglin 1975).

Clinical Manifestations

According to Davis and associates (1973), four distinct forms of clostridial gas-producing infections can be recognized.

Diffuse Spreading Clostridial Myonecrosis or True Gas Gangrene

After an accidental injury or an operation, usually after a few days and sometimes even after a few hours, a rapidly spreading wound infection is seen. The wound area is painful and body temperature rises quickly to about 40°C. The patient becomes seriously ill, somnolent or even comatose. The blood pressure may decrease, and in severe infections, jaundice develops as a sign of hemolysis. Gas bubbles escape from the wound and subcutaneous crepitation is palpable in the surrounding areas. The skin in the infected area develops a bronze discoloration with an erythematous border that advances rapidly. In a later stage, vesicles and bullae filled with reddish fluid can be seen on the skin. The wound has a most specific sickly sweet odor. The skin and underlying muscle undergo necrosis. The necrotic muscle varies from purplish-black to brick-red in color, may have a "cooked" appearance, and does not bleed when cut. Patients who survive the first 3 hyperbaric oxygen treatments usually overcome the clostridial infection (Heimbach et al. 1977).

Localized Clostridial Myonecrosis

The local wound appearance is similar to that seen in true gas gangrene, but except for fever there are no signs of systemic toxic reaction. Local excision and appropriate antibiotic treatment are usually sufficient to control this form of the disease.

Clostridial Cellulitis with Toxicity

Gas production is extremely abundant in this form of infection. The subcutaneous tissue undergoes necrosis whereas the underlying muscle remains uninvolved. Clostridial cellulitis can be accompanied by toxic symptoms similar to those seen in diffuse spreading myonecrosis, and it may have an equally grave prognosis. These patients must be treated in the same manner as those with true gas gangrene.

Clostridial Cellulitis without Toxicity

The symptoms and signs of this lesion are the same as in toxic cellulitis, except that the process remains more localized. Early decompression and drainage as well as appropriate intravenous antibiotic therapy are sufficient for treatment.

Diagnosis and Treatment

When a patient with a crepitant wound gangrene is admitted, the following schedule is pursued: the wound is inspected; remaining sutures are removed, the wound is opened widely and drained; clearly necrotic tissues are excised, and in cases with limb involvement fasciotomies are done; specimens for gram stain and bacterial cultures are taken from the wound exudate and necrotic tissue; and blood samples are taken for cultures and laboratory tests.

The presumptive diagnosis of clostridial wound gangrene is based on the clinical appearance of the patient and demonstration of gram-positive rods on smear. When this diagnosis has been made, hyperbaric oxygen therapy is begun without a delay by exposing the patient to pure oxygen at 2.5 to 3 atmospheres absolute (ATA) pressure—3 sessions of 2 hours during the first 24 hours; 2 sessions of 2 hours during the second 24 hours; and 2 sessions of 2 hours during the third 24 hours. Although the average number of treatments is seven, there is nothing sacrosanct in this number. Cures have been achieved with as few as 3 treatments, and in some cases 10 or more treatments have been required (Heimbach et al. 1977).

Oxygen tensions over 1500 mm Hg are bactericidal to clostridia (Kaye 1967). In infected lesions, the local pO_2 cannot be raised to such a high level. Studies from this institution indicate, however, that the pO_2 in tissues adjacent to clostridial infection may exceed 500 mm Hg during exposure to oxygen at 2.5 ATA pressure (Niinikoski and Aho 1983). At this level, a bacteriostatic effect is exerted against C. perfringens and the production of α toxin virtually ceases (van Unnik 1965).

The clinical improvement observed in patients after hyperbaric oxygen therapy is dramatic—the sensorium clears, pain is relieved and the heart rate and temperature return to normal. Spread of infection stops and necrotic areas become demarcated. After 2 or 3 exposures to hyperbaric oxygen, the patient can usually be returned to the operating room for more definitive debridement.

Antibiotic therapy is initiated with intravenous penicillin G, 20 to 40 million units per day. Because many of these processes are mixed infections, additional broad-spectrum antibiotic coverage is recommended, particularly against gram-negative organisms. For this purpose, the combination of clindamycin and gentamicin has been extensively used (Holland et al. 1975; Heimbach et al. 1977). Recently, metronidazole has been investigated as a first-line antibiotic in clostridial and other anaerobic infections (Serota and Feingold 1982). Piperacillin, a new broad-spectrum penicillin, in combination with an aminoglycoside may also be used in the treatment of these lesions.

Tetanus prophylaxis is administered according to the patient's preceding immunization history. Polyvalent gas gangrene antitoxin, of doubtful efficacy, is no longer available for administration.

All proven principles and methods of surgical intensive care must be efficiently applied in patients with clostridial wound gangrene. Vigilant monitoring of patient's cardiac, pulmonary and renal status is mandatory. Maintenance of normal blood volume is absolutely necessary to ensure adequate perfusion of organs and tissues. Fluid and electrolyte balance must be frequently evaluated, and proper intravenous fluid management and blood component therapy are given. The urine output should be maintained above the normal range keeping in mind that large amounts of potassium can be released from tissue destruction and hemolysis. No vasoconstrictive agents should be administered to patients in shock since vasoconstriction impedes oxygen supply to the affected tissues. Some of the clostridial exotoxins have a potent cardiodepressant effect; therefore, prompt digitalization of patients with signs of systemic toxicity is recommended.

Table 25.1 summarizes the essential features in the management of patients suspected of having clostridial wound gangrene.

NONCLOSTRIDIAL GAS-PRODUCING WOUND INFECTIONS

MacLennan (1943) and Altemeier and Culbertson (1948) were the first authors to stress the occurrence and potential severity of nonclostridial crepitant infections. Van Beek and colleagues (1974) as well as Nichols and Smith (1975) have thoroughly reviewed the medical literature concerning nonclostridial gas-producing infections.

Like clostridial organisms, nonclostridial gas-forming organisms may be contaminants in a wound, may cause local or diffuse cellulitis or spreading myositis mimicking clostridial myonecrosis (Skiles, Covert and Fletcher 1978). Thus the clinical differentiation between clostridial crepitant myonecrosis and that due to other organisms can be extremely difficult.

Nonclostridial crepitant infections are characterized by a rapidly spreading necrotizing infection of the skin and epifascial tissues of the perineum, abdominal wall, buttocks, hip, thorax, or neck, resulting from contamination by discharges from the intestinal, genitourinary, or respiratory tracts (Altemeier and Culbertson 1948). The process can spread rapidly over wide areas of the body, often without involvement of the structures beneath the deep fascia. The infection arises frequently in the perineum and extends beneath Scarpa's fascia into the inguinal region, abdominal wall, and flank (Himal, McLean and Duff 1974; Bubrick and Hitchcock 1979). Thrombosis of the nutrient vessels of the skin is a characteristic histological finding.

Factors that predispose to the development of these infections include lower extremity vascular disease and diabetes mellitus.

TABLE 25.1

Key Points in the Management of Clostridial Wound Gangrene

1. Maintain high index of suspicion.
2. Establish diagnosis, clinical picture, open and drain the wound, perform fasciotomy, gram stain specimens for culture.
3. Begin antibiotic therapy: give tetanus prophylaxis, treat diabetes or other underlying disorder.
4. Transfer immediately to hyperbaric facility (use air ambulance if necessary.
5. Administer hyperbaric oxygen treatment.
6. Administer intensive supportive therapy—repeated surgical debridements and topical wound care between hyperbaric exposures.
7. Perform final excision or amputation after demarcation of infection and diminished toxicity.
8. Perform reconstructive surgery.

DO NOT WASTE TIME!

Bacteriology

Both facultative aerobes and obligate anaerobes have been reported as etiologic organisms in nonclostridial crepitant infections. Anaerobic pathways of metabolism, such as denitrification, fermentation and deamination appear necessary for the production of insoluble gases, including hydrogen and nitrogen that form the gaseous collections in these infections (Stone and Martin 1972). The gas produced by the aerobic metabolic pathways is carbon dioxide, which is highly soluble and does not accumulate in tissues.

The nonclostridial bacteria that are capable of producing the infection often exert a synergistic effect. Most commonly they include some strains of the coliform group, particularly _Escherichia coli_; the anaerobic gram-negative bacilli, principally _Bacteroides fragilis_ and _Bacteroides melaninogenicus_; and the anaerobic _Streptococcus_. In infections associated with B. _melaninogenicus_, the involved tissues may show a gray or black discoloration (Altemeier 1982).

Diagnosis and Treatment

Definitive diagnosis of the organisms responsible for the gas infection requires a minimum of one to two days for bacteriological work-up. Because delays before the start of therapy cannot be tolerated if acceptable clinical results are to be expected, initial therapy should be begun immediately after specimens for gram stain have been collected and clinical inspection of the extent of the infection has been performed. The presumptive diagnosis is made on the basis of gram-stain results and the clinical appearance of the patient.

Adequate surgical debridement is fundamental to all types of nonclostridial gas-producing infections. The tissue losses can be kept minimal only by the rapidity of initial treatment.

Intravenous antibiotic therapy is adjunctive but important. The combination of clindamycin and gentamicin has been widely used for nonclostridial crepitant infections. If the definitive aerobic and anaerobic culture results differ from the presumptive diagnosis, antibiotic coverage can be changed at the time this information becomes available.

Hyperbaric oxygen therapy should be considered when quickly available, although this form of treatment is clearly of far less benefit in a nonclostridial infection (Skiles, Covert and Fletcher 1978). Slack, Hanson and Chew (1969) reported that hyperbaric oxygen therapy seems less effective in nonclostridial gas-producing infections but is a valuable diagnostic tool in their differentiation from clostridial infections.

Nonclostridial crepitant infections are more serious than has been realized. The mortality for patients with nonclostridial infections is generally greater than for those with clostridial infections (Slack, Hanson and Chew 1969; Skiles, Covert and Fletcher 1978).

All patients with serious gas infections should be treated in a surgical intensive care unit, where their clinical status and response to various modes of treatment can be properly monitored and controlled.

CLINICAL MATERIAL AND RESULTS

Clostridial Wound Infections

Between May 1971 and April 1983, 13 bacteriologically proven cases with clostridial crepitant wound infections were treated by the Department of Surgery of Turku University Central

Hospital, Finland. There were 11 males and two females ranging from 16 to 77 years of age, with a mean age of 43.8 years. Four cases were from this hospital while nine patients were transferred for hyperbaric oxygen therapy from other hospitals in Finland.

In 3 patients the infection was monomicrobial, with C. perfringens as the only organism encountered in the primary culture. In the remaining 10 patients, C. perfringens plus 1 to 3 additional types of bacteria were found (Table 25.2).

The patients were treated with strict adherence to the principles described. The hyperbaric oxygen therapy was given in a Vickers monoplace chamber. The patients received 1 to 9 two-hour treatments in pure oxygen at 2.5 ATA pressure, with an average of 5 treatments per patient.

Nine cases had diffuse spreading clostridial myonecrosis, eight of whom survived, and 4 patients had clostridial cellulitis with toxicity, all of whom survived (Table 25.3). Thus the overall mortality for these patients was 7.7%.

As shown in Table 25.4, nine of these infections developed postoperatively in surgical wounds while in four cases trauma was the antecedent cause. The trunk was involved in eight patients; one of them died. He was moribund prior to the treatment and died after the first exposure to hyperbaric oxygen. This patient developed a fulminant gas gangrene of the abdominal wall after rectal amputation. None of the five patients with the disease confined to the lower limb was lost. Three required amputation, two above and one below the knee.

Two patients had diabetes mellitus as a predisposing factor, one had a malignant tumor, and one had a debilitating mental disease as a contributing disorder.

TABLE 25.2

Organisms Encountered in the Primary Cultures of 13 Patients with Clostridial Crepitant Wound Infections

Organism	No. of Patients
Clostridium perfringens	13
Bacteroides spp.	3
Escherichia coli	4
Proteus spp.	4
Klebsiella	1
Streptococcus faecalis	5

TABLE 25.3

Patients with Clostridial Crepitant Wound Infections Treated with Hyperbaric Oxygen Therapy

Type of Infection	No. of Patients	Recovered	Died
Spreading myonecrosis	9	8	1
Cellulitis with toxicity	4	4	—
Total	13	12	1 (7.7%)

TABLE 25.4

Etiology and Site of Clostridial Crepitant Wound Infections in Patients Treated with Hyperbaric Oxygen Therapy

		Site of Involvement			
Etiology	No. of Patients	Abdominal Wall	Pelvis	Lower Limb and Trunk	Lower Limb
Postoperative	9	5 (1 died)	—	2	2
Posttraumatic	4	—	1	—	3
Total	13	5	1	2	5

Nonclostridial Gas-Producing Wound Infections

During the same 12-year period, three nonclostridial crepitant wound infections mimicking true gas gangrene were treated in Turku University Central Hospital (Table 25.5).

All patients were males. Each of these infections developed postoperatively in the abdominal wall, 2 after appendectomy and 1 after laparotomy for intestinal occlusion. The patients were treated with the same principles as patients with clostridial infections. Each patient received surgical debridement, antibiotic therapy, hyperbaric oxygen therapy, and full-scale supportive treatment in the intensive care unit.

The combination of *Escherichia coli* and *Bacteroides fragilis* was encountered in the primary culture of both appendectomy

TABLE 25.5

Patients with Nonclostridial Crepitant Wound Infections Treated with Hyperbaric Oxygen Therapy

Patient No. Age & Sex	Infection Location	Antecedent Cause	Tissues Involved in Necrotic Process	No. of HBO Treatments	Surgery	Organisms in Primary Culture	Result
No. 1 50; male	Abdominal wall	Appendectomy	Skin Subcutis Muscle	9	Excisions & drainage	*E. coli* *B. fragilis*	Died
No. 2 24; male	Abdominal wall	Appendectomy	Skin Subcutis	4	Incisions & drainage	*E. coli* *B. fragilis* *S. Faecalis*	Survived
No. 3 58; male	Abdominal wall	Laparotomy for intestinal obstruction	Skin Subcutis	8	Excisions & skin graftings	*B. distasonis* *B. thetaiotamicron* *Proteus vulgaris*	Survived

patients, whereas in the third patient *Bacteroides distasonis*, *Bacteroides thetaiotamicron*, and *Proteus vulgaris* were cultured from the wound exudate.

A 50-year-old patient, who developed massive, nonclostridial gas gangrene after appendectomy, failed to respond to treatment and died after having received nine two-hour treatments in hyperbaric oxygen. Severe calcification and stenosis of the aortic valve resulting in cardiac insufficiency contributed to the death of this patient.

SUMMARY

The addition of hyperbaric oxygen therapy to the treatment program of clostridial wound gangrene—although strictly adjunctive to surgery, antibiotics and intensive care—has dramatically changed the surgical approach to treatment. When hyperbaric oxygenation is available, the initial debridement can be limited to opening and drainage of the infected wound, excision of only clearly necrotic tissue, and fasciotomies in cases with limb involvement. Compromised but still viable tissue should be left in place, because hyperbaric oxygen therapy may return this tissue to normal. Final debridement can be delayed until clinical cure of clostridial infection has occurred.

Like clostridial organisms, nonclostridial gas-forming organisms may be contaminants in a wound, may cause cellulitis and subcutaneous infections or may cause a full blown myositis which closely resembles clostridial myonecrosis. Several groups of bacteria seem to be capable of producing these lesions, often exerting a synergistic effect. Nonclostridial gas-producing wound infections with fulminating, septic courses should receive prompt and radical surgical debridement combined with effective antibiotic therapy. Hyperbaric oxygen therapy is of far less benefit in a nonclostridial infection.

REFERENCES

Altemeier, WA. 1982. Diagnosis and treatment of necrotizing infections. Paper read at the postgraduate course Pre- and Postoperative Care: Surgical Infections, 68th Annual Clinical Congress, American College of Surgeons, October 24-29, 1982, Chicago. Manual pp. 97-103.

Altemeier, WA, and WR Culbertson. 1948. Acute non-clostridial crepitant cellulitis. Surg. Gynecol. Obstet. 87:206-212.

Altemeier, WA, and WD Fullen. 1971. Prevention and treatment of gas gangrene. JAMA 217:806-813.

Brummelkamp, WH, J Hogendijk and I Boerema. 1961. Treatment of anaerobic infections (clostridial myositis) by drenching the tissues with oxygen under high atmospheric pressure. Surgery 49:299-302.

Bubrick, MP, and CR Hitchcock. 1979. Necrotizing anorectal and perineal infections. Surgery 86:655-662.

Davis, JC, JM Dunn, CO Hagood, and BE Basset. 1973. Hyperbaric medicine in the U.S. Air Force. JAMA 224:205-209.

Demello, FJ, JJ Haglin, and CR Hitchcock. 1973. Comparative study of experimental Clostridium perfringens infection in dogs treated with antibiotics, surgery and hyperbaric oxygen. Surgery 73:936-941.

Heimbach, RD, I Boerema, WH Brummelkamp, and WG Wolfe. 1977. Current therapy of gas gangrene. In Hyperbaric Oxygen Therapy, edited by JC Davis and TK Hunt, pp. 153-176. Bethesda: Undersea Medical Society.

Himal, HS, APH McLean, and JH Duff. 1974. Gas gangrene of the scrotum and perineum. Surg. Gynecol. Obstet. 139: 176-178.

Hitchcock, CR, FJ Demello, and JJ Haglin. 1975. Gangrene infection: New approaches to an old disease. Surg. Clin. N. Am. 55:1403-1410.

Holland, JA, GB Hill, WG Wolfe, S Osterhout, HA Salzman, and JW Brown, Jr. 1975. Experimental and clinical experience with hyperbaric oxygen in the treatment of clostridial myonecrosis. Surgery 77:75-85.

Kaye, D. 1967. Effect of hyperbaric oxygen on clostridia in vitro and in vivo. Proc. Soc. Exp. Biol. Med. 124:360-366.

MacLennan, JD. 1943. Anaerobic infection of war wounds in Middle East. Lancet 2:63-66, 94-99, 123-126.

Nichols, RL, and JW Smith. 1975. Gas in the wound: what does it mean? Surg. Clin. N. Am. 55:1289-1296.

Niinikoski, J, and AJ Aho. 1983. Combination of hyperbaric oxygen, surgery, and antibiotics in the treatment of clostridial gas gangrene. Infections in Surgery 2:23-37.

Roding, B, PHA Groeneveld, and I Boerema. 1972. Ten years of experience in the treatment of gas gangrene with hyperbaric oxygen. Surg. Gynecol. Obstet. 134:579-585.

Serota, AJ, and SM Feingold. 1982. Necrotizing soft tissue infections following abdominal surgery. Infections in Surgery 1:50-60.

Skiles, MS, GK Covert, and HS Fletcher. 1978. Gas-producing clostridial and nonclostridial infections. Surg. Gynecol. Obstet. 147:65-67.

Slack, WK, GC Hanson, and HER Chew. 1969. Hyperbaric oxygen in the treatment of gas gangrene and clostridial infection. A report of 40 patients treated in a single-person hyperbaric oxygen chamber. Br. J. Surg. 56:505-510.

Stone, HH, and JD Martin, Jr. 1972. Synergistic necrotizing cellulitis. Ann. Surg. 175:702-711.

Van Beek, A, E Zook, P Yaw, R Gardner, R Smith, and JL Glover. 1974. Nonclostridial gas-forming infections. Arch. Surg. 108:552-557.

van Unnik, AJM. 1965. Inhibition of toxin production in Clostridium perfringens in vitro by hyperbaric oxygen. Antonie van Leeuwenhoek 31:181-186.

26
Quantitative Bacteriology and Inflammatory Mediators in Soft Tissue

Martin C. Robson and John P. Heggers

INTRODUCTION

Health is not a germ-free state. Rather, it is a delicate balance between bacteria and host resistance. There exists in soft tissue a delicate equilibrium between those factors which together contribute to host resistance and a myriad of bacterial species. If any of the bacterial species get out of balance and are allowed to multiply, the equilibrium is upset. This balance is dependent on many factors, of which, local and systemic host defense mechanisms play a major role.

LOCAL HOST DEFENSE MECHANISMS

The effect of the interaction between the bacteria and the host, although under systemic influence, is ultimately determined by local factors in the wound. Among these are necrotic tissue, foreign body, hematoma, dead space, and decreased local perfusion. Clinically each of these seems to alter host resistance and thus be capable of allowing infection to occur. Each of these local wound factors can be present at the time of wounding or can be added by the surgeon.

Howe has presented the concept that a wound represents a gradient of resistance at different points based upon the amount of tissue damage and the local blood supply.[28] Tissue damage, whether chemical, mechanical, or thermal may result in lowered resistance and a greater propensity for minor contamination to initiate an infection. Edlich et al. have stated that all devitalized soft tissues left in a wound, damage its defenses and encourage the development of infection. This capacity to enhance bacterial infection appears to be comparable for devitalized skin, fat, and muscle.[17]

Three mechanisms have been suggested by which devitalized tissue enhances infection.[17] The first is that it acts as an excellent culture medium and promotes bacterial growth. Secondly, it inhibits phagocytosis and subsequent intracellular killing by the leukocytes. Thirdly, it provides an anaerobic environment which, by lowering the oxygen tension decreases the efficiency of the leukocytes.

Foreign bodies, whether dirt and debris, or iatrogenic foreign bodies such as sutures and drains, have been associated with decreased host resistance. Rodeheaver et al. showed that the presence of as little as 5 milligrams of soil reduced the number of bacteria necessary to cause a wound infection in an experimental animal from one million to one hundred.[50] It appears from this research that in the presence of soil, leukocytes cannot ingest and kill bacteria, and nonspecific humoral factors seem to be less effective in controlling bacterial levels.[17]

The presence of a single silk suture was shown by Elek to decrease the number of staphylococci necessary to form a pustule in human volunteers from over a million to one hundred—a ten-thousand-fold decrease.[18] In a thorough study of contaminated wounds, Edlich and his associates have unequivocally documented the role of percutaneous sutures in causing wound infections.[17] Studies by Getzen and Jansen suggest that sutures may react as allergens and have correlated the incidence of wound complications with skin reactions to the suture materials themselves and increased blood eosinophil counts.[20]

Drains in wounds can act as foreign bodies and as such, may decrease local host resistance. The use of drains requires weighing the potential benefits against the harmful effects. No one would quarrel with the use of drains in a wound following drainage of loculated pus. When no localized collection is present, drains by definition are prophylactic and one must weigh the pros and cons. In the cooperative National Research Council prospective study, drains of any sort were associated with an 11.1% wound infection rate compared to 5% for non-drained wounds.[2,5,11]

In 1935 Meleney documented the clinical impressions of Kocher and Halsted when he reported an increased infection rate in wounds that developed hematoma.[40] Conolly et al. and May et al. reported that up to 30% of clinical wound infections were associated with hematomas.[10,39] When 5×10^7 E. coli organisms were injected subcutaneously in the absence of an experimental hematoma, the E. coli were effectively contained at the injection site by natural host defenses and blood stream cultures or tissue cultures from the lung, liver, spleen, and kidney remained at 10^5 organisms or fewer per/gram. However, when the same number of bacteria were injected into a hematoma, the bacterial counts in the blood and tissues began to rise precipitously within six hours. The counts reached levels greater than 10^5 organisms per/gram and 80% of the animals died. Thus the hematoma seemed to prevent the natural defense mechanisms from localizing the bacteria at the injection site.

Although studies by Davis and Yull have suggested that the hemoglobin fraction of the red blood cell may be the major etiology of decreased resistance seen with hematomas, dead space alone can be a problem.[12] Hunt et al. have developed an experimental rabbit model using wire mesh cylinders to make a reproducible dead space.[29] Using this model, they showed that dead space alone could increase the susceptibility of tissue to infection. deHoll similarly demonstrated that dead space potentiates infection in contaminated wounds. However, attempts at suture obliteration of the dead space increases the infection rate even more.[15] Closed suction drainage systems can decrease dead space and thereby minimize this local infection risk. Alexander et al. have shown that the wound fluid collecting in potential dead spaces becomes deficient in opsonic factors with time.[5] Removal of this fluid appears to be beneficial and allows more efficient neutrophil functioning in the presence of tissue bacteria. This advantage of a drain to decrease dead space must be weighed against the previously discussed hazards of a drain.

In addition to the previously mentioned local factors, there is documented evidence of increased susceptibility to infection due to decreased local wound perfusion. The location of the wound will reflect the potential of local defense mechanisms because of the variation in blood perfusion. The excellence of blood supply to the face and scalp provide inherently greater resistance than is present on the lower extremities. Conolly et al. have stated that a wound requires oxygen for collagen synthesis and healing and this requires local circulation.[11] Hunt et al. have shown that all wounds are hypoxic and, therefore, have only borderline circulation.[30] Consequently, if the local circulation becomes impaired, healing will be affected and infection increased.

Each of these local factors can upset the equilibrium. Circumstances are produced in which a normally subinfectious innoculum of bacteria may produce infection. The resultant quantitative increase in bacterial growth reflects these changes.

SYSTEMIC HOST DEFENSE MECHANISMS

The response of the host to an invader is governed by conditions operative at the portal of entry. Beyond that site the body fluids and cells provide the dynamic activities of protective resistance.[1] Host defense mechanisms can be categorized as specific or nonspecific. These mechanisms are complex, diversified, frequently interdependent and numerous. The specific host defense mechanisms are divided into two distinct entities. These are the humoral and cellular responses. The cellular components responsible for keeping the inner portals free of any foreign substances consist of neutrophils, eosinophils and monocytic macrophages. Other nonspecific defenses include temperature elevation (fever), pH of body tissues, nutrition and interferons which afford protection from viral infection and tumors.

Nonspecific Host Defense Response

The most important physical defenses which prevent exogenous as well as endogenous microorganisms from gaining access to the internal structures are the skin and the mucous membranes.

This is the first target to be breached in any assault, be it surgery or trauma. The character of the tissue, cell type, nature of local secretions, drainage, and tissue pH have all been shown to determine the ease with which the host barrier is broached. The dryness of the keratin layer of the skin provides protection against the staphylococci.[2,23] If this physical characteristic of the skin is changed by a wetting agent, such as an impermeable wet dressing, this barrier is lost and the skin surface is rapidly covered with folliculitis-minute staphylococcal abscesses. Also active at the skin portal are bactericidal and fungicidal fatty acids in the sebaceous secretions. These prevent massive invasion by the streptococci.[3,4,23] The laminated epidermal layer of nucleated cornified cells form an antibacterial environment for most organisms, except those considered to be "resident" flora such as Staphylococcus epidermidis, Corynebacteria, and Propionibacterium.[23]

In the lower respiratory tract, the cilia and mucous of the trachea and bronchi remove particulate matter, including bacteria. However, important as mucin is as a defense mechanism, an accumulation of this bronchial secretion can lower resistance by preventing phagocytosis. In the alimentary tract portals, pH has proved to be an important defense mechanism. The population of resident bacteria change and increase in numbers as we proceed distally. Peristaltic elimination of waste prevents overgrowth of the resident flora. Any interruption of this mobility may compromise the host by allowing microbial overgrowth.[23]

After penetrating the epithelial layer of the skin, respiratory, alimentary or genital tract, the bacteria are deposited in the intercellular spaces. With the onset of proliferation, the products of the bacteria cause injury to local tissue, thus evoking the inflammatory response. This response is initiated by vasoactive amines, such as histamine and serotonin, kinin polypeptides and other chemical mediators. These have been shown to cause a biphasic, vascular phenomenon consisting of constriction of the venular sphincters and dilation of the capillaries. In addition, the kallikrein-kinin system has been demonstrated to be responsible for increased vascular permeability along with the prostaglandins and the adherent properties of the venular endothelial surfaces.[45] The result of these initial vascular changes is that edema fluid and fibrinogen exude from the dilated permeable vessels, creating a fibrin network and thrombi which tend to localize the intruding bacteria. The adherent endothelial walls trap the phagocytic cells coming in contact with them and allow them to emigrate through the widened endothelial spaces. Menkin has described a chemotactic agent called "leukotaxine" which increases the migration of the phagocytic cells to the site of invasion. The "leukotaxis" has since been found to be mediated through the kinin system.[23]

As the nonspecific inflammatory response occurs and increased plasma or serum reaches the bacterium, the total complex of "nonspecific" resistance is brought into action. In addition to the kinin system, other factors or chemoattractants present in serum or plasma, such as products of complement activation and the fibrinolytic system are also responsible for chemotaxis.

The inflammatory process begins immediately post-trauma/ invasion. Certain tissue substances, mainly those of the arachidonic acid cascade, initiate along with the above mentioned products, the cardinal signs of the process known as the "inflammatory response."

Arachidonic acid provokes overt pain. Prostaglandin G_2 (PGG_2) and PGH_2 cause a modest hyperalgesia. Other prostaglandins such as PGI_2, PGE, and PGE_2 act synergistically with bradykinin and histamine in provoking hyperalgesia. Prostanoids, such as 12-L hydroperoxyeicosatetraenoic acid (12 HPETE) produce a hyperalgesic state greater than the PGEs, whereas $PGF_{2\alpha}$ antagonizes the effects of PGE_2 (Table 26.1).[43,60]

Fever can also be induced by arachidonic acid, PGE and PGE_2. These same substances at low doses, along with PGG_2, PGH_2, PGI_2 and $PGF_{1\alpha}$ can also potentiate carrageenan, bradykinin and histamine edema. However, PGE_1, PGE_2, and $PGF_{1\alpha}$ at high doses inhibit this activity. While most of those prostanoids potentiate edema, be it carrageenan, bradykinin, and histamine, PGG_2, PGH_2, and HPETE may potentiate phorbol

TABLE 26.1

Effects of Prostaglandins in Inflammation

Compound	Edema	Vascular Tone	Chemotaxis	Pain	Fever
Arachidonic acid	carrageenan	vasodilation	chemotactic	overt pain	fever
PGG_2, PGH_2 (endoperoxides)	weak, carrageenan, bradykinin and histamine	vasoconstriction if PGI pathway blocked	NE	hyperalgesia	none if stable products
PGI_2 (prostacyclin)	bradykinin and carrageenan	vasodilation	inhibits		NE
PGE_1		vasodilation	depresses chemokinesis	hyperalgesia synergistic with histamine and bradykinin	fever
PGE_2	low dose carrageenan histamine bradykinin	vasodilation	depresses chemokinesis	E. hyperalgesia E. synergistic with histamine and bradykinin	fever
$PGF_{1\alpha}$		vasodilation	chemokinesis enhanced	antagonizes effects of PGE_2	NE
TxA_2	NE	potent vasoconstriction	?	NE	NE
HPETE	may mediate PMA	vasoconstriction	related compounds are chemotactic	hyperalgesia $>PGE_2$	NE

Notes: NE = not established.

myristate acetate (PMA) edema through the oxygen-derived free radial formed during conversion (Table 26.1).[43,60]

Pure arachidonate is chemotactic, when corrections are made for chemokinesis, and this activity is enhanced when exposed to H_2O_2 or ultraviolet light. PGI_2 on the other hand, inhibits chemotaxis, and PGE_2 depresses chemokinesis. Again $PGF_{2\alpha}$ has the opposite effect of PGE_2 in that it enhances both chemokinesis and chemotaxis (Table 26.1).[43,60]

These tissue prostanoids also mediate vascular tone or permeability, and, therefore, reversibly affect the functions of cells involved in inflammation. Prostanoids of the E class, PGI_2, HPETE and arachidonic acid all provoke vasodilation, of which PGI_2 is the most potent one. Those that counterbalance vasodilation or are vasoconstrictors are $PGF_{2\alpha}$ and TxA_2. However TxA_2 is extremely more potent a vasoconstrictor than $PGF_{2\alpha}$ (Table 26.1).[60]

Skin and soft tissue are not the only cell populations that have the capacity of prostanoid production. Each of the mobile cells of the acute and chronic inflammatory process can transform arachidonic acid into its biological active derivatives. If human polymorphonuclear (PMN) leukocytes are exposed to a phagocytic stimulus, they respond with a well designed and programmed sequence of secretory events, which produces three classes of mediators. These are lysosomal hydrolases, active products derived from molecular oxygen which are not only microbicidal, but can indiscriminately damage nearby cells. The third are those of the prostanoid family. The PMN not only produces PGI_2, PGE, and PGE_2, and other stable prostanoids, but when activated produces 4 times as much TxA_2 than it does in the resting state.[60]

While PGI_2 and those of the E series increase vascular permeability, PGI_2 and PGE_1 also have the ability to abrogate the antiinflammatory response. If either are present prior to chemotactic stimuli, they can affix to an appropriate receptor site on the PMN membrane and align the receptor site with the inner membrane's adenyl cyclase, increasing membrane fluidity. When a chemotactic stimulus comes in contact with the PMN, these two components activate a quantum increase of cAMP over the normal production creating a negative feedback or shutoff which inhibits phagocytic activity, SRS-A release and lysosomal enzyme release during phagocytosis.[60]

The slow reacting substances of anaphylaxis (SRS-A) belong to a series of compounds called leukotrienes (LT) which are metabolites of the prostanoid cascade. They have 3 conjugated double bonds with a hydroxy group. The leukotrienes exist in three distinct forms: LTC_4, LTD_4, and LTE_4. LTC has a thioether linked to glycine and glutamic acid. LTD has the same bond but to glycine only and LTE to cysteine. LTD is 100 to 1000 times more potent than histamine on a weight basis; however muscle contractions are slower. These leukotrienes are metabolic by-products of arachidonic acid via the enzyme lipoxygenase.[60]

Leukotriene B4 is a potent chemotactin causing migration and accumulation of PMNs at the site of secretion (release). LTB_4 is also responsible for the enhancement of expression of C_3b receptors. Prostaglandin E_2 along with LTD_4, synergistically enhances the alteration in cutaneous microvascular permeability suggesting an interaction between the two separate pathways. Leukotriene metabolism is enhanced when a nonsteroidal antiinflammatory or a prostanoid inhibitor such as indomethacin is used.[60]

The lipoxygenase pathway leads to the production of potent spasmogenic, vascular and chemotactic factors. Leukotrienes and related lipoxygenase metabolites represent the first class of mediators that can regulate both cellular and humoral components of human allergic reactions and may prove to be more important in a broad range of acute and chronic hypersensitivity conditions (Fig. 26.1).[59,60]

With all the activities attributed to the prostanoids, one should consider them as modulators rather than mediators of the inflammatory process. While these prostanoids and leukotrienes modulate inflammation, PGE_2 in conjunction with c-AMP modulate the normal maturation process of the skin. PGE_2 also modulates the cellular immune response through establishment of a T suppressor cell which suppresses MIF, cytotoxic activity, lymphokine and monokine production and prolongation of skin graft survival.[59,60]

Specific Host Defense Response

One might consider that the final line of host defense lies with the immunological potential of the host, after all other defense mechanisms are breached. The immune system is a highly complex, specific and diversified organ system that can be divided into two major responses 1) the humoral immune response and 2) cellular immune response. The former is primarily B-cell mediated and the latter T-cell mediated. As stated previously, no system of host defense is entirely independent and when combined with the nonspecific arm of the host defense system, the immune system becomes the major component of the

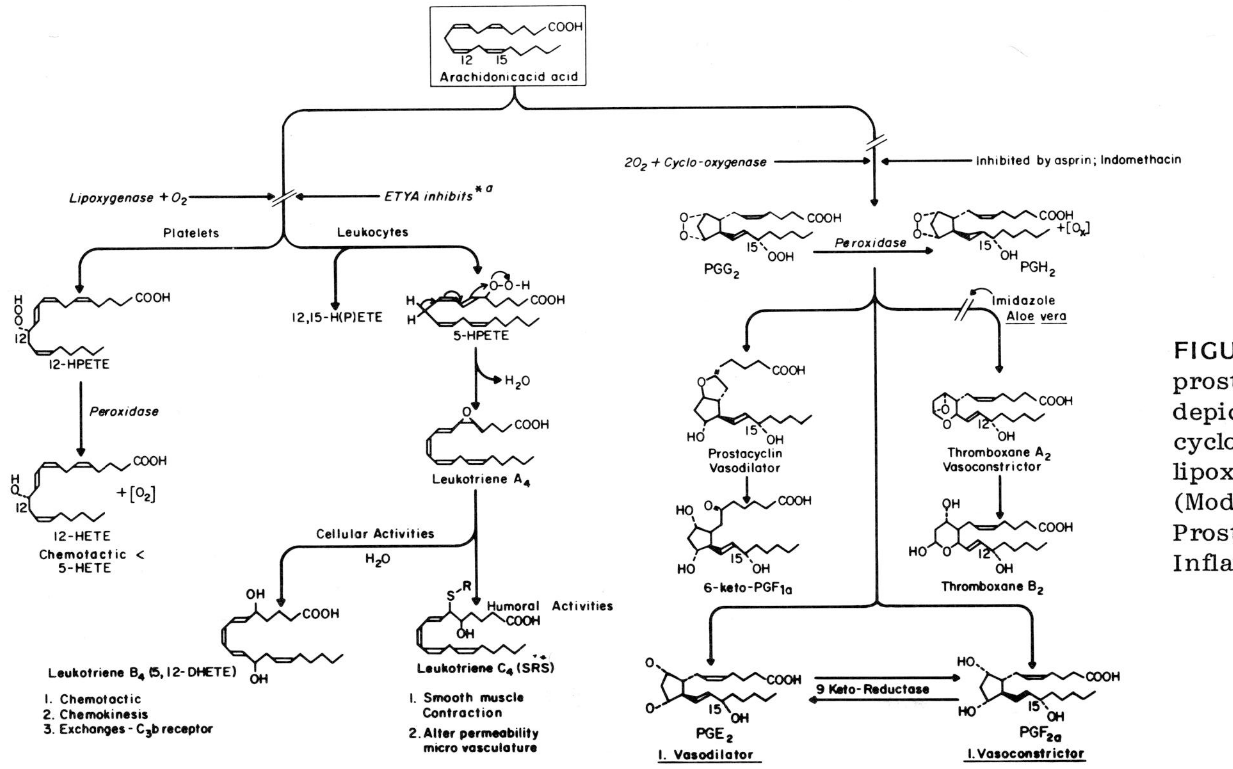

FIGURE 26.1 The prostanoic acid cascade, depicting both the cyclo-oxygenase and lipoxygenase pathways. (Modified, Weismann, Prostaglandins in Acute Inflammation, 1980. 60)

host's survival against bacterial invasion, as well as other invaders—that is, virus, tumors and parasites.[23]

The B-cell is the primary cell responsible for the humoral immune response. After receiving the antigenic message from the macrophage and some assistance from the T helper cell, the B-cell can be termed immunocompetent, thus producing plasma cells. These cells are responsible for producing specific antibodies which are directed against microbes or their by-products. There are five major classes of these immunoglobulins that are identified by their specific antigenicity. Of these three have been shown to have an effect on bacteria. They are IgG, IgM, and IgA. Their bactericidal capabilities are expressed by three methods. The first is neutralization of toxin. The responsible cell is the B cell which produces an antitoxin (IgG) directed at the specific toxic substance, such as that produced by Clostridium perfringens (welchii) or Corynebacterium diphtheriae. The second method is an activity directed against the cell wall components of gram-negative bacilli in the presence of complement, an interdependent action which causes bacteriolysis. Thirdly, is opsonization, which promotes and enhances the engulfment of the pathogen during phagocytosis.[23]

The cellular immune response which is T-cell mediated is somewhat more diverse in its actions. Once stimulated, the T-cell goes through a blastogenic change, the resultant offspring of which are a memory cell and activated T-effector cell. The T-effector cell initiates its predestined activity against the invader and the memory cell waits in reserve. As a reserve, it is a long lived cell population. This characteristic is particularly important in that it is a deterrent to reinfection. This mechanism is also inherent in the HIR cell population. The T-cell population also contains T-helper and suppressor cells. The helper cells are required to key B-cells for antibody production, whereas the T-suppressor regulates antibody production.[23]

The activated T-effector cells are capable of killing a variety of cells, an effect best demonstrated in allograft rejection and tumor immunity,[13] and also in being cytotoxic for cells infected by viruses. T-cell soluble mediators of lymphokines are non-antibody proteins which regulate both specific and nonspecific activities of leucocytes, macrophages and lymphocytes. These substances are produced by the T-lymphocyte upon stimulation. Some examples of lymphokines are migration, inhibition factor, skin reactive factor, macrophage activation and interferon.[23]

Recent studies have shown that delayed hypersensitivity skin testing, while invaluable in traumatic injuries are questionable in the thermal injury. A study of 110 patients showed that those patients who were relatively anergic to 6 skin recall antigens were no more susceptible to infection (66%) and to die (25%) than those patients considered normal (77% and 33% respectively).[25]

PROPERTIES AFFECTING THE PATHOGENICITY OR INVASIVENESS OF BACTERIA

An intact skin or mucous membrane barrier usually contains the microbial flora in a harmless, commensal balance. The bacteria only become truly parasitic when they actually invade the host and begin to survive at the host's expense. Parasitism can be divided into two categories, intracellular and extracellular. Bacteria that behave as intracellular parasites frequently give rise to relatively chronic diseases, such as tuberculosis. Extracellular parasites owe their invasiveness initially to a break in the membrane barrier, then to their antiphagocytic surface components, often demonstrable as definite capsules.[48,49]

Just what mechanisms make some microbes virulent and more invasive than others? How do the surface components of microorganisms contribute to their invasiveness? What are the criteria necessary for a microbe to cause infection? It must 1) enter the host, 2) multiply in host tissues, 3) resist and/or not stimulate host defenses, and 4) damage the host. The microbial products responsible for these processes are the determinants of virulence (pathogenicity). Some of these interactions occur solely between extracellular products such as toxins and antitoxins, but the majority are related to surface compounds.[48,49]

Though some microbes enter the host via an insect vector bite or trauma, most infections begin on the mucous membranes of the respiratory, alimentary and urogenital tracts. Usually the membrane surfaces are protected by mucous, moving lumen contents, and microbes of the commensal type. There are three basic methods of invasion upon these membranes. They are 1) attachment and multiplication without penetration, as seen with _Bordetella pertussis_ and _Vibrio cholerae_, 2) attachment and penetration of mucous membranes and localized multiplication with little or no spread—that is, shigellosis and influenza, and 3) attachment to, and penetration of the inner tissues either through or between the mucosal membranes as seen with _Streptococcus pyogenes_ and _Salmonella_ species.[52]

These surface components effect their invasion (attachment and penetration) by a series of activities. There are four major actions which determine the microbes virulence. They are 1) resisting the mechanical cleansing action of the mucous membranes (that is, moving lumen contents) by adherence to the epithelial surface, 2) competing for nutrients and space on the mucosal surface with commensals and antimicrobial resistance to the commensal's by-products, 3) by resisting the initial inflammatory response as well as the antimicrobial effects of humoral and cellular immune mechanisms, 4) in situ damage of the epithelial cells after penetration or invading and infecting of tissues after breaching the epithelial surfaces.[52]

The microbial adherence to surfaces of the mucosal membrane seems to be one of selectivity. In the buccal cavity, Streptococcus sanguis and mutans adhere to the teeth. To the tongue and buccal mucosa, we find Streptococcus salivarius and mitis, respectively. The attachment is effected by the production of high molecular weight glucose polymers such as dextran and glucan.

In the case of S. pyogenes adherence to the epithelium of the throat is a result of the cell wall protein.[19] Escherichia coli adheres to the ileum and the epithelial cells near the villous tips rather than the base.[52] Pseudomonas aeruginosa adherence is influenced by the viability of cells. Tracheal cells injured either by endotracheal intubation or an influenza infection are predisposed to P. aeruginosa adherence[47] as well as damaged heart valves.

The space on the mucosal membranes is prime real estate. The resident commensals are constantly in competition for their space with opportunistic and virulent microbes. Their position becomes even more compromised after the introduction of antimicrobial therapy. Stronger adherence mechanisms favor the virulent microbes, enabling them to evict the resident commensals--for example, Lactobacillus acidophilus is easily replaced by Neisseria gonorrhea because of its strong adherence properties.[38]

The human as a host has an elaborate defense system. The major defense mechanisms include the initial inflammatory response, the production of complement, humoral and cellular immune mechanisms. Staphylococcus aureus "M," encapsulated strains have cell wall peptoglycans and other cell wall components which are capable of inhibiting opsonization. They apparently mask the cell wall components, which in themselves mediate chemotaxigenesis, therefore enabling the encapsulated S. aureus M to evade the first line of cellular defense—phagocytosis.[13,41]

Lactoferrin, an iron-binding protein present in secretions that lubricate human mucosal tissues has been shown to have a bactericidal effect on some Streptococcus species, non-enterogenic E. coli, P. aeruginosa and Candida albicans. This protein is active in the iron-free state, and is a glycoprotein synthesized by neutrophils. However, Streptococcus pyogenes, S. aureus and epidermidis, E. coli (enteropathogenic 012:B16 and 0111) and Enterobacter cloacae are lactoferrin-resistant. This resistance has been attributed to the synthesis of iron chelators by the bacteria, which compete with lactoferrin or transferrin for the host's iron.[6]

Streptococcus pyogenes produces a leucotoxic factor which is called the cell-bound streptolysin S (SLS). When organisms containing copious amounts of this factor are ingested by or come in contact with human PMNs, the neutrophils are destroyed. The death of the PMN is associated with intracytoplasmic rupture of neutrophil granule.[48]

E. coli producing a complete lipopolysaccharide, such as 08 side chain moiety of lipopolysaccharide, and exopolysaccharide K antigens, enhances the strain's ability to evade the bactericidal effects of serum. This mechanism has been shown to be genetically controlled.[55]

Besides the capsular structures, many bacterial species elaborate extracellular enzymes that enhance their invasive (parasitic) properties. Such an enzyme is hyaluronidase, originally referred to as "spreading factor." This enzyme effects diffusion through connective tissue by depolymerizing hyaluronic acid. Several gram-positive bacteria elaborate hyaluronidase, especially Streptococcus pyogenes and Clostridium perfringens.[48]

The glycolipoprotein in the slime of P. aeruginosa is toxic and causes leukopenia, as well as preventing phagocytosis, which occurs in the course of lethal infection.[16]

Hemolysins dissolve red blood cells, whereas leukocidins attack the leukocytes. Streptolysin 0 is an example of a hemolysin of group A streptococci. Hemolysins are also produced by staphylococci, pneumococci and many gram-negative rods. Clostridia produce a wide variety of hemolysins. Among them, Davis et al. have described lecithinase, an enzyme capable of hydrolyzing lecithin in the cell wall.[12,14]

Some of the hemolysins of S. aureus have a necrotizing effect. The alpha toxin produces ischemic necrosis, whereas beta and delta toxins are less active, although they still have a dermonecrotic affect. The Panton-Valentine leukocidin (PVL) provokes a granulocytopenia.[13,41]

Virulence factors are not privy to bacteria alone. Viruses and fungi also are capable of adherence, competition with commensals, resistance to host defense mechanisms and penetration. Recent investigations with herpes simplex virus (HSV) have shown that prostaglandins E_2 and F_2 and cyclic AMP, while having no direct effect on HSV replication, could in fact indirectly enhance the growth of the virus by inhibiting the production of interferon.[57]

QUANTITATIVE BACTERIOLOGY

Peculiarities of various bacterial species have been shown to affect the organisms' ability to survive and multiply. Once bacterial survival occurs, infection becomes an expression of quantitative relationship between the bacteria and the local or systemic host resistance factors.

That the number of bacteria in a wound is of clinical import was suggested by French surgeons in 1917.[27] In war wounds more than 15 hours old, they performed wide debridement, cultured the wound, flooded it with Dakin's solution and packed it with gauze. The patient was evacuated to a base hospital accompanied by the culture plate of his wound. Upon arrival at the hospital, the plate was inspected. If no streptococci were present, and fewer than 5 colonies of other organisms had grown on the plate, the pack was removed from the wound and a delayed closure performed. If more than five colonies were present on the plate, the wound was left open and allowed to heal by secondary intention. This early quantitative evaluation suggested the importance of species peculiarities, since the streptococcus was considered more dangerous than other bacteria as it is today.

This early emphasis on the number of bacteria in a wound remained obscure after World War I, as attention shifted to the development of antimicrobials. However, in the late 1950s, several unrelated observations established the significance of quantitative bacteriology. Elek demonstrated that it required an average of 7.5×10^6 staphylococcal organisms to produce a pustule in normal human skin.[18] He also found that this number could be reduced 10,000-fold in the presence of a single silk suture.[18] While studying 2,000 people, Kass reported a quantitative relationship between bacteria in urine and symptoms of urinary tract infections. If these patients demonstrated symptoms, >100,000 organisms were always found.[31] The third report occurring at this time was by Liedburg et al.[36] They found that skin grafts were destroyed on rabbits when applied to beds inoculated with streptococci, pseudomonas or staphylococci in concentrations greater than 10^5 organisms/ml.

The fact that there appeared to be a critical number of bacteria which a host could handle before clinical infection ensue has been demonstrated in varied situations. Bendy et al., using a quantitative swab technique, showed that significant healing of decubiti occurred only when bacterial counts were $<10^6$ bacteria/ml.[7] They found that, despite the healthy appearance of the wound, healing did not occur if the bacterial level was greater than 10^6. Multiple studies from the United States Army Institute of Surgical Research have made invasive burn wound sepsis synonymous with a bacterial level of $>10^5$ organisms/gm of tissue.[54,56]

Reporting differences at first suggested that there was an apparently "critical number" of bacteria between 10^4 and 10^6 organisms which was significant. Closer perusal of the data has narrowed the range. Most reports state the significant number as $>10^5$ or 10^6 organisms. Therefore, the number seems to approximate 1 million organisms per gram of tissue or milliliter of biologic fluid. This number varies surprisingly little for the multitude of organisms that have been studied. The number also varies little despite a variety of quantitative culture techniques.[8,26,31,33,36,37,42,56]

The authors have used quantitative bacteriology routinely in both experimental and clinical situations. The initial technique of quantification was to cleanse the wound surface with isopropyl alcohol and obtain a biopsy tissue specimen. The specimen was aseptically weighed, flamed and homogenized after being diluted 1:10 with supplemented thioglycolate or Brain Heart infusion broth. Serial tube dilutions and then either pourplates or backplating were performed to arrive at an accurate bacterial count.[22,48,49]

Using this method, Krizek and Davis demonstrated quantitatively the level of bacteria necessary to cause fatal sepsis and the host's ability to localize bacteria to an injection site.[32] Following this, the technique was used to evaluate the quantitative relationship between bacteria and skin-graft survival in humans. In 50 granulating wounds requiring split-thickness grafts, various topical agents were evaluated for controlling bacteria in the wounds.[33] The evaluation was performed by quantitative bacterial cultures. All wounds underwent grafting when deemed clinically ready, as described by Pulaski.[44] When the bacterial counts were reviewed, it was found that the average skin-graft survival was 94% when the bacterial count was 10^5 or fewer organisms/gm of tissue and less than 20% when the bacterial count was greater than 10^5.

Delayed wound closures were similarly studied in a retrospective manner with quantitative tissue cultures.[43] During the period of delay, the open wound was treated with a variety of topical agents and the wound was closed on clinical criteria alone, without knowledge of the bacterial counts. Of the 40 wounds included in the initial study, 20 were wounds left open at the time of surgery for anticipated delayed closure. The other 20 were wounds resulting from primarily closed incisions which had been reopened to drain incisional abscesses. On reviewing the bacterial counts performed at the time of delayed wound closure, it was found that 28 of 30 wounds which contained 10^5 or fewer organisms progressed to uncomplicated healing, whereas none of the 10 wound closures performed on wounds containing $>10^5$ organisms/gm were successful. A complete historical review of these earlier quantitative bacterial studies has been presented.[48] In 1969, a technique was developed to rapidly predict if the critical number of bacteria were present.[22,48]

Employing the rapid slide technique in a prospective manner, the authors found that 89 of 93 wounds with delayed closure progressed to rapid uncomplicated healing when the rapid slide suggested a count of 10^5 or fewer. When used to determine the feasibility of reclosing incisional abscesses, the quantitative estimate resulted in an average 14.3-day decrease in hospitalization. Quantitative bacteriology is now used to determine graft bed receptiveness, test efficacy of topical antimicrobial agents, monitor the course of major burns, evaluate pulmonary infections, distinguish between contamination and infection in urine and predict the safety of closure of wounds in the emergency room.[48]

Since 1973, surgeons and microbiologists have developed many variations on "The Theme of Quantitative Bacteriology." Raahave[45,46] developed a velvet pad rinse (VPR) technique for bacteriological sampling. Sterile velvet pads 2.0 × 4.5 cm backed by aluminum foil, were used to sample wound surfaces, by imprinting the sterile pads on incisional wound. Then the pads were rinsed in physiological saline, centrifuged and resuspended and cultured on blood agar plates. Using this technique bacterial recovery was increased by 20-fold when compared to the velvet pad imprint (VPI) technique. The organism in clean operations was exclusively gram positive, with an overwhelming domination of <u>Staphylococcus epidermidis</u>. However, it contaminated operations, once the breakdown of the integument occurred, a precipitous rise in both gram positive and gram negative organisms was observed.

Since the Teplitz et al. 1964[56] demonstration of the pathogenesis of burn wound sepsis by progressive colonization, many modifications have been attempted. Brentano and Graven,[8] designed a gauze-capillary technique. After contact with the burn wound, it was implanted and sandwiched between two agar surfaces. Again the numerical value of greater than 10^5 correlated with burn wound sepsis. In 1974 Loebl et al.[37] reported on a comparison of surface contact plates (Rodac®) and skin biopsy technique. Their conclusion was that full-thickness wound biopsy cultures more accurately reflect burn wound colonization than do surface techniques. The mere presence of bacteria in a wound does not constitute an infection. A definite critical number of microbes are necessary to create soft-tissue wound infection.

Recently investigators have demonstrated histologic correlation between the depth of tissue invasion and quantitative counts demonstrating that the critical number of organisms required for burn wound sepsis was $>10^5$ organisms per gram of tissue.[42]

In 1976, Levine at al.[35] reported on a quantitative swab culture and smear technique. Using the swab in a similar manner to Raahave's VPI/VPR technique, the tip of a sterile cotton swab is twirled over one square centimeter area of an open wound for 5 seconds. The swab is transferred to one ml of transport medium. Serial dilutions are prepared and cultured on pour-plates. Two swabs are used simultaneously when the smear technique is required. According to the authors, this technique is linearly related to biopsy quantification of viable bacteria in the underlying tissue, and counts $>10^5$ are detrimental to wound closure and healing.

Though the quantitative approach of a single biopsy has been greater than 95% accurate, a true statistical analysis of one biopsy vs. multiple biopsies was not evaluated until 1979. Volenec and his co-workers[58] showed that the 95% confidence interval based on a single biopsy was determined SD ± 1.31. Therefore, they concluded that the wound biopsy is a reliable procedure for quantitating organisms in a wound.

However, there are researchers who advocate that quantitative bacteriology is of little value in assessing burn wound sepsis. Woolfrey and colleagues[61] reported that only 38% of the quantitative results might be expected to agree with the same $\log_{10}$ unit and 44% would be expected to differ by a factor of ± 2 $\log_{10}$ units or more. Therefore, their conclusion was that quantitative eschar cultures more often than not, provide significantly misleading quantitative information about burn wound microflora. These authors like so many other investigators fall into the same pitfall attempting quantitative assays without complete understanding of the previous literature. Teplitz et al.[56] distinctly describe the correct procedure for the collection of wound biopsies. If this procedure is not followed it is obvious why the authors fail to show a direct correlation between sepsis and the numbers of bacteria per gram of tissue.

Schneider and his co-workers[51] re-evaluated Volenec's earlier study on the statistical assessment of one biopsy vs. multiple biopsies. It is unique that they arrived at the same results but the opposite conclusion. Many serious deficiencies exist in their evaluation; 1) if one totals up all the samples for each individual subgroup, the total counts exceed $<10^5$/gm tissue, 2) tissue sizes evaluated for quantitation were exceptionally small, thus influencing the number of bacteria, 3) their method of homogenization has been shown to create alterations in viability and recovery of the bacteria.[53] In the final analysis, actual closure of the wound was not performed since the authors were biased from the outset. Apparently their statistical evaluation falls short of the final proof, successful wound closure.

Though the proponents of quantitative wound assessment employ a variety of techniques and these techniques correlate in numbers and linearity, it is our considered opinion that surface sampling does not give the surgeon a true indication of the dynamics of infection as it exists in deeper tissue, either in surgical or burn sepsis.

Although the significance of the number of bacteria present has been established, the species must also be identified. Because of individual species idiosyncrasies, qualitative bacteriology maintains its role. It is the combination of qualitative and quantitative bacterial analysis, performed under both aerobic and anaerobic conditions, which provides the maximum information. However, it should be mentioned that not every species of bacteria appears to adhere to the level of greater than 10^5 organisms to produce complications. In particular, the B-hemolytic streptococcus has been repeatedly demonstrated to be clinically significant at a much lower level.[48] This has been shown to be due to its specificities described in a previous section. To date, no other species has proved to be troublesome at a lower level, but this may be a chance phenomenon. In all situations described, it has been the practice of the authors not to perform a skin graft or close a wound in the presence of the B-hemolytic streptococcus, regardless of its quantitative level.

Another important finding directly related to quantitative bacteriology is the presence of septicemia. When surgical or burn wound counts exceed 10^5 organisms per gram of tissue, the probability of septicemia increases precipitously for log increases in the bacterial count over 10^5 (that is, 10^6/50%; 10^7/70%; 10^8/90%).[48]

An adjunctive therapeutic approach to the treatment of suspect septicemias is the evaluation of the blood glucose. If the parameters for septicemia exist—that is, fever, surgical or burn wound sepsis, and so on, blood glucose levels will give an indication of the etiological agent. Glucose levels above 130 mgm% are indicative of gram-positive septicemias and those levels under 110 mgm% are indicative of gram-negative infections.[34]

Thus, if septicemia is suspected on the basis of clinical findings and antibiotics are indicated, a gram-negative bactericidal agent is administered if the glucose level is less than 110 mgm% pending blood culture results. If the glucose level is greater than 130 mgm%, a gram-positive bactericidal agent is instituted.

CONTROL OF CERTAIN INFLAMMATORY MEDIATORS

In a recent experimental situation, microabscess formation was prevented by control of vasoconstrictive prostanoids ($PGF_{2\alpha}$ and TxA_2). If left unchecked, these prostanoids would seem detrimental to tissue control of bacterial growth. Production of vasoconstrictive prostanoids in soft tissue enhances bacterial growth in the experimental situation and results in 8.5×10^6 organisms/gram of tissue. This allows microabscess formation to be seen histologically. Prevention of excess production of the vasoconstrictor TxB maintained the bacterial count at 2.2×10^4 bacteria/gram of tissue (comparable to controls) and totally prevented the histologic appearance of microabscesses.[24]

In a recent investigation Gulbis and his co-workers reported that bacteria have the capability of producing prostanoid derivatives, particularly PGE_2.[21] This ability may account for ease with which certain bacteria species gain entrance into the sterile confines of the host. Since PGE_2 increases permeability, some bacteria may gain entrance to intra- and intervascular spaces and establish abcesses, thus forming a <u>locus minoris resistantiae</u> of minor inconsequence. However, when surgically penetrated, the organisms are freed to seed the host and multiply and eventually cause a septic episode.

The effects of TxA_2, a vasoconstrictor and mediator of dermal ischemia, can also predispose the host to a septic episode. Dead or dying tissue provides the appropriate nutrients for bacterial proliferation.[26] Recently investigators reported that PGI_2 and TxA_2 were mediators of the early hemodynamic events of sepsis.[9] Septic blood was evaluated for PGI_2 and TxA_2 levels by radioimmunoassay. Given that the platelet population would be producing TxA_2 to counteract the endothelial production of PGI_2, the elevated rise of TxA_2 observed, could also be accounted for by the production of TxA_2 by the PMNs which when activated not only secrete stable prostaglandins, but an inordinate amount of TxA_2.[26,60] This, in fact, could account for white blood cells sticking in the vasculature of the thermal injury and thus potentiating an infection by restricting the numbers of scavengers available to combat an infection. The author makes no mention of other prostanoids (PGE_2) which may potentiate the invasiveness of a microbial invader.

However, if tissue integrity is based on the equilibrium relationship between PGE_2 and $PGF_{2\alpha}$ and concomitantly maintaining the tissue viability, the control of the devastating prostanoid TxA_2 is essential.[26] If this occurs, the potential for a locus minoris resistantiae can be abrogated and sepsis can be prevented.

Thus, in maintaining the delicate balance between the host's resistance and the bacteria, it must be understood that the bacteria have established a territorial prerogative on earth long before man's conception. Therefore, man must learn to adapt to this environment as did his symbiotic friends and keep the checks and balances in order to exist. Man's whole existence is based on values, specifically normal values. If there is a deviation from the norm, a pathological condition exists, such as inflammation, infection, and so on. A rise in the white blood count indicates an infection. Bacteria isolated from the blood stream is indicative of a bacteremia or septicemia. A quantum rise of over 10^5 bacteria per gram of tissue in a surgical or burn wound is conclusive evidence that a septic situation does exist and appropriate measures must be taken to obviate the course of events which are inevitable if left unchecked.

NOTES

1. Adams, F. The Genuine Work of Hippocrates (trans.). New York: Wm. Wood (1849) Vol. 1.

2. Ad Hoc Committee of the Committee on Trauma, Division of Medical Sciences, National Research Council Report. Postoperative wound infections: The influences of ultraviolet irradiation of the operating room and the influence of various other factors. Ann. Surg. 160 (suppl.): (1964) 1-191.

3. Adler, JL, Burke, JP, Finland, M. Infection and antibiotic usage at Boston City Hospital, January 1970. Arch. Int. Med. 127: (1971), 460-465.

4. Alexander, JK, Dennis, EW, Smith, WG, Amad, KH, Duncan, WC, and Austin, RC. Blood volume, cardiac output, and distribution of systemic blood flow in extreme obesity. Cardiovas. Rest. Cent. Bull. 1: (1962) 39. Abstract.

5. Alexander, JW, Korelitz, J, Alexander, NS. Prevention of wound infections: A case for closed suction drainage to remove wound fluids deficient in opsonic proteins. Am. J. Surg. 132: (1976) 59-63.

6. Arnold, RR, Brewer, M, and Gauthier, JJ. Bactericidal activity in human lactoferrin: Sensitivity of a variety of microorganisms. Infect. Immun. 28: (1980) 893-898.

7. Bendy, RH, Nuccio, PA, Wolfe, E, Collins, B, Tamburro, C, Glass, W, and Martin, CM. Relationship of quantitative wound bacterial counts to healing of decubiti: Effect of topical gentamicin. Antimicrobial Agents and Chemother. 4: (1964) 147-155.

8. Brentano, L, and Gravens, DL. A method for the quantitation of bacteria in burn wounds. Appl. Microbiol. 15: (1967) 670-671.

9. Carmona, RH, Tsao, TC, and Trunkey, DD. The roles of prostacyclin and thromboxane in sepsis and septic shock. Arch. Surg. (1983) IN PRESS.

10. Conolly, WB, and Golovsky, D. Postoperative wound sepsis. MJ Australia 1: (1967) 643-645.

11. Conolly, WB, Hunt, TK, and Dunphy, JE. Management of contaminated surgical wounds. Surg., Gynec., and Obst. 129: (1969) 593-601.

12. Davis, JH, and Yull, AB. A possible toxic factor in abdominal injury. J. Trauma 1: (1961) 291-300.

13. Davis, JH. Staphylococcal disease. In Davis JH (ed), Current Concepts in Surgery, New York: McGraw-Hill Book Company. (1965).

14. Davis, BD, Dulbecco, R, Eisen, HN, Ginsberg, HS, and Wood, WB. Microbiology, 4th ed. New York: Hoeber Medical Division, Harper and Row, Publishers (1968).

15. deHoll, D. Potentiation of infection by suture closure of dead space. Am. J. Surg. 127: (1974) 716-720.

16. Dimitra-copoulos, G, and Bartell, PF. Slime glycoproteins and the pathogenicity of various strains of Pseudomonas aeruginosa in experimental infection. Infect. Immun. 30: (1980) 402-408.

17. Edlich, RF, Rodeheaver, GT, Thacker, JG, and Edgerton, NT. Technical factors in wound management. In Fundamentals of Wound Management in Surgery, Dunphy, JE, and Hunt, TK (eds). South Plainfield, New Jersey: Chirurgecom. (1977).

18. Elek, SD. Experimental staphylococcal infections in the skin of man. Ann. New York Acad. Sci. 65: (1956) 85-90.

19. Ellen, RP, and Gibbons, RJ. M. protein associated adherence of Streptococcus pyogenes to epithelial surfaces: Prerequisite for virulence. Infect. Immun. 5: (1972) 826-830.

20. Getzen, LC, and Jansen, GA. Correlation between allergy to suture material and postoperative wound infections. Surgery 60: (1966) 824-826.

21. Gulbis, E, Marion, AM, Dumont, JE, and Schell-Frederick, E. Prostaglandin formation in bacteria. Prostaglandins 18: (1979) 397-400.

22. Heggers, JP, Robson, MC, and Ristroph, JD. A rapid method of performing quantitative wound cultures. Military Med. 134: (1969) 666-667.

23. Heggers, JP. Natural host defense mechanisms. In Clinics in Plastic Surgery, Krizek, TJ and Robson, MC (eds). Philadelphia: W. B. Saunders (1979).

24. Heggers, JP, Robson, MC, and London, MC. Prevention of microabscess formation following thermal injury. J. Amer. Technol. 44: (1982) 215-218.

25. Heggers, JP, Robson, MC, Kucan, OC, Jellema, A, and Osborne, J. Skin testing: A valuable predictor in the thermal injury? Arch. Surgery (1983) IN PRESS.

26. Heggers, JP and Robson, MC. Chapter 5. Prostaglandins and thromboxanes. In Traumatic Injury—Infection and Other Immunologic Sequellae, J. Ninnemann (ed). Baltimore: University Park Press. (1983).

27. Hepburn, HH. Delayed primary suture of wounds. Brit. Med. J. 1: (1919) 181-183.

28. Howe, CW. Experimental studies on determinants of wound infection. II. Surgery 60: (1966) 1072-1076.

29. Hunt, TK, Jawetz, E, Hutchison, JGP, and Dunphy, JE. A new model for the study of wound infection. J. Trauma 7: (1967) 298-306.

30. Hunt, TK, Twomey, P, Zederfeldt, B, and Dunphy, JE. Respiratory gas tensions and pH in healing wounds. Am. J. Surg. 114: (1967) 302-307.

31. Kass, EH. Bacteriuria and the diagnosis of infections of the urinary tract. A.M.A. Arch. Int. Med. 100: (1957) 709.

32. Krizek, TJ, and Davis, JH. The role of the red cell in subcutaneous infection. J. Trauma 5: (1965) 85-95.

33. Krizek, TJ, Robson, MC, and Kho, E. Bacterial growth and skin graft survival. S. Forum 18: (1967) 518-519.

34. Kucan, JO, Heggers, JP, and Robson, MC. Blood glucose level as an aid in the diagnosis of septicemia burns. 6: (1979) 111-113.

35. Levine, NS, Lindberg, RB, Mason, AD, and Pruitt, BA, Jr. The quantitative swab culture and smear: A quick simple method for determining the number of viable aerobic bacteria on open wounds. J. Trauma 16: (1976) 89-94.

36. Liedberg, NCF, Reiss, E, and Artz, CP. The effect of bacteria on the take of split-thickness skin grafts in rabbits. Ann. Surg. 142: (1955) 92-96.

37. Loebl, EC, Marvin, JA, Heck, EL, Curreri, PW, and Baxter, CR. The method of quantitative burn wound biopsy cultures and its routine use in the after care of the burned patient. Ann. J. Clin. Path. 61: (1974) 20-24.

38. Mardh, PA, and Westrom, L. Adherence of bacteria to epithelial cells. Infect. Immun. 13: (1976) 661-666.

39. May, J, Chalmers, JP, Loewenthal, J, and Rountree, PM. Factors in the patient contributing to surgical sepsis. Surg., Gynec. & Obst. 122: (1966) 28-32.

40. Meleney, FL. Infection in clean operative wounds: A 9 year study. Surg. Gynec. & Obst. 60: (1935) 264-276.

41. Melly, MA, Duke, J, Liau, DF, and Hash, JH. Biological properties of the encapsulated Staphylococcus aureus M. Infect. Immun. 10: (1974) 389-397.

42. Neal, GD, Lindholm, GR, Lee, MJ, Marvin, JA, and Heimbach, DM. Burn wound histologic culture—a new technique of predicting burn wound sepsis. J. Burn Care of Rehab. 2: (1981) 35-39.

43. Penneys, NS. Prostaglandins in skin. In Current Concepts, A Scope Publication, Monograph, The Upjohn Co., Kalamazoo, MI (1980).

44. Pulaski, EJ. Surgical Infections. Springfield: Charles C. Thomas (1954), Chapter 3.

45. Raahave, D. Bacterial density in operation wounds. Acta Chir. Scand. 140: (1974) 585-593.

46. Raahave, D. A new technique for quantitative bacteriological sampling of wounds by velvet pads: Clinical sampling trial. J. Clin. Microbiol. 2: (1975) 277-280.

47. Ramphal, R, Small, PM, Shands Jr., JW, Fischlschweiger, W, and Small Jr, PA. Adherence of Pseudomonas aeruginosa to tracheal cells injured by influenza infection or by endotracheal intubation. Infect. Immun. 27: (1980) 614-619.

48. Robson, MC, Krizek, JJ, and Heggers, JP. Biology of surgical infection. In Current Problems in Surgery, Ravitch, MM (ed). Chicago: Year Book Publishers (1973).

49. Robson, MC. Infection in the surgical patient; imbalance in the normal equilibrium. In Clinics of Plastic Surgery, Krizek, TJ and Robson, MC (eds). Philadelphia: W. B. Saunders (1979).

50. Rodeheaver, G, Pettry, D, Turnbull, B, Edgerton, N, and Edlich, R. Identification of the wound infection - Potentiating factors in soil. Am. J. Surg. 128: (1974) 8-14.

51. Schneider, M, Vildozola, CW, and Brooks, S. Quantitative assessment of bacterial invasion of chronic ulcers. Amer. J. Surg. 145: (1983) 260-262.

52. Smith, H. Microbial surfaces in relation to pathogenicity. Bact. Rev. 41: (1977) 475-500.

53. Splenger, MD, Rodeheaver, GT and Edlich, RF. Technical considerations in quantitative bacteriology. J. Burn Care of Rehab. 2: (1981) 200-202.

54. Shuck, JM and Moncrief, JA. The management of burns, Part I. General considerations and sulfamylon method. In Current Problems of Surgery. Chicago: Year Book Medical Publishers, February (1969).

55. Taylor, PW, and Robinson, MK. Determinants that increase the serum resistance of Escherichia coli. Infect. Immun. 29: (1980) 278-280.

56. Teplitz, C, Davis, D, Mason, AD, Jr, and Moncrief, JA. Pseudomonas burn wound sepsis, I. Pathogenesis of experimental pseudomonas burn wound sepsis. J. Surg. Res. 4: (1964) 200-216.

57. Trofatter, KF, and Daniels, CA. Effect of prostaglandins and cyclic adenocyclic 3'5' monophosphate modulators on herpes simplex virus. Growth and interferon response in human cells. Infect. Immun. 27: (1980) 158-167.

58. Volenec, FJ, Clark, GM, Mani, MM, and Humphrey, LJ. Burn wound biopsy bacterial quantitation: A statistical analysis. Amer. J. Surg. 138: (1979) 695-697.

59. Webb, DR, Rogers, TJ, and Nowowiejski, I. Endogenous prostaglandin synthesis and the control of lymphocyte function. NYAS 332: (1979) 262-270.

60. Weismann, E. Prostaglandins in acute inflammation. In Current Concepts, A Scope Publication, Monograph, The Upjohn Co., Kalamazoo, MI (1980).

61. Woolfrey, BF, Fox, JM, and Quall, CO. An evaluation of burn wound quantitative microbiology I, quantitative eschar cultures. Amer. J. Clin. Path. 75: (1981) 532-537.

PART VIII
Growth and Repair

27
The Control of Regenerative Epidermal Hyperplastic Growth

Thomas S. Argyris and Rebecca Morris

INTRODUCTION

The production of an epidermal hyperplasia following wounding is one of the two major tissue reparative processes that occurs in wound repair. The other is the regeneration of the connective tissue, or granulation tissue formation. Granulation tissue formation is so massive that it usually over-shadows epidermal regeneration. Indeed, most people, when they think of wound repair, think only of the regeneration of the connective tissue. But in spite of the fact that epidermal regeneration is not as massive a process as granulation tissue formation, proper wound repair cannot occur without it. Thus, an understanding of how the production of a regenerative epidermal hyperplasia in wound repair is accomplished is central for our understanding of how wound repair is controlled. Clearly, it is worthy of serious investigation.

The principal histological characteristics of regenerative epidermal hyperplasia (Figures 27.1 and 27.2) are the thickening of the epidermis, enlargement of basal and suprabasal cells, a massive increase in cytoplasmic basophilia, and a large increase in nuclear and nucleolar size (for review, see Argyris, 1968; 1981a). These are morphological hallmarks for cells undergoing marked protein synthesis; and accordingly, there is a massive increase in epidermal ribosomal RNA (Argyris, 1978; 1980; 1981b). There is also an increase in the intercellular spacing in the epidermis. In deep wounds, the resting hair follicles adjacent

---

The authors' work was supported by NIH grants AM18219 and AG01324 to Thomas S. Argyris.

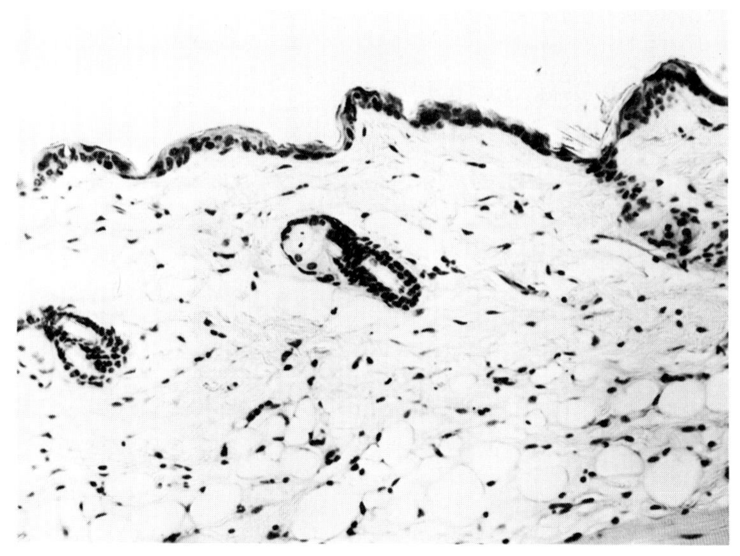

FIGURE 27.1 Normal mouse skin, x195, H&E.

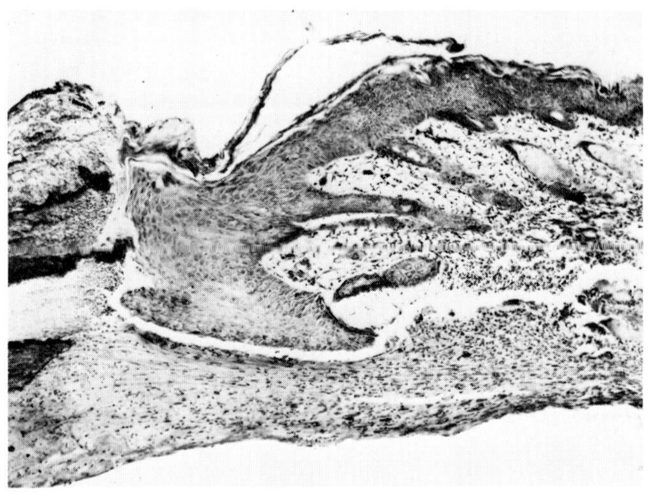

FIGURE 27.2 Mouse skin seven days after a full thickness wound has been made. Upper left is the scab. To the right is the hyperplastic epidermis. The granulation tissue is below the scab and extends to the right underneath the dermis and hair follicles, x195, H&E.

to the wound lose their sebaceous glands, and the hair follicles are converted into cords of enlarged cells which have a similar appearance to the cells in the hyperplastic epidermis (Figure 27.2). If the hair follicles adjacent to the wound are in the growth phase, then only the part of the hair follicles from about the level of the sebaceous gland upwards undergoes this transformation (for reviews see Argyris, 1968; 1981a).

As wound repair is accomplished, the epidermal hyperplasia begins to regress, eventually returning to its normal thickness (Argyris, 1968; 1981a). The mechanism by which the production and regression of the epidermal hyperplasia is regulated must be unraveled in order to understand wound repair, and thus hopefully influence its course.

To study the regulation of regenerative epidermal hyperplastic growth, we need to have a good model system for producing a regenerative epidermal hyperplasia, and a method for measuring the epidermal growth during its production and regression. The latter, strangely enough, has been ignored by students of skin regeneration, in contrast to those studying regeneration of other organs, such as liver and kidney, where the development of techniques for quantitatively measuring regenerative growth was the first order of business. We have developed a model system for studying regenerative epidermal hyperplasia, uncomplicated by massive granulation tissue formation, as well as a method for measuring the amount of epidermal growth.

TECHNIQUES FOR PRODUCING AND MEASURING REGENERATIVE EPIDERMAL HYPERPLASTIC GROWTH

The technique for producing a controlled regenerative epidermal hyperplasia has been described (Argyris, 1976; 1977, 1978). Briefly, mice are anesthetized with nembutal, their backs clipped, and the remaining hair stubble removed by the application of a depilatory. The epidermis is removed with a felt wheel mounted on a motor tool. Figure 27.3 shows two mice which have been abraded. Within 21 days, the epidermis is completely regenerated from the cells of the underlying hair follicles (Figure 27.4), now often called the intrafollicular epidermal cells (Klein-Szanto et al. 1980). Figure 27.5 shows the back skin two days after abrasion. The epidermis has been removed, and cells from the underlying hair follicles are beginning to spread out over the denuded surface. By 4-5 days, a marked hyperplasia is obvious (Figure 27.6). By 21 days, the epidermis has returned to its normal thickness (Figure 27.7).

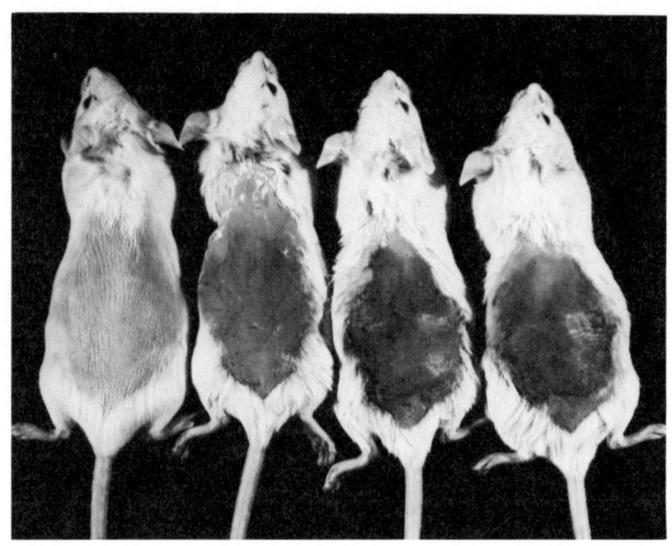

FIGURE 27.3 Induction of epidermal regeneration by abrasion. Mice three and four have been abraded. First mouse is the clipped control and mouse two a clipped and a depilatory control.

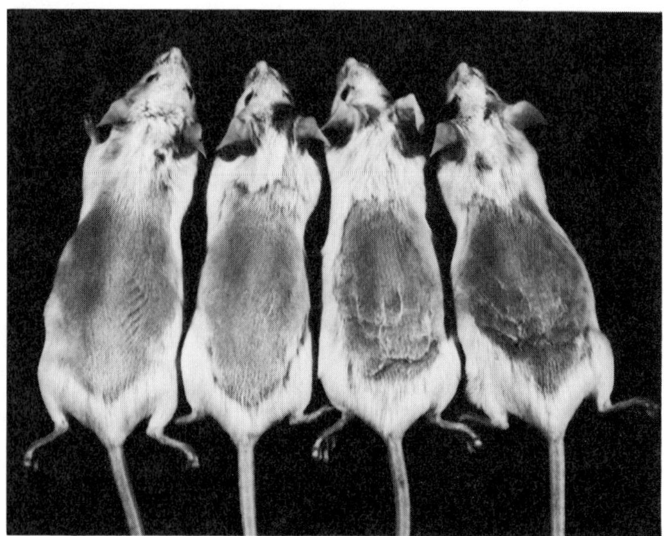

FIGURE 27.4 Mice three and four show that by 21 days the epidermis is completely regenerated. Mouse one is the clipped control and mouse two is the clipped and depilatory control.

FIGURE 27.5
Mouse skin two days after removal of the epidermis by abrasion. Note the absence of the epidermis. In some areas, nuclei of hair follicle cells are seen which have spread over the denuded skin, x195, H&E.

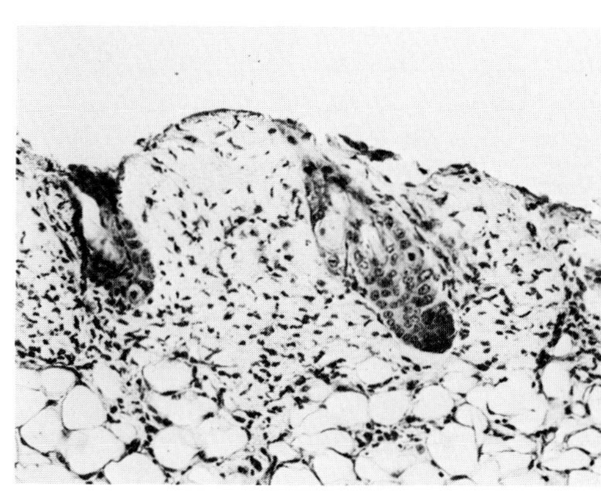

FIGURE 27.6
Hyperplastic epidermis seven days after abrasion, x195, H&E.

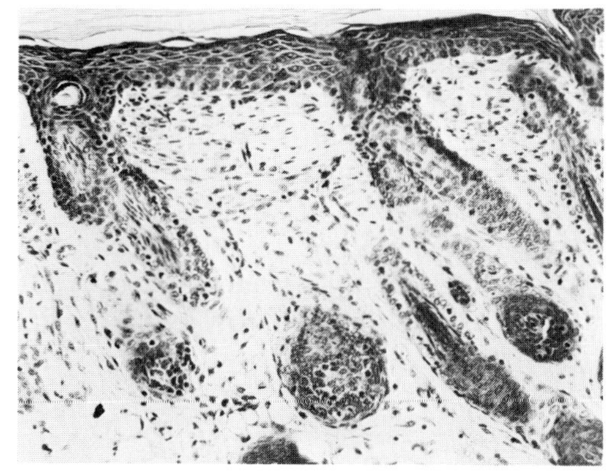

FIGURE 27.7
Regenerated epidermis about 18 days after abrasion. Note regression to normal thickness, x195, H&E.

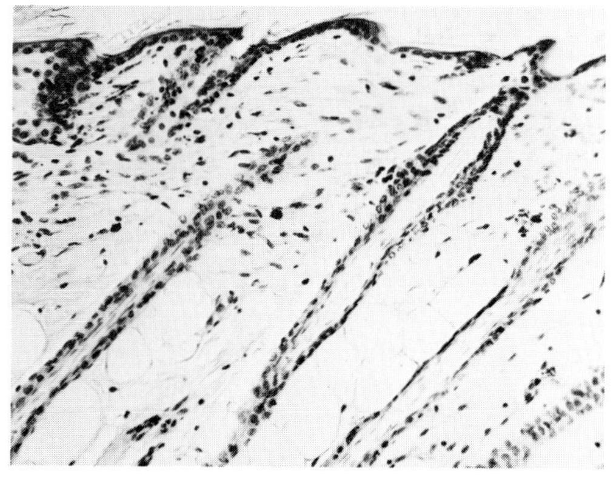

The technique for measuring the amount of epidermal growth has been published (Argyris, 1976; 1977; 1978). Briefly, mice are killed by cervical dislocation, clipped, and the hair stubble removed with a depilatory. The back skin in normal mice (about 17 cm^2) or the regenerated area in abraded mice (about 3 cm^2) is removed and placed in physiological saline at 4°C. The skin is placed epidermis side down on the cover of an ice-filled petri dish, and the subcutaneous tissue removed by scraping with a #10 Bard Parker blade. The scraped pieces of skin are then placed on a precooled translucent white plate glass resting on a light box, and covered with a piece of clear glass, the two plates of glass kept separate by folded pieces of paper toweling at either end. A piece of clear plastic acetate is then placed on top of the clear glass and the pieces of normal or regenerating skin traced with a felt pen. The traced areas are cut out and weighed. The epidermis is then removed by placing the skin dermis side down on the cover of a petri dish filled with ice and the epidermis is scraped off with a fresh #10 Bard Parker blade. The epidermis is dried in between filter paper and weighed. The area of skin from which the epidermis has been harvested is determined by converting the weight of the pieces of acetate to area in cm^2 by using a previously prepared standard curve relating weight of acetate to area. Knowing the area from which the epidermis is harvested, and the amount of epidermis harvested, we can calculate the amount of epidermis harvested per unit area of skin. For convenience, we normalize all our data to 100 cm^2 of skin.

KINETICS OF REGENERATIVE EPIDERMAL GROWTH FOLLOWING ABRASION

Epidermal wet weight—that is, gm epidermis/100 cm^2 skin—is already much increased from normal by 3 days after abrasion, the first time it can be measured (Figure 27.8). Prior to that, it is not possible to harvest enough epidermis to get a reliable measurement, partly because of a large scab which cannot be separated from the regenerating epidermis. Epidermal wet weight reaches its peak at 4 days, remains high for the next two days, and soon after seven days it begins to decrease, returning essentially to normal levels by day 20. This pattern of growth is similar to that reported in previous experiments (Argyris, 1977; 1978). Figure 27.8 also demonstrates a parallel increase in epidermal protein, indicating that the increase in epidermal wet weight is not simply due to an increase in water or some

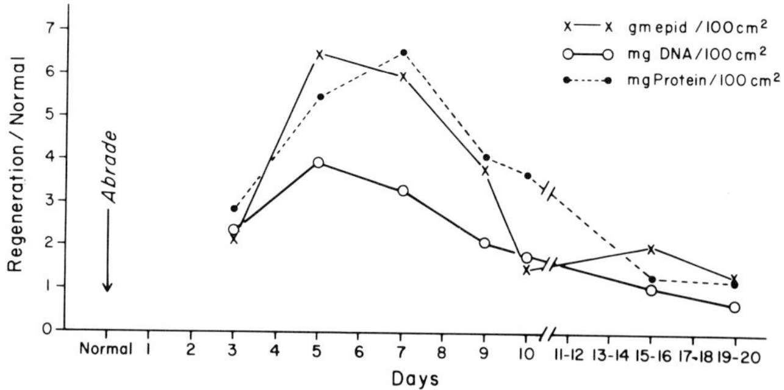

FIGURE 27.8 The changes in epidermal wet weight, total protein and DNA in the regenerating epidermis following abrasion. No data were obtained at 1 and 2 days after abrasion because of the intense inflammatory response and paucity of regenerating epidermis. The average ± standard error of the mean (SEM) of the normal value are: gm epidermis/100 cm^2, 0.153 ± 0.0043 (N = 6); mg DNA/100 cm^2, 0.691 ± 0.074 (N = 6); mg protein/100 cm^2, 14.9 ± 1.5 (N = 6).

other liquid substance. It is a real increase in epidermal protoplasmic mass. How are these changes in epidermal mass brought about?

The increase in DNA indicated in Figure 27.8 suggests that an increase in epidermal cell number plays a significant role in bringing about the increase in epidermal mass. This is confirmed by cell counts (Figure 27.9). The increase in epidermal cell number is due to an increase in the number of suprabasal cells. The basal cells actually decrease in number. During epidermal regression, the number of epidermal cells and the DNA/100 cm^2 return to normal values. Thus, it is clear that increases in cell number make a significant contribution to the increase in epidermal mass. How is the increase in cell numbers brought about? The epidermis is a renewing tissue. Its thickness is maintained by a balance between cell production in the basal layer, and cell loss or keratinization (terminal differentiation) in the suprabasal layers. Therefore, epidermal growth following abrasion could be brought about by an increase in epidermal cell proliferation and/or a decrease in epidermal cell loss. Therefore, the possible role of each of these processes to the produc-

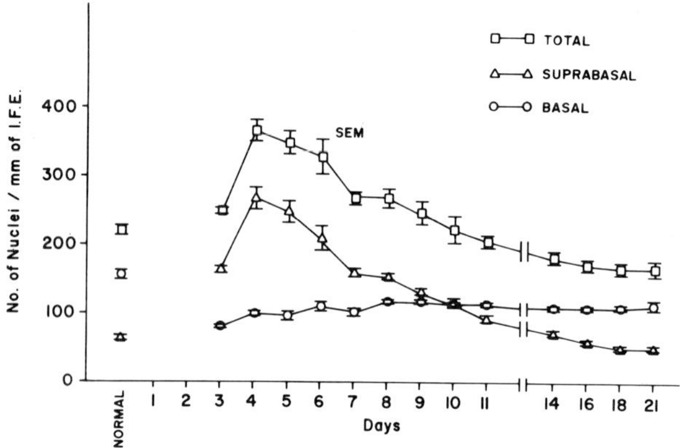

FIGURE 27.9 The average and standard error of the mean (SEM) of the number of basal, suprabasal, and total epidermal nuclei/mm of interfollicular (I.F.E.) epidermis following abrasion (N = 6).

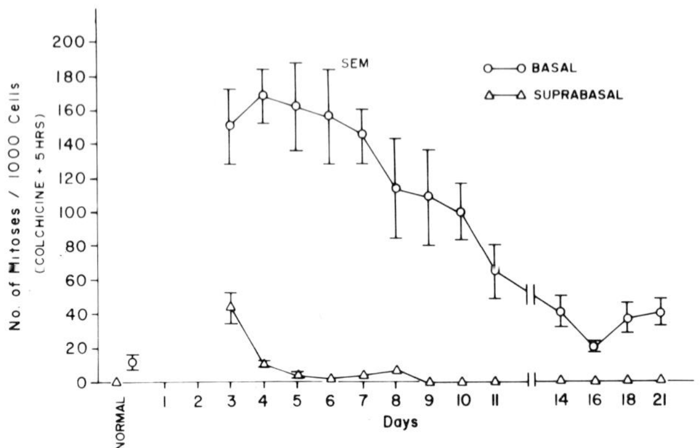

FIGURE 27.10 The average ± standard error of the mean (SEM) of the epidermal mitotic activity in regenerating mouse epidermis following abrasion. Six mice were sacrificed at each time point.

tion and regression of epidermal hyperplastic growth following abrasion has been examined.

But before doing so, we wish to point out in passing, that cell enlargement also contributes to the increase in epidermal mass. It is evident from Figure 27.6 that during epidermal hyperplastic growth, epidermal cells undergo considerable enlargement. Also, Figure 27.8 shows that the % increase in DNA/100 cm^2 is less than the protein/100 cm^2, consistent with an increase in epidermal protein per cell. During the regression of the epidermal hyperplasia, epidermal cell size returns to normal.

THE ROLE OF CELL PROLIFERATION IN EPIDERMAL HYPERPLASTIC GROWTH FOLLOWING ABRASION

Within 3 days after abrasion—the first time it can be measured—epidermal mitotic activity in the basal layer is at its peak (Figure 27.10). Epidermal mitotic activity remains high for the next few days and then slowly returns toward normal values. Thus, high epidermal mitotic activity is associated with the production and maintenance of the regenerative epidermal hyperplasia, and a return towards normal mitotic levels is associated with the period of regression of the epidermal hyperplasia. Clearly, changes in cell proliferation are important during epidermal hyperplastic growth.

The increase in epidermal cell proliferation may be brought about by an increase in the rate of epidermal cell proliferation and/or in the fraction of epidermal cells capable of proliferating. The latter is usually referred to as the "growth fraction." A significant increase in the growth fraction following abrasion is unlikely, since the growth fraction in normal epidermis is essentially 100% (Morris and Argyris, 1983; Potten, 1974). To be certain, we have measured the growth fraction in regenerating hyperplastic epidermis 3 days after abrasion and find it to be essentially 100% (Table 27.1). This is consistent with what has been reported for other forms of epidermal hyperplastic growth (for review, see Argyris, 1981a). This suggests that the increase in epidermal cell proliferative activity following abrasion is due to an increase in the rate of epidermal cell proliferation. The chief mechanism by which the rate of epidermal cell proliferation may be brought about is by a decrease in the time required for the epidermal cells to cycle. Therefore, we next measured the changes in the cell cycle time of epidermal cells during epi-

TABLE 27.1

Epidermal Labelling Indices Following Repeated Injection of Tritiated Thymidine Three Days Post-Abrasion or Three Days After Treatment with 17 Nmoles 12-0-tetradecanoyl-phorbol-13-acetate (TPA)

Hours of Labelling[a]	Number of Mice	Labelled Basal Nuclei per 1000 Basal Nuclei[b]
	Abrasion	
1	5	310 ± 104
5	6	326 ± 131
9	6	771 ± 204
13	4	922 ± 99.1
17	4	992 ± 10.0
	TPA	
1	6	124 ± 115
5	6	295 ± 27.8
9	6	326 ± 102
13	5	340 ± 103
17	6	452 ± 66.5
21	5	684 ± 204
25	5	817 ± 111

a 10 μCi of tritiated thymidine were injected every four hours; groups of mice were sacrificed one hour following each injection.

b Average ± Standard Deviation.

dermal regeneration by injecting groups of mice with 30 μCi of (^{3}H) thymidine, sacrificing them at hourly intervals, determining the number of labelled mitoses, and constructing percentage labelled mitoses (PLM) curves (Morris and Argyris; 1983). In instances when the rise in the second inflection of the percentage labelled mitoses was not sufficient enough to determine the length of the cell cycle, the cell cycle was determined by using three different formulae (Morris and Argyris, 1983), utilizing the labelling index as described by Steel (1977). In Table 27.2, it is seen that by 3 days after abrasion, the epidermal cell cycle time is only 11 hours, a drastic reduction from the normal value of 5-7 days. The cell cycle remains very short so long as the epidermis is hyperplastic. When the hyperplastic epidermis begins to regress, the length of the cell cycle increases and by 14 days after abrasion, it is almost back to normal. Table 27.2 also strongly suggests that the principal reason for the decrease in the cell cycle time is due to a decrease in the length of G_1. Therefore, it is clear that the principal mechanism for increasing epidermal cell proliferation during epidermal hyperplastic growth following abrasion is a dramatic shortening of the cell cycle time.

THE ROLE OF CELL LOSS IN EPIDERMAL HYPERPLASTIC GROWTH FOLLOWING ABRASION

The second major factor for controlling epidermal thickness is the rate of epidermal cell loss or terminal differentiation (keratinization). The usual way of measuring the rate of cell loss is by labelling the nuclei of the basal cells with [^{3}H] thymidine and following the movement of the labelled basal cells through the suprabasal layers until the labelled cells reach the

TABLE 27.2

The Cell Cycle Time of Basal Epidermal Cells in Normal and Regenerating CD-1 Female Mouse Epidermis

Days Post Abrasion	Cell Cycle Time	Hours		
		G_2 + 1/2 Mitosis	S	G_1
Normal	121-175[a]	5	9	107-161[b]
3	11	3	6	2
5	14	3	6	5
7	24-48[a]	3	7	14-38
14	96-120[a]	4	9	83-107

[a] The PLM curve lacked a defined second peak, therefore not permitting a direct estimate of the cell cycle time. Cell cycle time was estimated by using 3 different formulae, all well established for this purpose (for details, see Morris and Argyris, 1983).

[b] Length of G_1 based on the estimated cell cycle times.

outermost layer of the epidermis where they complete the process of keratinization and are transformed into corneum. The time required for the labelled basal cells to reach the uppermost layer of the epidermis and to become transformed into corneum is called the "transit time." Mouse epidermis has an ordered structure of epidermal columns (Christophers, 1972; Mackenzie, 1972; Potten, 1974). Accordingly, the suprabasal cells have been identified (Figure 27.11) as suprabasal 1, suprabasal nuclei in between columns; suprabasal 2, those in the lower portion of the column, suprabasal 3, those in the middle portion of the column; and suprabasal 4, those in the uppermost part of the column (Morris and Argyris, 1983). We have followed the movement of the labelled cells through the epidermal columns. In normal mouse epidermis, only 4-5 days are required for labelled nuclei to appear in suprabasal 1 position. Suprabasal 2 position shows labelled nuclei at 6 days, and suprabasal labelled nuclei in position 3 are seen by 7 days, and label is lost by 8 days (Table 27.3).

The rate of epidermal cell loss has been measured at 3, 5, 7, 10 and 14 days after abrasion. At 3 and 5 days after abrasion, the epidermal columnar organization is lost. It reappears

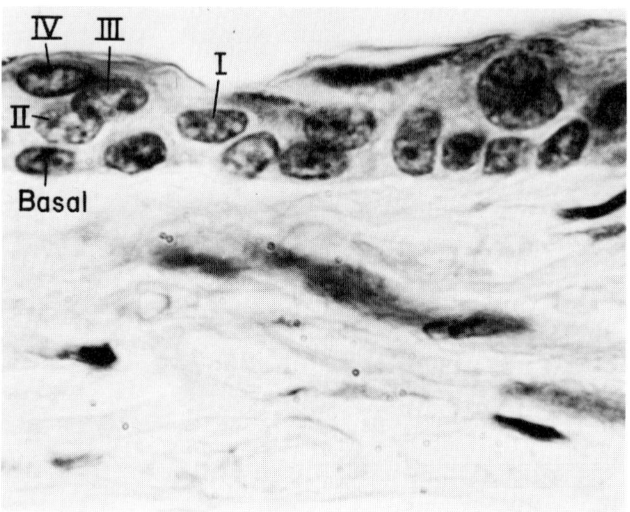

FIGURE 27.11 Epidermal columns in normal mouse epidermis. I, an intercolumnar cell. II, cell in the lower part of the column. III, cell in the middle portion of the column, and IV, cell in the uppermost part of the column. x960, H&E.

TABLE 27.3

Transit Time in Normal and Hyperplastic CD-1 Female Mouse Epidermis Following Abrasion or the Application of 17 Nmoles 12-0-tetra-decanoylphorbol-13-acetate (TPA)

Days Post Treatment	Days Required for Labelled Nuclei to Appear in Top Cell Layer of Epidermis	
	Abrasion	TPA
1 hour	—	2
3 days	2	4
5 days	2	5
7 days	4	—
10 days	—	5
14 days	6	—
Normal	8	

at approximately 7 days. As Table 27.3 indicates, 3 days after abrasion the transit time is drastically reduced from the normal value of 7-8 days to 1 day. By 5 days, the transit time is 2 days. By 7 days, it is 4 days. Recovery of normal epidermal column organization at this time raises the question of whether the displacement of labelled nuclei occurs serially through the columns as it does in normal epidermis. In fact, epidermal nuclei labelled at 7 days after abrasion do not appear in serial order from the lowermost portion of the column, to the uppermost part of the column; rather labelled nuclei are seen as they are 3 days after abrasion—that is, simultaneously in all columnar positions. By 14 days after abrasion when columnar organization is firmly re-established, the transit time is about 6 days. The displacement of labelled nuclei occurs as it normally does, serially, but is slightly faster than in normal epidermis. It appears, therefore, that the rate of epidermal cell loss is actually increased when the hyperplastic epidermis is being produced and so long as the hyperplastic state is maintained. This is also the time of highest proliferative activity. As the hyperplastic epidermis regresses, the transit time begins to increase and by 14 days after abrasion, it is almost normal. Thus, the increased thickness of the epidermis occurs in spite of an increased rate of cell loss, emphasizing the importance of the increased rate of cell proliferation in the production of the epidermal hyperplasia following abrasion.

CELL CYCLE KINETICS AND TRANSIT TIME IN EPIDERMAL HYPERPLASIA INDUCED BY 12-0-TETRADECANOYLPHORBOL-13-ACETATE (TPA)

The question may be raised if epidermal hyperplasias produced by means other than abrasion, also show similar changes in the cell cycle and transit time.

Application of 17 nmoles of 12-0-tetradecanoylphorbol-13-acetate (TPA), a powerful tumor promoter in mouse skin (for review see Boutwell, 1974), results in a marked epidermal hyperplasia (Figure 27.12). The overall kinetics of this epidermal hyperplastic growth are shown in Figures 27.13 and 27.14. It is clear that as after abrasion, TPA-induced epidermal growth is due mostly to an increase in epidermal cell number as indicated by the increases in total DNA (Figure 27.13) and in the number of epidermal nuclei/mm I.F.E., although an increase in cell size makes a contribution. Increased epidermal cell proliferation plays a significant role in bringing about the increase in cell numbers (Figure 27.15).

As after abrasion, in TPA-induced hyperplasia, the growth fraction is essentially 100% (Table 27.3)—that is, unchanged from normal. Thus, we must look to the changes in the length

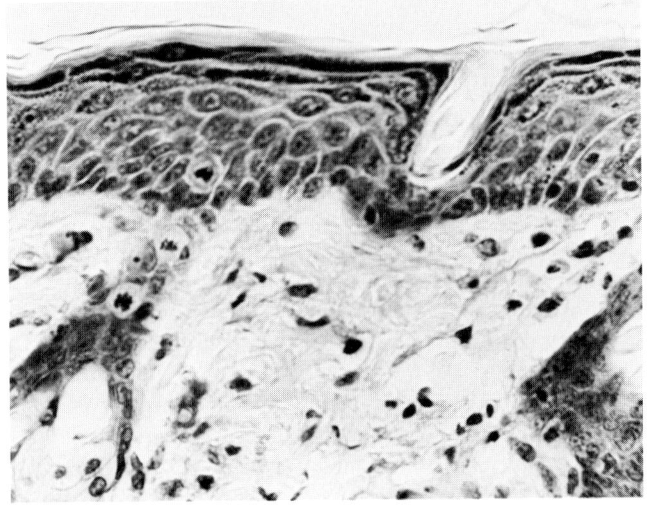

FIGURE 27.12 Hyperplastic epidermis 3 days after the application of 17 nmoles of 12-0-tetradecanoylphorbol-13-acetate (TPA) on the skin of mice, x495, H&E.

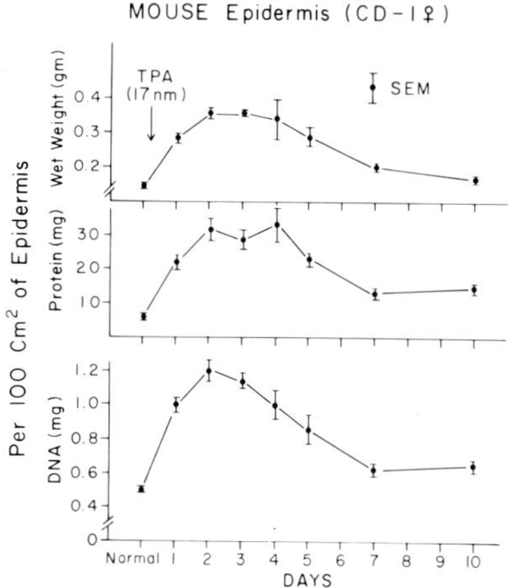

FIGURE 27.13 The epidermal wet weight, total protein and DNA following the application of 17 nmoles of 12-0-tetradecanoylphorbol-13-acetate (TPA) on the skin of mice. Bars are the standard error of the mean (SEM). N = 6.

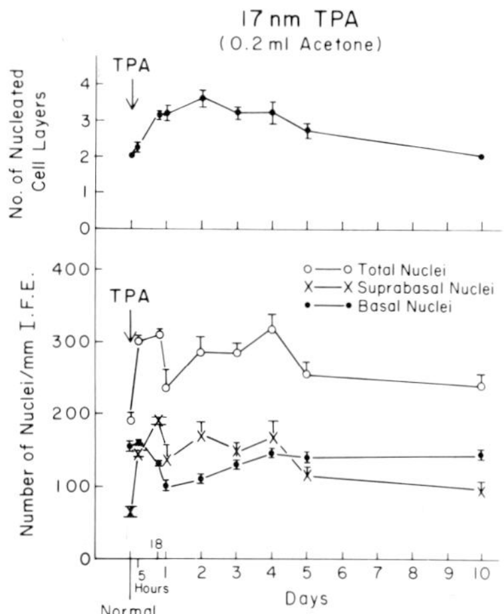

FIGURE 27.14 The number of nucleated cell layers and the number of epidermal nuclei/mm interfollicular epidermis (I.F.E.) following the application of 17 nmoles of 12-0-tetradecanoylphorbol-13-acetate on the skin of mice. Average ± standard error of the mean (SEM). N = 6.

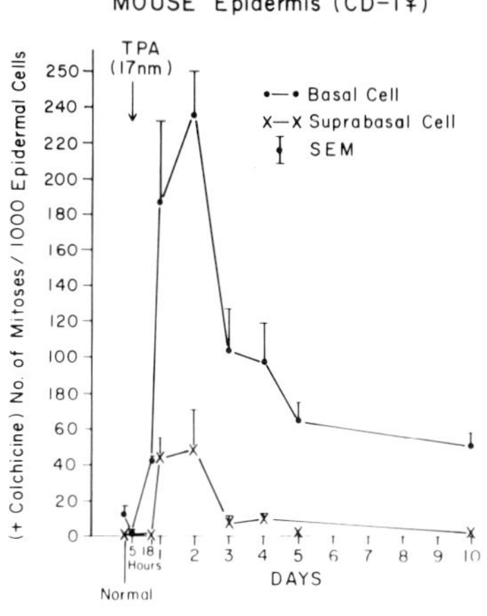

FIGURE 27.15 The epidermal mitotic activity following the application of 17 nmoles of 12-0-tetradecanoylphorbol-13-acetate (TPA) on the skin of mice. Average ± standard error of the mean (SEM). N = 6.

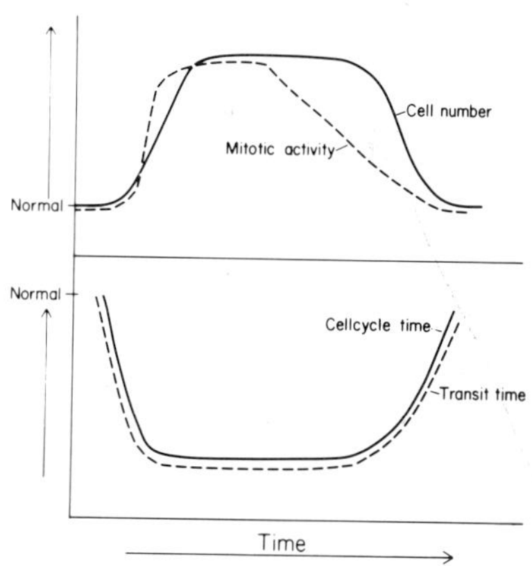

FIGURE 27.16 Diagrammatic representation of the changes in cell number, mitotic activity, cell cycle time and transit time, in mice following the induction of an epidermal hyperplasia by abrasion or the application of 17 nmoles 12-0-tetradecanoylphorbol-13-acetate.

TABLE 27.4

The Cell Cycle Time of Basal Epidermal Cells in CD-1 Female Mouse Skin Treated with a Single Topical Application of 17 Nmoles of 12-0-Tetradecanoyl-phorbol-13-acetate (TPA)

Time Post TPA	Cell Cycle Time	Hours		
		G_2 + 1/2 Mitosis	S	G_1
1 hour	16[a]	8	8	0
3 days	25[a]	3	6	16
5 days	48-72[b]	4	8	36-60
10 days	72-120[b]	4	8	60-108

[a] Because of considerable cell death following TPA, no mitoses are seen until 8 hours. Therefore, data are approximations.
[b] The PLM curve lacked a defined second peak, therefore not permitting a direct determination of the cell cycle time. Cell cycle time was estimated by using 3 different mathematical formulae, all well established for this purpose.

of the cell cycle time to account for the increased proliferative activity we see. Table 27.4 demonstrates that the cell cycle time dramatically shortens following TPA treatment, and that a shortened cell cycle time is associated with the maximum epidermal hyperplasia produced by TPA (Figures 27.13 and 27.14). As the hyperplasia regresses, the cell cycle time increases. A shortening of the G_1 phase of the cell cycle appears to largely account for the decrease in the cell cycle time.

Associated with the reduction in the cell cycle time following TPA administration, is an increase in the rate of epidermal cell loss as measured by the transit time (Table 27.3). As the TPA-induced hyperplasia regresses and the cell cycle increases, so does the transit time; that is to say, the rate of cell loss decreases. It appears that epidermal hyperplastic growth produced by TPA results in similar changes in cell cycle and transit time as occur following abrasion.

Thus, the changes in the cell cycle and transit time associated with abrasion-induced hyperplasia do not appear to be specific for it. It would be of considerable interest to determine if other chemical irritants such as acetic acid, mezerein, turpentine, and cantharidin which produce a regenerative epidermal hyperplasia, but are poor promoters (Boutwell, 1974; Mufson et al., 1981; Slaga et al. 1976) show similar changes in cell cycle and transit times during the production and regression of their induced hyperplasias.

GENERAL CONCLUSIONS

Figure 27.16 is a schematic representation summarizing our findings adapted from Morris and Argyris (1981). Induction of an epidermal hyperplasia by either abrasion or application of TPA results in an increase in epidermal cell number. This increase in epidermal cell number is primarily brought about by an increase in cell proliferation, although cell enlargement also plays a role. The increased cell proliferation is due to a shortening of the cell cycle primarily accomplished by a decrease in the G_1 phase of the cell cycle. The cell cycle is shortest when cell proliferation is the greatest. Associated with the decrease in cell cycle time is a marked increase in the rate of cell loss, as indicated by a decrease in the transit time. An increase in the rate of cell loss suggests that during epidermal hyperplastic growth, there is an increased rate of epidermal cell terminal differentiation or keratinization. This has been recently demonstrated following TPA administration (Reiners and Slaga, 1983) and indirectly suggested by the data of Astrup and Iversen (1981). During the regression of the epidermal hyperplasia, as cell number and proliferative activity decrease and return to normal levels, the length of the cell cycle also increases and returns to normal indicating a gradual lengthening of time spent in the cell cycle by epidermal cells. Also, a slowing down of the loss of epidermal cells, or keratinization occurs.

It seems that the length of the cell cycle not only controls the rate of cell proliferation, but it may also control at least in part, the rate of cell loss. This is suggested by the fact that all the suprabasal cells showing an increased rate of cell loss arose from cells which showed a decreased cycle time. It is as if once an epidermal cell is programmed to divide faster, the cell or its progeny are programmed to differentiate faster. If so, then how a reduced cell cycle time might result in enhanced epidermal differentiation becomes an exciting problem to investigate. Finally, how the stimulation of epidermal hyperplastic growth results in a reduction in the cell cycle time in the first place is also a critical problem which must be investigated to better understand how epidermal hyperplastic growth is controlled.

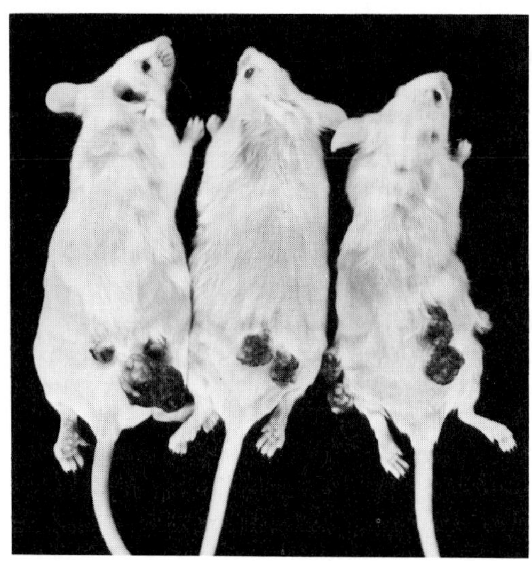

FIGURE 27.17 Papillomas produced by repeated abrasion of the backs of Sencar mice initiated with 100 nmoles of dimethylbenzanthracene.

FIGURE 27.18 Carcinomas produced by repeated abrasion of the backs of Sencar mice initiated with 100 nmoles of dimethylbenzanthracene.

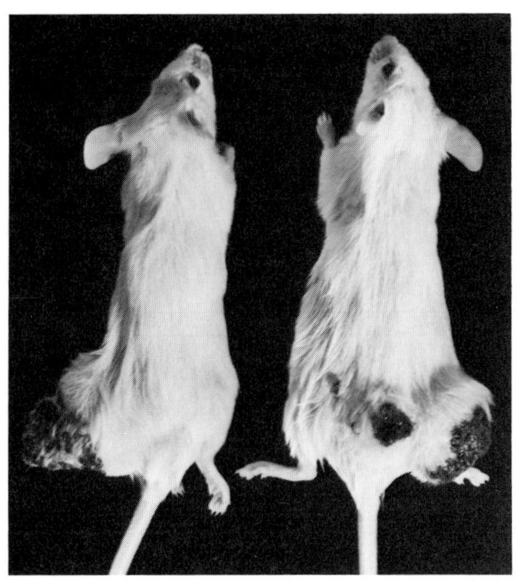

We have demonstrated that the epidermal hyperplasia produced by abrasion is similar to that produced by TPA, the powerful tumor promoter. (For review, see Argyris, 1981b.) Also, the changes in the cell cycle and rate of cell loss show a similar pattern in both of these hyperplasias. Therefore, the question may be raised whether abrasion-induced epidermal hyperplasia can promote epidermal carcinogenesis in the skin of mice appropriately initiated with dimethylbenzanthracene (DMBA), as does TPA.

Repeated epidermal regeneration induced by repeated abrasion of the skin of mice initiated with DMBA results in the promotion of papillomas (Figure 27.17) and carcinomas (Figure 27.18) (Argyris, 1980; Argyris and Slaga, 1981). Thus, an abrasion-induced regenerative epidermal hyperplasia is fully competent to promote epidermal tumorigenesis in the initiated skin of mice. This demonstrates that the epidermal hyperplasias produced by abrasion and TPA are biologically equivalent in so far as tumor promotion is concerned. Therefore, it also suggests that perhaps tumor promoters act by producing a chronic regenerative hyperplasia (Argyris, 1982; Frei and Stephens, 1968; Setala et al., 1959).

ACKNOWLEDGMENT

We thank Ms. Mary Gravante for the typing of our manuscript.

REFERENCES

Argyris, TS. 1968. Growth induced by damage. Adv. Morphog. 7:1-43.

Argyris, TS. 1976. Kinetics of epidermal production during regeneration following abrasion in mice. Am. J. Pathol. 83: 329-340.

Argyris, TS. 1977. Kinetics of regression of epidermal hyperplasia in the skin of mice following abrasion. Am. J. Pathol. 88:575-582.

Argyris, TS. 1978. Epidermal growth and ribosomal RNA accumulation in regenerating mouse epidermis following abrasion. J. Invest. Dermatol. 70:267-271.

Argyris, TS. 1980. Epidermal growth following a single application of 12-0-tetradecanoylphorbol-13-acetate in mice. Am. J. Pathol. 98:639-648.

Argyris, TS. 1981a. The regulation of epidermal hyperplastic growth. CRC Crit. Rev. Toxicol. 9:151-200.

Argyris, TS. 1981b. Ribosomal RNA synthesis throughout epidermal hyperplastic growth induced by abrasion or treatment with 12-0-tetradecanoylphorbol-13-acetate. J. Invest. Dermatol. 76:388-393.

Argyris, TS. 1982. Tumor promotion by degenerative epidermal hyperplasia in mouse skin. J. Cutaneous Pathol. 9:1-18.

Argyris, TS, and TJ Slaga. 1981. Promotion of carcinomas by repeated abrasion in initiated skin of mice. Cancer Res. 41:5193-5195.

Astrup, EG, and OH Iversen. 1981. Cell population kinetics in hairless mouse epidermis following a single topical application of 12-0-tetradecanoylphorbol-13-acetate. I. Carcinogenesis 2:999-1006.

Boutwell, RK. 1974. The function and mechanism of promoters of carcinogenesis. CRC Crit. Rev. Toxicol. 2:419-443.

Christophers, E. 1972. Kinetic aspects of epidermal healing. In Epidermal Wound Healing, Eds. HI Maibach and DT Rovee, pp. 53-69. Chicago: Year Book Publishers.

Frei, JV, and P Stephens. 1968. The correlation of promotion of tumor growth and of induction of hyperplasia in epidermal two-stage carcinogenesis. Br. J. Cancer 22:83-92.

Klein-Szanto, AJP, SK Major and TJ Slaga. 1980. Induction of dark keratinocytes by 12-0-tetradecanoylphorbol-13-acetate and mezerein as an indicator of tumor promoting efficiency. Carcinogenesis 1:399-406.

Mackenzie, IC. 1972. The ordered structure of mammalian epidermis. In Epidermal Wound Healing, Eds. HI Maibach and DT Rovee, pp. 5-25. Chicago: Yearbook Medical Publishers.

Morris, R, and T Argyris. 1983. Epidermal cell cycle and transit times during hyperplastic growth induced by abrasion or treatment with 12-0-tetradecanoylphorbol-13-acetate. Cancer Res. 43:4935-4942.

Mufson, AF, SM Fischer, AK Gleason, TJ Slaga, and RK Boutwell. 1979. Effects of 12-0-tetradecanoylphorbol-13-acetate and mezerein on epidermal ornithine decarboxylase activity, isoproterenol-stimulated levels of cyclic adenosine 3':5'-monophosphate, and induction of mouse skin tumors in vivo. Cancer Res. 39:4791-4795.

Potten, CS. 1974. The epidermal proliferative unit: The possible role of the central basal cell. Cell Tissue Kinet. 7:77-88.

Reiners, JJ, and TJ Slaga. 1983. Effects of tumor promoters on the rate and commitment to terminal differentiation of subpopulations of murine keratinocytes. Cell 32:247-255.

Setala, K, L Merenmies, L Stjernvall, Y Aho, and P Kajanne. 1959. Mechanism of experimental tumorigenesis. I. Epidermal hyperplasia in mouse caused by locally applied tumor initiator and dipole-type tumor promoter. J. Natl. Cancer Inst. 23: 925-951.

Slaga, T, GT Bowden, and RK Boutwell. 1975. Acetic acid, a potent stimulator of mouse epidermal macromolecular synthesis and hyperplasia but weak tumor-promoting ability. *J. Natl. Cancer Inst*. 55:983-987.

Steel, GG. 1977. *Growth Kinetics of Tumors*. Oxford: Oxford University Press, pp. 65-72.

28
The Role of Connective Tissue Matrix in Hypertrophic Scar Contracture

H. Paul Ehrlich

INTRODUCTION

Trauma initiates the repair process in soft tissue. In laboratory animals, full thickness skin excision or third degree burn injuries heal mostly by the process of "wound contraction." With rats, mice, guinea pigs and rabbits, surrounding normal skin will be pulled over the defect and a histological section through that once-damaged area will reveal normal skin.

In contrast, contraction plays a minor role in healing full thickness dermal wounds in humans although there are areas of the body such as the back of the neck and the buttocks where wound contraction does occur (Dunphy 1960). For the most part skin surrounding the defect is not pulled over the defect and the damaged area is repaired by filling in with scar tissue. Skin, like other mammalian organs, is very poor at regeneration and in addition to an inability to regenerate new skin dermis, there is an inability to cover that defect with normal skin by the process of "wound contraction." Histological sections of healed human wounds show scar tissue in the injured area. Scar tissue has both poor cosmetic appearance and functional ability.

In normal wound healing, the scar tissue is slowly restored to give a final near-normal appearance. However, in some circumstances—for example, third degree burns—when deep dermis is destroyed, the scar tissue does not resorb, but continues to proliferate becoming hypertrophic. Hypertrophic scar histologically has a rich vasculature which appears leaky. A number of plasma proteins have been identified within the interstitial space of hypertrophic scars (Cohen et al. 1975). The cause of this increased vascular permeability is not known. In addition, the fibroblast density in hypertrophic scars is greater than normal dermis and non-hypertrophic scar (Figure 28.1). The leaky vasculature may contribute to this increase in fibroblasts. The connective tissue matrix of hypertrophic scar contains swirls of collagen which make up a great deal of the increased connective tissue deposition.

Hence, hypertrophic scar with its enriched blood supply, elevated fibroblast density and more connective tissue matrix distinguishes it from normal skin. This hypertrophic scar tissue, is elevated, hard and tightly bound down to underlying skin surfaces. The fibrotic tissue is not static but undergoes a contractile process known as "scar contracture." In this process, contractile scar tissue causes distortion of surrounding skin. This can lead to loss of function and is responsible for the morbidity associated with the healing of third degree burns. The present clinical treatments for hypertrophic scar are surgical intervention and physical therapy.

The cause and mechanism of the contractile process associated with wound contraction and scar contractures is not known. For some time it was believed that the connective tissue collagen matrix was responsible for wound contraction. Then Abercrombie and his coworkers demonstrated the role of fibroblasts in the contractile process of wound contraction (Abercrombie et al. 1956), and at present these cells within the wound connective tissue matrix have been thought solely responsible for the contraction process. In this chapter I hope to present evidence showing that in the contractile process of repair, both wound contraction and scar contracture involve a cooperation between the mesenchymal cells and connective tissue matrix surrounding and deposited within the wound.

The controlling force for wound contraction may be the scar fibroblasts or the connective tissue matrix. I will now consider the evidence for each of these in turn.

FIBROBLASTS

The fibroblasts populating healing wounds and hypertrophic scar are sometimes called "myofibroblasts" based on their morphological appearance (Majno et al. 1971). It is believed that myofibroblasts are the specialized cells of the contractile process (Gabbiani et al. 1972). Myofibroblasts have a smooth muscle cell-like appearance (Ryan et al. 1974). They have abundant microfilaments and a folded and indented nucleus.

Are fibroblasts derived from hypertrophic scar better at the contractile process compared to normal skin-derived fibro-

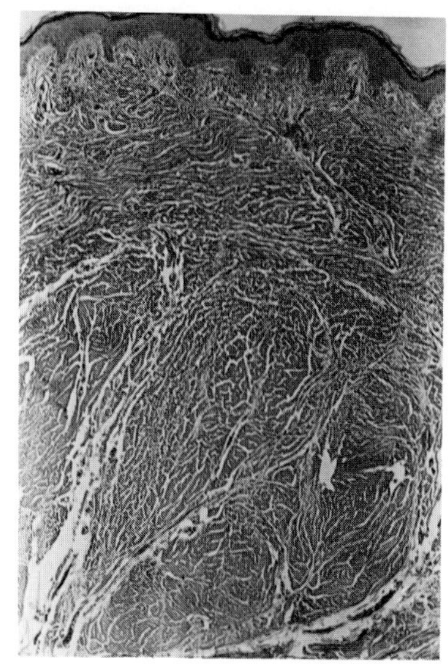

FIGURE 28.1 Histological section of human hypertrophic scar. A histological section from an excised 9-month-old hypertrophic scar stained with hematoxylin and eosin shows a high density of fibroblasts, a rich vascular bed and abundant collagen fibers throughout the tissue. A thickened epidermal layer covers its surface. The characteristic absence of any hair follicles or other dermal appendages within the scar are evident.

blasts? The model developed by Bell and coworkers (1979), a fibroblast populated collagen lattice (FPCL), is composed of serum containing culture medium, native collagen and freshly isolated cultured fibroblasts. When these components are mixed together under physiological conditions, fibroblasts are trapped within the polymerized collagen matrix. With time, fibroblasts entrapped within that FPCL change their morphology from rounded spherical cells to flattened elongated ones (Ehrlich et al. 1983). During this transition of cell shape, the entire FPCL undergoes a reduction in size. With time lattices show a loss of area which is referred to as "lattice contraction." Using this FPCL model system, a variety of fibroblasts were incorporated into the collagen lattice and their ability to contract that lattice was measured over a period of days. In general, the more cells incorporated into a FPCL the greater the rate and degree of lattice contraction (Bell et al. 1979). The greater the concentration of collagen the less the degree and rate of lattice contraction. Elimination or a reduction in serum concentration could reduce lattice contraction. Fetal bovine serum at 20% concentration appears an ideal concentration for maximal lattice contraction.

Steinberg and coworkers (1980), showed that normal fibroblasts were better at lattice contraction than transformed fibroblasts. With time, there are greater numbers of transformed cells in a FPCL compared to one containing normal cells because the normal cells do not proliferate as well as transformed cells (Buttle and Ehrlich, in press). Even with their greater cell density, transformed cells are poor at lattice contraction. Transformed cells proliferated as well within the collagen matrix as on tissue culture dish surfaces. Therefore, not all fibroblasts are identical in their ability to contract FPCL. Manufacturing collagen lattices with added keratinocytes or endothelial cells produced no lattice contraction. Thus it appears that normal fibroblasts are better at lattice contraction than transformed fibroblasts, epithelial or endothelial cells.

To obtain fibroblasts from hypertrophic scar and normal skin, small pieces of hypertrophic scar and normal human skin were tissue cultured as explants by standard procedures. Mesenchymal cells grew out from these explants, 5 forming primary hypertrophic scar-derived cell lines and 4 primary cell lines derived from normal skin were compared in FPCL lattice contraction studies. No differences in lattice contraction between hypertrophic scar-derived and normal skin-derived human fibroblasts could be documented (Figure 28.2A). When equal numbers of fibroblasts were incorporated into FPCL under identical conditions of collagen and serum containing medium, there were no differences in lattice contraction. Thus fibroblasts from normal skin and hypertrophic scar were identical in their ability to contract FPCL. We were unable to isolate a supercontractile cell from hypertrophic scars.

The possible reason for the failure to identify a difference between fibroblasts derived from normal skin and hypertrophic scar is that tissue culturing causes alterations in normal tissue fibroblasts. Tissue cultured fibroblasts show a difference in organization of contractile proteins compared to *in vivo* normal fibroblasts (Gabbiani et al. 1973). Transformed fibroblasts do not develop greatly organized contractile proteins and hence are shown to be poor at lattice contraction (Buttle and Ehrlich, in press).

We can assume that the environment of the fibroblast can alter its contractile protein organization. The environment of fibroblasts within hypertrophic scar may be different from the environment of fibroblasts within normal dermis. Smooth muscle cells derived from bovine aorta were also incorporated into a collagen lattice. Smooth muscle cells were not as capable of contracting lattices as an equal number of normal dermal fibroblasts (Figure 28.2B). It was estimated that it took 3 times the number of smooth muscle cells to contract a lattice as well as dermal fibroblasts. Therefore, fibroblasts derived from

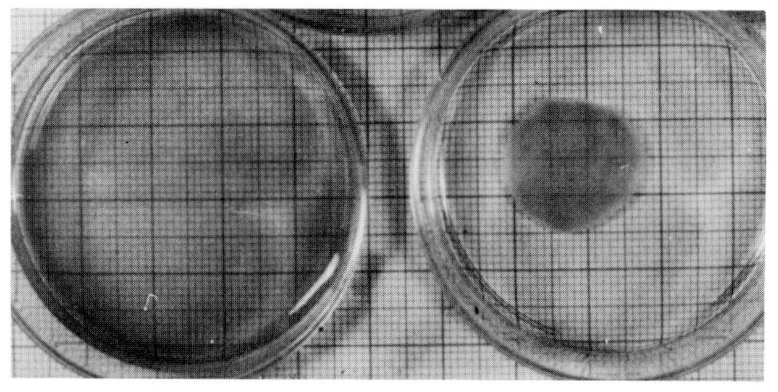

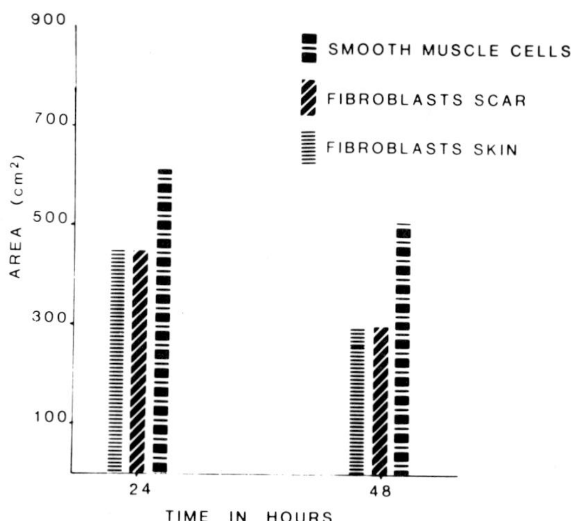

FIGURE 28.2 Fibroblasts and smooth muscle cell populated collagen lattices undergoing lattice contraction. A. FPCL at time 0 appears on the left. On the right an FPCL after 2 days in culture. The reduction in lattice size is referred to as lattice contraction. B. Graphs show the degree of lattice contraction on days 1 and 2. Equal numbers of fibroblasts derived from either normal human dermis or hypertrophic scar and smooth muscle cells derived from bovine aorta were incorporated into collagen lattices under identical conditions. Smooth muscle cell lattices showed a reduced ability at lattice contraction. These cells are poor at lattice contraction compared to fibroblasts. No differences exist between fibroblasts derived from either normal skin or hypertrophic scar.

normal dermis were better at contracting collagen lattices than blood vessel smooth muscle cells.

A diseased dermal fibroblast was identified which was defective at lattice contraction. The inheritable disease epidermolysis bullosa dystrophica recessive, EBdr, is characterized by skin blisters forming from minor trauma. This bullosa disease appears to be caused by defective fibroblasts within the dermis (Briggaman and Wheeler 1975). When equal numbers of age-matched fibroblasts derived from normals and EBdr patients were incorporated into collagen lattices, the patients' fibroblasts were defective at lattice contraction (Ehrlich et al. 1983). Morphologically, EBdr fibroblasts are unable to elongate and spread out as well as normal human dermal fibroblasts (Figure 28.3). This inability to elongate and spread out within collagen lattices was also noted with transformed fibroblasts incorporated into collagen lattices (Buttle and Ehrlich, in press). In general, it appears that cells such as EBdr fibroblasts, and transformed cells are not able to elongate and spread out as well as normal dermal fibroblasts. These affected cells do not contract collagen lattices as well as normal cells. Normal dermal-derived fibroblasts spread out and elongate as well as hypertrophic scar-derived fibroblasts and are identical in their contractile capabilities.

With third degree burn in rats there is a difference in the healing process compared to freeze produced wounds (Li et al. 1980). Burn wounds, like excised wounds, heal by wound contraction. On the other hand, freeze wounds do not heal by wound contraction (Figure 28.4). Fibroblasts within healing burn and freeze injuries appear to have similar morphologies. Freeze wounds may not contract because their fibroblasts are different from fibroblasts in healing burn wounds. One possibility is that healing burn wounds have myofibroblast-like fibroblasts and healing freeze wounds do not. Myofibroblast-like fibroblasts have a characteristic morphology. Using the electron microscope, healing freeze injuries have been shown to have fibroblasts identical to the myofibroblasts described by Gabbiani et al. (1972) in healing wounds.

Fibroblasts from healing freeze injury have abundant myofilaments, nuclear folds and indentations like those reported in myofibroblasts (Figure 28.5A). Another characteristic of the myofibroblasts in the healing wound is F-actin filaments staining within the cytoplasm in the form of stress fibers (Hirschel et al. 1971). The actin myosin of the mesenchymal cells may be responsible for contractile process in non-muscle cells (Majno 1979). The originally described actin staining of

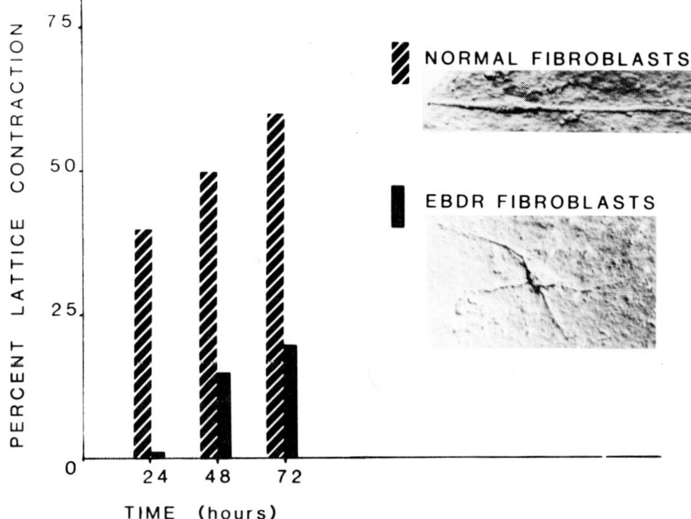

FIGURE 28.3 Collagen lattice contraction with normal and EBdr human fibroblasts. FPCL were made with equal numbers of EBdr patient fibroblasts and fibroblasts derived from age-matched normal individuals. With normal cells, lattice contraction continues over the 3 day period. With EBdr lattices contraction proceeds at a much slower rate. The insert at the right shows the typical morphology of fibroblasts within a collagen matrix. Normal fibroblasts are elongated and spread out as compared to EBdr fibroblasts which are rounded up and have a dendritic-like shape.

myofibroblasts used serum from patients with chronic hepatitis which contained anti-actin antibodies. Because of the hazards of using hepatitis sera for routine staining of these actin filaments, stress fibers, we have substituted fluorescent labelled phallacidin. Phallacidin, a toxin produced by the mushroom Amanita phalloides, specifically binds to F-actin (Barak et al. 1980). Fluorescent labelled phallacidin is an excellent probe because of its low molecular weight and its high specificity for F-actin. Within freeze-damaged healing wounds, actin staining cells are seen throughout the granulation tissue (Figure 28.5B). There is no actin staining cells in uninjured surrounding skin (Figure 28.5C). This staining pattern is identical to that seen

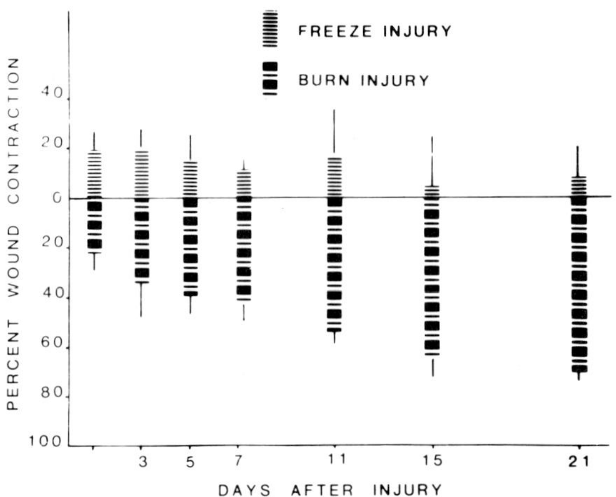

FIGURE 28.4 Comparative studies of healing burn or freeze injuries in rats. Rats were anesthesized with ether, their backs shaved and either a brass probe equilibrated in boiling water was applied to their back skin surface for 20 seconds or an identical size brass probe equilibrated in liquid nitrogen was applied to the skin surface for 45 seconds. The wound edges were tattooed and the wound size measured for a three-week period. Burn injured skin healed mostly by wound contraction. Freeze injuries skin did not undergo contraction. The lines represent the standard error of the means.

FIGURE 28.5 (opposite page) Fibroblast morphology from healing freeze injuries. Standard freeze injuries were made in rats. Wound specimens were taken at 14 days and processed for histological studies. Some specimens were prepared for electron microscope examination and others prepared for frozen section fluorescent examination.

A. (opposite left) Electron microscope picture of a characteristic fibroblast in a healing freeze injury is presented. There is an indented nucleus and the two cells shown in the micrograph are in very close contact to one another.

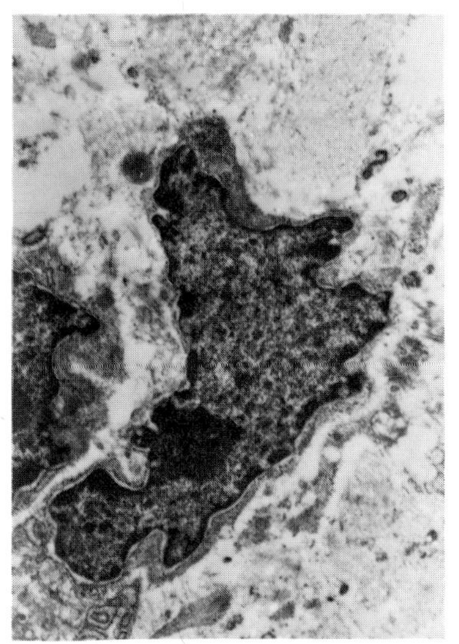

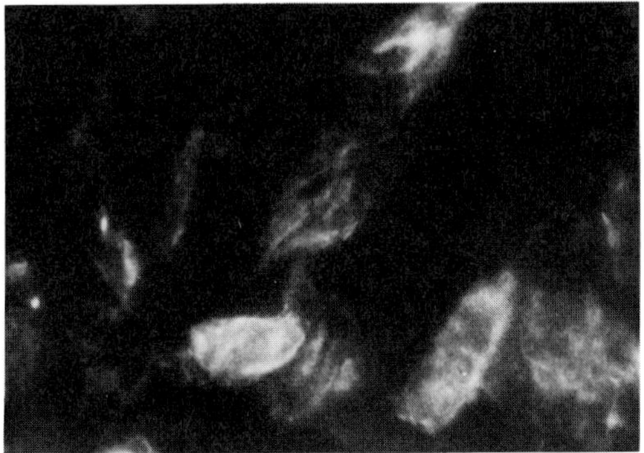

B. (above center) NBD phallacidin staining of actin filaments (stress fibers) in fibroblasts from freeze healing wounds. Most fibroblasts in these healing wounds have identifiable stress fibers, identical to cells from burn healing wounds.

C. (above right) NBD phallacidin staining of actin filaments in normal dermis adjacent to the freeze injury show that epidermal cells on the skin surface have actin staining but the normal fibroblasts within the dermis do not stain. Normal dermal fibroblasts have actin in the form of G-actin, while epidermal cells have their actin in the form of F-actin. Freeze healing fibroblasts have F-actin which is readily identifiable with NBD phallacidin staining.

with healing burn granulation tissue fibroblasts. Open wound granulation tissue has a similar histological appearance (Hirschel et al. 1971). Healing burn and freeze injuries have actin staining fibroblasts within their granulation tissue while there is no staining in the normal surrounding dermis. Therefore, the differences in wound contraction between freeze and burn do not appear to be due to a defect in morphology of resident fibroblasts.

CONNECTIVE TISSUE MATRIX

There are some unusual characteristics of the connective tissue matrix of hypertrophic scar. Hypertrophic scar collagen is laid down by the resident fibroblasts. Collagen composition of hypertrophic scar compared to normal skin is altered (Bailey et al. 1975; Hayakawa et al. 1979; Ehrlich and White 1981). There is more type III and type V collagen in hypertrophic scar. Hypertrophic scar is richer in type I trimer (unpublished work). Altered concentrations of the collagen types within hypertrophic scar may be important. Hypertrophic scar is richer in type III collagen. Collagen lattices are more easily contracted by fibroblasts when incorporated into type III FPCL.

Hypertrophic scar collagen is much more soluble than normal skin collagen (Table 28.1). Three times more pepsin solubilized collagen can be extracted from hypertrophic scar compared to normal skin. Based upon SDS polyacrylamide gel electrophoresis analysis, normal skin and hypertrophic scar have type V, III and I trimer collagens (Figure 28.6). Further characterization shows that the amino acid analysis of type V, III and I trimer collagens in hypertrophic scar is identical to that extracted from normal skin (Table 28.2). On the other hand, type I collagen from hypertrophic scar has reduced content of hydroxyproline; therefore hydroxyproline to proline ratio in hypertrophic scars is lower compared to normal skin. This lowered hydroxyproline content in type I hypertrophic scar collagen affects thermal stability. Viscosity measurement of type I collagen show that the melting temperature for hypertrophic scar type I collagen is 1.5 degrees Centigrade less than normal skin type I collagen (Figure 28.7). No differences in thermal stability of type III collagen extracted from either hypertrophic scar or normal skin were noted.

Is there a difference in the contractability of normal dermal collagen and hypertrophic scar collagen? The collagen composition of FPCL was studied using collagen extracted from either

TABLE 28.1

Collagen Extracts of Normal and Hypertrophic Scar

	EXTRACTED COLLAGENS	
	SKIN	HYPERTROPHIC SCAR
SOLUBILIZED	7%	41%
COLLAGEN		
TYPE I trimer	1%	4%
TYPE V	2%	4%
TYPE III	22%	34%
TYPE I	75%	59%

Note: Both skin and hypertrophic scar were pepsin treated and the collagen solubilized fractions fractionated by various sodium chloride salt precipitations. Collagen types were identified by SDS polyacrylamide gel electrophoresis of either denatured alpha chains or cyanogen bromide peptides. The percents given are based upon salt-free dry weights of each fraction.

TABLE 28.2

Amino Acid Composition of Collagen Alpha I Chains Extracted from Either Purified Normal Skin or Hypertrophic Scar

	Ratio of Hyroxyproline / Proline	
	Alpha Chain Skin	Alpha Chain Scar
TYPE (1)	0.68	0.58
TYPE (111)	0.91	0.92
TYPE (1) trimer	–	0.72

Note: Alpha I chain from type I trimer collagen and type III collagen alpha I chain are identical when comparing normal human skin and hypertrophic scar. The alpha 1 chain from type I collagen from hypertrophic scar is underhydroxylated compared to that extracted from normal skin.

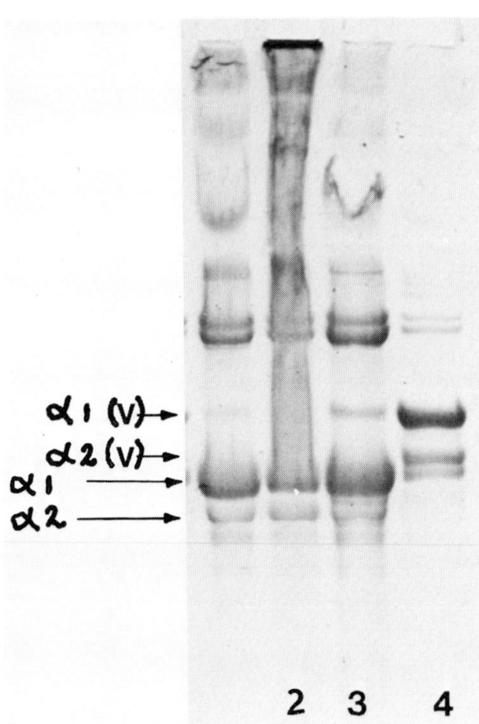

FIGURE 28.6 SDS polyacrylamide gel electrophoresis stained patterns of salt fractionated hypertrophic scar collagen extracts. Hypertrophic scar was treated with pepsin and solubilized collagen was fractionated with salt under neutral conditions. In lane 1, the lowest salt concentration, there is mostly alpha 1 chains which are mostly alpha 1 (III) chains from type III collagens. At the next higher salt concentration, lane 2, alpha 1 and alpha 2 chains are present. This appears to be type I collagen with alpha 1 (I) and alpha 2 (I) chains. In lane 3 the major band is alpha 1 chain which is alpha 1 (I) from type I trimer collagen. Also there is type V collagen alpha 1 (V) band present which shows type V collagen contamination of this type I trimer salt fraction. In lane 4 the highest salt concentration type V collagen chains are present as alpha 1 (V) and alpha 2 (V). Below alpha 2 (V) is a band of alpha 1 which appears to be alpha 1 (I) from type I trimer collagen contamination.

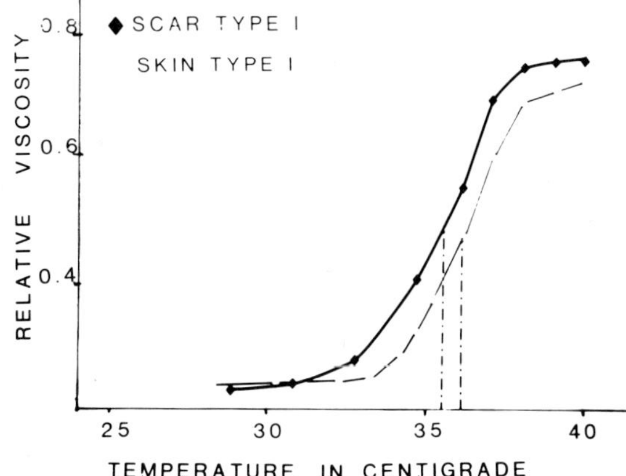

FIGURE 28.7 Melting temperature differences between type I collagen extracted from either normal skin or hypertrophic scar. Type I collagen from normal skin or hypertrophic scar were solubilized in 0.1 M acetic acid at 1.0 mg/ml. The viscosity measurement results are presented in terms of relative viscosity. The broken lines represent the denaturing or melting temperature for the collagen solutions. Hypertrophic scar collagen type I has a melting temperature of 35°C. Normal type I collagen has a melting temperature of 36.5°C which indicates that normal type I collagen is more stable than hypertrophic scar collagen.

normal human skin or hypertrophic scar. Hypertrophic scar and normal skin collagen were solubilized by limited pepsin digestion. Collagens were further purified by salt fractionation. FPCL made with unfractionated hypertrophic scar collagen extracts were more readily contracted compared to lattices made with unfractionated normal dermal collagen (Figure 28.8). FPCL made with salt fractionated types I, II or III collagens were compared. Lattice contraction was the least with type II collagen FPCL. There was more lattice contraction with type I collagen and the most with type III collagen. Hypertrophic scar is richer in type III collagen as compared to normal skin (Bailey et al. 1975; Hayakawa et al. 1979). These *in vitro* experiments show

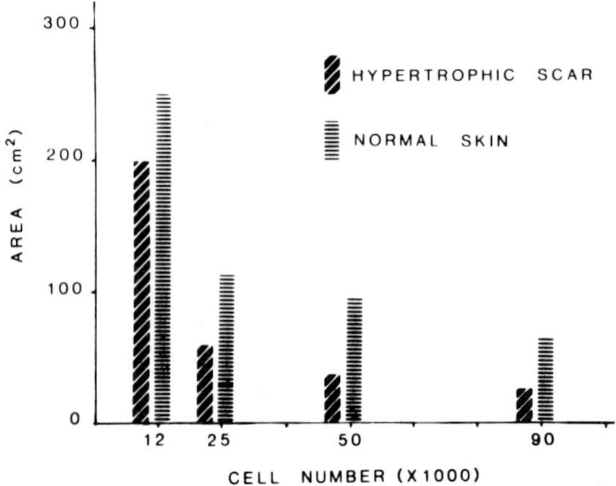

FIGURE 28.8 Fibroblast populated collagen lattices composed of either normal dermal or hypertrophic scar collagens. Equal numbers of normal human fibroblasts were incorporated into FPCL made with either normal skin or hypertrophic scar collagen extracts. With time, hypertrophic scar collagen FPCL showed a more rapid rate of lattice contraction compared to normal dermal collagen lattices.

that the source of collagen can alter the degree of lattice contraction. Collagen extracted from a hypertrophic scar can be more readily contracted by fibroblasts incorporated within it, compared to collagen extracted from normal dermis.

Evidence from in vivo experiments with rat freeze and burn injuries also suggests that the connective tissue matrix can control the contractile process of wound contraction. Histologically, freeze injuries produce an inflammatory cell response equivalent to burns. Vascular alterations were much greater with burn damage when compared to freeze damaged (Ehrlich et al. 1981). There are no patent blood vessels in the area of direct burn damage as demonstrated by yellow latex infusion. In contrast, freeze damaged skin 24 hours following injury, demonstrated patent vessels within the dead space. With 24-hour burn injury, more salt soluble collagen was extracted from the heat killed tissue (Figure 28.9). With freeze injury 24 hours old, less collagen was extracted from the freeze killed dermis. It appears that freeze trauma causes cellular necrosis, while

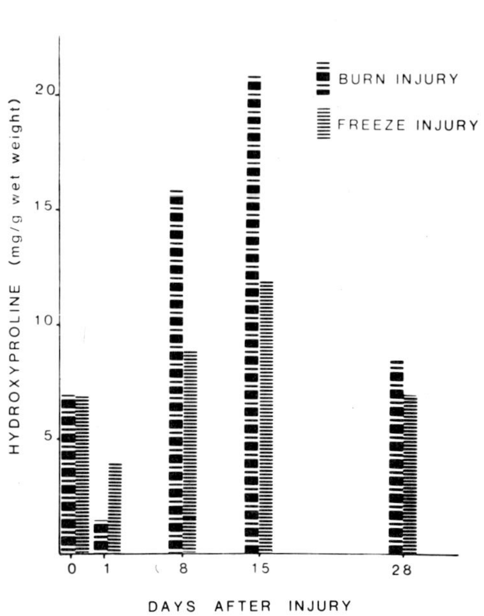

FIGURE 28.9 Hydroxyproline content of frozen or burn injured healing wounds. Standard burn or freeze injuries were made on rats as previously described. At various time points, wounds were excised and acid hydrolyzed. The hydroxyproline per gram of wet weight healing wound tissue initially was measured. Initially there is more hydroxyproline, collagen loss with burn injury. With time, burn healing wounds produces excessive amounts of collagen. With freeze damage, only a small loss of collagen initially appears and with time only a modest excess of new collagen synthesis occurs.

burn injury causes both necrosis and the complete destruction of the connective tissue matrix. With burn injury the connective tissue matrix is destroyed and nonfunctional. There is a loss of structural integrity. In freeze injury the structural integrity of the dermis survives, appearing similar to full thickness skin graft.

In humans, the majority of the skin surface is held down by underlying fascia (Brody et al. 1981). With laboratory animals, the skin is not held down as much and it is quite loose. When this loose skin is destroyed, healing occurs mostly by wound contraction. An *in vivo* model using a mouse with characteristic tightly held down skin has been used to study wound contraction. The tight skin mouse, TSK, is a genetic breed of mouse whose skin is held down tightly to the underlying hypodermis (Green et al. 1976). Open skin excisions in these mice do not have loose wound edges (Menton et al. 1978). Wound healing by wound contraction is initially delayed in these mice (Figure 28.10). Eventually wound contraction does proceed

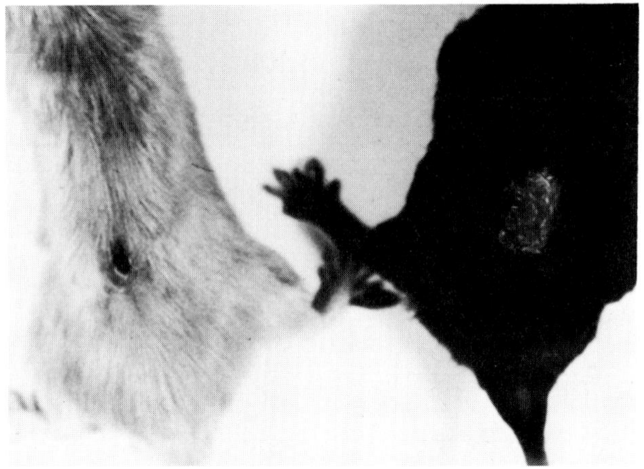

FIGURE 28.10 Wound healing in normal and tight skin mice. Standard full thickness open wounds were made on anesthesized normal or tight skin mice. After 17 days, mice were photographed. On the left, a normal litter mate has a tan coat color and shows a small remaining wound. This wound is almost totally closed by wound contraction. On the right, an affected litter mate with (TSK/+) genotype has black coat color and a tightly held down skin cover. Wound closure has been delayed compared to the normal litter mate.

(Figure 28.11). During this delay period, the density of fibroblasts in the granulation tissue of tight skin mouse wounds appears to be the same as that in normal litter mate skin wounds (Ehrlich and Needle, in press). The delay of wound contraction for two weeks with TSK mice appears to be related to the surrounding dermis which is not loose, much like that of normal human skin. At the end of this two week delay, TSK mouse wounds start to contract and proceed at a rate equivalent to that of normal litter mates. Histologically, two week old TSK wounds are hyperplastic with excessive connective tissue filling the dead space. This hyperplastic tissue mimics the appearance of human hypertrophic scar. When contraction eventually starts, the TSK mouse skin appears to free itself from the underlying hypodermis, normal skin is pulled over the defect and the excess hypertrophic scar like connective tissue matrix is resorbed. TSK wounds heal within 7 weeks with very small scars identical to that of their normal litter mates.

Thus, the contractile process seen in fibrotic matrices appears to involve a number of components. The force of the contractile process appears to be the resident mesenchymal cells, fibroblasts. The integrity of the surrounding skin not involved in the healing process and its association with underlying fascia appears to control the initiation of the contractile process of wound contraction. The connective tissue matrix laid down within the damaged area also can play a controlling

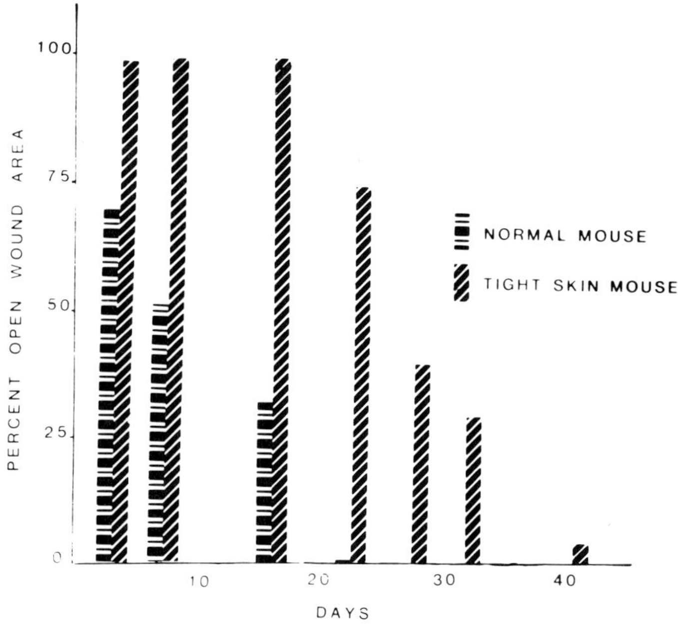

FIGURE 28.11 Wound contraction of normal and TSK mice. Normal mice heal open wounds by wound contraction which starts within a day after trauma. TSK mice heal wounds by wound contraction also but wound contraction does commence until more than 2 weeks after injury. It is proposed that TSK mice showed delayed wound contraction because skin at the wound edge is initially held down closely to the underlying surface. Eventually wound edges can be freed and wound contraction occurs.

role in the contractile process. The importance of the vascular supply to both the connective tissue matrix and fibroblasts within the healing wound could be related to maintaining the proliferative rate of resident fibroblasts, their ability to contract and type of collagen synthesized in the matrix. Hence, wound contraction and scar contractures appear as a cooperative effort between the vascular supply, resident fibroblast, and connective tissue matrix integrity around and within the healing wound. The search for means to alter any of these parameters within a hypertrophic scar may lead to a control of hypertrophic scar contractures and its associated morbidity.

REFERENCES

Abercrombie, M, Flint, MH, and Jones, DW. Wound contraction in relationship to collagen formation in scorbutic guinea pigs. J. Embryol. Exp. Morph. 4: (1956) 167-175.

Bailey, AJ, Bazin, S, Sims, TJ, LeLous, M, Nicoletis, C, and Delaunay, A. Characterization of the collagen of human hypertrophic and normal scars. Biochim. Biophys. Acta 405: (1975) 412-421.

Barak, LS, Yocum, RR, and Nothnagel, EA. Fluorescence staining of actin cytoskeleten in living cells wihth 7-nitrobenz-2-oxa-1,3-diazole-phallacidin. Proc. Nat. Acad. Sci. (USA) 77: (1980) 980-984.

Bell, E, Ivarrson, B, and Merrill, C. Production of a tissue-like structure by contraction of collagen lattices by human fibroblasts of different proliferative potential in vitro. Proc. Natl. Acad. Sci. (USA) 76: (1979) 1274-1278.

Briggaman, RA, and Wheeler, CE. Epidermolysis Bullosa dystrophica recessive; A possible role of anchoring fibrils in the pathogenesis. J. Invest. Derm. 65: (1975) 203-211.

Brody, GS, Peng, STJ, and Landel, RF. The etiology of hypertrophic scar contracture: Another view. Plast. Recon. Surg. 67: (1981) 673-679.

Buttle, DJ, and Ehrlich, HP. Studies of collagen lattice contraction utilizing a normal and a transformed cell line. J. Cell. Physiol. (in press).

Cohen, IK, Dieglmann, RF, and Bryant, CP. Alpha globulin collagenase inhibitors in keloid and hypertrophic scar. Surg. Forum 26: (1975) 61-62.

Dunphy, JE. On the nature and care of wounds. Ann. Roy. Col. Surg. Eng. 26: (1960) 69-78.

Ehrlich, HP, and White, BS. The identification of A and B collagen chains in hypertrophic scar. Exp. Mol. Path. 34: (1981) 1-8.

Ehrlich, HP, Trelstad, RL, and Fallon, JT. Dermal vascular patterns in response to burn or freeze injury in rats. Exp. Mol. Path. 34: (1981) 281-289.

Ehrlich, HP, Buttle, DJ, Trelstad, RL, and Hayashi, K. Epidermolysis Bullosa dystrophica recessive fibroblasts altered behavior within a collagen matrix. J. Invest. Derm. 80: (1983) 56-60.

Ehrlich, HP, and Needle, AL. Wound healing in tight skin mice; Delayed closure of excised wounds. Plas. Recon. Surg. (in press).

Gabbiani, G, Hirschel, BJ, Ryan, GB, Statkov, PR, and Majno, G. Granulation tissue as a contractile organ. A study of structure and function. J. Exp. Med. 135: (1972) 719-734.

Gabbiani, G, Majno, G, and Ryan, GB. The fibroblast as a contractile cell: the myofibroblast. In E. Kulanon and J. Pikkarainen, Biology of Fibroblast. New York: Academic Press. (1973). pp. 139-154.

Green, M, Sweet, HO, and Bunker, LE. Tight-skin, a new mutation of the mouse causing excess growth of connective tissue and skeleton. Am. J. Path. 82: (1976) 493-512.

Hayakawa, T, Hashimoto, Y, Myokei, Y, Aoyana, M, and Izawa, Y. Changes in type of collagen during the development of human post-burn hypertrophic scar. Clin. Chim. Acta 93: (1979) 119-126.

Hirschel, BJ, Gabbiani, G, Ryan, GB, and Majno, G. Fibroblasts of granulation tissue: Immunofluorescent staining with anti smooth muscle serum. Proc. Soc. Exp. Biol. Med. 138: (1971) 466-469.

Li, AKC, Ehrlich, HP, Trelstad, RL, Koroly, MJ, Shattenkerk, ME, and Malt, RA. Differences in healing of skin wounds caused by burn and freeze injuries. Ann. Surg. 191: (1980) 244-248.

Majno, G, Gabbiani, G, Hirschel, BJ, Ryan, GB, and Statkov, PR. Contraction of granulation tissue in vitro: Similarity to smooth muscle. Science 173: (1971) 548-550.

Majno, G. The study of the myofibroblast. Am. J. Surg. Path. 3: (1979) 535-542.

Menton, DN, Hess, RA, Lichenstein, JR, and Eisen, AZ. The structure and tensile properties of the skin of tight skin (TSK) mutant mice. J. Invest. Derm. 70: (1978) 4-10.

Ryan, GB, Cliff, WJ, Gabbiani, G, Irl'e, C, Montandon, D, Statkov, PR, and Majno, G. Myofibroblasts in human granulation tissue. Hum. Path. 5: (1974) 55-67.

Steinberg, BM, Smith, K, Colozzo, M, and Pollack, R. Establishment and transformation diminish the ability of fibroblasts to contract a native collagen gel. J. Cell Biol. 87: (1980) 304-308.

29
Epimorphic Regeneration in Mammals

Richard J. Goss

INTRODUCTION

The spectrum of regeneration embraces many developmental phenomena. Physiological regeneration, for example, involves the turnover of molecules and cells to counteract everyday wear and tear. Related to this is the process of compensatory growth. Exhibited by most internal organs and tissues, this is a mechanism whereby bodily parts may increase in size to compensate for reductions in mass or increases in functional load. It is achieved by either hyperplasia or hypertrophy of the cells involved. It is a morphological adaptation to physiological deficiencies (Goss 1978). Wound healing is a third kind of regeneration. Unlike physiological turnover and compensatory growth, it is a localized reaction to injury. Virtually all tissues and organs in the body (except teeth) are capable of repair (McMinn 1969). It is accompanied by cellular migration, proliferation (where possible), and differentiation. Tissue repair is a stopgap measure designed to complete the continuity of interrupted tissues.

The foregoing developmental processes are ubiquitous. They are found in all tissues and in all multicellular animals. A fourth category of regeneration, however, is not universal. Epimorphic regeneration, the process by which amputated appendages are regrown *in situ*, occurs here and there in the animal kingdom. For unaccountable reasons, some groups are richly endowed with regenerative abilities while in others they

---

The author is grateful to the Whitehall Foundation for grant support of research partly reported herein.

are singularly lacking (Goss 1969). There has been a gradual extinction of epimorphic regenerative abilities during vertebrate evolution, but some lower forms, including many invertebrates, are as regeneratively incompetent as mammals. Regeneration is presumably adaptive, but to what conditions its presence or absence has adapted is a rich field for speculation.

THE MECHANISM OF REGENERATION

The success of epimorphic regeneration depends upon a number of conditions (Wallace 1981). Although the actual loss of an appendage is not required, there must nevertheless be a transverse exposure of an appendage stump. An appendage may be defined as a histologically complex array of tissues enveloped in an integument. Thus, epidermal wound healing is an essential condition for the initiation of regeneration. Since the replacement of an appendage is limited to the anatomical territory of that structure, amputation must leave behind a source of cells from which the regenerate can develop. Following wound healing, the injured mesodermal tissues at the stump undergo varying degrees of dedifferentiation. This provides a pool of cells from which the blastema can form. These dedifferentiated cells migrate distally where they accumulate under the wound epidermis. They lose all overt signs of their previous states of differentiation, and their numbers are amplified by proliferation to sustain an apical growth zone. Physiological conditions conducive to the functional competence of the regenerate are usually required for blastema production.

Morphogenetic information must be communicated to the blastema, either brought with the cells into the regenerate, or secondarily transferred to them once the blastema has become established. In either case, morphogenesis is initiated by the differentiation of blastema cells into extensions of the tissues present in the stump. Differentiation unfolds in a distal direction, accounting for the sequential replacement of the anatomical parts of the appendage. It ceases only when the last cells have differentiated. The regeneration process typically replaces a lost appendage with precisely what was amputated.

REGENERATION VERSUS REPAIR

It must be asked if epimorphic regeneration can be interpreted as an extension of tissue repair. Each of the tissues represented in an amputation stump is itself capable of repair. Could regeneration represent the sum of these component repair processes, or is it a distinct and separate process?

Similarities

Both events are initiated by an injury, either the amputation of an appendage or a lesion in a tissue (for example, bone fracture). Such injuries interrupt the continuity of tissues, eliciting reactions designed to restore, to varying degrees, the original morphological integrity.

In each case, a remnant must exist from which renewed growth can proceed. Amputation of an entire appendage, removing all of the regeneration territory, is not followed by regeneration. Excision of a whole bone or muscle yields no provision for repair of the missing tissue. A source of cells must remain for regeneration or repair to occur.

Cell migration is an integral part of epimorphic regeneration and tissue repair. Cells stream toward the site of injury. Here they aggregate, proliferate and differentiate into tissues in continuity with the remnants from which they were derived.

Both phenomena are local reactions to injury. Both give rise to new components similar to those from which they are derived. Both recapitulate the ontogenies of their original modes of development. But this is as far as the similarities go. They are far outnumbered by the differences.

Differences

Epimorphic regeneration depends upon epidermal wound healing as a prelude to blastema formation. In fact, there are no examples of epimorphic regeneration in nature that are not initiated in an epidermal wound. Tissue repair, except in the skin itself, takes place internally without involvement of wound epidermis.

Dedifferentiation is an important step in epimorphic regeneration. It involves the complete morphologic disappearance of those specializations in cells upon which their identities depend. As a result, it is impossible to distinguish the exact origins of dedifferentiated cells in an amputation blastema. The cells adjacent to a tissue lesion likewise undergo a decrease in specialization, at least sufficient to enable them to migrate and proliferate. There is reason to believe, however, that the altered states of differentiation in these cases are of considerably less magnitude than in epimorphic regeneration. Indeed, these are probably more akin to cellular modulation inasmuch as the cells redifferentiate into the same kinds of tissues from which they were derived.

Whatever the extents of their loss of specialization, both appendage and tissue cells aggregate in the injured region. In epimorphic regeneration, this results in the establishment of a blastema. A blastema is a mass of dedifferentiated cells from diverse origins. It is organized beneath the wound epidermis and adjacent to the underlying tissues of the stump from which its cells emigrated. It possesses proximo-distal polarity.

In the case of tissue repair, the aggregate of unspecialized cells fills the region of injury. In fractured bones, it is referred to as a callus. In the dermis, it is granulation tissue. In other mesodermal structures such as tendons or muscles, comparable clusters of cells form. These "repair aggregates" differ from blastemas in that the differentiative potentials of their constituent cells are restricted to the tissue to be healed. They are not associated with wound epidermis. They lack proximo-distal polarity.

Parenthetically, it must be noted that in some examples of epimorphic regeneration (for example, fish fins and barbels, amphibian limbs), blastema formation cannot occur in the absence of adequate innervation. Tail regeneration may depend on the presence of a spinal cord. These neurotrophic influences are examples of the utilitarian imperative by which the regeneration of nonfunctional appendages is avoided. In cases of tissue repair, nerves are not required for cellular aggregation and differentiation to take place. Even in the case of skeletal muscle, proliferation and differentiation occur, although hypertrophy of the myofibers may be lacking.

Differentiation of cells in a blastema need not necessarily reflect their tissues of origin. While metaplasia is a difficult phenomenon to prove, there is reason to believe that it can occur in a developing blastema, whether or not it ordinarily does so. It is this potential that is the basis upon which dedifferentiation is defined in an amputation stump. The absence of metaplasia in tissue repair testifies to the less complete extent of dedifferentiation that prevails in this process.

Morphogenesis takes place to vastly differing degrees in epimorphic regeneration and tissue repair. In the former, the severed tissues in the stump are not only completed, but entirely new ones arise. Beyond each articulation, new skeletal elements develop. New muscles originate and insert on these bones. This is the essence of epimorphic regeneration. It goes beyond merely completing the continuity of interrupted tissues. It gives rise to wholly new anatomical structures. In tissue repair, the severed ends may become reunited (if they are not too far apart), but nothing really new is formed in the process.

Finally, it is worth noting that a blastema exhibits proximodistal polarity, as did the appendage it is destined to replace. Its morphogenesis is spatially and temporally coordinated so that the more proximal structures develop earlier than the more distal ones. In tissue repair, no such polarization is evident except insofar as differentiation immediately adjacent to the margins may precede that in the middle of the lesion.

Tissue repair inevitably includes some replacement of tissue. The degree to which this is achieved, however, is conspicuously deficient by epimorphic standards. Only enough tissue to reestablish continuity between the margins of the interrupted parts is produced. Tissue repair is therefore a very limited kind of development, well suited to the need to bridge a gap but not designed actually to replace substantial amounts of missing parts. It is interesting to note that these limitations of tissue repair apply as much to lower vertebrates as to higher ones, irrespective of their capacities for epimorphic regeneration. A bone may heal a fracture by forming a callus, but if the entire skeletal element is removed there is no provision for its replacement. Even in salamanders, whose limbs are so readily equipped to replace amputated parts, missing bones or muscles from otherwise intact limbs are replaced no better than in higher forms.

It would appear that tissue repair is such an important necessity of life that it has never been eliminated by natural selection. Epimorphic regeneration exhibits a spotty distribution suggesting that, however convenient it may be, it is not an indispensable requirement for survival.

On the basis of the above comparisons, it is concluded that epimorphic regeneration differs from tissue repair in kind, not just in degree. There are a number of events that both processes share in common, but their differences outnumber their similarities. Further, some of these differences (for example, epidermal wound healing, dedifferentiation, blastema formation) are of such fundamental significance as to be diagnostic of epimorphic regeneration. This distinction is of importance in the interpretation of how mammalian appendages react to amputation.

PHYLOGENETIC EXTINCTION OF REGENERATION

What might have been the factors that have influenced the acquisition or loss of epimorphic regeneration in the different appendages of various vertebrates? The general distribution of regeneration would seem to correlate with the metabolic characteristics of animals. Cold-blooded vertebrates replace missing appendages but warm-blooded ones usually do not. Even if higher vertebrates could replace lost limbs, would this be of selective advantage? Being warm-blooded commits an animal to the maintenance of a high metabolic rate. Such animals are in jeopardy of starving to death much sooner than were their cold-blooded ancestors. The loss of a leg, for example, would probably incapacitate mammals enough to insure their demise. Crippled predators would starve if unable to capture prey. Handicapped herbivores would be vulnerable to predation. Even if limbs could regenerate in mammals, this would probably require at least several months, a period of time that surpasses the survival period without food (not to mention water). Thus, the capacity to regenerate would seem to have been of little selective advantage among warm-blooded vertebrates even if it had evolved somewhere along the line.

Concomitant with the evolution of birds and mammals has been the impressive development of their central nervous systems. This has equipped these animals with mental capacities far in excess of their cold-blooded forebears. Being more intelligent, they are presumably better equipped to avoid the loss of appendages in the first place. Again, such a trend would be expected to counteract any selective pressure in favor of regeneration. This is particularly true with respect to vitally essential appendages because the ability to regenerate is of little use if the animal cannot survive long enough to achieve it.

It follows that body parts that are not vitally essential might have occasionally become favored with regenerative abilities. Loss or damage to such structures would not endanger the life of the animal. Yet if certain appendages were sufficiently important (without being vital) there may well have been some selective advantage in evolving mechanisms for their replacement. This may account for the capacity for certain mammalian structures, such as bat wings, rabbit ears, and deer antlers, to grow back missing parts (Goss 1980). Of these, the case of the deer antlers is the most striking exception to the rule that mammals are not supposed to be able to regenerate.

THE SIGNIFICANCE OF DEER ANTLERS

Antlers (Figure 29.1) are the only mammalian appendages capable of complete regeneration (Brown 1983; Goss 1983). As such, their histogenesis and mechanisms of growth and morphogenesis could have significant implications for our understanding of how tissues and organs in the body repair themselves, and why mammals are so incapable of regrowing entire appendages following their loss.

It is axiomatic that nothing regenerates unless something has been lost. The reason for this is more than semantic. It is that regeneration must always be initiated in a healing epidermal wound. Yet in the first antlers produced by a fawn or yearling, elongation of the pedicle and antler is not preceded by loss of a precursor nor by a lesion in the integument. The initial antler growth in the young deer, therefore, is as unique an exception to the rules of regeneration as is the annual replacement of antlers by adult bucks.

A Fawn's First Antlers

In most deer, the first set of antlers is grown by yearlings. In a few species, however, they are produced more precociously by fawns. Reindeer and caribou calves actually begin to grow their first sets of antlers within a few weeks after birth.

These develop into short spike antlers during the summer months. Reindeer and caribou of both sexes, therefore, go into their first winter equipped with a pair of unbranched antlers. These are of obvious advantage in competing for limited resources with other members of the herd. Infant antlers have also been reported in moose, roe deer, and mule and white-tailed deer. These first antlers, if they are produced at all, are small knobs usually less than a centimeter high. They develop during the deer's first autumn, shedding their velvet in winter. In the following spring, these small bony "buttons" are cast when renewed growth is initiated in the yearling.

It is perhaps significant that all species of the deer known to grow antlers as fawns are native to northern latitudes where it is important for the young animals to become mature enough by fall to survive early and severe winters. The development of precocious antlers in these species may therefore have been a consequence of the early maturation that evolved in animals adapted to the harsh climates of arctic and high northern latitudes. Closer to the equator, where less severe climates prevail,

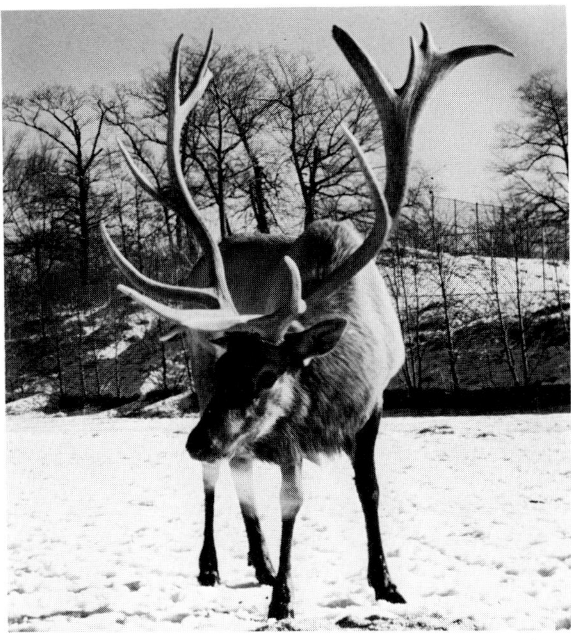

FIGURE 29.1 American elk, or wapiti, with antlers that attain lengths in excess of one meter. These antlers are regenerated in 3-4 months each year.

deer may mature at a more leisurely pace, postponing the onset of antler growth until they become yearlings.

Histogenesis

Before an antler can grow, a pedicle must first develop. The precise histogenesis of antlers per se remains to be determined. The histogenesis of the pedicles from which they develop, however, has been revealed through a series of deletion and transplantation experiments by Hartwig. Working on three-week old roe deer fawns, he transplanted skin from the region of the scalp overlying the prospective antler site to the thigh. No antlers developed from such transplants (Hartwig 1967). When the skin was removed from the antler site of young deer, healing subsequently took place and antler formation proceeded almost normally (Goss, Severinghaus and Free 1964; Hartwig, 1967).

Beneath the skin lies the periosteum of the frontal bone. This periosteum is extra thick in the presumptive antler region. If it is excised, with or without a slice of underlying frontal bone, subsequent development of the pedicle and antler is precluded, even though the overlying scalp may remain intact (Goss, Severinghaus and Free 1964; Hartwig 1968). Indeed, when Hartwig (1968) shifted the location of this antlerogenic periosteum to the center of the forehead, an ectopic antler sprouted from this graft site. In an even more ambitious experiment, Hartwig and Schrudde (1974) transplanted antlerogenic periosteum to the metacarpal bone beneath the skin of the foreleg. Even in this strange location, there developed a pedicle surmounted by a short length of antler. The latter ossified, shed its velvet, and was replaced in succeeding years. These experiments clearly demonstrated that the frontal periosteum is the source of both pedicle and antler, and that it is capable of inducing antlerogenic transformation in skin elsewhere on the body. This induction of velvet from ordinary skin takes place across a considerable thickness of subcutaneous connective tissue and dermis. By what developmental mechanisms such a long-range induction occurs is not known.

The histological sequence of events by which the original pedicle and antler arise bears out the important role of the frontal periosteum as elucidated in experimental investigations. In the young fawn the architecture of the frontal bone in the site from which the antler is destined to develop is little different from that elsewhere in the skull. The layers of bone are parallel to the surface. The only clue that a pedicle and antler will eventually develop is the thickening of the periosteum in this location (Figure 29.2).

When the protuberance begins to grow, the originally parallel layers of bone become disorganized at this site. As the incipient antler pedicle pushes upward, the bone of which it is composed develops as a cancellous knob of ossified tissue. The constituent trabeculae appear to arise from the overlying periosteum. In due course, the exostosis of spongy bone gradually becomes capped with a layer of cartilagenous columns continuous with their more proximal bony counterparts. These also appear to arise from the original periosteum, which is thereby transformed into a perichondrium. The apparent confluence of the bony and cartilaginous trabeculae suggests that they may originate from the same sources. The occasional presence of multinucleate cells (presumed to be chondroclasts) suggests that in the course of subsequent development the original cartilagenous trabeculae may be eroded and replaced by bony ones in an endochondral manner.

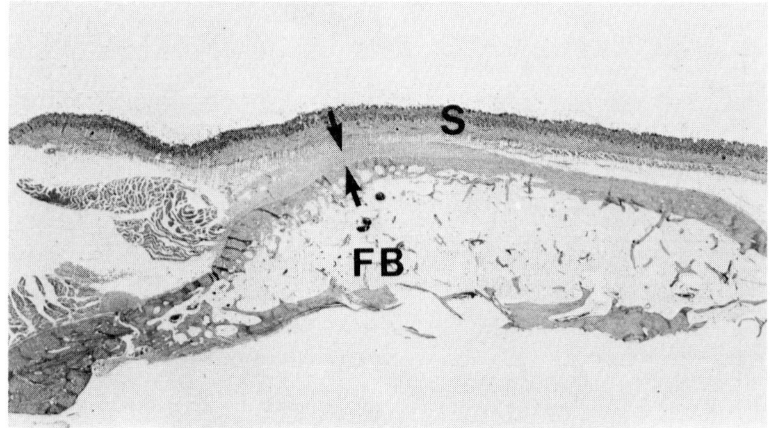

FIGURE 29.2 Sagittal section through the presumptive antler site on the skull of a fallow deer fawn. The periosteum (between arrows) is approximately 1 mm thick where it is sandwiched between the frontal bone (FB) and scalp (S).

The pedicle continues its growth for some months without overt signs of antler formation at its apex. The pedicle-antler transformation is a gradual one. As summer approaches, however, the thick fur on the scalp that covers the developing pedicle becomes progressively sparse at the growing tip, eventually giving rise to the typical antler-type velvet made up of hairs protruding perpendicular to the surface of the skin. By this time, the underlying tissues have acquired the typical zones of growth and differentiation that characterize the growing tips of antlers (Fig. 29.3). The perichondrium beneath the dermis becomes thickened into a highly proliferative cap of tissue made up of seemingly undifferentiated cells. At deeper levels, one recognizes successive stages of chondrogenesis with continued production of vertically oriented cartilaginous trabeculae. These are interspersed with blood vessels that channel the copious blood supply from the apex of the antler to the base of the pedicle. Still deeper in the developing antler are the bony trabeculae that replace their cartilaginous precursors.

If this mechanism by which the first antlers are grown by young deer represents a case of regeneration, it is not associated with a healing epidermal wound as is true in all other known examples of epimorphic regeneration. It will be important, therefore, for future investigators to pay close attention to possible interactions between the proliferating perichondrium

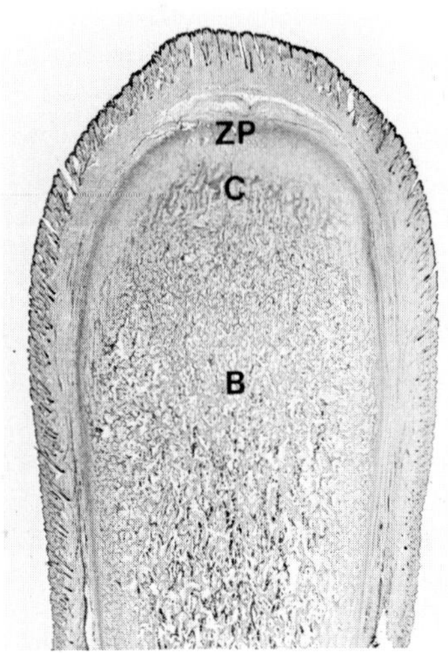

FIGURE 29.3 Sectioned antler pedicle of a fallow yearling as it appears in the spring. The scalp on the apex is beginning to transform into the velvet of the prospective antler. A zone of proliferation (ZP) provides cells that differentiate into cartilaginous columns (C). These are later replaced by bony trabeculae (B) in more proximal regions.

and its overlying integument. By some unknown mechanism, the differentiated skin of the scalp becomes transformed into the velvet of the growing antler. Histochemical analyses of this process are greatly to be desired.

Inasmuch as most antlers remain in velvet for approximately the same length of time, overall rates of elongation depend on how big the antlers are. In any case, their growth profiles describe a typical S-shaped curve, starting out slowly, accelerating to maximal rates in midseason before slowing down as the final dimensions are approached (Goss 1970). At the steepest inflection of the growth curve, the antlers of larger species, such as wapiti or caribou, may grow over 1.5 cm per day. In the extinct Irish elk (Megaceros), with antlers approximately 2 m long, maximal rates of elongation must have been 3-4 cm per day!

In many species of deer, the onset of new growth coincides with the casting of the old antlers. In some deer (for example, reindeer, white-tailed deer) casting may precede renewed growth by up to several months. Thus, these two events would seem not to be causally related. They could each be triggered by similar stimuli, however, such as decreased testosterone secretion.

The casting mechanism itself is presumed to be mediated by the erosion of bone by osteoclasts at the junction between the living bone of the pedicle and the dead bone of the antler. Unfortunately, there exists no detailed description of this process in the literature. Nevertheless, it is a remarkably rapid phenomenon judging from the fact that the antlers that drop off of their own weight were sufficiently firmly attached several days earlier to resist all attempts to break them off manually. Although the detached antler base typically remains free of blood, considerable hemorrhaging occurs from the raw surface of the pedicle. This leads to the formation of a scab beneath which migrating epidermis and associated mesodermal tissues advance in the process of wound healing. Even before the old antlers have been lost, the tumescent pedicle skin around the base of the antler forecasts the regenerative events soon to be initiated.

The healing of a wound in the skin is an indispensable event in the initiation of antler regeneration (as opposed to the development of the original antler in the yearling). For example, if full-thickness skin is sutured over the stump of the pedicle, antler growth can be effectively prevented (Goss 1972). In this respect, antlers resemble epimorphic regeneration in other animals.

It is not known specifically from what tissues the regenerating antler is derived. Histologically, cells from the dermis and periosteum of the pedicle appear to stream into the incipient antler bud. Experiments designed to pinpoint the source of antler-forming cells, however, have not yielded clear-cut evidence. Deletion experiments are plagued by the inconvenient efficiency with which the skin or bone of the pedicle is regenerated following its surgical excision. Antlers persist in developing even after relatively radical deletions of skin and/or bone from the pedicle and the surrounding regions of the head (Jaczewski 1955; Bubenik and Pavlansky 1956; Goss 1961). The antler-forming territory would seem to be widely distributed in and around the pedicle region.

Transplantation experiments have been equally inconclusive. If skin is grafted from the pedicle or velvet antler to other parts of the body, such as the scalp or ears, it may survive indefinitely but does not give rise to antler tissues _per se_ in such ectopic locations. On the other hand, when ear skin is grafted in place of pedicle skin, regeneration occurs even though ear skin is the only source of epidermis available (Goss 1964). Finally, there have been a few successful attempts to graft growing antler buds to other regions of the head (Jaczewski 1956a, b, 1958, 1961; Pavlansky and Bubenik 1960). Such transplants may give rise to typical antler appendages that mature and are replaced in synchrony with the normal ones. The implications are that antler cells _per se_ may survive from year to year as a source of renewed growth. Which cells they are, however, is not known.

The antler bud that rounds up from the healed pedicle is composed of seemingly undifferentiated cells in a high state of proliferation. These cells appear to have much in common with fibroblasts judging from the quantity of collagen fibers that are in association with them. Early in the process of bud formation, the epidermal configuration at the apex exhibits long tongues of epidermal cells protruding deeply into the underlying mesodermal tissues (Figure 29.4). This is reminiscent of the apical epidermal caps and ridges identified by embryologists in the limb and wing buds of developing embryos or the blastemas of regenerating amphibian appendages. Whatever its significance, it is a transient phenomenon that disappears once the developing antler starts to elongate and produce branches.

The velvet that enveloped the growing antler is a unique kind of skin because of its capacity to differentiate hair follicles de novo. These make their appearance in the growing tip, forming as downgrowths of epidermal cells that organize themselves into rudimentary hair follicles. Such follicles differentiate papillae at their lower ends, and sebaceous glands from their shafts. The hairs of the velvet differ from those elsewhere on the body in that they lack arrector pili muscles, the ones normally responsible for adjusting the angle of the hair where it protrudes from the skin. The pelage of the antler velvet stands out at right angles from the surface of the skin. In some species, during the early rapid phase of antler growth, one can detect longitudinal stripes in the velvet that resemble the grain in wood (Figure 29.5). The significance and origin of these "contour lines" has not been investigated.

Immediately beneath the epidermis on the end of the growing antler there is a zone of hyperplastic undifferentiated cells more or less continuous with the perichondrium and periosteum along the sides of the antler. This hyperplastic perichondrium is comparable to the blastema of other regenerating appendages. It is laced with collagen fibers that become arranged both circumferentially and longitudinally in peripheral regions (Speer 1983). As the antler increases in length by the addition of new cells in the growth zone, chondrogenesis can be observed in slightly more proximal (and older) regions (Banks and Newbrey 1983). The resulting cartilage becomes organized into vertically oriented columns interspersed with numerous vascular channels that drain blood from the growing tip. It is this cartilaginous zone that endows the velvet antler with the flexible and rubbery consistency typical of apical regions.

Farther down, however, calcification of the cartilage occurs presumably as an antecedent to its eventual erosion by chondro-

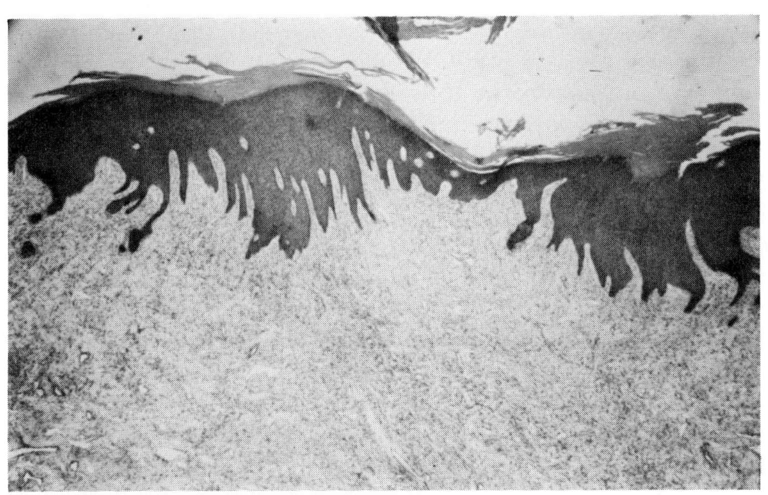

FIGURE 29.4 Vertical section through apex of an antler bud (sika deer), illustrating the conspicuous tongues of epidermis that extend down into the underlying mesoderm.

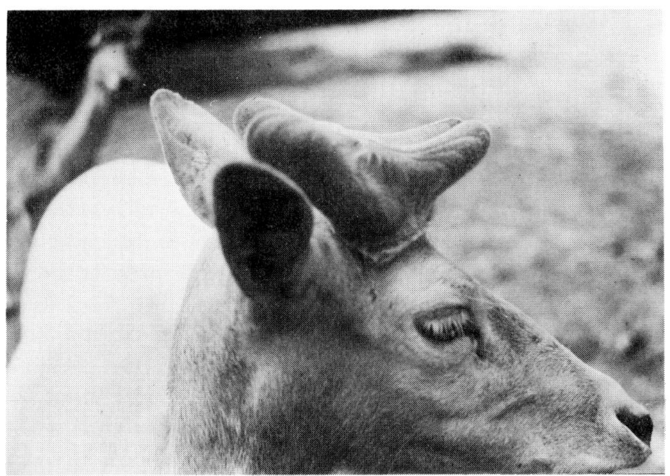

FIGURE 29.5 Photograph of a fallow deer with rapidly growing antlers. The striped pattern visible in the velvet pelage may represent growth increments in the elongating antlers.

clasts and replacement by bone. The zone of calcified cartilage, or primary spongiosa, gradually gives way to the secondary spongiosa made up of bony trabeculae. Remnants of cartilaginous matrix may persist in the innermost areas of these trabeculae, but this tends to disappear as ossification progresses. In the more proximal parts of the growing antler, the spongy bone becomes increasingly solid as osteoblasts deposit new layers of mineralized matrix on the original trabeculae, thereby reducing the dimensions of the intervening vascular spaces. It is this curtailment of the vasculature that eventually contributes to the demise of the mature antler and shedding of its velvet. Maturation of the antler, which occurs typically in the late summer as the day lengths decrease, is promoted by increasingly high levels of testosterone secreted in anticipation of the forthcoming reproductive season.

The Growth of Horns

In general, it is worth noting that deer antlers, in contrast to the horns of other ungulates, originate as an apophysis, that is, a direct outgrowth from the skull. Horns, on the other hand, arise as a separate center of ossification in the subcutaneous connective tissue, a structure more akin to an epiphysis. This *os cornu* subsequently fuses to the underlying skull while growing out into the horn core enveloped in cornified epidermis.

Experiments have identified another important difference between horns and antlers. As described above, the first pedicles and antlers grown by young deer originate in the periosteum of the frontal bone. The overlying skin is not necessarily specific for antler formation. Horns, on the other hand, originate in the integument. If this is removed no horn develops (Dove 1935), though the underlying periosteum may remain intact. If presumptive horn skin is grafted elsewhere, correspondingly ectopic horns, including the bone cores, differentiate.

Horns and antlers, therefore, are developmentally and phylogenetically very different structures notwithstanding the similar uses to which they are put. They are both hard cephalic appendages adapted for combat. Their hardness derives either from the epidermis as in horns, or the internal bone as in antlers. Needless to say, horns do not branch while antlers usually do. (Even in the pronghorn antelope, the prongs are only superficial configurations of the horn sheath. The underlying bony core remains tapered and unbranched.) Finally, the most obvious difference between horns and antlers is the fact that the latter are replaced annually while the former persist throughout the animal's life. (Although the pronghorn antelope sheds and replaces its horn sheath each year, the bone core and its enveloping layer of skin remain intact as a source from which the new sheath differentiates each year.)

Scars Versus Blastemas

The relationship between antler growth and the phenomenon of regeneration in lower vertebrates is interesting from the point of view of how these processes may have evolved. Although mammals are not supposed to be able to regenerate missing appendages, the annual replacement of antlers is an interesting exception to this rule. It is believed that antler regeneration is made possible by the special way in which the skin heals the wound on the end of the pedicle. Elsewhere on the body, one finds that in addition to wound contraction and epidermal migration there differentiates a thick scar of collagenous fibers that represents the regenerated dermis. This scar constitutes an effective barrier to regeneration. It could be evidence that higher vertebrates may have sacrificed the capacity for regeneration in favor of more efficient and complete integumental wound healing. Such a trade-off would be of obvious advantage to warm-blooded animals whose tissues are so conducive to the culture of bacteria.

How, then, does one account for antler regeneration? First of all, there is little or no wound contraction on the end of the pedicle when antler regeneration is initiated. Healing of the pedicle is achieved almost exclusively by epidermal migration. Secondly, the dermal tissues of the pedicle skin appear to give rise to the mass of undifferentiated and hyperplastic cells of which the antler bud is composed. Instead of giving rise to a scar on the end of the pedicle, they become deflected in the direction of blastema formation. Thus, the very tissues that elsewhere on the body are responsible for scar formation may be the ones that give rise to the new outgrowth. In this perspective, the mesodermal components of the antler may be an exaggerated version of what would otherwise have been a scar.

It was concluded earlier that epimorphic regeneration is in general qualitatively different from tissue repair. This was based on the fact that the differences between these two processes outnumber their similarities. The most basic difference is the involvement of wound epidermis and blastema formation in epimorphic regeneration. A blastema, like the appendage it replaces, is by definition enveloped in epidermis. The only tissue with which epidermis is otherwise in contact is the dermis. When dermis undergoes tissue repair, it is normally subjacent to epidermis. Regenerating dermis, therefore, resembles a regenerating blastema in that both are covered by wound epidermis. Yet dermis typically completes its continuity only with a scar, not a blastema. This is why some amputated appendages do not regenerate and others do. In the former, the stump is sealed with scar tissue instead of producing a regeneratively competent blastema. Although blastemas are ordinarily derived from a variety of stump tissues, there seems little reason why dermis alone could not give rise to a blastema on the end of a stump, especially if it were the chief source of cells available. Such may be the case in antler regeneration.

The antler pedicle consists of a solid core of bone surrounded by layers of periosteum, dermis, and epidermis. The source of the cells that make up the antler bud has not been precisely identified, but the dermis is almost certainly the major contributor. As such, one wonders why its cells congregate into a blastema instead of a scar over the end of the pedicle. If the regenerating antler is actually an extension of dermal scar formation, then it lies at the interface between tissue repair and epimorphic regeneration. The mechanism by which deer antlers regrow each year focuses attention on the problem of scars versus blastemas as the key to understanding how the regrowth of tissues and of appendages relate to each other. They are quite different processes except in the case of one tissue, the dermis. When the dermis repairs itself it is in a position to permit or inhibit epimorphic regeneration. Therein lies the secret of why mammalian appendages do not normally regenerate. Until we learn why scars are sometimes supplanted by blastemas, the answer is not likely to be forthcoming.

REFERENCES

Banks, WJ, and JW Newbrey. 1983. Antler development as a unique modification of mammalian endochondral ossification. In Antler Development in Cervidae, edited by Robert D. Brown, pp. 279-306. Kingsville, Texas: Caesar Kleberg Wildlife Research Institute.

Brown, RD (ed). 1983. Antler Development in Cervidae. Kingsville, Texas: Caesar Kelberg Wildlife Research Institute.

Bubenik, A, and R Pavlansky. 1956. Von welchem gewebe geht der eigentliche reitz zur geweihentwicklung aus? II. Mitteilung: Operative eingriffe auf den rosenstöcken der rehböcke, Capreolus capreolus (Linné, 1758). Saugetierk. Mitt. 4:97-103.

Dove, WF. 1935. The physiology of horn growth: A study of the morphogenesis, the interaction of tissues, and the evolutionary processes of a Mendelian recessive character by means of transplantation of tissues. J. Exp. Zool. 69: 347-406.

Goss, RJ. 1961. Experimental investigations of morphogenesis in the growing antler. J. Embryol. Exp. Morph. 9:342-354.

Goss, RJ. 1964. The role of skin in antler regeneration. In Advances in Biology of Skin. Wound Healing, edited by W. Montagna and R. E. Billingham, Vol. 5, pp. 194-207. New York: Pergamon Press.

Goss, RJ, CW Severinghaus, and S Free. 1964. Tissue relationships in the development of pedicles and antlers in the Virginia deer. J. Mammal. 45:61-68.

Goss, RJ. 1969. Principles of Regeneration. New York: Academic Press.

Goss, RJ. 1970. Problems of antlerogenesis. Clin. Orthopaed. Rel. Res. 69:227-238.

Goss, RJ. 1972. Wound healing and antler regeneration. In Epidermal Wound Healing, edited by H. I. Maibach and D. T. Rovee, pp. 219-228. Chicago: Year Book Med. Publ.

Goss, RJ. 1978. The Physiology of Growth. New York: Academic Press.

Goss, RJ. 1980. Prospects for regeneration in man. Clin. Orthopaed. Rel. Res. 151:270-282.

Goss, RJ. 1983. Deer Antlers: Regeneration, Function, and Evolution. New York: Academic Press.

Hartwig, H. 1967. Experimentelle Untersuchungen zur Entwicklungsphysiologie der Stangenbildung beim Reh (Capreolus c. capreolus L. 1758). Roux Arch. f. Entwmech., 158:358-384.

Hartwig, H. 1968. Verhinderung der Rosenstock und Stangenbildung beim Reh, Capreolus capreolus, durch Periostausschaltung. Zool. Garten 35:252-255.

Hartwig, H, and J Schrudde. 1974. Experimentelle Untersuchungen zur Bildung der primären Stirnauswuchse beim Reh (Capreolus capreolus L.). Z. Jagdwiss. 20:1-13.

Jaczewski, Z. 1955. Regeneration of antlers in red deer, Cervus elaphus L. Bull. Acad. Polon. Sci., Ser. 2, 3:273-278.

Jaczewski, Z. 1956a. Free transplantation of antler in red deer (Cervus elaphus L.). Bull. Acad. Polon. Sci., Ser. 2, 4:107-110.

Jaczewski, Z. 1956b. Further observations on transplantation of antler in red deer (Cervus elaphus L.). Bull. Acad. Polon. Sci., Ser. 2, 4:289-291.

Jaczewski, Z. 1958. Free transplantation and regeneration of antlers in fallow deer [Cervus Dama (L.)]. Bull. Acad. Polon. Sci. 6:179-182.

Jaczewski, Z. 1961. Observations on the regeneration and transplantation of antlers in deer Cervidae. Folia Biol. 9: 47-99.

McMinn, RMH. 1969. Tissue Repair. New York: Academic Press.

Pavlansky, R, and A Bubenik. 1960. Von welchem Gewebe geht der eigentliche Reiz zur Geweihentwicklung aus? IV. Mitteilung: Versuch mit Auto- und Homotransplantation des Geweihzapfens. Saugetierk. Mitt. 8:32-37.

Speer, DP. 1983. The collagenous architecture of antler velvet. In Antler Development in Cervidae, edited by Robert D. Brown, pp. 273-278. Kingsville, Texas: Caesar Kleberg Wildlife Research Institute.

Wallace, H. 1981. Vertebrate Limb Regeneration. New York: John Wiley & Sons.

30
Measurement of Human Repair: An Overview

William H. Goodson, Thomas K. Hunt, Finn Gottrup, Kent Jonsson, Ning Chang, Richard Firmin and Judith M. West

INTRODUCTION

Most advances in the understanding of wound healing have been based upon animal research. There are, however, pressing reasons to develop methods to study healing in human subjects. First, some clinical situations are difficult if not impossible to reconstruct in animal models, and therefore must be studied in human subjects. Second, information gained in the laboratory should ultimately be applied to patient care.

For twelve years the Wound Healing Laboratory at University of California, San Francisco, has been studying various aspects of the repair process in human subjects. These studies developed as an extension of the animal work by Hunt[1] who found the oxygen tension in subcutaneous wounds in the rabbit was lower than simultaneous arterial tension. Subsequently, Silver et al.[2] showed that wound tissue oxygen tension is high near arterioles and capillaries, and that the tissue oxygen tension rapidly decreases in proportion to the distance from the nearest blood vessel. Since the leading edge of new tissue growing into a wound is avascular, it is relatively far from the nearest capillary; therefore, the oxygen tension in this area is significantly lower than arterial oxygen tension.

These and other animal observations demonstrated that the net oxygen tension in the central portion of a wound is a complex function, dependent on many things: 1) arterial oxygen tension or pO_2—if there is an increase in the oxygen tension of arterial blood there will be a concurrent increase in the oxygen tension, and vice versa; 2) blood flow—if there is a decrease in blood flow in the area of the wound, there will be a decrease in wound oxygen tension because less oxygen is brought to the area of the wound; 3) wound module growth—as wound cells grow between the point of measurement and the nearest capillary, there will be increased consumption of oxygen by these cells and therefore a decrease in the amount of oxygen which reaches the point of measurement.

In 1972, Niinikoski and Hunt[3] first measured oxygen tension in small, subcutaneous wounds in humans. The study wound was made in a standardized fashion in a standard location, usually the upper arm. Therefore, the results were influenced primarily by changes in the subject, rather than changes in the technique.

In 1979, Goodson et al.[4] demonstrated that oxygen tension in this small, standardized arm wound varies in the same manner as oxygen tension in an operative incision in the same patient. Oxygen tension in the operative incision is usually slightly lower than in the needle wound in the arm; there is more disruption of the local vasculature by the trauma of the major surgical procedure than the small needle wound. Because the oxygen tension in the main operative incision and that in the arm wound change in tandem, a tissue oxygen monitor placed in the arm wound also monitors the efficiency of oxygen delivery to the operative incision.

A wound with adequate oxygen supply is assumed to be adequately perfused by blood, which brings the oxygen to the wound. Tissue oxygen tension therefore becomes a nearly direct measurement of tissue perfusion. Our clinical studies found that adequate tissue perfusion is not guaranteed by maintenance of adequate blood pressure and/or urine output.[5] The direct measurement or tissue oxygen perfusion provides an invaluable physiologic endpoint, that is, adequate wound perfusion, to guide fluid replacement, rather than the common standard of maintaining "normal" pressure in the vascular system or "normal" loss of fluid through the kidneys.

Since 1978, we have also evaluated hydroxyproline accumulation in similar needle wounds in the upper arms of human volunteers. Previous work by Viljanto[6] demonstrated that cellular material and trace amounts of collagen could be collected in small tubes left in operative wounds. Accumulation of connective tissue in subcutaneous sponges and cylinders had already been shown to be proportional to wound tensile strength.[7] We used a strong, porous material, expanded polytetrafluoroethylene (PTFE), and found that reproducible amounts of hydroxyproline could be retrieved from small, standardized arm wounds. The porous catheter placed in the upper extremity provided, for the first time, a minimally invasive method of studying human wound healing. It allowed participation by subjects who were not undergoing operative procedures and who would otherwise decline more traditional methods such as implanted wound cylinders or experimental disruption of incised wounds.

We evaluated this method by demonstrating a lower accumulation of hydroxyproline in patients who had had major illness before or at the time of surgery.[8] This is similar to results in animal wounds in cases of malnutrition, severe systemic illness or impeded healing. Subsequently, we found that patients on chronic hemodialysis accumulate hydroxyproline at a slower rate than nonuremic, normal controls.[9] After adrenalectomy for Cushing's disease, patients accumulate less hydroxyproline than those undergoing adrenalectomy for other reasons. A preliminary study of juvenile-type diabetics compared to normal controls showed that the diabetics do not have decreased hydroxyproline accumulation. At first, we were surprised by this result, but reappraisal of previous animal experimental data show that this result is actually quite predictable.

All of the studies of tissue oxygen tension and the studies of wound hydroxyproline accumulation have been carried out in the subcutaneous tissue. This is particularly appropriate because the subcutaneous tissue is where healing most frequently fails. If there is wound infection, usually the skin and fascia heal initially and the skin must be reopened to drain the subcutaneous area. If a skin defect must close by second intention, it is the subcutaneous tissue which must give rise to the wound module.

Studies such as these offer promise for a clearer understanding of healing problems in human subjects and a better understanding of ways to monitor postoperative patients.

MEASUREMENT OF TISSUE OXYGEN TENSION

Tissue oxygen tension is measured with a Silastic® catheter placed in a small, upper arm needle wound. The catheter is oxygen-permeable; the oxygen inside the catheter rapidly equilibrates with the surrounding tissue by diffusion of O_2. The initial measurements of tissue oxygen tension in humans were obtained by placing saline in the catheter and allowing the O_2 of the saline to equilibrate with that of the subcutaneous tissue and measuring the resulting pO_2 of the saline. This is an indirect measurement.

We started with a continuous flow method in which saline, which had been equilibrated with nitrogen to lower its pO_2, was passed through the subcutaneous catheter, collected in a nylon (oxygen-impermeable) tube, and passed directly to a Radiometer Copenhagen blood gas machine. It was quickly learned that a discontinuous flow could also be used.[10] Most of the early studies were conducted by collecting the effluent from the tissue oxygen catheter in sealed glass tubes which were then carried back to the laboratory for measurement.

Recently, Gottrup et al.[11] developed a technique to place a miniature electrode within a Silastic® catheter. This provides a direct measurement of subcutaneous wound tissue oxygen tension. Medical grade Silastic® tubing is attached at one end to a modified 19 g spinal needle and fitted at the other end to a catheter which fits a standard syringe. The needle is passed into the skin, through the subcutaneous tissue for a distance of 5 cm, and brought out through the skin again. This threads the catheter through the subcutaneous tissue. The catheter is secured in place with an adhesive plastic covering. Oxygen measurement is obtained by placing a reference, silver-silver chloride electrode in one end of the catheter and a miniature platinum electrode in the other. The catheter must be flushed at intervals with an electrolyte solution to maintain a contact between the two points. A picoammeter measures "oxygen" as the current between the two electrodes when a fixed potential is applied across them. Altogether, these methods have been used in more than 200 persons. There have been no infections and no significant complications.

The observed tissue oxygen tension while a patient is breathing room air or supplemental oxygen is a function of the length of the time that the catheter has been in place. If it has been in place for a long time, the measured oxygen tension in the central portion of the wound will be decreased. Cells collect around the catheter in the small needle wound. These cells consume oxygen. As this wound heals, more cells accumulate between the catheter and the nearest capillary; they consume oxygen and less oxygen reaches the catheter to be measured. Thus, normal healing around the catheter explains the gradual fall in observed oxygen tension over five to seven days after catheter insertion. Other factors also influence tissue oxygen. When tissue perfusion is compromised, the wound tissue oxygen tension decreases. There is less oxygen brought by blood flow; thus, patients who are hypoperfused have a lower tissue oxygen tension than would be expected.

In a large number of simultaneous wound oxygen tension and arterial oxygen tension measurements we found that there was a "normal" relationship between tissue and arterial oxygen.[5] This normal relationship defines a curve (Figure 30.1) and

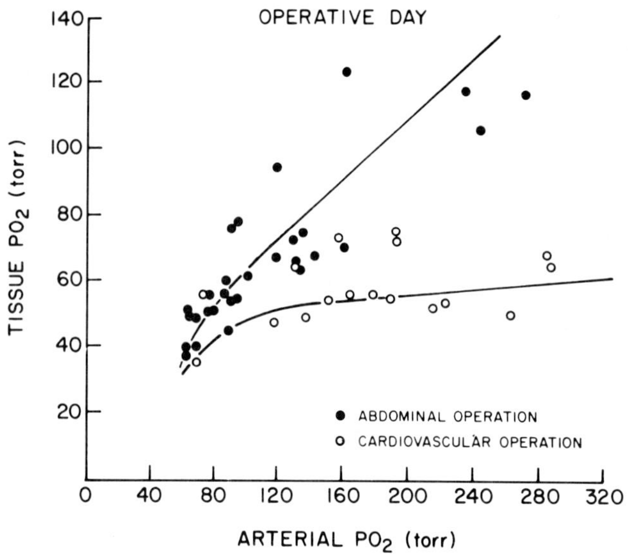

FIGURE 30.1

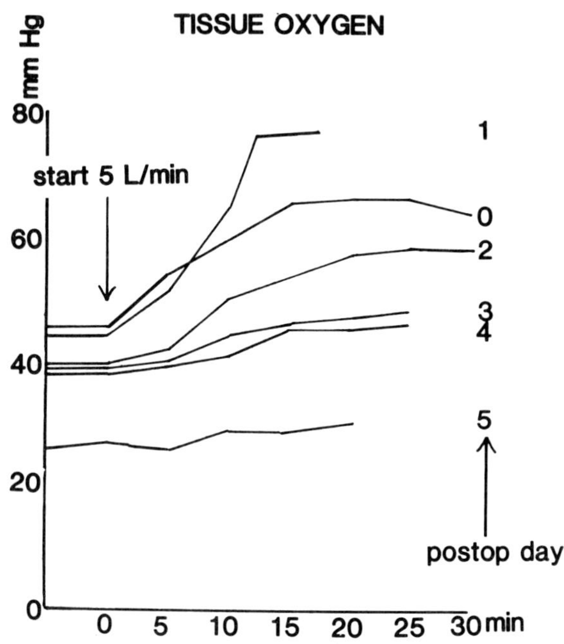

FIGURE 30.2

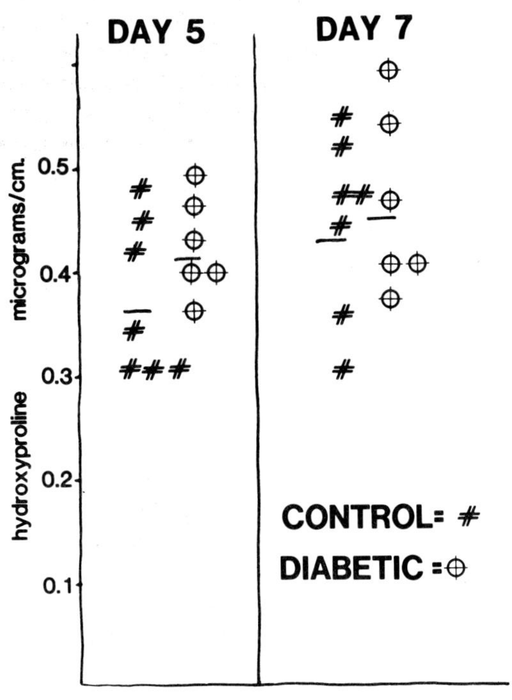

FIGURE 30.3

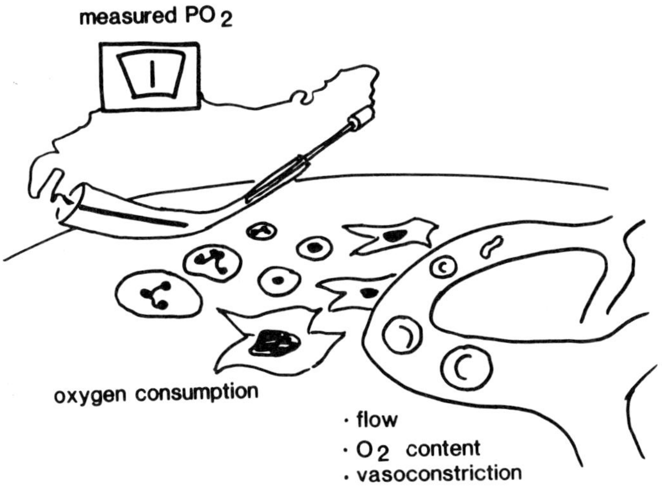

FIGURE 30.4

provides the basis of a test of tissue perfusion, as well as of oxygen delivery. If tissue oxygen tension is low, we measure arterial pO_2. We then plot the point corresponding to the measured tissue and arterial oxygen tension and compare it to the normal curve. If the point is on the line and both tissue and arterial oxygen are low, then appropriate therapy is initiated to improve pulmonary function to increase arterial oxygen. If, however, the point is below the "normal" curve, we know there is enough oxygen in the blood, but it is not reaching the wound tissue. This is a problem of perfusion which frequently responds to supplemental intravenous fluid. We have studied several patients who had lower tissue oxygen tension than expected. A fluid infusion, most frequently 500 ml normal saline, increased tissue oxygen tension in most of these.[12]

Diuretics given in doses sufficient to cause significant diuresis have been observed to decrease tissue oxygen tension by decreasing peripheral vascular volume. Similar studies have shown that during partial exchange transfusions, sickle cell patients experience a marked reduction in tissue oxygen delivery at the time a unit of blood is removed to begin the exchange.

Operative stress decreases tissue oxygen tension, presumably an effect of the catecholamines which circulate at a high level in the immediate postoperative period. Catecholamines cause vasoconstriction and reduce subcutaneous blood flow. Tissue oxygen tension is even more depressed in patients who have been on cardiopulmonary bypass. They are particularly refractory to efforts to increase tissue oxygen tension by increasing systemic arterial oxygen tension, probably because of their very high catecholamine levels.[5]

Continuous direct measurement of tissue oxygen tension allows not only measurement of an absolute number, but also observation of the rate at which this number (tissue oxygen) increases when the patient switches to breathing supplemental oxygen (5 L/min) by face mask. We have observed that the rate or increase is also a function of the length of time the catheter has been in place. The longer it has been in place, the more slowly the oxygen tension will rise (Figure 30.2). Our current hypothesis is that this reflects the increased consumption, and possibly also the increased oxygen debt, experienced by cells located between the last capillary and the tissue oxygen tonometer. These cells will consume the surplus oxygen for a longer time before increased oxygen is measured within the catheter.

STUDIES OF HYDROXYPROLINE ACCUMULATION IN HUMAN WOUNDS

We used expanded PTFE catheters, 1 mm in diameter and 7 cm in length. The material is handled with gloves to avoid surface contamination and steam-autoclaved. A large needle-with-trochar is passed into the subcutaneous tissue of the upper arm, through the subcutaneous tissue for 7 cm, and back out through the skin. The trochar is removed and the catheter inserted into the end opposite the handle of the needle. The PTFE tubing is very soft and requires a stylette to assist in insertion. Once the tubing has been placed in the needle, the end of the tubing is held and the needle withdrawn in the opposite direction. The tubing is thus left in the subcutaneous space. It is secured in place with a nylon stitch. The exposed end is covered with antiseptic ointment and a Bandaid® dressing. The tubing is removed a specified number of days later. We have left catheters in hospitalized patients for up to eight days, but not for longer than seven in ambulating, healthy persons. Even after only seven days several catheters have been difficult to remove, although none have become permanently stuck.

At the time of removal 0.5 cm of the tubing is separated and placed immediately into formalin fixative for histological study. The length of the remainder is measured and the tubing frozen at 4°C until analysis. For analysis, the catheter is washed with water, dried by lyophilization, and hydrolyzed for 18 hr in 6 N HCl at 118°C. An aliquot of the hydrolysate is dried in vacuum over sodium hydroxide, and then dissolved in water. Hydroxyproline is measured using an autoanalyzer. Results are expressed as micrograms of hydroxyproline per centimeter of tubing.

There is a random accumulation of hydroxyproline in the first three or four days after catheter insertion. During this time some values are very high and some very low, and the standard deviation of all groups evaluated thus far has been quite large. Beginning on the fifth day, data are much more predictable, and the standard deviation has consistently been less than 30% of the mean. The mark of good healing, according to this test, has been a satisfactory accumulation of hydroxyproline on the fifth day and an increase between the fifth and seventh days. We now study all subjects with two catheters which are removed at five and seven days, respectively.

Hydroxyproline is decreased in patients who have severe preoperative pathology. Our initial studies focused on patients with severe malnutrition, extensive metastatic carcinoma, severe

Cushing's disease, and other causes of major preoperative debility.[8] The method has also been useful for evaluating several other clinical problems which could not readily be interpreted on the basis of laboratory studies.

There has been a strong clinical impression that uremic patients heal poorly. Laboratory animals, made uremic by partial nephrectomy or use of toxic substances, have decreased healing. However, it was observed that such animals also lose weight. For this reason, it was postulated that the effect of the uremia was on appetite, and that therefore weight loss was the cause of the poor healing.[13] We studied uremic patients who were on chronic hemodialysis.[9] All had had stable weight for several months prior to the study, and none were obese. There was less hydroxyproline accumulation in these persons compared to normal, nonoperated controls on days three, five and seven. These results show that uremic patients do have decreased subcutaneous healing and help to clarify a question which could not be resolved with animal experiments.

The most significant question, and that for which this method was originally developed, concerns wound healing in diabetic patients. There is a very strong impression that diabetic patients have difficulty with healing, but little clinical data to support it. Numerous laboratory studies have shown that there is deficient healing in diabetic animals. We repeated these studies in rats and then demonstrated that insulin has a crucial role only in the early phases of healing. We interpreted this to mean that insulin was most necessary in the inflammatory and cell-proliferative phases of healing.[14] Seifter et al.[15] confirmed our hypotheses when they showed that supplementation of the inflammatory response by vitamin A also improved healing in diabetic rats.[13] It was, however, still difficult to relate these studies to patient care.

We recently studied a preliminary group of six juvenile-type diabetics and compared them to seven nondiabetic controls. In the respective groups, mean ages were 29 and 31, triceps skinfold thickness 12 and 12 mm, suprailiac skinfold thickness 20 and 23 mm, percent overweight 1.6 and zero, and, for the diabetic group, hemoglobin AIC 8.3% (range 6.7-13.1%, normal up to 6.9%). The results of this study, instead of showing a defect in the diabetic groups, showed a slightly higher hydroxyproline accumulation for them on day five (0.41 ± 0.03 μg/cm, vs. 0.36 ± 0.06 μg/cm), and very similar values for both groups on day seven (0.45 ± 0.07, vs. 0.43 ± 0.07 μg/cm). Day 7 values exceeded day 5 values in both groups. According to these data, well-controlled diabetics would have the same potential healing capacity in terms of wound hydroxyproline accumulation as nondiabetic controls.

At first this would seem to contradict all the previous experimental data, which have consistently shown deficient healing in diabetic animals. However, all previous studies observed that once-a-day insulin restored healing in diabetic animals, but made no significant effort to control diabetes more closely. In contrast, all of the patients in this series took twice-a-day (morning and evening) insulin. All monitored their own urine glucose at home, and two monitored their own blood glucose. Thus, these subjects were very well-controlled and as such are comparable to insulin-treated animals, not to the untreated group. Like animals who healed well with insulin replacement, diabetics should be expected to have normal subcutaneous healing ability when their disease is closely controlled.

These data suggest that healing in diabetic patients is not limited by factors such as microvascular disease. Diabetics do have more wound problems, but these problems are likely to be due to the known increased risk of infection, the results of severe lack of control precipitated by injury, infection or other illness, or abuse of tissue made anesthesic by neuropathy and macrovascular disease.[16]

SUMMARY

We have performed extensive studies of wound healing in humans, evaluating tissue perfusion and hydroxyproline accumulation in standardized, small, subcutaneous needle wounds in the upper arm. Studies of oxygen tension in these wounds suggested new methods of monitoring wound perfusion and, indeed, the vascular volume and circulatory status of the entire patient. Studies of hydroxyproline accumulation have given new insight into the healing defect found in persons on chronic hemodialysis and suggest that well-controlled diabetics may not have a healing defect.

NOTES

1. Hunt TK. A new method of determining tissue oxygen tension. Lancet 2:1370, 1964.

2. Silver IA. The physiology of wound healing. In Hunt TK (ed). Wound Healing and Wound Infection: Theory and Surgical Practice, pp. 11-31. New York: Appleton-Century-Crofts, 1980.

3. Niinikoski J, Hunt TK. Measurement of wound oxygen with implanted Silastic® tube. Surgery 71:22, 1972.

4. Goodson WH III, Andrews WJ, Thakral KK, Hunt TK. Wound oxygen tension in large vs. small wounds in man. Surg Forum 30:92, 1979.

5. Chang N, Goodson WH III, Gottrup F, Hunt TK. Direct measurement of wound and tissue oxygen tension in postoperative patients. Ann Surg 197:470, 1983.

6. Viljanto J. Wound healing in children as assessed by the Cellstic method. J Ped Surg 11:43, 1976.

7. Viljanto J. Biochemical basis of tensile strength in wound healing: An experimental study with viscose cellulose sponges in rats. Acta Clin Scand (suppl) 333:1, 1964.

8. Goodson WH III, Hunt TK. Development of a new miniature method for the study of wound healing in human subjects. J Surg Res 33:394, 1982.

9. Goodson WH III, Lindenfeld SM, Omachi R, Hunt TK. Chronic uremia does cause poor healing. Surg Forum 33:54, 1982.

10. Kivissari J, Niinikoski J. Use of Silastic® tube and capillary sampling technic in the measurement of tissue pO_2 and pCO_2. Am J Surg 125:623, 1973.

11. Gottrup F, Firmin R, Chang N, Goodson WH III, Hunt TK. Continuous direct tissue oxygen tension measurement by a new method using an implantable Silastic® tonometer and oxygen polarography. Am J Surg (in press), 1983.

12. Chang N, Goodson WH III, Gottrup F, Hunt TK. Direct measurement of tissue oxygen in postoperative patients. Surg Forum 33:52, 1982.

13. Kursh ED, Shaffer J, Klein L, Persky L. Role of nutrition in wound healing in uremia. Surg Forum 28:104-106, 1977.

14. Goodson WH III, Hunt TK. Studies of wound healing in experimental diabetes mellitus. J Surg Res 22:221, 1977.

15. Seifter E, Rettura G, Padawes J, Stratford F, et al. Impaired wound healing in streptozotocin diabetes, prevention by supplemental vitamin A. Ann Surg 194:42, 1981.

16. Goodson WH III, Hunt TK. Wound healing and the diabetic patient. Surg Gynec Obstet 149:600, 1978.

31
The Inhibition of Scar After Tendon and Nerve Injury

F. William Bora, Jr., and Anthony Unger

INTRODUCTION

The hand is a complex, mobile organ in which tendons and other structures must glide to perform the coordinate movements required for skilled work. Most injuries to the flexor tendons of the hand result in peritendinous scars which limit tendon gliding. For this reason, surgical results are "satisfactory" in only about 50% of patients who have lacerations of the flexor tendons in the digital sheaths, and less than 1% of these patients recover normal function. Treatment of injuries to peripheral nerves is also disappointing. In one study, only 13% of patients with a nerve laceration recovered completely normal function and essentially none recovered normal sensation.[1]

Injuries of tendons and nerves are among the most common injuries among workmen, and the economic consequences of such injuries are costly. For example, injuries of the hand and fingers were the most common injuries reported by the Department of Labor of Pennsylvania in August 1975; they accounted for 2,522 of the 11,175 injuries that month.[2] The economic consequences of such injuries is reflected in the fact that many people who sustain these hand injuries are out of work for at least 50 days. In 1969, a total of 200,000 work days were lost because of hand injuries to workers in the state of Pennsylvania.[3] Comparable data for the state of New York indicate that in one year (1968) 33,887 injuries of the hand were reported, and the payments made for Workers' Compensation (exclusive of the cost of medical care) were $29 million.[4]

Although a variety of problems exist in the treatment of patients with injuries and diseases of the hand, a major problem compromising results is the formation of excessive amounts of scar tissue. It seems clear that, in order to improve the results obtained in the surgical management of injuries to tendons and nerves, we will need more information about the biochemical and cellular reactions which occur in and around these tissues following injury. Since scar tissue consists almost entirely of collagen, we will especially need to know more about collagen synthesis in these situations.

As described below, we have data showing that the use of proline analogs may be of great benefit because they reduce scar formation following tendon and nerve injury. The development of techniques to administer proline analogs locally will probably focus this effect on the local area of injury without systemic effects and have direct application to clinical situations. It should also be noted, however, that if proline analogs are beneficial in the clinical management of such injuries, they may prove to be useful in other clinical situations such as strictures of the esophagus or ureters, adhesions of the intestine, keloids, arachnoiditis and burn contractures.

The inhibition of collagen synthesis by proline analogs involves a highly unusual principle. We have now extensively confirmed the original observations indicating that the several analogs we have studied do not alter collagen synthesis by a direct action as drugs or anti-metabolites.[5-11] Instead, their effect on the process occurs after the analogs are incorporated into the polypeptide chains of collagen in the positions normally occupied by either proline or hydroxyproline. The presence of the proline analogs in the newly synthesized polypeptide chains prevents the chains from folding into the normal triple-helical structure of collagen.[12-15] Because the chains do not fold into a triple helix, they cannot be used for the assembly of collagen fibers and they remain as totally non-functional polypeptide chains.

The unusual mechanism by which proline analogs alter collagen synthesis in itself provides strong presumptive evidence that the effects on collagen might be highly specific, even though our results, as well as earlier observations by other laboratories clearly demonstrate that the analogs are incorporated into all proteins in place of proline.[16,17] Two general considerations here are pertinent:

(1) Collagen is unusual among proteins in that it is large and contains a large amount of proline and hydroxyproline.[18-21] On this basis alone, one can say that, if a proline analog were administered in a dose sufficient to replace 0.5% of the proline sites in newly synthesized proteins, only one hemoglobin polypeptide chain out of 25 would on the average contain a residue of analog but essentially all the collagen polypeptide chains would contain at least one residue of analog.

(2) Proline is generally regarded as a "helix-breaker" in terms of the alpha-helix found in most globular proteins and it is found only[22-24] in non-helical sequences or at the C-terminal end of such sequences. Therefore, if a proline analog is inserted at a proline site in a globular protein, it should have little effect on the conformation of the protein. In contrast, such a substitution clearly decreases the conformational stability of collagen triple helix.[26-28]

Several studies have demonstrated that the systemic administration of cis-hydroxyproline, a proline analog, will inhibit scar formation.[29,30] Using a rat tendon model in which scar was created by the placement of a silk suture in the tendon, cis-hydroxyproline was noted to decrease the biomechanical force that was necessary to flex the digits. The conclusion drawn was that the drug will reduce the tensile strength of peritendinous adhesions. Peripheral nerve regeneration was superior to controls when cis-hydroxyproline was administered to rats after nerve laceration and suture; in these animals the fibrous tissue was less in the neuroma in the treated animals. Furthermore, the cis-hydroxyproline-treated animals had no changes in the contralateral normal sciatic nerves suggesting that the drug does not interfere with peripheral nerve physiology.

Several other agents have been shown to reduce scar formation and a comparison of four agents, alpha-alpha-dipyridyl, beta-amino-propionitrile, D-pencillamine, and cis-hydroxyproline were all found to decrease the amount of scar after flexor tendon injury when they were administered parenterally.[32] Alpha-alpha-dipyridyl showed significant toxic effects, beta-amino-propionitrile showed moderate toxic effects and D-pencillamine showed minimum toxic effects. Cis-hydroxyproline showed no toxic effect in our experiments and significantly decreased the amount of force necessary to flex the digit after scarring the flexor tendon when compared to the control. The parenteral administration of cis-hydroxyproline is incorporated in the fibroblasts and prevents the peptide change necessary for the triple helix formation. The extrusion of the immature (non-triple helix) chains from the cell make them susceptible to the degrading enzymes in the extracellular space.

It became clear with the above experiments that the development of a local route of administration of the drug would be cheaper, decrease potential systemic toxicity and increase the drug concentration in local areas of increased fibrosis. For these reasons, the last five years of this study have been directed to developing a local route of administration for cis-hydroxyproline.

A local hydrogel tube consisting of hydroxyethylmethacrylate (HEMA) was impregnated with trans-hydroxyproline and cis-hydroxyproline and measured for its drug release characteristics in physiologic solutions. A reproducible, significant diffusion rate was not found and the effort was discontinued. pH fluctuations and bacteria growth were thought to be possible causes of the difficulties, but no identifiable reasons were uncovered. Because of the difficulty in obtaining reproducible diffusion rates from the hydrogel, a biodegradable polymeric vehicle was studied. A report on the study of biodegradable systems for the sustained release of pharmacological agents was published by the World Health Organization and a polymer known as Alzamer™ was described as one of the most elegant of all new local vehicles for drug delivery.[33] This hydrophobic, biodegradable polymer (U.S. Patent #3,983209) was impregnated with 10% and 20% of cis-hydroxyproline and delivered in a liquid, sterile state. It was injected into the digit of rats after they were exposed to our suture scar model. Results showed that the amount of work required to flex the digit in those treated with cis-hydroxyproline was less, but not significantly less than the control groups. The main problem in this experiment was the fact that the liquid drug diffused out of the area of tendon injury and it was felt that if the vehicle could be made in solid form, its effect might be more predictable.

Alzamer™, a biodegradable vehicle, is a glassy polyester which can be fabricated into a variety of physical shapes. The matrix cradles the drug and as the polymer is eroded, the drug is released by diffusion. The vehicle is hydrophobic and is eroded by hydrolysis and the breakdown products, which are nontoxic, are excreted in the urine and incorporated into the Krebs cycle and used for energy.

Consequently, the Alza Corporation has produced a solid form of the biodegradable polymer. This vehicle was impregnated with cis-hydroxyproline in a 10% weight concentration and supplied in the form of a tube. A peripheral nerve scar model was developed to study this vehicle.

Scar around peripheral nerve was studied because the use of the surgical technique, neurolysis, is being reported with increasing frequency. Many favorable reports have appeared in the surgical journals, but questions have been raised about this procedure from writings in the neurological literature. A report from London, Ontario, specifically reports neurolysis following carpal tunnel release causes conduction block and questions the value of this procedure. It is well recognized that the surgical manipulation of a nerve, especially incisions

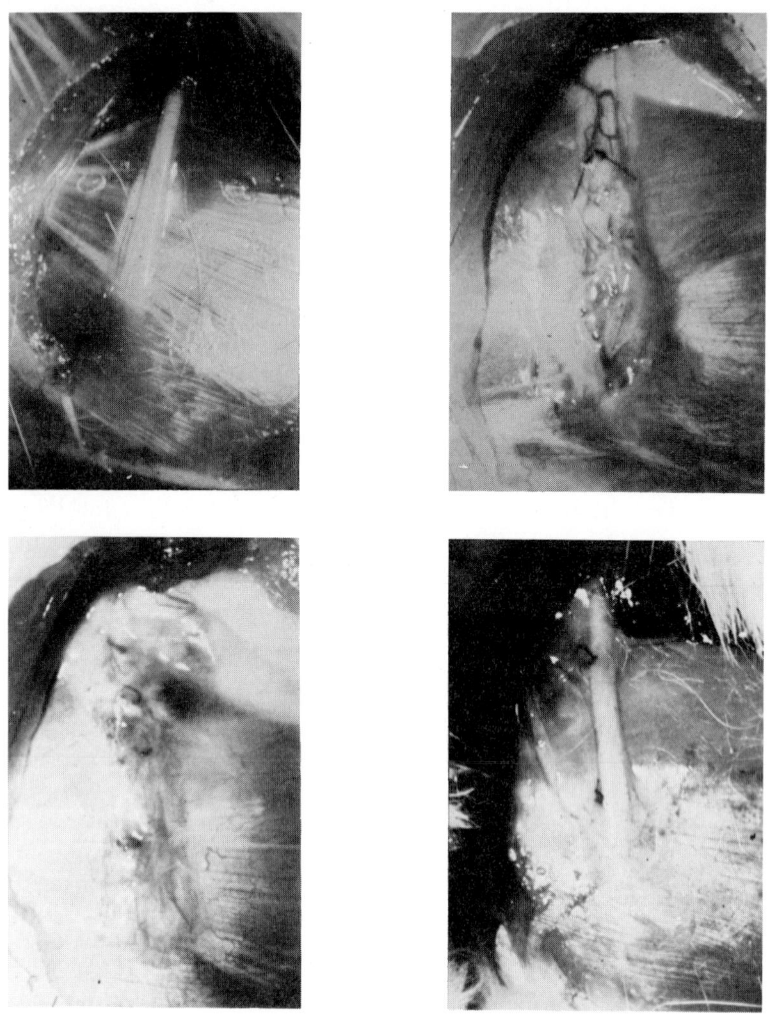

FIGURE 31.1 The gross appearance of perineural fibrosis when observed in the various groups at three weeks. A (top left), unoperated normal. B (top right), a nerve treated with carrageenan. C (bottom left), a nerve treated with carrageenan and Alzamer™. D (bottom right), a nerve treated with carrageenan, Alzamer™ and cis-hydroxyproline.

and dissections of the epineurium, provokes scar tissue. If the response from the surgical manipulation could be neutralized by an effective local inhibitor of scar formation, a significant improvement in the nerve function following Neurolysis could be anticipated.

The experimental work was performed in the following manner: Twenty seven 3 kg New Zealand male rabbits were randomized into three groups: (1) all control; (2) a vehicle without cis-hydroxyproline; and (3) a vehicle with cis-hydroxyproline. The common peroneal nerve of the rabbits was exposed and a specific length (1 cm) marked by perineural suture. Nerve scar was created in a reproducible manner by the injection of carrageenan, a potent scar provoker. The three animal groups were as follows: (1) the control group received the scar agent only; (2) the second group received the scar agent plus the vehicle (Alzamer™); and (3) the third group received the scar agent plus the vehicle (Alzamer™) with the collagen inhibitor, cis-hydroxyproline. The vehicle (Alzamer™) was in the form of a tube which was wrapped around the nerve at the same time the scar agent was injected in the nerve. The rabbits were followed for three weeks and then killed. Sacrifice was at three weeks because the vehicle was designed to be eroded between seven and 21 days after implantation. It has been shown in this model that collagen accumulation is maximal at three weeks.

TABLE 31.1

The Results of Biochemical Studies of the Neural Fibrosis in the Three Groups Studied

	CARAGEENAN	CARAGEENAN + VEHICLE WITHOUT CIS OH PRO	CARAGEENAN + VEHICLE WITH CIS OH PRO	
		($\bar{x}$ ± SEM)		
	N=8	N=10	N=9	
Collagen Content of Neural Fibrosis	250.8 ±44.5 p < 0.02	220.0 ±44.1 p < 0.05	145.3 ± 24.1	Δ μg OH PRO / 5mm segment
Dry Wt of Neural Fibrosis	7.57 ± 1.28 p < 0.01	10.39 ± 1.83 p < 0.01	3.51 ± 0.84	Δ mg Dry Wt
Protein Content of Neural Fibrosis	26.7 ± 4.6 p <0.01	27.4 ± 4.0 p < 0.01	14.4 ± 2.7	Δ α Amino Acid

In each animal the right extremity had the above procedures and the left was studied as an internal, contralateral control for each animal in each group.

Rabbit function was observed daily and serial electrodiagnostic studies were used to evaluate nerve function. Gross and histologic studies of the nerves were made after sacrifice. Biochemical analyses of the amount of scar in and around the nerve were calculated as follows: Hydroxyproline, a measure of the total collagen, was calculated by the Woessner technique; the amino acid content, a measure of total protein, was calculated by the Rosen technique.

At three weeks, there was a significant gross and histologic decrease in the amount of scar around the nerve in the group treated by cis-hydroxyproline and the vehicle Alzamer™ (Figure 31.1). Biochemically, the amount of scar tissue around the nerves treated by cis-hydroxyproline and the vehicle Alzamer™ was reduced by 40% when compared to the other two groups (Table 31.1). The vehicle <u>without</u> cis-hydroxyproline had <u>no</u> effect on scarring. Electrical diagnostic studies showed normal nerve function in the group treated with cis-hydroxyproline and the vehicle Alzamer™.

In conclusion, perineural scar formation is significantly reduced by the local administration of cis-hydroxyproline when delivered in the biodegradable vehicle, Alzamer™. Previous studies have shown that this system is satisfactory in reducing scar in tenolysis situations (unpublished). We feel the future of this drug-delivery system, Alzamer™ carrying cis-hydroxyproline, should be tried in clinical situations where excessive scar compromises function results after injury and disease.

NOTES

1. Grabb, W. Management of nerve injuries in the forearm and hand. Orthop. Clinics of N.A. 1:419-431, 1970.

2. Bulletin of the Department of Labor and Industry, Commonwealth of Pennsylvania, August 9, 1975.

3. Bulletin of the Bureau of Research and Statistics, Commonwealth of Pennsylvania, 1970.

4. Research and Statistics Bulletin No. 23, Workmen's Compensation Board, State of New York, 1968.

5. Takeuchi, T, and Prockop, DJ. Biosynthesis of abnormal collagens with amino acid analogues, 1. Incorporation of L-azetidine. 2. Carboxylic acid and cis-4-fluoro-L-proline into protocollagen and collagen. Biochim. Biophys. Acta 175: 142-155, 1969.

6. Takeuchi, T, Rosenbloom, J, and Prockop, DJ. Biosynthesis of abnormal collagens with amino acid analogues. II. Inability of cartilage cells to extrude collagen polypeptides containing L-azetidine-2-carboxylic acid or cis-4-fluoro-L-proline. Biochim. Biophys. Acta 175:156-164, 1969.

7. Lane, JM, and Prockop, DJ. Inhibition of collagen synthesis in chick embryos by the proline analogue L-azetidine-2-carboxylic acid. Arthritis Rheum. 13:331, 1970.

8. Lane, JM, and Dehm, P, and Prockop, DJ. Effect of the proline analog azetidine-2-carboxylic acid on collagen synthesis in vivo. I. Arrest of collagen accumulation in growing chick embryos. Biochim. Biophys. Acta 236:517-527, 1971.

9. Lane, JM, Parkes, LJ, and Prockop, DJ. Effect of the proline analog azetidine-2-carboxylic acid on collagen synthesis in vivo. II. Morphological & physical properties of collagen containing the analogue. Biochim. Biophys. Acta 236:528-541, 1971.

10. Rosenbloom, J, and Prockop, DJ. Incorporation of cis-hydroxyproline into protocollagen and collagen. J. Biol. Chem. 246:1549-1555, 1971.

11. Jimenez, SA, and Prockop, DJ. Specific inhibition of collagen synthesis in rat granulomas by incorporation of the proline analog cis-4-hydroxyproline into intracellular collagen. J. Clin. Invest. 50:49a, 1971.

12. Uitto, J, Dehm, P, and Prockop, DJ. Incorporation of cis-hydroxyproline into collagen by tendon cells. Failure of the intracellular collagen to assume a triple-helical conformation. Biochim. Biophys. Acta 278:601-605, 1972.

13. Uitto, J, and Prockop, DJ. Incorporation of proline analogues into collagen polypeptides. Effects on the production

of extracellular procollagen & on the stability of the triple-helical structure of the molecule. Biochim. Biophys. Acta 336: 234-251, 1974.

14. Uitto, J, and Prockop, DJ. Inhibition of collagen accumulation by proline analogues. The mechanism of their action. In Collagen Metabolism in the Liver, pp. 139-148, edited by H Popper and K Becker, Stratton Intercontinental Medical Book Corporation, New York, 1975.

15. Fowden, L, and Richmond, MH. Replacement of proline by azetidine-2-carboxylic acid during biosynthesis of protein. Biochim. Biophys. Acta 71:459-461, 1963.

16. Fowden, L, Lewis, D, and Tristram, H. Toxic amino acids: Their action as antimetabolites. Adv. in Enzymol. 29: 89-163, 1967.

17. Cleland, R, and Olson, AC. Direct incorporation of hydroxyproline into avena coleoptile proteins. Biochemistry 7: 1745-1751, 1968.

18. Grant, ME, and Prockop, DJ. The biosynthesis of collagen. New England J. Med. 286:194-199, 1972.

19. Traub, W, and Piez, KA. The chemistry and structure of collagen. Adv. Protein Chem. 25:243-352, 1971.

20. Ramachandran, GN. Molecular structure. In Biochemistry of Collagen, pp. 45-84, edited by GM Ramachandran and AH Reddi. Plenum Publishing Corp., New York, 1976.

21. Prockop, DJ, Berg, RA, Kivirikko, KI, and Uitto, J. Intracellular steps in the biosynthesis of collagen. In Biochemistry of Collagen, pp. 163-273, edited by GM Ramachandran and AH Reddi. Plenum Publishing Corp., New York, 1976.

22. Dehm, P, and Prockop, DJ. Biosynthesis of cartilage procollagen. Eur. J. Biochem. 35:159-166, 1973.

23. Morris, H, and Schlesinger, MJ. Effects of proline analogues on the formation of alkaline phosphatase in Escherichia coli. J. Bacteriology 111:203-210, 1972.

24. Galbraight, DB, and Kollar, EJ. Effects of L-azetidine-2-carboxylic acid, a proline analogue on the invitro development of mouse tooth germs. Arch. Oral Biol. 19:1171-1176, 1974.

25. Alescio, T. Effect of a proline analogue, azetidine-2-carboxylic acid on the morphogenesis invitro of mouse embryonic lung. J. Embryol. Exp. Morph. 29:439-451, 1973.

26. Berman, HM, McGandy, EL, Burgner, JW, and Van Etten, RL. The crystal & molecular structure of L-azetidine-2-carboxylic acid. A naturally occurring homolog of proline. J. Am. Chem. Soc. 91:6177-6182, 1973.

27. Daly, JM, Steiger, E, Prockop, DJ, and Dudrick, JJ. Inhibition of collagen synthesis by the proline analogue cis-4-hydroxyproline. Surg. Res. 14:551-555, 1973.

28. Rojkind, M. Inhibition of liver fibrosis by L-azetidine-2-carboxylic acid in rats treated with carbon tetrachloride. J. Clin. Invest. 52:2451-2456, 1973.

29. Lane, JM, Bora, FW, Prockop, DJ, Heppenstall, RB, and Black, J. Inhibition of scar formation by the proline analog cis-hydroxyproline. J. Surg. Res. 13:135-137, 1972.

30. Lane, JM, Bora, FW, Black, J. Cis-hydroxyproline limits work necessary to flex a digit after tendon injury. Clin. Orthop. 109:193-200, 1975.

31. Pleasure, D, Bora, FW, Lane, JM, and Prockop, D. Regeneration after nerve transection: Effect on inhibition of collagen synthesis. Exp. Neuro. 45:72-78, 1974.

32. Bora, FW, Lane, JM, Prockop, DJ. Inhibitors of collagen, biosynthesis as a means of controlling scar formation in tendon injury. J. Bone and Joint Surg. 54A, 1501-1508, 1972.

33. Benagiano, G, and Gabelnick, HL. World Health Organization Special Program of Research, Development and Training in Human Reproduction, Geneva, Switzerland.

Index

List of Contributors

HAROLD ALEXANDER, Ph.D., UMDNJ-New Jersey Medical School, The George L. Schultz Laboratories for Orthopaedic Research, Newark, New Jersey

WALTER ANDREWS, M.D., University of California, School of Medicine, Department of Surgery, San Francisco, California

THOMAS S. ARGYRIS, Ph.D., Upstate Medical Center, S.U.N.Y., Department of Pathology, Syracuse, New York

MICHAEL BANDA, Ph.D., University of California, San Francisco, School of Medicine, Department of Radiology, San Francisco, California

ROLAND BARON, D.D.S., Ph.D., Yale University School of Medicine, New Haven, Connecticut

ELSIE BARR, University of Kentucky, Wenner-Gren Research Laboratory and Department of Anatomy, Lexington, Kentucky

JIRI T. BERANEK, M.D., University of Nice, School of Medicine, Department of Immunology, Nice, France

CHARLES N. BERTOLAMI, D.D.S., D.M.Sc., Massachusetts General Hospital, Department of Oral and Maxillofacial Surgery, Boston, Massachusetts

F. WILLIAM BORA JR., M.D., University of Pennsylvania, School of Medicine, Department of Orthopaedic Surgery, Philadelphia, Pennsylvania

CARL T. BRIGHTON, M.D., Ph.D., University of Pennsylvania, School of Medicine, Department of Orthopaedic Surgery, Philadelphia, Pennsylvania

JOHN F. BURKE, M.D., Harvard Medical School, Massachusetts General Hospital, Boston, Massachusetts

NING CHANG, M.D., University of California, San Francisco, School of Medicine, Department of Surgery, San Francisco, California

I. KELMAN COHEN, M.D., Medical College of Virginia, Division of Plastic Surgery, Richmond, Virginia

CAROLYN COMPTON, M.D., University of Massachusetts, Department of Pathology, Worcester, Massachusetts

ROBERT F. DIEGELMANN, Ph.D., Medical College of Virginia, Division of Plastic Surgery, Richmond, Virginia

ANDREW C. DOGANIS, M.D., Yale University School of Medicine, New Haven, Connecticut

WILLIAM H. EAGLSTEIN, M.D., University of Pittsburgh School of Medicine, Department of Dermatology, Pittsburgh, Pennsylvania

H. PAUL EHRLICH, Ph.D., Shriners Burn Institute, Wound Healing Laboratory, Boxton, Massachusetts

MAGDALENA EISINGER, D.V.M., Memorial Sloan-Kettering Cancer Center, New York, New York

R. SCOTT ESTES, University of Kentucky, Wenner-Gren Research Laboratory and Department of Anatomy, Lexington, Kentucky

W. PAGE FAULK, M.D., University of Nice, School of Medicine, Department of Immunology, Nice, France

RICHARD FIRMIN, M.D., University of California, San Francisco, School of Medicine, Department of Surgery, San Francisco, California

JOSEPH G. FORTNER, M.D., Memorial Sloan-Kettering Cancer Center, New York, New York

GARY E. FRIEDLAENDER, M.D., Yale University School of Medicine, Department of Orthopaedic Surgery. New Haven, Connecticut

GREGORY GALLICO, M.D., Shriners Burns Institute and Massachusetts General Hospital, Boston, Massachusetts

RENATE GAY, M.D., University of Alabama Medical Center, Department of Medicine, Birmingham, Alabama

STEFFEN GAY, M.D., University of Alabama Medical Center, Department of Medicine, Birmingham, Alabama

JULIE GLOWACKI, Ph.D., Harvard Medical School and Children's Hospital Medical Center, Department of Surgery, Boston, Massachusetts

WILLIAM H. GOODSON III, M.D., University of California, San Francisco, School of Medicine, Department of Surgery, San Francisco, California

RICHARD J. GOSS, Ph.D., Division of Biology and Medicine, Brown University, Providence, Rhode Island

FINN GOTTRUP, M.D., Institute of Anatomy, University of Aarhus, Aarhus, Denmark

MARTIN F. GRAHAM, M.D., Children's Medical Center, Medical College of Virginia, Department of Pediatrics, Richmond, Virginia

HOWARD GREEN, M.D., Harvard Medical School, Department of Physiology and Biophysics, Boston, Massachusetts

GARY R. GROTENDORST, Ph.D, Laboratory of Developmental Biology and Anomalies, National Institute of Dental Research, National Institutes of Health, Bethesda, Maryland

BETTY HALLIDAY, B.A., University of California, San Francisco, School of Medicine, San Francisco, California

JOHN P. HEGGERS, Ph.D., Wayne State University, School of Medicine, Division of Plastic Surgery, Detroit, Michigan

R. BRUCE HEPPENSTALL, M.D., University of Pennsylvania Medical School of Medicine, Department of Orthopaedic Surgery, Philadelphia, Pennsylvania

DAVID C. HOHN, M.D., University of California, San Francisco, School of Medicine, Department of Surgery, San Francisco, California

B. L. HSI, Ph.D., University of Nice, School of Medicine, Department of Immunology, Nice, France

THOMAS K. HUNT, M.D., University of California, San Francisco, School of Medicine, Department of Surgery, San Francisco, California

DAVID S. JACKSON, Ph.D., Wound Care Research, Johnson & Johnson Products, Inc., New Brunswick, New Jersey

KENT JONSSON, M.D., University of California, San Francisco, School of Medicine, Department of Surgery, San Francisco, California

LEONARD B. KABAN, D.M.D., M.D., Harvard Medical School and Children's Hospital Medical Center, Department of Surgery, Boston, Massachusetts

LOLA KAMP, B.S., Wound Care Research, Johnson & Johnson Products, Inc., New Brunswick, New Jersey

OLANIYI KEHINDE, B.S., Harvard Medical School, Department of Physiology and Biophysics, Boston, Massachusetts

DAVID R. KNIGHTON, M.D., University of California, San Francisco, School of Medicine, Department of Surgery, San Francisco, California

EDWARD R. KRAFT, B.S., Memorial Sloan-Kettering Cancer Center, New York, New York

SAMUEL JOSEPH LEIBOVICH, Ph.D., Northwestern University, The Dental School, Department of Oral Biology, Chicago, Illinois

WILLIAM J. LINDBLAD, Ph.D., Medical College of Virginia, Division of Plastic Surgery, Richmond, Virginia

GEORGE R. MARTIN, Ph.D., Laboratory of Developmental Biology and Anomalies, National Institute of Dental Research, National Institutes of Health, Bethesda, Maryland

STEPHEN J. MATHES, M.D., University of California, San Francisco, School of Medicine, Department of Surgery, San Francisco

BARBARA MATLAGA, B.S., Ethicon, Inc., Somerville, New Jersey

PATRICIA M. MERTZ, B.A., University of Pittsburgh School of Medicine, Department of Dermatology, Pittsburgh, Pennsylvania

DOV MICHAELI, M.D., Ph.D., University of California, San Francisco, School of Medicine, Department of Surgery, San Francisco, California

REBECCA MORRIS, Ph.D., University of Texas System Cancer Center, Smithville, Texas

JOHN B. MULLIKEN, M.D., Harvard Medical School and Children's Hospital Medical Center, Department of Surgery, Boston, Massachusetts

JUHA NIINIKOSKI, M.D., Department of Surgery, University of Turku, Turku, Finland.

NICHOLAS E. O'CONNOR, M.D., Shriners Burns Institute and Brigham and Women's Hospital, Boston, Massachusetts

CHARLES E. OLSEN, Ph.D., Wound Care Research, Johnson & Johnson Products, Inc., New Brunswick, New Jersey

SVEN OREDSSON, B.S., University of California, San Francisco, School of Medicine, Department of Surgery, San Francisco, California

JEAN P. ORTONNE, M.D., University of Nice, School of Medicine, Department of Dermatology, Nice, France

JOHN R. PARSONS, Ph.D., UMDNJ-New Jersey Medical School, The George L. Schultz Laboratories for Orthopaedic Research, Newark, New Jersey

RICHARD R. PELKER, M.D., Ph.D., Yale University School of Medicine, New Haven, Connecticut

DOBROMIR PENCEV, Ph.D., Laboratory of Developmental Biology and Anomalies, National Institute of Dental Research, National Institutes of Health, Bethesda, Maryland

ELI PINES, Ph.D., Wound Care Research, Johnson & Johnson Products, Inc., New Brunswick, New Jersey

DAVID C. PRICE, M.D., University of California, San Francisco, School of Medicine, Department of Surgery, San Francisco, California

A. HARI REDDI, Ph.D., Bone Cell Biology Section, Mineralized Tissue Research Branch, National Institute of Dental Research, National Institutes of Health, Bethesda, Maryland

MARTIN C. ROBSON, M.D., Wayne State University, School of Medicine, Division of Plastic Surgery, Detroit, Michigan

LAWRENCE ROSENBERG, M.D., Montefiore Medical Center, Orthopaedic Research Laboratories, Bronx, New York

ROBERT K. ROSENTHAL, M.D., Harvard Medical School and Children's Hospital Medical Center, Department of Surgery, Boston, Massachusetts

DAVID T. ROVEE, Ph.D., Wound Care Research, Johnson & Johnson Products, Inc., New Brunswick, New Jersey

W. DOUGLAS SHEFFIELD, D.V.M., Ph.D., Ethicon, Inc., Somerville, New Jersey

IAN A. SILVER, D.V.M., University of Bristol Medical School, Department of Pathology, Bristol, England

BETTY F. SISKEN, Ph.D., University of Kentucky, Wenner-Gren Research Laboratory and Department of Anatomy, Lexington, Kentucky

JARO SODEK, D.D.S., University of Toronto, Faculty of Dentistry, Toronto, Canada

STEPHEN T. SONIS, D.M.D., D.M.Sc., Harvard Medical School and Children's Hospital Medical Center, Department of Surgery, Boston, Massachusetts

K. K. THAKRAL, M.D., University of California, San Francisco, School of Medicine, Department of Surgery, San Francisco, California

ANTHONY UNGER, M.D., University of Pennsylvania, School of Medicine, Department of Orthopaedic Surgery, Philadelphia, Pennsylvania

ANDREW B. WEISS, M.D., UMDNJ-New Jersey Medical School, The George L. Schultz Laboratories for Orthopaedic Research, Newark, New Jersey

JUDITH M. WEST, R.N., M.N., University of California, San Francisco, School of Medicine, San Francisco, California